Nutrition and Health

Series Editors

Adrianne Bendich, Wellington, FL, USA

Connie W. Bales, Duke University School of Medicine
Durham VA Medical Center
Durham, NC, USA

The Nutrition and Health series has an overriding mission in providing health professionals with texts that are considered essential since each is edited by the leading researchers in their respective fields. Each volume includes: 1) a synthesis of the state of the science, 2) timely, in-depth reviews, 3) extensive, up-to-date fully annotated reference lists, 4) a detailed index, 5) relevant tables and figures, 6) identification of paradigm shifts and consequences, 7) virtually no overlap of information between chapters, but targeted, inter-chapter referrals, 8) suggestions of areas for future research and 9) balanced, data driven answers to patient/health professionals questions which are based upon the totality of evidence rather than the findings of a single study.

Nutrition and Health is a major resource of relevant, clinically based nutrition volumes for the professional that serve as a reliable source of data-driven reviews and practice guidelines.

Crystal D. Karakochuk
Michael B. Zimmermann
Diego Moretti • Klaus Kraemer
Editors

Nutritional Anemia

Second Edition

Springer

Editors
Crystal D. Karakochuk
Human Nutrition
The University of British Columbia
Vancouver, BC, Canada

Michael B. Zimmermann
Institute of Food Nutrition and Health
ETH Zurich
Zürich, Zürich, Switzerland

Diego Moretti
Department of Health
University of Applied Sciences of South Switzerland (SUPSI) and Swiss Distance University of Applied Sciences (FFHS)
Zürich, Zürich, Switzerland

Klaus Kraemer
International Health
Sight and Life Foundation and Johns Hopkins School of Public Health
Basel, Switzerland

ISSN 2628-197X ISSN 2628-1961 (electronic)
Nutrition and Health
ISBN 978-3-031-14523-0 ISBN 978-3-031-14521-6 (eBook)
https://doi.org/10.1007/978-3-031-14521-6

This Springer imprint is published by the registered company Springer Nature Switzerland AG
The registered company address is: Gewerbestrasse 11, 6330 Cham, Switzerland

Preface

Anemia is a worldwide public health problem affecting 1.62 billion people, or ~25% of the global population [1]. The highest prevalence of anemia occurs in children aged 6–59 months (40%, or ~269 million globally) and importantly, the largest group of affected individuals (30%, or ~571 million globally) is women of reproductive age (15–49 years) [2]. Reduction of anemia in women of reproductive age is a target of Goal 2 (zero hunger) of the 17 Sustainable Development Goals (SDGs), which are an urgent call to action by all countries to achieve a better and more sustainable future for all. In contrast to women, targets for anemia reduction in infants and children have yet to be set.

Anemia is defined as a hemoglobin concentration below a defined threshold established for a specific age, sex, or life stage. In children, anemia can impair cognitive development, decrease learning potential, and have long-term implications on overall quality of life. In adults, it can impair work capacity and productivity and increase the risk of adverse pregnancy outcomes (e.g., low birth weight). Causes of anemia can include micronutrient deficiencies (e.g., iron and folic acid), infection and disease, and genetic hemoglobin disorders (e.g., sickle cell disease), which are autosomal recessive disorders that result in a decreased or defective hemoglobin production. Understanding the causes of anemia is critical to inform appropriate strategies to prevent and treat anemia, particularly to reduce the risk of anemia and the burden of disease.

The 2007 first edition text concluded that despite a great deal of programmatic experience, scientific data and new information on iron metabolism and the role of other nutrients in the etiology of nutritional anemia, there has unfortunately been little documented success in addressing the problem at a public health level. Now, 15 years later, the release of this second edition text, which has been comprehensively expanded to 27 chapters, further highlights the complexity of the topic and the phenomenal advances we have observed in science during this timeframe. Unfortunately, despite this, these phenomenal advances have not yet been translated into anemia reduction. This second edition text addresses some of the potential reasons why these advances in discovery and implementation have not resulted in acceptable progress in anemia reduction. Anemia prevalence among women and children remains unacceptably high in most regions of the world, despite the global and national attention and the plethora of policies, interventions, and programs designed to treat, prevent, and reduce anemia.

Chapter authors of this second edition text are leading global experts in nutrition and health. The introductory chapters provide an overview of the worldwide prevalence and the progress in anemia reduction, iron biology and homeostasis, laboratory methods for anemia and iron deficiency surveillance, and interpretation of biomarkers associated with nutritional anemia. Subsequent chapters highlight new evidence on anemia among special populations, the role of other micronutrients in the etiology of anemia, hepcidin homeostasis and the emerging association between hepcidin and vitamin D, iron and the human gut microbiota, and novel approaches to oral iron supplementation. The summarizing chapters highlight program and policy approaches to treat, prevent, and reduce anemia in the global context, including food-based approaches, policy considerations of food fortification, and designing effective programs for anemia reduction.

This landmark publication aims to inform government, NGO, and international agencies on how to effectively measure, treat, prevent, and reduce anemia globally. We hope this second edition text will be a current and comprehensive resource on anemia for all those involved in global health and nutrition policy, strategy, programming, or research, and, ultimately, helps to facilitate meaningful progress in anemia reduction globally.

Vancouver, BC, Canada — Crystal D. Karakochuk
Zürich, Switzerland — Diego Moretti
Basel, Switzerland — Klaus Kraemer
Zürich, Switzerland — Michael B. Zimmermann

References

1. World Health Organization. Worldwide prevalence of anaemia 1993-2005: WHO Global Database on Anaemia. Geneva: World Health Organization; 2008.
2. Stevens GA, et al. National, regional, and global estimates of anaemia by severity in women and children for 2000-19: a pooled analysis of population-representative data. Lancet Glob Health. 2022;10(5): E627–39.

Contents

Part I

Prevalence, Biology, Lab Methods and Interpretation of Biomarkers

1 Anaemia: Worldwide Prevalence and Progress in Reduction

Andrew Baldi and Sant-Rayn Pasricha

Keywords

Haemoglobin · Anaemia · Chronic hypoxia
Iron deficiency · Myelodysplastic syndrome
Haemolysis

Introduction

Anaemia remains one of the most common health conditions and has a wide range of causes including nutritional deficiencies, infections and genetic factors. Especially when moderate or severe, anaemia results in significant morbidity and impaired functioning, particularly among women of reproductive age and children in low- and middle-income countries. Further, anaemia is a risk factor for mortality from a range of health conditions.

This chapter will provide an overview of anaemia, including haemoglobin thresholds used to define anaemia, and key determinants of anaemia especially in the public health context. It will summarise global estimates of the prevalence of anaemia, explain methodologies of these estimates and discuss how anaemia prevalence has changed over time.

Defining Anaemia

Anaemia is defined as a reduction in the circulating red blood cell mass such that oxygen-carrying capacity is insufficient to meet the body's physiological needs. Typically, anaemia is identified when the haemoglobin concentration falls below a defined threshold, generally specific to the sex and age (and pregnancy status) of the individual and adjusted for residence at an elevation above sea level (>1000 m) [1, 2].

An individual with anaemia may experience symptoms related to inadequate tissue oxygen delivery and the physiological response to this state. While some individuals with anaemia may be asymptomatic, common signs and symptoms

A. Baldi
Population Health and Immunity Division, The Walter and Eliza Hall Institute of Medical Research, Parkville, VIC, Australia

Department of Medical Biology, The University of Melbourne, Parkville, VIC, Australia

Clinical Haematology, The Royal Children's Hospital, Parkville, VIC, Australia

S.-R. Pasricha (✉)
Population Health and Immunity Division, The Walter and Eliza Hall Institute of Medical Research, Parkville, VIC, Australia

Department of Medical Biology, The University of Melbourne, Parkville, VIC, Australia

Diagnostic Haematology, The Royal Melbourne Hospital; and Clinical Haematology, The Peter MacCallum Cancer Centre and The Royal Melbourne Hospital, Melbourne, VIC, Australia
e-mail: pasricha.s@wehi.edu.au

C. D. Karakochuk et al. (eds.), *Nutritional Anemia*, Nutrition and Health,
https://doi.org/10.1007/978-3-031-14521-6_1

include pallor, tiredness and fatigue, headache, shortness of breath (especially on exertion), an increase in heart rate and/or reduced exertional tolerance. Anaemia may cause decompensation of medical conditions such as ischaemic heart disease and congestive cardiac failure [3]. Anaemia is recognised as an important risk factor for mortality in patients with other health conditions such as chronic kidney disease and chronic heart failure and prior to major surgery [3–5]. Other consequences of anaemia include effects in pregnancy such as increased maternal mortality, reduced birth weight and increased preterm birth [6]. Anaemia in pregnancy may result in reduced neonatal iron stores and therefore predispose to anaemia in infancy and childhood [7–9]. Anaemia is also responsible for reduced productivity and therefore adversely impacts income generation [10]. Iron supplementation to infants does not improve neurodevelopmental outcomes [11].

Definitions of Anaemia

Anaemia is defined and categorised by the World Health Organization (WHO) using thresholds that vary depending on age, sex and pregnancy status (Table 1.1) [1].

Chronic hypoxia will cause reduced oxygen tension and elevations in haemoglobin concentration, and thus physiological haemoglobin thresholds are also adjusted for residence at elevation above sea level (>1000 m) and smoking status [1].

Haemoglobin reference ranges and anaemia cut-offs published by other groups demonstrate differences from the WHO definitions in approaches to subgroup selection and/or the haemoglobin cut-offs themselves. The US Centers for Disease Control and Prevention (CDC), for example, recommends a higher haemoglobin cut-off of 135 g/L for adult men and also subdivides children into narrower categories, each providing a different haemoglobin threshold [14].

The evidence base for haemoglobin thresholds continues to evolve, and the applicability of WHO cut-offs to the global population has been challenged by several more recent studies of healthy individuals. Two recent studies have obtained and analysed haemoglobin data among healthy individuals and have both proposed haemoglobin thresholds lower than those in the current WHO guidelines. For pregnant women, a prospective study examined maternal haemoglobin with respect to gestational age [15]. A nadir of haemoglobin was observed between 31 and 32 weeks' gestation in this healthy pregnant population, which was similar to WHO data. Its proposed definition of anaemia was a measurement below the third centile for gestational age, and at all time points, the cut-off was lower than the corresponding measurement in the WHO guidelines—however, this study did not exclude individuals with iron deficiency, limiting the utility of these thresholds.

Similar studies have sought to refine haemoglobin thresholds in other populations. A large

Table 1.1 WHO recommendations for haemoglobin thresholds to define anaemia [12]

	Mild anaemia (g/L)	Moderate anaemia (g/L)	Severe anaemia (g/L)
Males ≥15 years	110–129	80–109	<80
Females ≥15 years	110–119	80–109	<80
Pregnant women	100–109[a]	70–99	<70
Children 6–59 months	100–109	70–99	<70
Children 5–11 years	110–114	80–109	<80
Children 12–14 years	110–119	80–109	<80

[a] Anaemia has been defined in some WHO guidelines in the second trimester of pregnancy as haemoglobin <105 g/L [13]

study of children in India conducted between 2016 and 2018 determined its own haemoglobin cut-offs and noted these were also lower than the WHO definitions across all age groups and would result in a 19.2% lower prevalence of anaemia [16]. However, these thresholds are derived from secondary analyses of population surveys in settings where there is a high prevalence of undetected concurrent or recent inflammation or infection and likely do not represent a healthy population. Further validation in clinically selected healthy populations is needed to establish if lower thresholds are appropriate. Changes in accepted haemoglobin thresholds for defining anaemia would have considerable implications for policymakers and resource allocation.

Differences in haemoglobin thresholds also exist between clinical laboratories [17] and between guidelines produced by different professional societies and other reference sources [18]. Varying thresholds for defining anaemia may have important implications for treatment of individuals, for estimating population prevalence and for devising and implementing policy to reduce anaemia.

Causes of Anaemia

Broadly, anaemia is caused by one or several of reduced red cell production, reduced red cell survival (either due to abnormal production or increased destruction), blood loss, or red cell sequestration [19]. Table 1.2 lists specific causes within these categories, with important contributors to global anaemia prevalence underlined. Anaemia may be attributable to more than one cause in a given individual.

A physiologic reduction in haemoglobin concentration occurs during pregnancy due to haemodilution (increased plasma volume exceeding increased red blood cell production) [19].

Among causes of anaemia due to reduced red cell production, iron deficiency is a common

Table 1.2 Causes of anaemia

Mechanism of anaemia	Potential causes
Reduced red cell production	• *Iron deficiency (including from poor nutrition and poor iron absorption)—see* Table 1.3 • *Vitamin B12, folate, vitamin A, zinc deficiency* • Bone marrow failure (e.g. due to aplastic anaemia, viral infection such as parvovirus B19 causing pure red cell aplasia, bone marrow infiltration due to haematologic malignancy (e.g. acute leukaemia), bone marrow fibrosis, metastatic cancer, infection, irradiation, antineoplastic chemotherapy) • Medications (immunosuppressants, e.g. methotrexate, or idiosyncratic responses) • *Inflammation (functional iron deficiency) including malarial infection* [20][a] • Myelodysplastic syndrome • Reduced erythropoietin production, e.g. kidney failure • Inherited conditions, e.g. Diamond-Blackfan anaemia
Reduced red cell survival (including blood loss)	• *Haemoglobinopathy, e.g. thalassaemia major or intermedia, sickle cell disease (ineffective erythropoiesis)* • *Haemoglobinopathy trait* • Haemolysis: e.g. autoimmune haemolysis; inherited red cell membrane conditions, e.g. hereditary spherocytosis; inherited red cell enzyme disorders, e.g. *G6PD deficiency*; microangiopathic haemolysis • *Acute blood loss/haemorrhage* • *Chronic blood loss including menstrual blood loss and helminth infections* (usually causes anaemia via iron deficiency)

Adapted from [21]

[a] Malaria can result in anaemia through anaemia of inflammation, intravascular haemolysis, haemolysis of non-parasitised red cells and splenic sequestration

underlying factor (Table 1.3). Iron is required for synthesis of the haem component of haemoglobin, and in the setting of iron deficiency, the body initially produces red blood cells with a lower haemoglobin content. With ongoing iron deficiency and depleted body iron stores, red cell production is further impaired, resulting in anaemia [22].

Iron availability to the bone marrow may also be restricted because iron is withheld from the plasma (even if total body iron stores are not depleted)—this typically occurs during inflammation or infection and is termed 'functional iron deficiency' [23]. Functional iron deficiency is an important driver of anaemia of inflammation.

Mean corpuscular volume (MCV) is a red cell parameter that is often useful in stratifying the cause of anaemia and guiding additional investigations to determine the underlying cause of anaemia (Table 1.4). This parameter is reported in a full blood count when a blood sample is analysed by an automated haematology analyser instrument, but is not available from point-of-care instruments that measure haemoglobin concentration alone [24, 25].

Table 1.3 Potential causes of absolute iron deficiency

Mechanism of iron deficiency	Potential cause
Inadequate iron uptake	Inadequate nutritional iron intake • Inadequate dietary iron content • Inadequate nutritional iron absorption (including concomitant consumption of inhibitors of iron absorption (e.g. phytate, tannins), inadequate stomach acidification, intestinal mucosal dysfunction, obesity, inappropriately increased hepcidin concentrations preventing iron absorption (e.g. during chronic inflammation or iron-refractory iron deficiency anaemia caused by *TMPRSS6* genetic mutations)
Increased iron requirements	• Growth (e.g. during early childhood and adolescence) • Pregnancy • Physiological blood losses exceeding iron intake • Erythropoiesis stimulating agent therapy
Blood loss	• Gastrointestinal blood loss • Gynaecological bleeding • Menstrual • Urinary tract • Respiratory bleeding • Blood donation (especially whole blood donation) • Excess iatrogenic blood losses (e.g. excessive blood collection for diagnostic testing and iron losses during haemodialysis)
Exercise	Multifactorial: reduced iron absorption due to exercise-related inflammation, increased losses in sweat, gastrointestinal bleeding and haemolysis with haemoglobinuria (rhabdomyolysis)

Adapted from [23]

Table 1.4 Causes of anaemia divided by low, normal and increased mean corpuscular volume (MCV)

Low MCV (Microcytic anaemia)	Iron deficiency – Inadequate nutritional intake/malabsorption – Blood loss Thalassaemia (carrier state, compound heterozygous or homozygous) Lead poisoning Sideroblastic anaemia
Normal MCV (Normocytic anaemia)	Acute blood loss Anaemia of inflammation Haemolytic anaemia Bone marrow infiltration (e.g. from malignancy) Myelodysplasia Aplastic anaemia
Increased MCV (Macrocytic anaemia)	Vitamin B12 deficiency (profound increase in MCV, megaloblastic anaemia) Folate deficiency (profound increase in MCV, megaloblastic anaemia) Anaemia with reticulocytosis Hypothyroidism Myelodysplasia

Based on [19]

The Global Prevalence of Anaemia

There are systematic analyses by groups including WHO and the Global Burden of Disease to quantify the global prevalence of anaemia using models derived from national and sub-national prevalence data. Key data sources include national surveys of anaemia prevalence, often undertaken through the Demographic and Health Survey (DHS) programme, which has been measuring capillary haemoglobin concentration using HemoCue devices in survey participants across many countries [26]. These data are summarised in the WHO Vitamin and Mineral Nutrition Information System [27].

World Health Organization

In 2008, WHO published an estimate of the global prevalence of anaemia using prevalence data measured between 1993 and 2005 [28]. This was among the first efforts to synthesise national and regional data to develop global estimates.

According to this analysis, global prevalence of anaemia was 24.8%, or 1.62 billion people (95% CI, 1.50–1.74 billion), over this period. The data demonstrated that anaemia disproportionately affects women (especially pregnant women) and preschool children.

Subsequent WHO estimates have focused on anaemia prevalence in these high-risk populations: children 6 months to 5 years of age, pregnant women and non-pregnant women of reproductive age. The WHO estimated that anaemia affected 273 million preschool children, 496 million non-pregnant women and 32 million pregnant women globally in 2011. Estimates of the prevalence of severe anaemia (defined as haemoglobin below 70 g/L in pregnant women and children 6–59 months of age and below 80 g/L for other population groups) were included (Table 1.5) [29].

The Global Health Observatory (GHO) is a WHO database containing information relating to a wide range of health indicators for the 194 WHO member states. Data is compiled using methods specific to the health indicator. It is pre-

Table 1.5 Global prevalence of anaemia by demographic group (2011 estimate)

Demographic group	Percentage (95% CI) of population with anaemia	Number (95% CI) of people with anaemia (millions)	Percentage (95% CI) of population with severe anaemia	Number (95%CI) of people with severe anaemia (millions)
Children aged 6–59 months	42.6 (37.7–47.4)	273.2 (241.8–303.7)	1.5 (1.0–2.2)	9.6 (6.9–14.1)
Pregnant women aged 15–49 years	38.2 (33.5–42.6)	32.4 (28.41–36.2)	0.9 (0.6–1.3)	0.8 (0.5–1.1)
Non-pregnant women aged 15–49 years	29.0 (23.9–34.8	496.3 (409.3–595.1)	1.1 (0.7–1.7)	19.4 (12.7–29.4)

Adapted from [29]

Table 1.6 Anaemia prevalence by population group in each WHO region, *2004 and 2019 Global Health Observatory data* [28, 30–32]

	Preschool-aged children %, (95% CI)		Pregnant women %, (95% CI)		Non-pregnant women (15–49 years) %, (95% CI)	
WHO region	2004	2019	2004	2019	2004	2019
Africa	67.9 (65.3–70.2)	60.2 (56.6–63.7)	49.7 (47.9–51.5)	45.8 (43.1–48.4)	44.1 (40.5–47.7)	39.8 (36.0–43.9)
Americas	22.3 (19.5–25.3)	16.5 (13.4–20.1)	22.3 (18.5–26.4)	18.9 (14.1–24.8)	17.8 (15.0–20.4)	15.3 (11.8–19.5)
Southeast Asia	59.0 (52.6–64.2)	49.0 (39.2–57.9)	50.2 (46.8–53.0)	47.8 (43.1–51.3)	46.5 (41.1–51.5)	46.5 (39.3–53.2)
Europe	22.7 (18.3–27.8)	20.3 (14.5–27.4)	24.3 (19.3–29.8)	23.5 (17.5–30.4)	18.2 (14.7–22.6)	18.6 (14.3–23.9)
Eastern Mediterranean	48.6 (43.7–53.4)	42.7 (35.5–49.7)	40.9 (36.9–44.5)	36.8 (30.7–42.1)	35.8 (31.9–39.9)	34.8 (29.3–40.0)
Western Pacific	24.5 (16.7–34.0)	19.4 (10.8–31.7)	28.1 (22.5–33.7)	21.3 (14.6–30.6)	19.5 (15.1–24.5)	16.2 (11.2–23.5)
Global	45.5 (42.8–48.1)	39.8 (36.0–43.8)	39.9 (38.1–41.6)	36.5 (34.0–39.1)	29.6 (27.4–31.9)	29.6 (26.6–32.5)

sented in a manner that allows comparison between countries, as well as changes over time. It regularly releases anaemia prevalence data for women and children, most recently for 2019 [30–32].

WHO and other groups also demonstrate regional variation in anaemia prevalence, demonstrating the increased prevalence of anaemia in Africa and Southeast Asia. WHO estimates of anaemia prevalence by region are outlined in Table 1.6.

WHO defines the severity of anaemia as a public health problem according to the prevalence of anaemia among groups of interest. A prevalence exceeding 40% is considered a 'severe' public health problem; a prevalence between 20 and 39.9% a moderate public health problem; and a prevalence from 5 to 19.9% a mild public health problem [33]. Using this classification approach, anaemia is considered a severe public health problem in preschool-aged children, pregnant women and non-pregnant women in Africa and Southeast Asia [28].

Other Groups

In 2013 the Nutrition Impact Model Study Group (Anaemia) published an analysis of anaemia prevalence trends between 1995 and 2011 [34]. The analysis used data from 107 countries and modelled changes in anaemia prevalence in children, pregnant women and non-pregnant women. Sources included summary data from the WHO

Table 1.7 Nutrition Impact Model Study Group (Anaemia) estimates of 2011 anaemia prevalence [34]

	Mean haemoglobin g/L, (95% CI)	Anaemia %, (95% credibility interval)	Severe anaemia %, (95% credibility interval)
Children <5 years	111 (110–113)	43 (38–47)	1.5 (1.1–2.2)
Non-pregnant women (15–49 years)	126 (124–128)	29 (24–35)	1.1 (0.7–1.7)
Pregnant women (15–49 years)	114 (112–116)	38 (34–43)	0.9 (0.6–1.3)

Vitamin and Mineral Nutrition Information System as well as national and other international surveys and databases. For example, to compile anaemia data for Malawi, the authors drew upon DHS data from 2004 and 2010, as well as results from the 2010 Malawi National Malaria Indicator Survey (MIS), which included national-level anaemia prevalence figures for children under 5 [27, 35]. The 2011 prevalence estimate (Table 1.7) shows anaemia prevalence of 43% among preschool children, 38% among pregnant women and 29% among non-pregnant women of reproductive age.

Global Burden of Disease

The Global Burden of Disease (GBD) undertakes an ongoing systematic summary of the prevalence of anaemia (among many other diseases) across all countries. The GBD summarises disease burden through successive large-scale collaborative projects that have used a multitude of data sources to examine morbidity and mortality caused by conditions, injuries and other risk factors [36, 37]. The 2019 global anaemia prevalence was estimated by GBD at 23.67% [38]. The GBD will be discussed further in the next section.

Global Determinants of Anaemia

Much of the global burden of anaemia is attributable to iron deficiency, thalassaemias and other haemoglobinopathies and infections such as malaria [39, 40].

Causes of anaemia in low- and middle-income countries (LMICs) may be complex and multifactorial [41]. In many cases regions with high anaemia prevalence are also areas with relatively low socioeconomic status, and in these settings, anaemia may be a marker of disadvantage in domains including food security, water quality, sanitation and hygiene (WASH) status and may reflect poor access to health care (Fig. 1.1). These areas may also have high rates of endemic pathogens such as malaria and soil-transmitted helminths and other pathogens causing recurrent respiratory and gastrointestinal infections. As highlighted previously, anaemia in women of reproductive age in environments that predispose to iron deficiency may have follow-on effects in pregnancy and on infants born to these women [42].

Finally, physiological states that result in increased iron requirements disproportionately affect certain demographic groups, placing them at increased risk of iron deficiency anaemia. These include preschool-aged children, premenopausal women and pregnant women. For children, periods of rapid growth demand higher amounts of iron from the diet. Similarly, pregnancy is a physiological state of relatively increased iron requirements. Menstrual losses that deplete iron stores in excess of dietary iron intake will also result in iron deficiency in premenopausal women [23].

Several studies have estimated the proportion of anaemia attributable to different causes. The proportion of anaemia attributable to iron deficiency appears to vary according to the region of the world and the demographic of the group of interest. For example, WHO estimated that half of anaemia cases globally were attributable to iron deficiency, though this varies by age and region. Globally, the proportion of anaemia cases amendable to iron interventions is estimated at

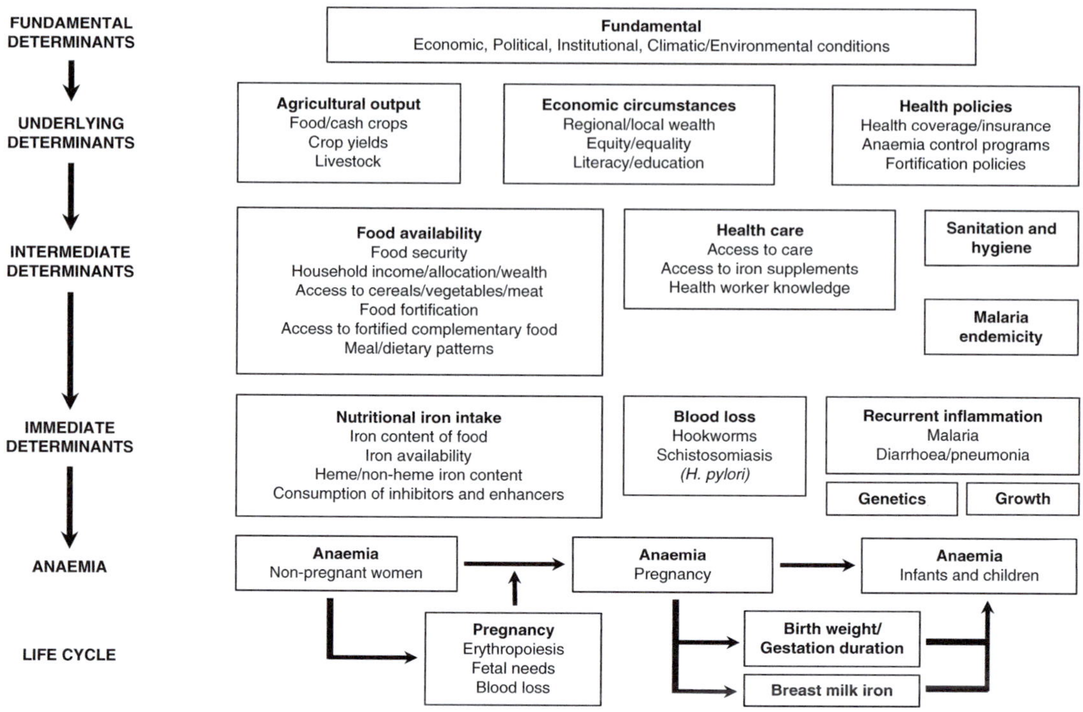

Fig. 1.1 Determinants of iron deficiency anaemia. Adapted from [42]

42% (95% CI 38–46%) for preschool children, 49% (43–53%) for non-pregnant women of reproductive age and 50% (47–53%) for pregnant women. In some regions this figure is lower; for example, in the WHO African Region, these estimates are 32% (30–34%), 41% (36–46%) and 44% (42–47%), respectively [29]. Overall, the proportion of anaemia attributable to iron deficiency is highest in cases of severe anaemia and in settings where other key causes such as endemic infections are less prevalent [34].

Subsequent meta-analyses of national population studies suggest the contribution of iron deficiency to anaemia may be smaller than previously reported: 25% in preschool-aged children and 37% in non-pregnant women of reproductive age [43]. These figures were found to be even lower in countries with anaemia prevalence greater than 40% (14 and 16%, respectively) and with high burden of inflammation (20 and 25%, respectively) [43].

The Biomarkers Reflecting Inflammation and Nutritional Determinants of Anemia (BRINDA) Project has also estimated the proportion of anaemia attributable to iron deficiency in women of reproductive age and preschool children. BRINDA incorporated their model for correcting for infection and inflammation when assessing ferritin and sTfR concentrations and body iron stores. For both demographic groups, it was found that infection burden had an influence on the proportion of anaemia caused by iron deficiency. Among women of reproductive age, iron deficiency was estimated to be present in 35% of women with anaemia in areas with high infection burden, but at higher levels in anaemic women living in areas with moderate and low infection burdens (65 and 71%, respectively) [44]. Among preschool children with anaemia, iron deficiency ranged from 50% in areas with low infection to 58% in areas with very high prevalence of infection [45].

Global Burden of Disease Attributable to Anaemia

In order to ascertain the burden of a particular disease or condition, it is necessary to quantify its contribution to both mortality and morbidity. The burden of a disease is defined through the Disability Adjusted Life Years (DALYs) attributable to it. DALYs are the sum of the ongoing morbidity associated with a condition (Years Lived with Disability, YLDs), where the severity of the suffering is estimated by the 'disability weight' and the years of life lost (YLLs) from early mortality due to a condition. Thus, diseases that induce a long duration of suffering but do not cause death will produce DALYs via a large number of YLDs but not YLLs, whereas a short-lasting illness which causes premature mortality will produce the opposite impact. Disability weights assigned to anaemia in the GBD 2010 study are shown in Table 1.8. Disability weights assigned (through international population surveys) to mild anaemia are relatively low, whereas moderate and especially severe anaemia have been assigned much higher disability weights.

Mortality attributable to anaemia is rare. However, the enormous prevalence of anaemia and its long duration mean that anaemia continues to exert a substantial contribution to the overall global burden of disease. In particular, anaemia of moderate severity, which has a higher disability weight and is also prevalent in many countries, is an important contributor to the overall burden of anaemia [47]. GBD 2019 reported that anaemia was responsible for 50.3 million YLDs (33.5–73.4 million) out of a total of 861 million (641–1107 million), representing 5.8% of all YLDs [38].

Table 1.8 Disability weights for anaemia GBD 2010 [46]

	Disability weight (95% uncertainty interval)[a]
Mild anaemia	0.005 (0.002–0.011)
Moderate anaemia	0.058 (0.038–0.086)
Severe anaemia	0.164 (0.112–0.228)

[a] Disability weight values range from 0 to 1, where 0 signifies a fully healthy state and 1 is the equivalent of death

Anaemia Reduction Targets

There are international targets to reduce the global burden of anaemia. Table 1.9 summarises key global policy frameworks and targets relevant to anaemia reduction efforts.

Table 1.9 International targets relevant to anaemia reduction

Policy framework	Year endorsed	Targets(s) relevant to anaemia
WHO Global Nutrition Targets 2025 [48, 49]	2012	Target 2: 50% reduction of anaemia in women of reproductive age WHO recommendations for prevention, control and treatment of anaemia in women: • Intermittent iron and folic acid supplementation is advised in menstruating women living in settings where the prevalence of anaemia is 20% or higher • Daily oral iron and folic acid supplementation is recommended as part of antenatal care, to reduce the risk of low birth weight, maternal anaemia and iron deficiency. In addition to iron and folic acid, supplements may be formulated to include other vitamins and minerals, according to the United Nations International Multiple Micronutrient Antenatal Preparation (UNIMMAP), to overcome other possible maternal micronutrient deficiencies • In areas where the prevalence of anaemia among pregnant women is lower than 20%, intermittent iron and folic acid supplementation in non-anaemic, pregnant women is advised, to prevent anaemia and to improve pregnancy outcomes • In the postpartum period, iron supplementation, either alone or in combination with folic acid, for at least 3 months, may reduce the risk of anaemia by improving the iron status of the mother • Fortification of wheat and maize flours with iron, folic acid and other micronutrients is advised in settings where these foods are major staples • In malaria-endemic areas, the provision of iron and folic acid supplements should be made in conjunction with public health measures to prevent, diagnose and treat malaria • In emergencies, pregnant and lactating women should be given the United Nations International Children's Emergency Fund (UNICEF)/WHO micronutrient supplement providing one RNI (recommended nutrient intake) of micronutrients daily (including 27 mg iron), whether or not they receive fortified rations. Iron and folic acid supplements, when already provided, should be continued[a] • All pregnant women with active tuberculosis should receive multiple micronutrient supplements that contain iron and folic acid and other vitamins and minerals, according to the UNIMMAP, to complement their maternal micronutrient needs • Multiple micronutrient supplements offer important benefits to pregnant women in poor settings, particularly for pregnant women with HIV to reach recommended levels • Exclusive breastfeeding of infants for up to 6 months of age should be protected, promoted and supported. The beneficiaries include the infant and the mother (i.e. longer amenorrhoea, increased birth spacing), as well as the newborn (an important source of iron, which is very well absorbed in breast milk)
UN Sustainable Development Goals (SDGs) [50, 51]	2015	Goal 2: End hunger, achieve food security and improved nutrition and promote sustainable agriculture Target 2.2: By 2030, end all forms of malnutrition, including achieving, by 2025, the internationally agreed targets on stunting and wasting in children under 5 years of age, and address the nutritional needs of adolescent girls, pregnant and lactating women and older persons Indicator 2.2.3: Prevalence of anaemia in women aged 15–49 years, by pregnancy status (percentage)
UN Decade for Action on Nutrition [52]	2016	Nutrition focus (micronutrient deficiencies)

[a] Joint statement by WHO, World Food Programme and UNICEF [53]

Progress in Anaemia Reduction

Anaemia in women and preschool children reduced globally over the period from 1995 to 2011, from 33% to 29% of non-pregnant women of reproductive age and from 47% to 43% of preschool children (Table 1.10) [34, 54]. This global trend, however, was not uniform between geographic areas. While anaemia in women overall over this time period showed modest reduction in particular regions including Latin America, East Africa and East and Southeast Asia, in other regions there was no improvement, especially in central and west Africa (for non-pregnant women) and in South Asia (for pregnant women). In children, despite global improvement in mean haemoglobin and reduction in anaemia, anaemia prevalence in Southern Africa has likely *increased* over this same period (Table 1.11).

Over the period 2011–2016, annual data published by the Global Nutrition Report shows a plateauing of anaemia prevalence in women of reproductive age, with 2016 prevalence similar to that from 2006 [55]. According to the 2020 Global Nutrition Report, no country is presently on track to meet its anaemia target of a 50% reduction in anaemia in women of reproductive age for the year 2025 [56, 57]. Indeed, just a quarter of countries (49 out of 194) had made 'some progress'—as opposed to no progress or deteriorating anaemia prevalence—towards the target [57].

Despite this limited reduction in overall anaemia, the prevalence of severe anaemia has declined considerably in all regions, with 2011 prevalence under 2.5% in all regions with the exception of preschool children in central and west Africa (from 9.7% [95% credibility interval 7.4–12.1%] in 1995 to 4.9% [3.8–6.2%] in 2011) [34].

GBD-compiled anaemia data from 1990, 2010 and 2019 demonstrates modest reductions in prevalence (as a percentage of the population) and YLDs over time, but again shows slowing progress in the last decade (Table 1.12).

Table 1.10 Global mean haemoglobin, anaemia and severe anaemia among key population groups (1995 and 2011)

	1995			2011		
	Mean haemoglobin (g/L)	Anaemia (%)	Severe anaemia (%)	Mean haemoglobin (g/L)	Anaemia (%)	Severe anaemia (%)
Children <5 years	109 (107–111)	47 (43–51)	3.7 (2.8–4.7)	111 (110–113)	43 (38–47)	1.5 (1.1–2.2)
Non-pregnant women (15–49 years)	125 (123–126)	33 (29–37)	1.8 (1.3–2.3)	126 (124–128)	29 (24–35)	1.1 (0.7–1.7)
Pregnant women (15–49 years)	112 (111–113)	43 (39–47)	2.0 (1.5–2.6)	114 (112–116)	38 (34–43)	0.9 (0.6–1.3)

Table 1.11 Mean haemoglobin and anaemia prevalence in selected regions and population groups (1995 and 2011)

	1995			2011		
	Mean haemoglobin (g/L)	Anaemia (%)	Severe anaemia (%)	Mean haemoglobin (g/L)	Anaemia (%)	Severe anaemia (%)
Southern Africa						
Children <5 years	116 (111–119)	30 (21–42)	1.1 (0.3–2.3)	110 (105–116)	46 (31–62)	0.9 (0.3–2.4)
Central and west Africa						
Non-pregnant women (15–49 years)	118 (114–123)	52 (39–61)	2.8 (1.8–4.1)	119 (115–123)	48 (37–58)	2.2 (1.4–4.0)
South Asia						
Pregnant women (15–49 years)	108 (104–111)	53 (43–63)	2.9 (1.8–4.4)	108 (105–113)	52 (40–63)	1.3 (0.7–2.4)

(95% credibility intervals in parentheses.) Adapted from [34]

Table 1.12 Anaemia figures based on GBD data

	1990	2010	2019
Prevalence (number)	1.44 billion	1.64 billion	1.76 billion
Prevalence (%)	27.94	24.48	23.67
YLDs (number due to anaemia)	65.5 million	68.4 million	50.3 million
YLDs (% due to anaemia)	11.2	8.8	5.82

Derived from [38]

The GBD programme also provides longitudinal estimates of iron deficiency burden as a nutritional risk factor. According to this data, iron deficiency remains a significant health risk in terms of percentage of DALYs, with little overall improvement between 1990 and 2019 (annualised rate of change from 1990 to 2019 of −0.50% [−0.65 to −0.38%]) [58]. Nutritional iron deficiency remains the top risk factor among people aged 10–24 years. There has, however, been a net reduction in number of DALYs attributable to iron deficiency in this age group over the same period (−0.9% change in DALYs [−11.4 to 9.5], with age-adjusted rate −17.6% [−26.4 to −8.8]) [58].

Progress in 2020 and Beyond

Given the modest rate of progress in anaemia reduction, additional strategies are clearly required to reach the nutrition targets set in the last decade and to ensure that anaemia interventions adequately address the needs of people at highest risk of anaemia. The causes of anaemia are complex and differ according to region and population group. Regional factors including local nutritional data and infection burden must be considered so that interventions can be tailored appropriately. Increased recognition of non-iron deficiency causes of anaemia, including the contribution to the prevalence of anaemia from carrier states or milder forms of haemoglobinopathies and thalassaemia, will become increasingly important in developing more nuanced anaemia control policies.

COVID-19 Pandemic

The COVID-19 pandemic has had wide-ranging effects on global health, and anaemia reduction efforts have not been spared from this impact. Further progress in combating anaemia continues to be threatened by the pandemic through its effects on exacerbating poverty and food insecurity [59]. The 2020 SDG report highlights the devastating disruption to all SDGs caused by the pandemic [50]. The virus and the actions taken to limit transmission have resulted in the first increase in global poverty since 1998 [50]. The pandemic has been strongly linked to worsening food insecurity through poverty-related changes in food consumption and through disruptions to the food supply chain [50, 60].

According to the UN, the number of people undernourished in 2019 was 60 million more than it was in 2014, and it projects an additional 132 million people may be affected in 2020 [50]. COVID-19 and related disruptions have been estimated to result in 2.1 million additional cases of maternal anaemia by 2022 [61]. While these impacts disproportionately affect already-vulnerable groups in LMICs, COVID-19 responses including stay-at-home orders have exacerbated risks of food insecurity even in previously relatively food secure populations [62, 63]. Finally, progress in malaria reduction had already stalled in the latter part of the 2010s, and COVID-19-related impacts on malaria control measures may impair further progress. Indeed, modelling has predicted significant increases in cases and up to a doubling of mortality, with follow-on effects beyond 2020 [50, 64].

References

1. World Health Organization. Haemoglobin concentrations for the diagnosis of anaemia and assessment of severity. Geneva: World Health Organization; 2011. http://www.who.int/vmnis/indicators/haemoglobin.pdf.
2. Pasricha S-R, Colman K, Centeno-Tablante E, Garcia-Casal M-N, Peña-Rosas J-P. Revisiting WHO haemoglobin thresholds to define anaemia in clinical medicine and public health. Lancet Haematol. 2018;5(2):e60–e2.
3. Komajda M, Anker SD, Charlesworth A, Okonko D, Metra M, Di Lenarda A, et al. The impact of new onset anaemia on morbidity and mortality in chronic heart failure: results from COMET. Eur Heart J. 2006;27(12):1440–6.
4. Musallam KM, Tamim HM, Richards T, Spahn DR, Rosendaal FR, Habbal A, et al. Preoperative anaemia and postoperative outcomes in non-cardiac surgery: a retrospective cohort study. Lancet. 2011;378(9800):1396–407.
5. Kovesdy CP, Trivedi BK, Kalantar-Zadeh K, Anderson JE. Association of anemia with outcomes in men with moderate and severe chronic kidney disease. Kidney Int. 2006;69(3):560–4.
6. Daru J, Zamora J, Fernández-Félix BM, Vogel J, Oladapo OT, Morisaki N, et al. Risk of maternal mortality in women with severe anaemia during pregnancy and post partum: a multilevel analysis. Lancet Glob Health. 2018;6(5):e548–e54.
7. Rahman MM, Abe SK, Rahman MS, Kanda M, Narita S, Bilano V, et al. Maternal anemia and risk of adverse birth and health outcomes in low- and middle-income countries: systematic review and meta-analysis. Am J Clin Nutr. 2016;103(2):495–504.
8. Haider BA, Olofin I, Wang M, Spiegelman D, Ezzati M, Fawzi WW, et al. Anaemia, prenatal iron use, and risk of adverse pregnancy outcomes: systematic review and meta-analysis. BMJ. 2013;346:f3443.
9. World Health Organization. WHO Global Anaemia estimates, 2021 Edition. Geneva: World Health Organization; 2021. https://www.who.int/data/gho/data/themes/topics/anaemia_in_women_and_children.
10. Haas JD, Brownlie T. Iron deficiency and reduced work capacity: a critical review of the research to determine a causal relationship. J Nutr. 2001;131(2s-2):676S–88S; discussion 88S–90S.
11. Pasricha SR, Hasan MI, Braat S, Larson LM, Tipu SMM, Hossain SJ, et al. Benefits and Risks of Iron Interventions in Infants in Rural Bangladesh. N Engl J Med. 2021;385(11):982–95.
12. World Health Organization. Nutritional anaemias: tools for effective prevention and control. Geneva: World Health Organization; 2017. https://www.who.int/publications/i/item/9789241513067.
13. World Health Organization. WHO recommendations on antenatal care for a positive pregnancy experience. Geneva: World Health Organization; 2016. https://www.who.int/publications/i/item/9789241549912.
14. Centers for Disease Control and Prevention. Recommendations to prevent and control iron deficiency in the United States. Atlanta, GA: Centers for Disease Control and Prevention; 1998. https://www.cdc.gov/mmwr/preview/mmwrhtml/00051880.htm.
15. Ohuma EO, Young MF, Martorell R, Ismail LC, Pena-Rosas JP, Purwar M, et al. International values for haemoglobin distributions in healthy pregnant women. EClinicalMedicine. 2020;29-30:100660.
16. Sachdev HS, Porwal A, Acharya R, Ashraf S, Ramesh S, Khan N, et al. Haemoglobin thresholds to define anaemia in a national sample of healthy children and adolescents aged 1–19 years in India: a population-based study. Lancet Glob Health. 2021;9(6):e822–e31.
17. Colman KS, Wood EM, De La Salle B, Stanworth SJ, Pasricha SR. Heterogeneous hemoglobin lower thresholds in clinical laboratories. Am J Hematol. 2018;93(6):E142–E4.
18. Pasricha SR, Colman K, Centeno-Tablante E, Garcia-Casal MN, Pena-Rosas JP. Revisiting WHO haemoglobin thresholds to define anaemia in clinical medicine and public health. Lancet Haematol. 2018;5(2):e60–e2.
19. Lewis S, Bain B, Bates I. Dacie and Lewis practical haematology. 12th ed. London: Elsevier; 2017.
20. Muriuki JM, Mentzer AJ, Mitchell R, Webb EL, Etyang AO, Kyobutungi C, et al. Malaria is a cause of iron deficiency in African children. Nat Med. 2021;27(4):653–8.
21. Baldi AJ, Larson LM, Pasricha SR. Balancing safety and potential for impact in universal iron interventions. Nestle Nutr Inst Workshop Ser. 2020;93:51–62.
22. Bain B. Blood cells: a practical guide. Wiley Blackwell; 2015.
23. Pasricha S-R, Tye-Din J, Muckenthaler MU, Swinkels DW. Iron deficiency. Lancet. 2021;397(10270):233–48.
24. Sanchis-Gomar F, Cortell-Ballester J, Pareja-Galeano H, Banfi G, Lippi G. Hemoglobin point-of-care testing: the HemoCue system. J Lab Autom. 2013;18(3):198–205.
25. Neufeld LM, Larson LM, Kurpad A, Mburu S, Martorell R, Brown KH. Hemoglobin concentration and anemia diagnosis in venous and capillary blood: biological basis and policy implications. Ann N Y Acad Sci. 2019;1450(1):172–89.
26. United States Agency for International Development. The Demographic and Health Surveys (DHS) Program. 2021. https://dhsprogram.com/.
27. World Health Organization. Vitamin and Mineral Nutrition Information System (VMNIS). 2021. https://www.who.int/teams/nutrition-and-food-safety/databases/vitamin-and-mineral-nutrition-information-system.

28. World Health Organization. Worldwide prevalence of anaemia 1993–2005: WHO Global Database on Anaemia. Geneva: World Health Organization; 2008. https://apps.who.int/iris/handle/10665/43894.
29. World Health Organization. The global prevalence of anaemia in 2011. Geneva: World Health Organization; 2015. https://apps.who.int/iris/handle/10665/177094.
30. World Health Organization. Global Health Observatory data repository. Prevalence of anaemia in children under 5 years (%). Geneva: World Health Organization; 2021. https://apps.who.int/gho/data/view.main.ANAEMIACHILDRENREG.
31. World Health Organization. Global Health Observatory data repository. Prevalence of anaemia in pregnant women. Geneva: World Health Organization; 2021. https://apps.who.int/gho/data/view.main.ANAEMIAWOMENPWREG.
32. World Health Organization. Global Health Observatory data repository. Prevalence of anaemia in non-pregnant women. Geneva: World Health Organization; 2021. https://apps.who.int/gho/data/view.main.ANAEMIAWOMENNPWREG.
33. World Health Organization. Iron deficiency anaemia: assessment, prevention and control, a guide for program managers. Geneva: World Health Organization, UNICEF, UNU; 2001.
34. Stevens GA, Finucane MM, De-Regil LM, Paciorek CJ, Flaxman SR, Branca F, et al. Global, regional, and national trends in haemoglobin concentration and prevalence of total and severe anaemia in children and pregnant and non-pregnant women for 1995–2011: a systematic analysis of population-representative data. Lancet Glob Health. 2013;1(1):e16–25.
35. Government of Malawi MoH. Malawi National Malaria Indicator Survey 2010. Lilongwe: Ministry of Health; 2010. https://files.givewell.org/files/DWDA%202009/AMF/Malawi_MIS_2010_Final.pdf.
36. Lozano R, Naghavi M, Foreman K, Lim S, Shibuya K, Aboyans V, et al. Global and regional mortality from 235 causes of death for 20 age groups in 1990 and 2010: a systematic analysis for the Global Burden of Disease Study 2010. Lancet. 2012;380(9859):2095–128.
37. Murray CJL, Ezzati M, Flaxman AD, Lim S, Lozano R, Michaud C, et al. GBD 2010: design, definitions, and metrics. 2012. p. 2063–6.
38. Institute for Health Metrics and Evaluation. GBD Compare Data Visualization Seattle. WA: IHME, University of Washington; 2020. https://vizhub.healthdata.org/gbd-compare/.
39. World Health Organization. Anaemia. Geneva: World Health Organization; 2020. https://www.who.int/health-topics/anaemia.
40. Chaparro CM, Suchdev PS. Anemia epidemiology, pathophysiology, and etiology in low- and middle-income countries. Ann N Y Acad Sci. 2019;1450(1):15–31.
41. Kassebaum NJ, Jasrasaria R, Naghavi M, Wulf SK, Johns N, Lozano R, et al. A systematic analysis of global anemia burden from 1990 to 2010. Blood. 2014;123(5):615–24.
42. Pasricha SR, Drakesmith H, Black J, Hipgrave D, Biggs BA. Control of iron deficiency anemia in low- and middle-income countries. Blood. 2013;121(14):2607–17.
43. Petry N, Olofin I, Hurrell RF, Boy E, Wirth JP, Moursi M, et al. The proportion of anemia associated with iron deficiency in low, medium, and high human development index countries: a systematic analysis of national surveys. Nutrients. 2016;8(11)
44. Wirth JP, Woodruff BA, Engle-Stone R, Namaste SM, Temple VJ, Petry N, et al. Predictors of anemia in women of reproductive age: Biomarkers Reflecting Inflammation and Nutritional Determinants of Anemia (BRINDA) project. Am J Clin Nutr. 2017;106(suppl_1):416S–27S.
45. Engle-Stone R, Aaron GJ, Huang J, Wirth JP, Namaste SM, Williams AM, et al. Predictors of anemia in preschool children: Biomarkers Reflecting Inflammation and Nutritional Determinants of Anemia (BRINDA) project. Am J Clin Nutr. 2017;106(suppl_1):402S–15S.
46. Salomon JA, Vos T, Hogan DR, Gagnon M, Naghavi M, Mokdad A, et al. Common values in assessing health outcomes from disease and injury: disability weights measurement study for the Global Burden of Disease Study 2010. Lancet. 2012;380(9859):2129–43.
47. Pasricha SR, Gheorghe A, Sakr-Ashour F, Arcot A, Neufeld L, Murray-Kolb LE, et al. Net benefit and cost-effectiveness of universal iron-containing multiple micronutrient powders for young children in 78 countries: a microsimulation study. Lancet Glob Health. 2020;8(8):e1071–e80.
48. World Health Organization. Global Targets 2025: to improve maternal, infant and young child nutrition. Geneva: World Health Organization; 2014. https://www.who.int/teams/nutrition-and-food-safety/global-targets-2025.
49. World Health Organization. Global Targets 2025: anaemia policy brief. Geneva: World Health Organization; 2014. https://apps.who.int/iris/handle/10665/148556.
50. United Nations. The Sustainable Development Goals Report 2020. United Nations; 2020. https://unstats.un.org/sdgs/report/2020/.
51. United Nations. SDG indicators: global indicator framework for the Sustainable Development Goals and targets of the 2030 Agenda for Sustainable Development. New York: United Nations; 2021. https://unstats.un.org/sdgs/indicators/indicators-list/.
52. United Nations System Standing Committee on Nutrition. The Decade of Action on Nutrition 2016–2025. United Nations; 2016. https://www.unscn.org/en/topics/un-decade-of-action-on-nutrition.
53. World Health Organization. Preventing and controlling micronutrient deficiencies in populations

affected by an emergency: multiple vitamin and mineral supplements for pregnant and lactating women, and for children aged 6 to 59 months: joint statement by the World Health Organization, the World Food Programme and the United Nations Children's Fund. Geneva: World Health Organization; 2007. https://www.who.int/publications/m/item/WHO-WFP-UNICEF-statement-micronutrients-deficiencies-emergency.
54. 2020 Global Nutrition Report: action on equity to end malnutrition (Executive Summary). Bristol, UK: Development Initiatives; 2020. https://globalnutritionreport.org/reports/2020-global-nutrition-report/executive-summary/.
55. Global Nutrition Report: Country Nutrition Profiles. Bristol, UK: Development Initiatives; 2021. https://globalnutritionreport.org/resources/nutrition-profiles/.
56. World Health Organization. Global anaemia reduction efforts among women of reproductive age: impact, achievement of targets and the way forward for optimizing efforts. Geneva: World Health Organization; 2020.
57. 2020 Global Nutrition Report: Action on equity to end malnutrition (Inequalities in the global burden of malnutrition). Bristol, UK: Development Initiatives; 2020. https://globalnutritionreport.org/reports/2020-global-nutrition-report/inequalities-global-burden-malnutrition/.
58. Murray CJL, Aravkin AY, Zheng P, Abbafati C, Abbas KM, Abbasi-Kangevari M, et al. Global burden of 87 risk factors in 204 countries and territories, 1990–2019: a systematic analysis for the Global Burden of Disease Study 2019. Lancet. 2020;396(10258):1223–49.
59. The Lancet D, Endocrinology. Food policies: in times of COVID-19 and beyond. Lancet Diabetes Endocrinol 2021;9(6).
60. Laborde Debuquet D, Martin W, Vos R. IFPRI Discussion Paper 01993 December 2020: impacts of COVID-19 on Global Poverty, Food Security and Diets. Washington, DC: International Food Policy Research Institute; 2020. https://doi.org/10.2499/p15738coll2.134229.
61. Osendarp S, Akuoku JK, Black RE, Headey D, Ruel M, Scott N, et al. The COVID-19 crisis will exacerbate maternal and child undernutrition and child mortality in low- and middle-income countries. Nature Food. 2021;2(7):476–84.
62. Hamadani JD, Hasan MI, Baldi AJ, Hossain SJ, Shiraji S, Bhuiyan MSA, et al. Immediate impact of stay-at-home orders to control COVID-19 transmission on socioeconomic conditions, food insecurity, mental health, and intimate partner violence in Bangladeshi women and their families: an interrupted time series. Lancet Glob Health. 2020;8(11):e1380–e9.
63. International Food Policy Research Institute. 2021 Global Food Policy Report: Transforming Food Systems after COVID-19. Washington, DC: IFPRI; 2021. https://doi.org/10.2499/9780896293991.
64. Weiss DJ, Bertozzi-Villa A, Rumisha SF, Amratia P, Arambepola R, Battle KE, et al. Indirect effects of the COVID-19 pandemic on malaria intervention coverage, morbidity, and mortality in Africa: a geospatial modelling analysis. Lancet Infect Dis. 2020.

2 Iron Biology: Metabolism and Homeostasis

Tomas Ganz

Keywords

Hepcidin · Ferroportin · Iron overload
Anemia · Interleukin-6 · Inflammation
Heme · Hemoglobin · Erythroferrone

Introduction

This is an overview of systemic iron regulation focused predominantly on human physiology and its disorders and laboratory rodent models that are informative about human pathophysiology. A complementary discussion of these topics is available in other recent reviews [1, 2].

Biological Roles of Iron

Iron is an essential trace element for nearly every living organism. Because it readily accepts or donates electrons, iron is a versatile catalyst of biochemical reactions but is also potentially toxic. In biological organisms, its chemical reactivity is controlled by its association with prosthetic groups (iron-sulfur clusters or heme) or with protein amino acid side chains. Iron-containing proteins carry or store oxygen (e.g., hemoglobin or myoglobin); catalyze metabolic, signaling-related, and antimicrobial redox reactions (e.g., cytochromes, ribonucleotide reductase, nitric oxide synthase, NADPH oxidase, myeloperoxidase); and transport or store iron (e.g., transferrin, lactoferrin, or ferritin). Iron-containing proteins are essential for energy metabolism and intermediary metabolism including nucleotide synthesis and play a role in signaling pathways as well as host defense.

The Iron Economy

Despite the abundance of iron on the Earth, most organisms commonly experience iron scarcity, a paradox attributable to the low solubility of oxidized forms of iron. For humans, iron is inefficiently absorbable from plant-based foods, and this is reflected in the high prevalence of iron deficiency in human populations that consume meat-poor or vegetarian diets. Heme iron from animal flesh is more efficiently absorbed, but these foods are scarce in many areas of the world. In this environment, humans and other animals evolved ways of efficiently conserving and recycling iron. At the other extreme, most consumers of high-iron diets in prosperous countries physiologically limit dietary absorption of iron and avoid the toxicity of excessive iron accumulation.

T. Ganz (✉)
Departments of Medicine and Pathology, David Geffen School of Medicine, University of California, Los Angeles, CA, USA
e-mail: TGanz@mednet.ucla.edu

C. D. Karakochuk et al. (eds.), *Nutritional Anemia*, Nutrition and Health,
https://doi.org/10.1007/978-3-031-14521-6_2

The iron economy of the adult human is summarized in Fig. 2.1. The average adult human contains about 3–4 g of iron, about 2–3 g of which is in erythrocyte hemoglobin. Other iron-rich tissues include the liver and the spleen, the major reserve organs for iron, where iron is stored in macrophages and hepatocytes in a specialized cytoplasmic iron storage protein, ferritin. Muscle contains iron predominantly in myoglobin, an oxygen storage protein. All cells contain smaller concentrations of iron-containing proteins essential for energy production, synthetic metabolism, and other important functions. Iron is distributed to tissues through blood plasma, which contains only 2–4 mg of iron, bound by the iron transport protein transferrin, whose iron-binding sites are normally only 20–45% filled. Plasma iron turns over every few hours, as about 20–25 mg of iron a day move through this compartment. Of all cells, erythrocytes have the highest concentration of iron, about 1 mg/mL packed volume. Although smaller amounts of iron from other cell types are

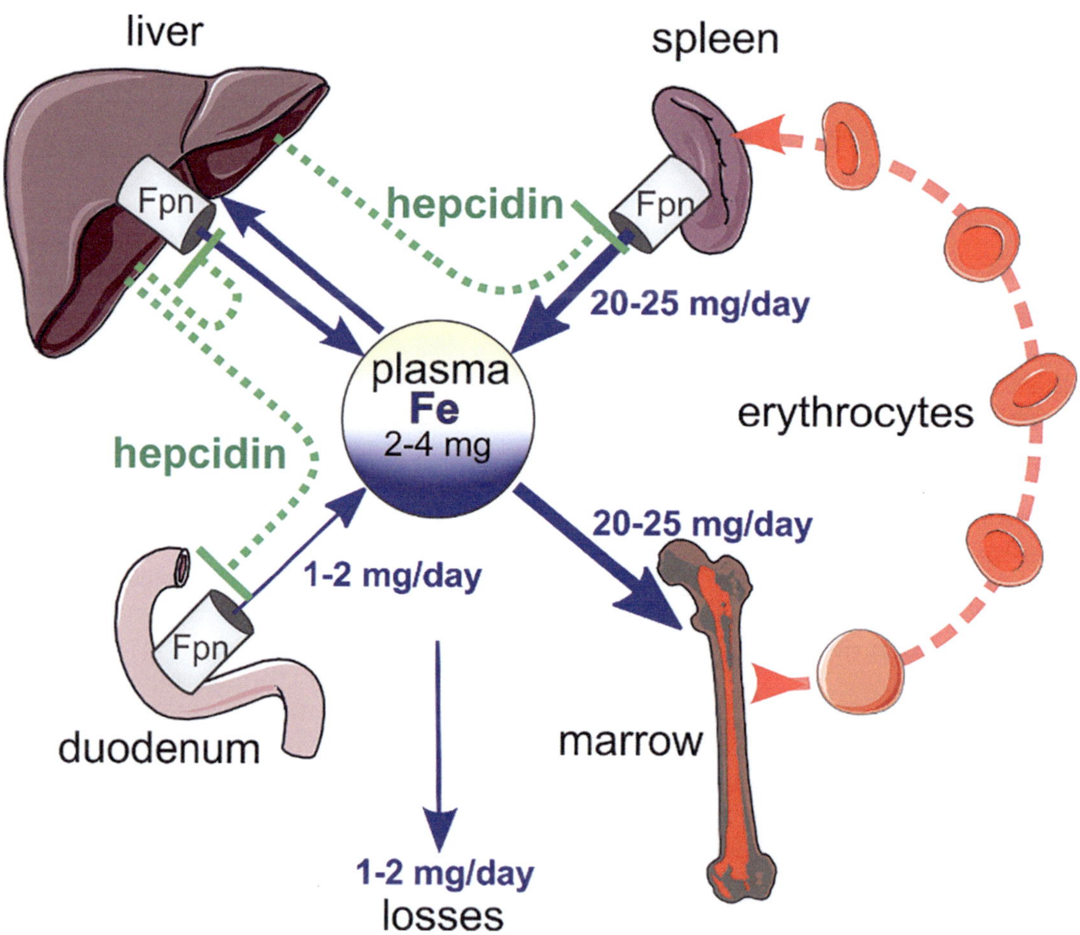

Fig. 2.1 Major iron flows and their regulation by hepcidin and ferroportin. Iron in transferrin is indicated in solid blue, iron in erythrocytes in dashed red. Hepcidin (green dashes) produced by hepatocytes controls the flow iron into plasma by blocking iron export through ferroportin (Fpn) in the duodenal enterocytes, hepatocytes, and splenic and hepatic macrophages. Aged erythrocytes (~120 days in humans) undergo erythrophagocytosis by macrophages in the spleen (and the liver), and their iron content is recycled through the small plasma iron pool and used mainly by the marrow for the production of new erythrocytes. Normally, iron absorption in the duodenum is sufficient to replace small losses of iron through minor bleeding and loss of epithelial cells from body surfaces. The liver functions as the main storage organ for iron

also recovered by macrophages, most plasma iron is derived from aged erythrocytes that are recycled by macrophages in the spleen and other organs. As the lifespan of human erythrocytes is about 120 days, about 0.8% (or about 15–25 mg) of all erythrocyte iron must be recycled every day. In turn, iron is extracted from the plasma compartment mostly for hemoglobin synthesis by erythrocyte precursors. Despite rapid turnover and changes in iron utilization, plasma iron concentrations are generally stable, indicating that the delivery of iron from recycling macrophages into plasma is homeostatically controlled.

Iron losses from the body are only 1–2 mg/day mainly from desquamation of epithelial surfaces. Under normal circumstances the losses are balanced by dietary iron absorption, primarily in the proximal duodenum. Because losses of iron from the body are not significantly modulated by systemic iron deficiency or excess, regulation of the iron content of the body is completely dependent on close control of dietary iron absorption.

Iron Homeostasis: Tissues and Cellular Transporters

Tissues, Cells, and Fluxes

The three key cell types involved in postnatal iron homeostasis are duodenal enterocytes which absorb dietary iron, macrophages which recycle iron from erythrocytes and other cells, and hepatocytes which store iron and can release it when needed. During fetal development, the placental syncytiotrophoblast transfers iron from the mother to the fetus. The main regulated step in all iron-transporting tissues is the transfer of iron from these cells to plasma. The iron-regulatory hormone hepcidin is produced by hepatocytes (including fetal hepatocytes) and controls the transfer of iron to plasma from enterocytes, macrophages, hepatocytes, and syncytiotrophoblast. Iron not transferred to plasma is retained in macrophages and hepatocytes, where it functions as a cellular storage compartment (Fig. 2.1). Iron retained in enterocytes is rapidly lost from the body because these cells turn over every 2–5 days in humans and are sloughed into the fecal stream along with any iron that had not been transferred to plasma. Accordingly, the partitioning of iron between duodenal enterocytes (the mucosa) and the plasma effectively determines the body iron content.

The predominant forms of iron in the human diet are ferric iron, heme, and ferritin all complexed with other macromolecules. The acidic environment of the stomach and exposure to digestive enzymes cause a partial release of these iron forms from the digestate. The transport of inorganic iron is well understood, but little is known about the transport and metabolism of heme and ferritin in the enterocyte. It appears that iron from ferritin or heme exits the enterocyte by the same route and in the same form as inorganic dietary iron (Fig. 2.2).

Most of the iron flux in the body is generated by macrophages recycling senescent erythrocytes. The phagolysosome digests the erythrocyte and its hemoglobin, releasing heme, which is then degraded by the inducible heme oxygenase-1 (HO-1), freeing iron for cytoplasmic storage or export to blood plasma. The presence of a heme transporter (heme responsive gene-1, HRG-1) in the phagolysosomal membrane and the consequences of its ablation favor a model in which heme is transported across the phagosomal membrane and then degraded within the cell outside the phagolysosome [3, 4] (Fig. 2.2). This model was recently challenged by evidence that senescent erythrocytes may lyse in the spleen just prior to erythrophagocytosis, in which case haptoglobin-hemoglobin complexes would be the main species recycled by macrophages into iron [5]. Although normally most iron is exported to plasma across the macrophage cell membrane, during hemolytic stress heme may be exported intact by heme transporters and then bound to hemopexin, a plasma heme carrier.

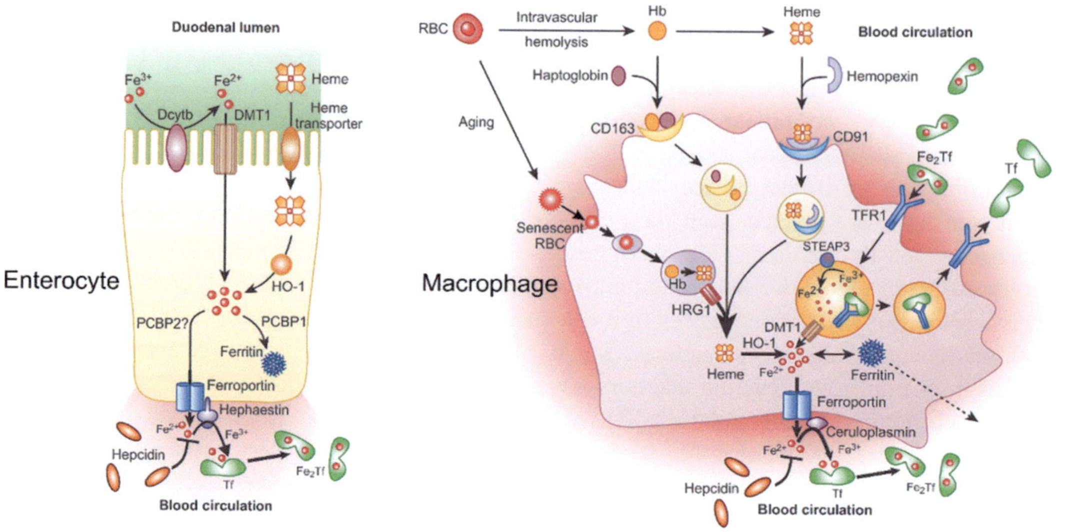

Fig. 2.2 Transport of iron by enterocytes and macrophages. Iron uptake takes place at the apical brush border of enterocytes, mainly by DMT1 and an unknown heme transporter. Ferric reductase dCytB at the apical surface facilitates the conversion from the predominant dietary form, Fe^{3+} to Fe^{2+}, which is then transported by DMT1 into the cytoplasm. The heme transporter must be coupled to a cytoplasmic heme oxygenase (HO) which extracts iron from heme. Cytoplasmic iron transport to ferritin and ferroportin is mediated by chaperones PCBP1 and PCBP2. Intracellular iron is stored in ferritin. Basolateral iron (Fe^{2+}) export is solely mediated by ferroportin, but before it can be loaded onto the iron carrier transferrin (Tf), it is converted to Fe^{3+} by the oxygen-dependent ferroxidase hephaestin. Iron-transporting macrophages take up iron predominantly in the form of senescent erythrocytes which undergo proteolysis in the phagolysosome, followed by heme and iron transport into the cytoplasm. Macrophages can also take up iron through the conventional transferrin/TfR1-mediated uptake mechanism. During hemolytic episodes, macrophages can process hemoglobin/haptoglobin and heme/hemopexin complexes endocytosed by CD163 and CD91 receptors, respectively. Macrophage export of iron to plasma transferrin is dependent on ferroportin and ceruloplasmin. Hepcidin controls iron export by both enterocytes and macrophages. Macrophages and hepatocytes are the predominant cells secreting ferritin into plasma

Cellular Iron Homeostasis

Each cell regulates its own iron content and subcellular distribution by sensing internal iron concentrations and regulating its iron uptake, storage, utilization, and export. The best characterized sensing systems involve the iron-regulatory proteins IRP1 and IRP2 which during cellular iron deficiency bind to many mRNAs that encode proteins involved in cellular iron metabolism. When IRPs bind to mRNAs with iron-regulatory elements (IREs) in the 5′ end, they inhibit their translation. When bound to mRNAs with IREs in the 3′ end, they stabilize them against degradation so these mRNAs become more abundant. During cellular iron deficiency, as the IRP concentration increases, the production of the iron-importing transferrin receptor TfR1 also increases because its mRNA has 3’ IREs, but the synthesis of the iron storage protein ferritin is blocked because its mRNA has a 5’ IRE. The rich biology of this system is summarized elsewhere [6].

Iron Import

In the enterocyte (Fig. 2.2), the apical uptake transporter of inorganic iron is the divalent metal transporter DMT1 which imports ferrous iron (reviewed in [7]). DMT1 is found on the brush border membrane of duodenal enterocytes and also abundant in erythrocyte precursors where it colocalizes with transferrin in recycling endosomes. In erythrocyte precursors and other cell types dependent on transferrin for their iron supply, DMT1 transports iron released from transferrin in acidified endosomes to the cytoplasm. DMT1 and a related molecule, natural resistance-associated macrophage protein-1 (Nramp1), are also involved in iron transport in macrophages, but their specific function in these cells remains uncertain. Intestine-specific DMT1 knockout mice develop postnatal anemia and systemic iron deficiency but can be rescued by parenteral iron administration bypassing the intestinal tract, demonstrating the essential role of DMT1 in intestinal iron transport. DMT1 is dispensable for absorption of other divalent metals.

DMT1 is a proton-coupled Fe^{2+} transporter [8], found in at least four isoforms with differing transcription initiation sites and exon splicing. The mRNAs for some of the isoforms contain a 3′ iron-responsive element (3'IRE) that binds iron-regulatory proteins 1 and 2 to stabilize the mRNA and increase DMT1 synthesis when cellular iron concentrations are low. The 3'IRE+ forms are predominantly expressed in epithelial cells, while DMT1 mRNAs in erythroid cells lack the 3'IRE [7].

Effective iron transport by DMT1 depends on the concentration of ferrous iron and on the cotransport of protons. Duodenal cytochrome B (dcytB) contributes to the reduction of luminal ferric iron but is not required for DMT1 function, perhaps because other ferric reductase activities contribute as well. The intestinal Na^+/H^+ exchangers NHE3, and to a lesser extent NHE2, appear to be responsible for generating the proton concentrations necessary for DMT1 to function, a role previously ascribed to acid secretions generated in the stomach.

Heme Import

Iron can also be transported as heme, a form appearing either as a synthetic intermediate or generated by degradation of heme-containing proteins. The best documented mammalian heme uptake transporter, heme responsive gene-1, was cloned by homology to heme transporters identified in the heme auxotroph *C. elegans*. It localizes to the phagolysosomes of macrophages [9] and is required for the transport of heme recovered from senescent erythrocytes [3] and its recycling for iron (Fig. 2.2).

Ferritin and Cytoplasmic Storage

Ferritin is a spherical protein composed of 24 subunits of heavy (H) or light (L) type, with the capacity to store large amounts of iron in its interior. The H-ferritin subunits function as ferroxidases to facilitate the conversion of cytoplasmic Fe^{2+} to an oxidized mineral form for storage. Targeted deletion of the H-subunit in the intestine caused systemic iron dysregulation with increased intestinal iron absorption and mild systemic iron overload manifested by increased plasma and hepatic iron concentrations. The ability of the ferritin compartment to store iron in enterocytes may be required for controlled delivery of iron to the basolateral iron exporters.

Ferrous iron is delivered to ferritin by cytoplasmic chaperones, chiefly poly (rC)-binding protein 1 (PCBP1) [10]. Exit of iron from ferritin may occur through gated pores but mainly by the autophagy and lysosomal degradation of ferritin. The ferritin cargo receptor NCOA4 delivers ferritin to the autophagic system [11]. The transit of iron from ferritin to iron exporters may be mediated by PCBP2 [12], a protein closely related to and functionally interacting with PCBP1.

A soluble, relatively iron-poor form of ferritin is found in blood plasma. This form is a 24-subunit polymer containing mostly L-ferritin and is derived primarily from macrophages and hepatocytes. Recent studies indicate that ferritin may be released from cells by an unusual secretory pathway as a mixture of variably iron-loaded ferritin molecules, with subsequent receptor-mediated selective reuptake of iron-rich ferritin by neighboring cells, so that only iron-poor ferritin remains in circulation [13]. As the iron stores in macrophages generally reflect the total iron stored in hepatocytes and macrophages, serum concentrations of ferritin correlate with total iron stores [14], with exceptions reflecting pathological situations in which the macrophages are much less or much more iron-loaded than hepatocytes or situations where ferritin synthesis is primarily driven by inflammation.

Iron Exporters

The sole known mammalian cellular iron exporter is ferroportin (also called Slc40a1). It is expressed at all sites involved in iron transfer to plasma (Fig. 2.1), i.e., the basolateral membranes of duodenal enterocytes [15], the membranes of macrophages, the sinusoidal surfaces of hepatocytes, and the basal surface of the placental syncytiotrophoblast facing the fetal circulation [15]. Like DMT1, ferroportin is a 12-transmembrane domain protein with both termini in the cytoplasm. Structural analyses of ferroportin are converging on a model in which an N-terminal bundle of six helical segments connects by a loose cytoplasmic domain to the C-terminal bundle of six helices, effectively forming a cup that can alternate between "open in" and "open out" conformations. Ferrous iron, possibly complexed with a small organic molecule, binds to one or both small cavities, respectively, located in the C-terminal and N-terminal lobes of "open in" ferroportin, triggering a conformational change to an "open out" configuration which releases the iron to the extracellular space [16, 17]. The cytoplasmic domain connecting the two halves of the structure is thought to have a regulatory function controlled by ubiquitination [18]. Ferroportin is encoded by two tissue-specific differentially spliced transcripts, FPN1A and FPN1B, that encode the same protein but differ in the presence (FPN1A) or absence (FPN1B) of a 5'IRE that functions to translationally repress ferroportin synthesis when cellular iron is scarce. FPN1B is highly expressed in the duodenum and in erythroid precursors, allowing perhaps for altruistic export of iron by these cells even when they sense iron deficiency.

Cellular iron export is dependent on members of a family of copper-containing ferroxidases, including ceruloplasmin, hephaestin, and perhaps also zyklopen [19, 20], that use molecular oxygen to oxidize ferrous to ferric iron (Fig. 2.2). Hephaestin-deficient mice (sex-linked anemia or *sla*) manifest iron deficiency anemia with accumulation of iron in enterocytes [19], indicating that the basolateral transfer of iron to plasma is defective. Ceruloplasmin deficiency impedes both intestinal iron absorption and the release of iron from macrophages and causes accumulation of iron in the brain and in hepatocytes. Although detailed characterization of the respective tissue-specific roles of these ferroxidases remains to be done, it is likely that they facilitate ferroportin-mediated Fe^{2+} efflux by oxidizing iron to its ferric form Fe^{3+}, allowing its uptake by apotransferrin and thereby maintaining a low concentration of Fe^{2+} at the cell surface and Fe^{2+} gradient to the extracellular face of ferroportin that can drive iron transport. It remains to be established how the four known ferroxidase forms cooperate to provide ferroxidase function for enterocytes, macrophages, hepatocytes, and the placenta.

Heme Exporters

Feline leukemia virus, type C, receptor 1 (FLVCR1) is the sole known heme exporter. Its ablation in mice causes a severe fetal anemia lethal in mid-gestation [21]. Recent studies reveal that there are two functional isoforms of FLVCR1. FLVCR1b contains only the C-terminal half of FLVCR, is expressed in mitochondria, and may mediate heme export from mitochondria to the cytoplasm of erythrocyte precursors and other cells with active heme synthesis [22]. FLVCR1b is required for erythroid development and differentiation, presumably because without it heme does not reach the cytoplasm and is not incorporated into hemoglobin, but does not appear to be involved in systemic iron homeostasis. The full-length form of FLVCR1a is found in the plasma membrane and is not required for erythroid development.

Extracellular Iron Carriers

Ferric iron exported from cells becomes bound to the plasma iron carrier, transferrin, a protein that can carry up to two ferric ions and deliver them to target tissues for uptake by the transferrin receptor-1 (TfR1). The essential role of transferrin in delivering iron for erythropoiesis is revealed by the severe anemia in genetic hypotransferrinemia, or atransferrinemia, in humans and in mice. Paradoxically, the disorder results in systemic iron overload, showing that other tissues can take up non-transferrin-bound iron (NTBI). In atransferrinemia, or if iron enters plasma in excess of the carrying capacity of transferrin, iron becomes complexed to citrate, other organic acids, and albumin. These NTBI forms are taken up by hepatocytes via the manganese transporter Zip14, with alternative, less well-characterized mechanisms that import NTBI in other tissues susceptible to iron overload [23]. Plasma ferritin may also deliver iron to some tissues [13], but the relative physiologic contribution of this process is not understood. In addition to carriers that bind inorganic iron, hemopexin and haptoglobin are plasma proteins that bind free heme and free hemoglobin, respectively, limiting their toxic effects and scavenging them for recycling into iron [24, 25]. Hemopexin and haptoglobin have an important homeostatic role during hemolytic stress and diseases. These systems are overwhelmed during rapid hemolysis, such as a hemolytic transfusion reaction, where unchaperoned heme and hemoglobin can cause systemic and pulmonary hypertension, renal injury, abdominal pain, activation of the clotting system, and systemic inflammation [26].

Hormonal Control of Iron Homeostasis by Hepcidin and Its Receptor Ferroportin

Hepcidin

Despite fluctuations in the iron content of human diets and occasional blood loss, most adult humans maintain plasma iron concentrations of 10–30 μM and iron reserves of about 0.2–1 g [14]. Iron absorption is increased in mice or humans during periods of iron deficiency, and absorption is decreased by parenteral iron overload. These observations have led to the expectation that a systemically acting hormone regulates the major flows of iron (history reviewed in [27]).

The iron-regulatory hormone hepcidin is a small (25-amino acid) peptide synthesized and secreted by hepatocytes. Hepcidin circulates in blood plasma mostly free, and is filtered by the kidneys. The nine-amino acid N-terminal hepcidin segment is highly conserved and essential for the iron-regulatory function of hepcidin and its interaction with its receptor ferroportin [28]. In addition to the 25-amino acid form of hepcidin, less bioactive N-terminally truncated shorter forms (22 and 20 amino acids) are also found in human urine and the 20-amino acid form in human plasma, generally at much lower concentrations.

Mechanism of Action of Hepcidin

Hepcidin acts by posttranslationally controlling the membrane concentration of the cellular iron exporter ferroportin [29]. Hepcidin can also directly occlude the transport of iron by ferroportin, but this mechanism may require higher concentrations of hepcidin [16]. A recent structural analysis of the ferroportin-hepcidin complex reveals a potential modulatory role of iron wherein the interaction of ferroportin and hepcidin is stabilized by an iron atom [30]. The hepcidin-ferroportin interaction effectively controls the flux of iron into plasma and the iron supply available to all the iron-consuming tissues. Injection of 1–2 μg/g of synthetic hepcidin into mice elicits a profound decrease in serum iron concentrations within 1 h, and the hypoferremic effect persists for many hours. Similar effects have been reported in early human trials of therapeutic formulations of hepcidin or hepcidin agonists. Chronic overproduction of hepcidin causes iron deficiency anemia in mouse models and humans, both by inhibiting iron absorption and restricting the release of stored iron. Transgenic hepcidin overexpression during fetal life can impair iron transfer to the fetus, causing severe iron deficiency anemia at birth, with most mice dying perinatally. However, this model is not reflective of the role of hepcidin in fetal iron regulation because fetal hepcidin concentrations are normally extremely low [31]. Hepcidin deficiency in mice or humans causes hyperabsorption of iron and iron overload in parenchymal organs including the liver, pancreas, and the heart, coupled with the paradoxical loss of macrophage iron stores [32, 33]. These effects of hepcidin excess or deficiency are evidence of the fundamental role of hepcidin in the control of iron absorption and the release of recycled iron from macrophages. Importantly, the phenotype of hepcidin deficiency is mimicked by heterozygous human ferroportin mutations that interfere with hepcidin binding [34], confirming the critical role of the hepcidin-ferroportin interaction in iron homeostasis and suggesting that ferroportin may be the sole target of hepcidin.

The identification of the binding interface between hepcidin and ferroportin was achieved by studying the effects of natural and experimental mutations in both partners [16, 28]. The N-terminus of hepcidin (~9 amino acids) is sufficient for ferroportin binding and internalization [35]. Recent advances in the structural characterization of ferroportin [17] helped identify a likely hepcidin-binding site in the cavity formed in the open-out conformation of ferroportin [16, 30]. The binding of hepcidin to ferroportin is followed within minutes by the ubiquitination of lysines in a cytoplasmic loop of ferroportin [18] which appears to be required for the subsequent endocytosis of ferroportin.

Hepcidin-Independent Homeostatic Mechanisms

Although ferroportin is evolutionarily ancient with conserved sequences in plants, worms, and other multicellular animals, its ligand hepcidin is found only in vertebrates, with the possible exception of birds. The absence of hepcidin in invertebrates suggests that alternative mechanisms for systemic regulation of ferroportin may exist in invertebrates and persist in vertebrates, although they may not be sufficiently effective to compensate for pathological situations in which hepcidin is deficient or excessive. In the mouse, duodenal ferroportin mRNA is increased by hypoxia and iron deficiency, and hypoxia and anemia increase ferroportin mRNA in macrophages but not hepatocytes. These tissue-specific effects may be mediated by hypoxia-inducible factors, especially HIF-2α [36], regulating the transcription of ferroportin. The degradation of HIFs by prolyl hydroxylases is dependent on both iron and oxygen, so HIF-2α concentrations could be increased by cellular iron deficiency or hypoxia alone. It should be noted that a potential counterregulatory mechanism could decrease ferroportin during cellular iron deficiency. One isoform of ferroportin mRNA contains a 5'IRE and could undergo translational repression during iron deficiency, but the alternative splice form of ferroportin abundant in the duodenum and lacking the 5'IRE would evade this effect. Iron deficiency may also repress HIF-2α translation through the interaction of iron-regulatory proteins (IRP1 and 2) with the iron-regulatory element (IRE) in the 5′ region of the HIF-2α mRNA. Other components of the iron transport machinery in the duodenum, including DMT1 and dcytB, are also targets of HIF-2α, and their mRNAs are increased during hypoxia and iron deficiency. In the duodenum, these cell-autonomous mechanisms may function to coordinate apical iron absorption by DMT1 with basolateral iron export by ferroportin.

Regulation of Hepcidin by Iron

Dual Regulation of Hepcidin by Extracellular Iron and Iron Stores

The relative stability of plasma iron concentrations despite rapid turnover of iron suggests feedback regulation of hepcidin by plasma iron (Fig. 2.3). Experimentally, regulation of hepcidin by plasma iron concentrations was detected in human volunteers [37] given small doses of iron sufficient to raise plasma iron concentrations transiently but too small to contribute significantly to iron stores. Serum hepcidin levels were observed to rise dramatically in response to transient increases in plasma iron with a delay of

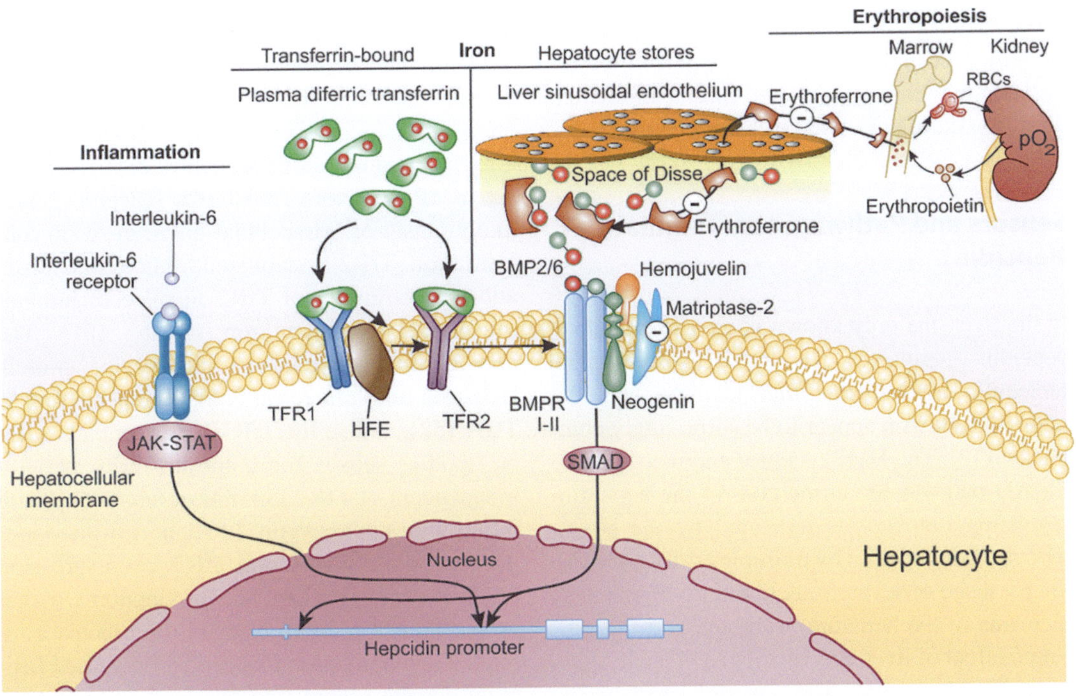

Fig. 2.3 Molecular pathways regulating hepcidin transcription. Iron stores and plasma iron (diferric transferrin) concentrations regulate hepcidin transcription through the BMPR-SMAD pathway. The BMPR ligands BMP2/6 are secreted by the hepatic sinusoidal endothelial cells into the space of Disse, a narrow gap separating these cells from hepatocytes. BMP2/6 production is proportional to hepatic iron stores. The activity of the BMPR-SMAD pathway is modulated by adaptors specific to its iron-regulatory function: hemojuvelin, matriptase-2, and neogenin. Hepcidin transcription in response to plasma iron is stimulated by the putative plasma iron-sensing complex of TfR1, HFE, and TfR2 through enhanced BMP signaling. The main activator of the inflammatory pathway is interleukin-6 acting through its receptor and the JAK-STAT pathway. During active erythropoiesis, hepcidin transcription is suppressed by erythropoietin-stimulated erythroblasts that inhibit BMP signaling by secreting erythroferrone. Erythroferrone acts by trapping BMP2/6 heterodimers and preventing them from activating the BMP receptor

about 8 h [37]. The relatively narrow distributions of estimated body iron stores in men and women on varied diets suggest that body stores could regulate hepcidin independently of the short-term effects of plasma iron concentrations [14]. In humans, observations that support hepcidin regulation by iron stores include the correlation between hepcidin mRNA and iron stores in human liver biopsies [38] and the strong correlation between serum ferritin, a recognized marker of iron stores, and serum hepcidin [37]. In mouse models, convincing evidence has been developed that plasma iron and hepatic iron stores regulate hepcidin independently. Hepcidin regulation by plasma iron and by tissue iron stores appears to operate on different time scales (hours vs. days), and this could allow the two regulators to function in parallel.

Tissues Involved in Hepcidin Regulation

Hepatocytes are the predominant producers of hepcidin, and this source of hepcidin is both necessary and sufficient for systemic iron homeostasis [39]. However, recent studies indicate that another hepatic cell type, sinusoidal endothelial cells, is also essential for the regulation of hepcidin production [40, 41]. Cardiac myocytes, macrophages, and adipocytes contain much lower concentrations of hepcidin mRNA than hepatocytes. In murine models, autocrine effects of hepcidin have been documented in cardiac myocytes [42] and may serve to preserve cardiac mitochondrial iron during systemic iron deficiency.

Sensors and Pathways that Regulate Hepcidin

In the liver, the only known mode of hepatocyte hepcidin regulation is transcriptional. The molecular mechanisms that mediate hepcidin regulation by iron appear to be surprisingly complicated [2]. The BMP receptor and its canonical SMAD pathway are at the core of the hepcidin-regulating complex as indicated by the strong induction of hepcidin by multiple BMPs [43, 44], the presence of several functional BMP response elements in the hepcidin promoter, and the profound effect of liver-specific SMAD4 ablation on hepcidin expression. The specific form of the BMP receptor used for iron-related hepcidin regulation in hepatocytes includes Alk2 or Alk3 as type I subunits and predominantly ActRIIA and BMPR2 as the type II subunit. Another hepatic cell type, the sinusoidal endothelial cell, provides essential input into iron and hepcidin regulation by secreting the two required hepcidin-regulating ligands of the BMP receptor, BMP6 and BMP2 [40, 41], that must cross the narrow perisinusoidal space to interact with BMP receptors on hepatocytes. Of the two distinct modes of hepcidin regulation, by extracellular iron concentration and intracellular liver iron stores, only the accumulation of iron in the liver regulates the expression of BMP6 and BMP2. Liver iron loading increases BMP6 about fourfold [45, 46] but affects BMP2 much less [47]. BMP2 and BMP6 may act physiologically as a heterodimeric ligand of the iron-relevant BMP receptor.

The GPI-linked protein hemojuvelin is an essential co-receptor for activation of the BMP receptor for iron-related signaling. Its ablation leads to severe hepcidin deficiency and severe iron overload in humans (early-onset, juvenile form of hereditary hemochromatosis) and in mice [48–50]. The hepatic form of hemojuvelin appears to be essential for hepcidin regulation, while the muscle form is dispensable.

Regulation of hepcidin by extracellular iron concentrations involves the same BMP pathway through modulation of signaling at the level of the BMP receptor. Transferrin receptor 2 is a likely sensor of extracellular holotransferrin concentration. TfR2 is stabilized by holotransferrin, and the disruption of TfR2 in mice or humans impairs extracellular iron sensing [51]. The hemochromatosis-related membrane protein HFE and holotransferrin compete for binding to TfR1 [52], and so the TfR1/HFE complex could be another sensor for holotransferrin, perhaps independent of TfR2 [53, 54] or interacting with it and with hemojuvelin. In support of the independent roles of HFE and TfR2, overexpression of HFE stimulates hepcidin production whether or not Tfr2 is present. Neogenin promotes iron-related signaling as evidenced by decreased hepcidin despite severe iron overload in mice with neogenin-attenuating retrotransposon insertion, but the mechanism of this effect is uncertain. Finally, a membrane serine protease matriptase-2 (also called TMPRSS6) functions as a negative regulator of hepcidin-related BMP signaling, acting by cleaving and inactivating the BMP agonist hemojuvelin [55–58]. Genetic loss of matriptase-2 (transmembrane serine protease 6, TMPRSS6) activity in mice or humans causes iron-refractory iron deficiency anemia by stimulating excessive hepcidin synthesis that leads to sequestration of iron in macrophages and decreased dietary iron absorption.

Regulation of Hepcidin by Erythropoiesis

Intestinal iron absorption is greatly increased in response to hemorrhage or erythropoietin leading to the hypothesis that an "erythroid regulator" modulates intestinal iron absorption [59], assuring adequate supply of iron when needed for accelerated erythropoiesis (Fig. 2.3). Patients with ineffective erythropoiesis (e.g., in β-thalassemia), whose erythroid precursor populations are greatly expanded but fail to mature into functional erythrocytes, also have increased intestinal iron absorption despite often severe systemic iron overload [60]. Although required blood transfusions (e.g., in β-thalassemia major) contribute to the lethal iron overload in ineffective erythropoiesis, many patients (exemplified by β-thalassemia intermedia) who receive few or no transfusions can still become severely iron-overloaded.

After the discovery of hepcidin, the erythroid regulator concept was modified from that of a direct regulator of iron absorption to a regulator of hepcidin. The preponderance of data now supports a model in which the bone marrow produces a hepcidin suppressor, in response to erythropoietin. A similar suppressive substance has been postulated in anemias with ineffective erythropoiesis where hepcidin is decreased despite iron overload, even in the absence of transfusions [61]. GDF-15, a BMP family member whose serum concentrations are greatly increased in iron-loading anemias, has been proposed as a hepcidin suppressor in β-thalassemia and in congenital dyserythropoietic anemias, but its contribution to hepcidin suppression and iron overload in these conditions remains uncertain. Based on studies in blood donors, GDF-15 is unlikely to function as the physiologic suppressor of hepcidin after blood loss [62].

A systematic search for mRNAs in murine bone marrow that were induced within hours after hemorrhage and encoded secreted proteins led to a glycoprotein member of the TNFα-C1q superfamily with the systematic name Fam132b, which was renamed erythroferrone. Erythroferrone has all the attributes postulated for the erythroid regulator: erythroferrone mRNA and protein secretion is induced by erythropoietin or blood loss within hours and before hepcidin is suppressed [63, 64]; recombinant murine and human erythroferrone suppresses hepcidin mRNA and protein concentrations produced by hepatocytes in vitro and in mouse models [63]; erythroferrone is secreted by erythropoietin-stimulated erythroblasts [63]; and ablation of erythroferrone in a mouse model nearly completely blunts the acute suppression of hepcidin by hemorrhage or erythropoietin administration [63]. After multiple unsuccessful searches for a hepatic erythroferrone receptor, evidence has been accumulating that erythroferrone acts by interfering with the access of BMP2/6 to the hepatocyte BMP receptor [65, 66].

Serum erythroferrone concentrations are pathologically increased in the mouse model of β-thalassemia intermedia with hepcidin suppression and iron overload [67], and the ablation of erythroferrone in this model corrects their hepcidin deficiency and partly alleviates their iron overload. In patients with β-thalassemia, serum erythroferrone concentrations inversely correlate with serum hepcidin [64]. In patients receiving transfusions, erythroferrone levels are high before transfusion and decrease after transfusion, as would be expected from the effect of transfusion on the production of erythropoietin, a direct regulator of erythroferrone [64]. Erythroferrone concentrations are also increased in patients with other anemias with ineffective erythropoiesis, including MDS with SF3B1 mutations and in congenital dyserythropoietic anemia type II. In these settings, high erythroferrone concentrations in plasma are secreted by erythropoietin-stimulated and greatly expanded but dead-end erythroblast populations.

Hepcidin in Inflammation, Liver Injury, and Host Defense

Hepcidin Is Induced by Infections and Inflammation

Initial studies of hepcidin revealed its intrinsic antimicrobial activity. Subsequently, microbial molecules, the plant-derived inflammatory agent turpentine, and cytokines were shown to be potent inducers of hepcidin synthesis. Interleukin-6 (IL-6) is the main hepcidin-inducing cytokine in vivo [68], but other cytokines may also contribute. In multiple myeloma, a plasma cell malignancy which almost invariably causes anemia, serum hepcidin is greatly increased and both BMP4 and IL-6 were implicated as its pathogenic inducers [69]. The stimulatory effects of inflammation are mediated by the dual and in some cases synergistic [69] regulation of hepcidin transcription by SMAD and STAT3 transcription factors.

The Role of Hepcidin in Host Defense

Specific evidence for the role of hepcidin in host defense has only recently been provided. Remarkably, mice that lack hepcidin are exquisitely susceptible to rapid death after infection with certain gram-negative bacteria, including *Vibrio vulnificus, Yersinia enterocolitica, Klebsiella pneumoniae*, and *Escherichia coli* [70, 71], infections to which wild-type mice are highly resistant. Death appears to be caused by the extremely rapid proliferation of bacteria. The hepcidin-ablated mice can be partially or completely rescued by iron depletion or by administration of hepcidin analogs. In vitro studies indicate that it may not be hypoferremia per se that protects the host but hepcidin-mediated suppression of non-transferrin-bound iron (NTBI) generation, as gram-negative bacteria utilize NTBI for rapid growth [72]. Patients with hereditary hemochromatosis, nearly all of whom have absolute or relative hepcidin deficiency, are known to be more susceptible to such infections, e.g., *Vibrio vulnificus, Yersinia enterocolitica, and Listeria monocytogenes*. The involvement of hepcidin and iron in resistance to other microbial infections is less obvious and remains an active area of investigation. There is evidence that induction of hepcidin during erythrocyte infection with malaria interferes with superinfection with another strain by redistributing iron from hepatocytes to macrophages, thus inhibiting the early hepatic phase of superinfecting malaria. However, such protective effects of hepcidin may not be applicable to all infections. Under some conditions, hepcidin-induced iron redistribution from extracellular spaces and hepatocytes to macrophage cytoplasm could even favor the growth of certain intracellular microbes, depending on the specific subcellular compartment they utilize and the effect of hepcidin on its local iron concentrations.

Genetic Disorders of the Hepcidin-Ferroportin System

Mutations in the genes encoding hepcidin, its various regulators, or its molecular target ferroportin may manifest as disorders of iron regulation [1, 73]. Hepcidin deficiency or ferroportin resistance to the effect of hepcidin results in hereditary hemochromatosis, a group of diseases characterized by systemic iron overload due to hyperabsorption of dietary iron, with subsequent injury to iron-overloaded tissues [74]. Although the pathogenesis of iron-mediated toxicity is not well understood, in part because current rodent models are resistant to iron-induced injury, the ability of iron to catalyze the production of reactive oxygen species is the main suspect in this process. The destructive process may affect the liver, causing cirrhosis and liver cancer; the heart, leading to heart failure; and endocrine glands where the effects are wide-ranging, including delayed growth and sexual development in the juvenile forms of the disease and diabetes mellitus in the juvenile and adult forms. The age of onset and the rate of disease progression correlate roughly with the severity of the hepcidin deficiency but are likely to be modulated by genes not yet identified as part of the iron-regulatory system, as well as alcohol use and abuse, dietary factors, and blood loss through menstruation. The epidemiology, diagnosis, and treatment of hereditary hemochromatosis are well covered in other reviews [74].

At the opposite end of the spectrum of genetic iron disorders are conditions in which the production and blood concentrations of hepcidin are inappropriately high or the membrane concentration or iron-transporting capacity of ferroportin is decreased. Genetic lesions in the negative hepcidin regulator matriptase-2 (TMPRSS6), affecting both of its alleles, cause hepcidin overproduction resulting in iron deficiency anemia due to decreased iron absorption and sequestration of iron in macrophages [75]. Treatment with parenteral iron can bypass the block of iron absorption but does not fully overcome the iron-restrictive effect of the block to macrophage iron export.

Heterozygous loss-of-function mutations in the ferroportin gene result in decreased membrane concentrations of ferroportin or its diminished ability to transport iron. The disorder, named "ferroportin disease" [76], is manifested by trapping of iron in macrophages, high serum ferritin levels, and a tendency to anemia when therapeutic iron removal by venesection is attempted. If iron loading is limited to macrophages, the disorder rarely causes clinically significant disease. "Ferroportin disease" is distinct from the manifestations of ferroportin gain-of-function mutations that cause parenchymal iron loading, attributable to partial or complete resistance to hepcidin binding or defective subsequent internalization of ferroportin [16, 34, 77, 78]. Certain ferroportin mutations may induce a combined resistance to hepcidin and a loss of transport function resulting in mixed or complex phenotypes. A puzzling feature of all forms of ferroportin disease is that it invariably involves heterozygous missense mutations acting in a dominant manner, so it cannot be attributed to simple haploinsufficiency. Although mistrafficking of ferroportin multimers containing both wild-type and mutant forms of ferroportin could explain the dominant negative effect, the existence and importance of ferroportin multimerization have been contested.

Conclusion

Iron is an essential trace element whose stores in the body and concentrations in tissues are closely regulated by the hepatic hormone hepcidin and its receptor ferroportin. Genetic and acquired disorders of this system are common, with manifestations ranging from anemia caused by inadequate iron supply to tissue injury and carcinogenesis from excess iron.

References

1. Camaschella C, Nai A, Silvestri L. Iron metabolism and iron disorders revisited in the hepcidin era. Haematologica. 2020;105(2):260–72.
2. Wang CY, Babitt JL. Liver iron sensing and body iron homeostasis. Blood. 2019;133(1):18–29.
3. Pek RH, Yuan X, Rietzschel N, Zhang J, Jackson L, Nishibori E, et al. Hemozoin produced by mammals confers heme tolerance. Elife. 2019:8.
4. Korolnek T, Hamza I. Like iron in the blood of the people: the requirement for heme trafficking in iron metabolism. Front Pharmacol. 2014;5:126.
5. Klei TRL, Dalimot J, Nota B, Veldthuis M, Mul FPJ, Rademakers T, et al. Hemolysis in the spleen drives erythrocyte turnover. Blood. 2020;136(14):1579–89.
6. Wilkinson N, Pantopoulos K. The IRP/IRE system in vivo: insights from mouse models. Front Pharmacol. 2014;5:176.
7. Shawki A, Knight PB, Maliken BD, Niespodzany EJ, Mackenzie B. H(+)-coupled divalent metal-ion transporter-1: functional properties, physiological roles and therapeutics. Curr Top Membr. 2012;70:169–214.
8. Shawki A, Engevik MA, Kim RS, Knight PB, Baik RA, Anthony SR, et al. Intestinal brush-border Na+/H+ exchanger-3 drives H+-coupled iron absorption in the mouse. Am J Physiol Gastrointest Liver Physiol. 2016;311(3):G423–30.
9. Delaby C, Rondeau C, Pouzet C, Willemetz A, Pilard N, Desjardins M, et al. Subcellular localization of iron and heme metabolism related proteins at early stages of erythrophagocytosis. PLoS One. 2012;7(7):e42199.
10. Shi H, Bencze KZ, Stemmler TL, Philpott CC. A cytosolic iron chaperone that delivers iron to ferritin. Science. 2008;320(5880):1207–10.
11. Mancias JD, Wang X, Gygi SP, Harper JW, Kimmelman AC. Quantitative proteomics identifies NCOA4 as the cargo receptor mediating ferritinophagy. Nature. 2014;509(7498):105–9.
12. Yanatori I, Richardson DR, Imada K, Kishi F. Iron export through the transporter ferroportin 1 is modulated by the iron chaperone PCBP2. J Biol Chem. 2016;291(33):17303–18.
13. Truman-Rosentsvit M, Berenbaum D, Spektor L, Cohen LA, Belizowsky-Moshe S, Lifshitz L, et al. Ferritin is secreted via 2 distinct nonclassical vesicular pathways. Blood. 2018;131(3):342–52.
14. Cook JD, Flowers CH, Skikne BS. The quantitative assessment of body iron. Blood. 2003;101(9):3359–63.
15. Donovan A, Brownlie A, Zhou Y, Shepard J, Pratt SJ, Moynihan J, et al. Positional cloning of zebrafish ferroportin1 identifies a conserved vertebrate iron exporter. Nature. 2000;403(6771):776–81.
16. Aschemeyer S, Qiao B, Stefanova D, Valore EV, Sek AC, Ruwe TA, et al. Structure-function analysis of ferroportin defines the binding site and an alternative mechanism of action of hepcidin. Blood. 2018;131(8):899–910.

17. Deshpande CN, Ruwe TA, Shawki A, Xin V, Vieth KR, Valore EV, et al. Calcium is an essential cofactor for metal efflux by the ferroportin transporter family. Nat Commun. 2018;9(1):3075.
18. Qiao B, Sugianto P, Fung E, del Castillo-Rueda A, Moran-Jimenez MJ, Ganz T, et al. Hepcidin-induced endocytosis of ferroportin is dependent on ferroportin ubiquitination. Cell Metab. 2012;15(6):918–24.
19. Vulpe CD, Kuo YM, Murphy TL, Cowley L, Askwith C, Libina N, et al. Hephaestin, a ceruloplasmin homologue implicated in intestinal iron transport, is defective in the sla mouse. Nat Genet. 1999;21(2):195–9.
20. Cherukuri S, Potla R, Sarkar J, Nurko S, Harris ZL, Fox PL. Unexpected role of ceruloplasmin in intestinal iron absorption. Cell Metab. 2005;2(5):309–19.
21. Keel SB, Doty RT, Yang Z, Quigley JG, Chen J, Knoblaugh S, et al. A heme export protein is required for red blood cell differentiation and iron homeostasis. Science. 2008;319(5864):825–8.
22. Chiabrando D, Marro S, Mercurio S, Giorgi C, Petrillo S, Vinchi F, et al. The mitochondrial heme exporter FLVCR1b mediates erythroid differentiation. J Clin Invest. 2012;122(12):4569–79.
23. Knutson MD. Non-transferrin-bound iron transporters. Free Radic Biol Med. 2019;133:101–11.
24. Hvidberg V, Maniecki MB, Jacobsen C, Hojrup P, Moller HJ, Moestrup SK. Identification of the receptor scavenging hemopexin-heme complexes. Blood. 2005;106(7):2572–9.
25. Kristiansen M, Graversen JH, Jacobsen C, Sonne O, Hoffman HJ, Law SK, et al. Identification of the haemoglobin scavenger receptor. Nature. 2001;409(6817):198–201.
26. Rother RP, Bell L, Hillmen P, Gladwin MT. The clinical sequelae of intravascular hemolysis and extracellular plasma hemoglobin: a novel mechanism of human disease. JAMA. 2005;293(13):1653–62.
27. Ganz T. The discovery of the iron-regulatory hormone hepcidin. Clin Chem. 2019;65(10):1330–1.
28. Nemeth E, Preza GC, Jung CL, Kaplan J, Waring AJ, Ganz T. The N-terminus of hepcidin is essential for its interaction with ferroportin: structure-function study. Blood. 2006;107(1):328–33.
29. Nemeth E, Tuttle MS, Powelson J, Vaughn MB, Donovan A, Ward DM, et al. Hepcidin regulates cellular iron efflux by binding to ferroportin and inducing its internalization. Science. 2004;306(5704):2090–3.
30. Billesbolle CB, Azumaya CM, Kretsch RC, Powers AS, Gonen S, Schneider S, et al. Structure of hepcidin-bound ferroportin reveals iron homeostatic mechanisms. Nature. 2020;586(7831):807–11.
31. Sangkhae V, Fisher AL, Wong S, Koenig MD, Tussing-Humphreys L, Chu A, et al. Effects of maternal iron status on placental and fetal iron homeostasis. J Clin Invest. 2020;130(2):625–40.
32. Lesbordes-Brion JC, Viatte L, Bennoun M, Lou DQ, Ramey G, Houbron C, et al. Targeted disruption of the hepcidin 1 gene results in severe hemochromatosis. Blood. 2006;108(4):1402–5.
33. Roetto A, Papanikolaou G, Politou M, Alberti F, Girelli D, Christakis J, et al. Mutant antimicrobial peptide hepcidin is associated with severe juvenile hemochromatosis. Nat Genet. 2003;33(1):21–2.
34. Sham RL, Phatak PD, Nemeth E, Ganz T. Hereditary hemochromatosis due to resistance to hepcidin: high hepcidin concentrations in a family with C326S ferroportin mutation. Blood. 2009;114(2):493–4.
35. Preza GC, Ruchala P, Pinon R, Ramos E, Qiao B, Peralta MA, et al. Minihepcidins are rationally designed small peptides that mimic hepcidin activity in mice and may be useful for the treatment of iron overload. J Clin Investig. 2011;121(12):4880–8.
36. Taylor M, Qu A, Anderson ER, Matsubara T, Martin A, Gonzalez FJ, et al. Hypoxia-inducible factor-2alpha mediates the adaptive increase of intestinal ferroportin during iron deficiency in mice. Gastroenterology. 2011;140(7):2044–55.
37. Ganz T, Olbina G, Girelli D, Nemeth E, Westerman M. Immunoassay for human serum hepcidin. Blood. 2008;112(10):4292–7.
38. Detivaud L, Nemeth E, Boudjema K, Turlin B, Troadec MB, Leroyer P, et al. Hepcidin levels in humans are correlated with hepatic iron stores, hemoglobin levels, and hepatic function. Blood. 2005;106(2):746–8.
39. Zumerle S, Mathieu JR, Delga S, Heinis M, Viatte L, Vaulont S, et al. Targeted disruption of hepcidin in the liver recapitulates the hemochromatotic phenotype. Blood. 2014;123(23):3646–50.
40. Canali S, Zumbrennen-Bullough KB, Core AB, Wang CY, Nairz M, Bouley R, et al. Endothelial cells produce bone morphogenetic protein 6 required for iron homeostasis in mice. Blood. 2017;129(4):405–14.
41. Koch PS, Olsavszky V, Ulbrich F, Sticht C, Demory A, Leibing T, et al. Angiocrine Bmp2 signaling in murine liver controls normal iron homeostasis. Blood. 2017;129(4):415–9.
42. Lakhal-Littleton S. Cardiomyocyte hepcidin: from intracellular iron homeostasis to physiological function. Vitam Horm. 2019;110:189–200.
43. Babitt JL, Huang FW, Xia Y, Sidis Y, Andrews NC, Lin HY. Modulation of bone morphogenetic protein signaling in vivo regulates systemic iron balance. J Clin Invest. 2007;117(7):1933–9.
44. Silvestri L, Nai A, Dulja A, Pagani A. Hepcidin and the BMP-SMAD pathway: an unexpected liaison. Vitam Horm. 2019;110:71–99.
45. Ramos E, Kautz L, Rodriguez R, Hansen M, Gabayan V, Ginzburg Y, et al. Evidence for distinct pathways of hepcidin regulation by acute and chronic iron loading in mice. Hepatology. 2011;53(4):1333–41.
46. Corradini E, Meynard D, Wu Q, Chen S, Ventura P, Pietrangelo A, et al. Serum and liver iron differently regulate the bone morphogenetic protein 6 (BMP6)-SMAD signaling pathway in mice. Hepatology. 2011;54(1):273–84.
47. Wang CY, Canali S, Bayer A, Dev S, Agarwal A, Babitt JL. Iron, erythropoietin, and inflammation regulate hepcidin in Bmp2-deficient mice, but serum iron

fails to induce hepcidin in Bmp6-deficient mice. Am J Hematol. 2019;94(2):240–8.
48. Papanikolaou G, Samuels ME, Ludwig EH, MacDonald ML, Franchini PL, Dube MP, et al. Mutations in HFE2 cause iron overload in chromosome 1q-linked juvenile hemochromatosis. Nat Genet. 2004;36(1):77–82.
49. Niederkofler V, Salie R, Arber S. Hemojuvelin is essential for dietary iron sensing, and its mutation leads to severe iron overload. J ClinInvest. 2005;115(8):2180–6.
50. Huang FW, Pinkus JL, Pinkus GS, Fleming MD, Andrews NC. A mouse model of juvenile hemochromatosis. J Clin Invest. 2005;115(8):2187–91.
51. Johnson MB, Chen J, Murchison N, Green FA, Enns CA. Transferrin receptor 2: evidence for ligand-induced stabilization and redirection to a recycling pathway. Mol Biol Cell. 2007;18(3):743–54.
52. Lebron JA, West J, Bjorkman PJ. The hemochromatosis protein HFE competes with transferrin for binding to the transferrin receptor. J Mol Biol. 1999;294(1):239–45.
53. Schmidt PJ, Fleming MD. Transgenic HFE-dependent induction of hepcidin in mice does not require transferrin receptor-2. Am J Hematol. 2012;87(6):588–95.
54. Wallace DF, Summerville L, Crampton EM, Frazer DM, Anderson GJ, Subramaniam VN. Combined deletion of Hfe and transferrin receptor 2 in mice leads to marked dysregulation of hepcidin and iron overload. Hepatology. 2009;50(6):1992–2000.
55. Finberg KE, Whittlesey RL, Fleming MD, Andrews NC. Down-regulation of Bmp/Smad signaling by Tmprss6 is required for maintenance of systemic iron homeostasis. Blood. 2010;115(18):3817–26.
56. Finberg KE, Heeney MM, Campagna DR, Aydinok Y, Pearson HA, Hartman KR, et al. Mutations in TMPRSS6 cause iron-refractory iron deficiency anemia (IRIDA). Nat Genet. 2008;40(5):569–71.
57. Silvestri L, Pagani A, Nai A, De Domenico I, Kaplan J, Camaschella C. The serine protease matriptase-2 (TMPRSS6) inhibits hepcidin activation by cleaving membrane hemojuvelin. Cell Metab. 2008;8(6):502–11.
58. Du X, She E, Gelbart T, Truksa J, Lee P, Xia Y, et al. The serine protease TMPRSS6 is required to sense iron deficiency. Science. 2008;320(5879):1088–92.
59. Finch C. Regulators of iron balance in humans. Blood. 1994;84(6):1697–702.
60. Cazzola M, Finch CA. Iron balance in thalassemia. Prog Clin Biol Res. 1989;309:93–100.
61. Origa R, Galanello R, Ganz T, Giagu N, Maccioni L, Faa G, et al. Liver iron concentrations and urinary hepcidin in beta-thalassemia. Haematologica. 2007;92(5):583–8.
62. Tanno T, Rabel A, Lee YT, Yau YY, Leitman SF, Miller JL. Expression of growth differentiation factor 15 is not elevated in individuals with iron deficiency secondary to volunteer blood donation. Transfusion. 2010;50(7):1532–5.
63. Kautz L, Jung G, Valore EV, Rivella S, Nemeth E, Ganz T. Identification of erythroferrone as an erythroid regulator of iron metabolism. Nat Genet. 2014;46(7):678–84.
64. Ganz T, Jung G, Naeim A, Ginzburg Y, Pakbaz Z, Walter PB, et al. Immunoassay for human serum erythroferrone. Blood. 2017;130(10):1243–6.
65. Arezes J, Foy N, McHugh K, Sawant A, Quinkert D, Terraube V, et al. Erythroferrone inhibits the induction of hepcidin by BMP6. Blood. 2018;132(14):1473–7.
66. Wang CY, Xu Y, Traeger L, Dogan DY, Xiao X, Steinbicker AU, et al. Erythroferrone lowers hepcidin by sequestering BMP2/6 heterodimer from binding to the BMP type I receptor ALK3. Blood. 2020;135(6):453–6.
67. Kautz L, Jung G, Du X, Gabayan V, Chapman J, Nasoff M, et al. Erythroferrone contributes to hepcidin suppression and iron overload in a mouse model of beta-thalassemia. Blood. 2015;126(17):2031–7.
68. Nemeth E, Rivera S, Gabayan V, Keller C, Taudorf S, Pedersen BK, et al. IL-6 mediates hypoferremia of inflammation by inducing the synthesis of the iron regulatory hormone hepcidin. J Clin Invest. 2004;113(9):1271–6.
69. Maes K, Nemeth E, Roodman GD, Huston A, Esteve F, Freytes C, et al. In anemia of multiple myeloma, hepcidin is induced by increased bone morphogenetic protein 2. Blood. 2010;116(18):3635–44.
70. Stefanova D, Raychev A, Deville J, Humphries R, Campeau S, Ruchala P, et al. Hepcidin protects against lethal escherichia coli sepsis in mice inoculated with isolates from septic patients. Infect Immun. 2018;86(7).
71. Arezes J, Jung G, Gabayan V, Valore E, Ruchala P, Gulig PA, et al. Hepcidin-induced hypoferremia is a critical host defense mechanism against the siderophilic bacterium Vibrio vulnificus. Cell Host Microbe. 2015;17(1):47–57.
72. Stefanova D, Raychev A, Arezes J, Ruchala P, Gabayan V, Skurnik M, et al. Endogenous hepcidin and its agonist mediate resistance to selected infections by clearing non-transferrin-bound iron. Blood. 2017;130(3):245–57.
73. Coffey R, Ganz T. Iron homeostasis: an anthropocentric perspective. J Biol Chem. 2017;292(31):12727–34.
74. Brissot P, Cavey T, Ropert M, Guggenbuhl P, Loreal O. Genetic hemochromatosis: pathophysiology, diagnostic and therapeutic management. Presse Med. 2017;46(12 Pt 2):e288–e95.
75. Finberg KE. Iron-refractory iron deficiency anemia. Semin Hematol. 2009;46(4):378–86.
76. Pietrangelo A. The ferroportin disease. Blood Cell Mol Dis. 2004;32(1):131–8.
77. Drakesmith H, Schimanski LM, Ormerod E, Merryweather-Clarke AT, Viprakasit V, Edwards JP, et al. Resistance to hepcidin is conferred by hemochromatosis-associated mutations of ferroportin. Blood. 2005;106(3):1092–7.
78. Fernandes A, Preza GC, Phung Y, De Domenico I, Kaplan J, Ganz T, et al. The molecular basis of hepcidin-resistant hereditary hemochromatosis. Blood. 2009;114(2):437–43.

3 Measurement Methods for Anemia and Iron Status Surveillance

Sorrel Namaste, Eleanor Brindle, and Dean Garrett

Keywords

Anemia assessment · Ferritin · Hepcidin
Hemoglobin · Iron · Iron assessment
Laboratory methods · Transferrin
Point-of-care testing

Introduction

Anemia, iron deficiency, and iron excess all result in poor health outcomes, which in turn lead to negative economic consequences [1]. Assessing anemia and iron status at the individual and population level can inform policies, programs, and interventions within food and health systems. The information on anemia and iron status is used to develop cost-effective strategies that target the most at-risk populations, improve preventive and treatment-based healthcare, evaluate the impact of interventions, and track prevalence trends.

Accurate, yet simple and inexpensive methods to assess anemia and iron status are critical. This is especially pertinent in low- and middle-income countries (LMIC), where these conditions are highly prevalent and there are greater cost and infrastructure constraints. This chapter focuses on measurement methods for biomarkers to assess anemia and iron status that are suitable for use in clinical laboratories and field settings in low-resource environments (Boxes 3.1 and 3.2).

> **Box 3.1 Selection of Seminal Reviews and WHO Documents on Methods to Assess Anemia and Iron Status**
>
> *Biomarkers of Nutrition for Development (BOND)—Iron Review* [2].
>
> *Measurement and interpretation of hemoglobin concentration in clinical and field settings: A narrative review* [3].
>
> *WHO Guideline on Use of Ferritin Concentrations to Assess Iron Status in Individual Populations* [4].
>
> *WHO Haemoglobin concentrations for the diagnosis of anaemia and assessment of severity* [5].
>
> *WHO Serum transferrin receptor levels for the assessment of iron status and iron deficiency in populations* [6].

S. Namaste (✉)
The DHS Program, ICF, Rockville, MD, USA
e-mail: Sorrel.Namaste@icf.com

E. Brindle · D. Garrett
PATH, Seattle, WA, USA
e-mail: ebrindle@path.org

C. D. Karakochuk et al. (eds.), *Nutritional Anemia*, Nutrition and Health,
https://doi.org/10.1007/978-3-031-14521-6_3

Box 3.2 Source of Anemia and Iron Status Surveillance Data at the Population Level

The DHS Program serves as the largest global source of hemoglobin data. As of 2022, the protocol for Hb assessment has remained relatively consistent since testing was first introduced into The DHS Program in 1996 to maintain comparability [7]. The protocol consists of testing a single drop of capillary blood in the Hb-201+ device. In rare cases, the Hb-301 device has been used.

While anemia testing has been carried out on a large scale in several surveys, facilitated by field friendly point-of-care Hb testing, iron status surveillance remains less common.

Iron status data is typically collected in a stand-alone micronutrient survey but has also been collected as part of multi-topic, agriculture, nutrition, and other surveys. Better harmonized data collection, processing, and analysis procedures would improve comparability across surveys.

Anemia Assessment

Anemia is a condition where the physiological demand for oxygen in the body is not met which results from impaired production, turnover, loss, or destruction of red blood cells (RBCs). Anemia is often accompanied by a decreased concentration of hemoglobin (Hb), a protein contained in red blood cells that delivers oxygen to the tissues, and changes in RBC morphology.

The following section describes methods for assessing anemia. Hb is the most common hematologic measure used to define anemia. Thus, the greatest attention is given to the point-of-care (POC) hemoglobinometer device which is used to measure Hb concentrations in the blood. While performed less frequently than Hb alone, other RBC parameters are measured to diagnose the type of anemia in a clinical setting. This is typically done on an automated hematology analyzer as part of a complete blood cell count (CBC) along with a peripheral blood smear for morphology. Less sophisticated methods used in clinical practice covered in this section include the WHO Haemoglobin Colour Scale and clinical pallor.

Hemoglobinometers

POC devices for Hb measurement, or hemoglobinometers, are well suited for use in the field and in primary healthcare clinics. They are portable, relatively inexpensive, and easy to use and can be powered by batteries. Use of POC devices in the field setting allows for the immediate return of results to survey participants and the ability to refer participants to a health clinic. In a healthcare setting, the POC devices provide an opportunity to diagnose and make clinical decisions while the patient is still present, which is especially important in LMIC where distance and time can be barriers to accessing care.

Instrumentation and Methodology. The HemoCue® (HemoCue AB, Angelholm, Sweden) model of hemoglobinometers is the most widely used hemoglobinometer. The HemoCue® models currently on the market include the Hb-201+ introduced in 1990, followed by the release of modified versions, the Hb-301 and the Hb-801. The testing principle of the Hb-201+ analyzer differs from the Hb-301 and Hb-801 analyzers.

The measurement of Hb by the Hb-201+ analyzer is based on the hemiglobincyanide (HiCN) method, where potassium cyanide is replaced with sodium azide. Whole blood is mixed with sodium deoxycholate which lyses the RBCs, releasing heme. Heme, in the presence of sodium nitrite, is oxidized to the ferric state to form methemoglobin. Methemoglobin reacts sodium azide to form the stable colored complex, azide methemoglobin which has an absorbance maximum at 570 nm. The azide method is attractive to many users because it obviates the use of cyanide, a highly toxic chemical. Further, the azide methemoglobin complex is stable, and its absorbance maximum is similar to that of hemiglobincyanide. The photometer uses a measuring wavelength of 570 nm and a reference wavelength of 880 nm to compensate for turbidity in the sample. The azide method adheres to the Beer-Lambert Law.

Unlike the Hb-201+ analyzer, the Hb- 301+ analyzer uses filter photometry to measure Hb in whole blood. The principle of the Hb-301+ method is based on scattering measurement of whole blood at the isosbestic point of HHb/HbO2. The concentration of Hb in whole blood at its isosbestic point is independent of oxygen saturation. The analyzer uses a measuring wavelength of 506 nm and a reference wavelength of 880 nm which compensates for turbidity in the sample.

The HemoCue® analyzers are factory calibrated against the HiCN method of the International Council for Standardization in Hematology [8]. The devices need to be sent back to the manufacturer when problems are detected for recalibration. Internal quality control is possible using liquid quality control solutions, although not required according to the manufacturer [9].

Collection Procedures. The hemoglobinometers require approximately 10 μL of peripheral whole blood. If the Hb measurement will be performed elsewhere, or if a larger volume of blood is required to perform additional tests, the blood should be collected into a tube containing an anticoagulant. Collection tubes containing potassium ethylenediaminetetraacetic acid (K_2 or K_3EDTA) or lithium heparin in solid form should be used. Blood samples should not be collected in tubes containing sodium fluoride as an anticoagulant (HemoCue AB, Angelholm, Sweden). Sodium fluoride is used commonly to inhibit glycolysis in blood samples for glucose measurement but is also known to promote hemolysis [10].

The blood can be loaded into a microcuvette directly from the finger/heel (or tube) or placed on an intermediate surface and then loaded into the microcuvette. The microcuvette must be filled completely in one continuous process and void of air bubbles (Fig. 3.1). The outside of the microcuvette is wiped clean of excess blood and inserted into the photometer. Results are generated within 60 s (or less depending on the model).

Factors Affecting Hb Measurements. The HemoCue® device is generally considered to provide accurate and precise measurements of Hb concentration when used properly. There are, however, several pre-analytical, analytical, and post-analytical aspects to consider (Table 3.1).

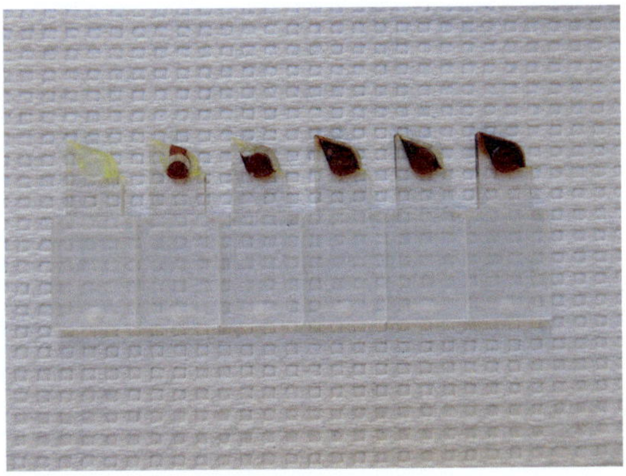

Fig. 3.1 Hb-201+ microcuvettes. Far right is a correctly filled cuvette. Far left is a cuvette with the dry reagent (in yellow) prior to filling the cuvette with the blood specimen. Exposure of the cuvette to heat or moisture results in deterioration of the chemicals in the microcuvette and results in false increases in Hb concentrations. The cuvettes in the middle are examples of incorrect filling of the cavity. Air bubbles lower the concentration of red blood cells in the cuvette resulting in false decreases in Hb concentrations, and incomplete filling does not allow the chemicals in microcuvette to mix properly with the reagents resulting in false decreases in Hb concentrations. © Ellie Brindle

The blood source and quality of the blood sample are two notable pre-analytical factors that can impact the Hb concentration. Venous blood is considered the reference sample for hematological measurements. While there are indications that testing Hb concentrations using venous blood gives lower Hb values compared to capillary blood, mean differences have been within acceptable levels (threshold of ±7%) in a more controlled environment [11]. However, poor blood collection technique can lead to a compromised capillary sample (Table 3.1), and inherent variation in Hb concentration between capillary blood drops on the same individual has been observed [12]. In a survey context, substantially lower Hb values and consequently higher anemia estimates have been shown in surveys using capillary blood compared to surveys using venous blood matched by country and time [13].

Table 3.1 Factors influencing point-of-care and laboratory-based assessment of hemoglobin and anemia at different stages of testing

Methods	Sample collection and processing	Measurement and assessment
Hemoglobinometers	• Venous preferable to capillary blood • Capillary sampling technique should avoid “milking” or squeezing the finger • Microcuvette must be filled correctly • Outside of microcuvette should be cleaned before placement in device	• HemoCue® model type • Proper storage and use of microcuvettes required to maintain integrity, humidity, and temperature • Maintenance of cuvette holder and optical lens required • Manufacturer calibrated
Clinical auto analyzer	• Whole blood needs to be refrigerated and tested within 6–8 h	• Automated process • High sample throughput • Regular maintenance and technical service required
WHO Haemoglobin Colour Scale	• Sufficient blood spot (neither deficient or excessive blood volume) • Quality ambient lighting • Follow appropriate readout times	• Readings are subjective • Limited to semi-quantitative results in intervals of 1 g/dL
Clinical pallor	• Some sites influenced by dark skin color • Affected by presence of cyanosis or jaundice • Avoid fluorescent lighting	• Highly subjective

Analytical considerations associated with the testing method include the performance of the HemoCue® device, model type, and environmental factors (Table 3.1). Comparisons of the HemoCue® device to an automated hematology analyzer (reference method) have generally found an allowable degree of variation (threshold of ±7%) even though the Hb-301 and 201+ devices tend to give higher Hb values [11]. In addition, the Hb-201+ device tends to read slightly lower than the Hb-301 device [3]. Use of the same model in all surveys is preferable, especially between surveys in the same country, although the extent to which these differences will impact anemia trends is likely minimal.

The performance of the HemoCue® hemoglobinometers is influenced by temperature and humidity and the integrity of the microcuvettes used for blood sampling. For optimal performance, the recommended storage and operating temperature of the Hb-201+ hemoglobinometer is 15–35 °C and for the Hb-301 and Hb-801, 10–40 °C. The active reagents in the Hb-201+ microcuvettes are sensitive to high temperature and high humidity, making them prone to degradation once a canister of microcuvettes is opened. Using degraded microcuvettes (reagents) can lead to higher Hb concentrations. The impact of the environment on the Hb-201+ microcuvette function can potentially be mitigated by limiting exposure of the device and microcuvettes to temperatures that fall outside the operating range and high humidity [14]. The Hb-301 and Hb-801 models use reagent-free cuvettes, offering greater stability in extreme weather conditions, but have been shown to result in artificial increases in Hb concentrations if the Hb readings are not performed within 20–30 s [11, 14].

At the postanalytical phase, transcription of results is usually recorded by the technician, although there is the potential to digitally transmit the results from the measurement device over a Bluetooth bridge. To define anemia, WHO recommended cutoffs are applied to Hb concentrations that are dependent on age, sex, and pregnancy status [5]. Prior to applying cutoffs, hypoxic conditions are accounted for by adjusting for altitude in populations living at high altitudes and for smoking status. There is also some evidence that Hb concentrations vary by ethnicity, but adjustments for this have not been universally adopted [15]. Additional information on the definition of anemia is provided in Chap. 4.

Automated Hematology Analyzer

The automated hematology analyzer is the most common method used in clinical laboratories (Table 3.1). In addition to Hb, the analyzer provides measures that are helpful in the evaluation of anemia for clinical purposes. These parameters, collectively known as a CBC, include hematocrit, mean corpuscular Hb, mean cell volume, RBC count, red cell distribution width, and reticulocyte count. Information on the interpretation of these biochemical indicators can be found in Lynch et al. and Karakochuk et al. [2, 3].

Blood is aspirated directly from a sample tube and mechanically diluted in an RBC lysis buffer and the concentration of Hb measured colorimetrically. Most instruments operate using the Coulter Principle whereby particles and cells suspended in fluid are forced through a small aperture between electrodes and the change in electrical impedance is measured. The instrument may be paired with a system for automatically capturing clinical data, or it may be necessary to manually enter results into a database.

The automated hematology analyzer is not ideal for use in primary and secondary level healthcare laboratories because operating the instrument is not cost-effective for laboratories with small sample loads. Further, operating these instruments requires a constant source of electricity, routine maintenance and calibration, and the resources to procure required reagents and supplies. Countries are often constrained by the cost of purchasing and maintaining equipment and the availability of experienced operators; investments to foster improvements in laboratory medicine are needed [16].

WHO Haemoglobin Colour Scale

The WHO Haemoglobin Colour Scale (HCS) is a semi-quantitative method that measures the Hb concentration in whole blood by comparing the color of the blood samples to a color on the scale with a known Hb value (Table 3.1). Its intended use is to diagnose anemia in primary healthcare settings that lack the capacity or resources to measure Hb using an automated system or a POC device. To determine the Hb concentration using the Colour Scale, a drop of blood is placed on chromatography filter paper and its color compared against shades of red on the Colour Scale that correspond to different Hb levels (i.e., 4, 6, 8, 10, 12, and 14 g/dL) [17]. The quality of the blood spot, ambient lighting, and timing of readings can impact the test results, but overall it is found to be simple to administer [18]. The HCS performs better than clinical assessment alone, but a cost-benefit analysis of the added advantage of the HCS in improving clinical care would better inform its use [19].

Clinical Pallor

A physical examination can be used to detect anemia by assessing the pallor of the skin or mucous membrane (Table 3.1). Sites where capillary blood vessels are close to the surface are examined. The palms, conjunctiva, and nail beds are the most frequent sites and are appropriate regardless of skin pigmentation.

The sensitivity and specificity of clinical pallor for diagnosing anemia vary across studies but overall appear to have limited ability to detect anemia. This applies in particular to milder cases of anemia and to settings where anemia is highly prevalent [20]. These findings are based on a small number of studies mostly in Africa; thus, the extent to which clinical pallor can support health management decisions requires further exploration.

Use of clinical pallor is imperfect but is a common anemia assessment approach. The WHO-UNICEF Integrated Management of Childhood Illness (IMCI) guidelines, a cornerstone of pediatric care, include use of palmar (palm of the hand) pallor to check for anemia and provide treatment and, in severe cases, referral to a hospital. Clinical pallor will likely continue to be an assessment approach used in healthcare settings when hematologic measures are not available.

Biochemical Iron Indicators

Iron status assessment generally aims to measure the body's iron stores. Stainable iron in bone marrow is the best measure of iron reserves, but is too invasive for broad use and is mainly limited to clinical settings. Ferritin and soluble transferrin receptor (sTfR) are the most widely used biochemical indicators in surveys that measure iron status. These biomarkers capture different facets of iron biology, and indices using the ratio of sTfR to ferritin have also been used [2, 21, 22]. Threshold values for identifying iron deficiency using either the individual biomarkers or their combination are dependent on the assays used, and the influence of inflammation and infection on the biomarkers should be considered whether they are used individually or in construction of the indices (Boxes 3.3 and 3.4). Regulation of iron absorption may also be informative and can be assessed by measuring hepcidin. Strengths and limitations of these commonly used indicators, and the laboratory methods for measuring them, are discussed in greater detail below (Table 3.2). There are several other circulating iron biomarkers, notably serum iron and its carrier protein transferrin, which can be informative, but variability in their levels across the day limits their use in surveillance of iron status. A comprehensive discussion of these and other biochemical indicators of iron status not considered in detail here can be found in Lynch et al. (2018) [2].

Table 3.2 Factors influencing laboratory-based assessment of iron status at different stages of testing

Iron status biomarkers	Sample collection, processing, and storage	Laboratory testing challenges
Ferritin	• Venous preferable to capillary blood • Stable for 3 freeze-thaw cycles • Hemolysis a major consideration	• Immunoassay using clinical analyzers or manual immunoassay kits • Clinical analyzers require expensive equipment; manual assay kits (ELISA) require plate reader, plate washer, and other basic lab equipment
sTfR	• Serum or heparin plasma preferable to EDTA plasma • Can be measured in dried blood spots	• Poor comparability between assays, including both clinical analyzer assays and manual ELISA kits
Hepcidin	• Serum or plasma	• Difficult to produce antibodies; results in challenges in assay kit development • Assay standardization to secondary reference material under development

Blood Specimen Collection

The type of blood specimen collected is determined by both the site of the collection (e.g., from the arm, the finger, or the heel) and the vessel into which it is collected. Venipuncture blood samples are the biologic specimen of choice to assess iron status, and venous collection is often required to have sufficient blood to test the analytes. While even the most restrictive guidelines for safety allow maximum volumes of approximately 1 mL of blood per kg of body weight to be drawn for research [23, 24], collecting 5 mL of whole blood yields approximately 2 mL of serum or plasma, which is enough for multiple laboratory tests. Although in most cases certified phlebotomists can perform venous draws relatively easily and safely, well-trained and experienced phlebotomists are needed for infants and young children because their veins are not as well developed in the antecubital areas. An alternative blood source is capillary blood sampling using a lancet to create a small incision in either the finger or, for infants less than 12 months of age, in the heel and collecting blood into capillary tubes. Capillary blood collection has its own challenges including being more painful than venous collection and requiring careful training. Phlebotomists are less likely to be familiar with capillary blood collection, and poor technique can significantly influence sample quality. Improperly collected capillary blood is more likely than venous blood to be compromised by hemolysis or mixing with interstitial fluid during the collection process. The volume of blood obtained is also significantly smaller than for venous blood: capillary whole blood volume collected is generally 0.25–0.5 mL, and the resulting recovered serum or plasma volumes after separating blood components are approximately 0.125–0.25 mL.

Phlebotomy supplies are relatively inexpensive and widely available. Venous blood can be collected into tubes with or without additives that speed clotting, prevent clotting, or aid in separation of the blood components. The type of blood collection tube required is determined by the specific laboratory assay protocols to be used. Often, either serum or plasma is acceptable, although serum is generally the sample of choice for biochemical analyses, as it is devoid of anticoagulants, cellular material, and most clotting proteins which have potential to interfere with assays. EDTA, a common anticoagulant used for tests that require whole blood (i.e., hematology) and in plasma preparation, has been found to interfere with some sTfR assays [25].

Blood Specimen Processing and Storage

Blood specimen processing and storage require equipment and can pose logistical challenges for field collection. After collection, the blood specimens must be centrifuged to separate the components of the blood, and the serum or plasma fractions must be removed from the collection tubes into storage tubes using a pipette. The fractionation must be done within a specific window of time dictated by the type of collection tube used and the laboratory protocols (ideally within hours of collection).

A power source is needed for processing samples into blood components, and an unbroken cold chain is required from the point of collection through transportation to the lab. Refrigeration at 2–10 °C is required before blood fractions have been separated to prevent hemolysis. Once the samples have been processed, they are stored frozen (generally −20 °C) while still in the field. Electronic temperature monitoring devices, electronic data loggers, and digital thermometers can be used to monitor and record temperatures. Once samples reach the central laboratory, they are stored frozen (ideally −70 °C or colder) until analysis or shipment. Freeze-thaw cycles should be kept to a minimum. While portable power sources for operating centrifuges and portable means of refrigeration and freezing are available, these are heavy and require regular recharging and thus present difficulties for blood collection in remote field locations.

Where the difficulties of processing whole blood and storing serum or plasma are barriers to data collection, dried blood spots (DBS) may be a viable alternative [26]. DBS are prepared from a finger or heel prick by collecting free-flowing blood drops onto a special filter paper card. The samples do not require processing in the field, and while there may still be a need for a cold chain, storage temperature requirements are more permissive. Despite the ease of collection, the use of DBS in biochemical assays has its own limitations, and they have only been used rarely to measure sTfR. DBS ferritin is not interpretable because the sample contains a mixture of ferritin from serum and from the red blood cells. It has not yet been determined whether hepcidin measurement in DBS may offer a reliable alternative.

Biomarkers of Iron Status

Ferritin. Ferritin is an iron-binding protein that is used to assess iron stores and is one of the most widely used biomarkers [4]. However, ferritin is an acute-phase protein that increases with inflammation, so it must be measured in conjunction with inflammation biomarkers. Ferritin is present in relatively low concentrations in serum, and assays used in identifying iron deficiency must have adequate sensitivity to accurately quantify the physiologic range observed in individuals with low body iron stores. Serum or plasma may be assayed without dilution, which increases the volume of sample required for testing. The relatively large sample volume and the sensitivity of serum ferritin assays to hemolysis can be obstacles to the use of capillary collected blood for ferritin measurement.

Ferritin is measured using a variety of immunoassay methods, including both manual ELISA that require relatively basic laboratory equipment (Fig. 3.2) and more expensive clinical autoanalyzer methods. In micronutrient surveys, a few notable methods have been used more than others. Many have relied upon an assay described by Erhardt et al. used for testing in the VitMin Laboratory, but not currently in use elsewhere [27]. A commonly used manual ELISA for ferritin (Ramco Spectro Ferritin, Webster, TX) is no longer available. Other notable methods for ferritin measurement rely upon clinical laboratory equipment, including the ferritin immunoturbidimetry assay for the Roche Cobas 6000 system used by the US CDC [28]. The WHO considers immunoassay methods acceptable if the assays are calibrated against the WHO international reference material [29]. Application of common threshold values for determining iron deficiency should be approached with caution, and assay-specific reference ranges or harmonization may be required [30] (see *Reference Materials and Harmonization* below).

Soluble transferrin receptor. Soluble transferrin receptor (sTfR) circulates in the bloodstream at concentrations that vary depending on erythropoietic activity, which can be reflective of the body's demand for iron [6]. Increased sTfR indicates that the body iron stores are inadequate to meet demand and has been shown to correlate to stainable iron in bone marrow [31], which is the site of primary body iron demand for utilization in erythroid maturation. An advantage of sTfR is that concentrations may not be directly affected by inflammation, but sTfR has still been found to be weakly associated with inflammation biomarkers and is also impacted by other factors that cause erythropoiesis [22, 32].

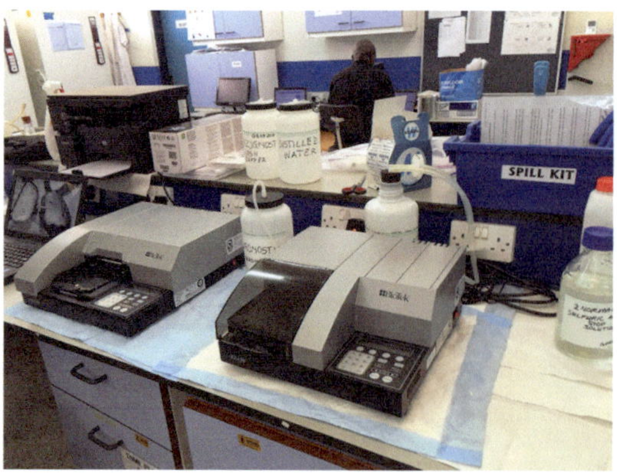

Fig. 3.2 Major equipment required for manual ELISA; a microtiter plate reader for quantifying colorimetric signal intensity (left) and a microtiter plate washer (right)

Like for ferritin, measurement of sTfR is done using immunoassays, either in the form of clinical analyzers or manual ELISA. Also, like ferritin, sTfR has commonly been measured in the VitMin lab using the Erhardt et al. method [27]. Manual ELISAs have been supplied by a few manufacturers, and these have used different forms of native sTfR in kit standards, causing some significant discrepancies in calibration. For example, the material supplied for calibration in the Ramco sTfR ELISA kit (now discontinued) used sTfR of placental origin, which reacts differently in ELISA than the sTfR calibration material derived from serum that was used in the R&D Systems ELISA kit [33]. Therefore, as described in Box 3.4, the use of an assay needs to be considered carefully before applying sTfR cutoffs and a conversion factor applied to account for use of different methods [34].

A WHO reference material is available for sTfR, but has poor commutability, meaning it reacts differently depending on the assay used. The issue of commutability of reference materials, discussed in more detail below, is of concern generally for biochemical tests, but sTfR assays seem to be particularly susceptible to these problems, and this has led to poor comparability between studies that have measured sTfR.

Hepcidin. Hepcidin is a hormone that plays an important role in regulating iron homeostasis; its expression is induced by inflammatory cytokines in response to iron or infection and is reduced in response to erythropoiesis, anemia, and hypoxia. Hepcidin shows promise as an iron biomarker as it regulates the absorption of iron and thereby regulates the body's iron stores [2]. Increasing hepcidin levels reduce absorption of iron, indicating either adequate iron stores or a response to inflammation [35]. While hepcidin is raised in an inflammatory state, it is not adjusted for inflammation because its intended use is to better understand iron absorption and mobilization. Hepcidin can be measured by time-of-flight mass spectrometry, but immunoassay, either using a clinical analyzer or manual ELISA kit, is a more readily available and affordable method. To date, a major limitation is the lack of a standardized assay or international reference materials. However, significant progress has recently been made toward harmonizing hepcidin assays [36, 37].

Box 3.3 Assessment of Other Biomarkers to Aid in the Interpretation of Iron Biomarkers from a Laboratory Perspective

Biomarkers of inflammation are measured in conjunction with iron status biomarkers in populations and settings with high levels of inflammation or infections to support the interpretation of ferritin and sTfR. The most common inflammatory biomarkers measured are C-reactive protein (CRP) and α 1-acid glycoprotein (AGP) to capture acute and chronic inflammation, respectively. Both CRP and AGP are measured using immunoassay, either with manual ELISA or clinical analyzer assays, and comparability is generally good across assays. International reference materials are available for both analytes, and the blood sample volumes required are relatively small. CRP assays may be described as "high sensitivity" or hsCRP, but in the laboratory, this distinction is somewhat arbitrary and reflects the interest in chronic, slight elevation of CRP as an indicator of cardiovascular disease risk.

In a clinical context, a higher ferritin cutoff can be used for individuals with inflammation [4]. At the population level, those with inflammation can be excluded or an arithmetic or regression adjustment applied to ferritin and sTfR [4, 32]. Use of the regression correction approach has the advantage of adjusting the iron biomarkers across the full physiological range of inflammation [38]. From a method perspective, this means accurate and precise CRP and AGP values across this range are needed, including at low concentrations, which has been an issue for some assays [39].

Adjustments to sTfR for the presence of malaria have also been proposed using microscopy and/or rapid diagnostic tests to diagnose malaria status [32, 40]. The added value of measuring malaria for adjustment purposes is likely minimal given that after adjusting for AGP the influence of malaria on prevalence estimates has been insignificant.

Additional information on adjustments to iron biomarkers can be found in Chap. 5.

Standard Reference Materials

Reference materials are prepared with the support of the WHO and other organizing bodies for use in the validation and standardization of new assays, to assess inter-laboratories' performance, and for periodic recalibration of assays which are increasingly recognized as important if the reagent of equipment for a commercial assay has changed since initially being calibrated. Reference materials are typically assigned a value by measurement using a method recognized as the gold standard for the specific analyte. In the absence of a clear gold standard, a value is assigned based on a consensus process in which a material is measured repeatedly by a number of methods in a number of laboratories (see Thorpe et al. (1997) for an example of this process [41]). There can be considerable variation in the measured values used to assign a concentration to the reference material. The National Institute for Biological Standards and Control

(NIBSC) has issued a WHO International Standard for Hb (98/708) and ferritin (94/572) and a WHO reference reagent for sTfR (07/202) to assist laboratories in validating analytical measurements [42]. Reference materials that allow harmonization of hepcidin assays have also been developed [36, 37, 43]. The supply and lifespan of reference materials are finite, and they are periodically replaced with new materials with different concentration values and sometimes made by different means. These production source differences can affect the potency of the reference material in immunoassays. For example, native ferritin from liver, spleen, and serum may react differently in immunoassays, and marked differences have been noted between sTfR from serum and placental sources [33]. The current ferritin reference material, 94/572, a recombinant protein produced in *E. coli*, is over two decades old and is now in short supply, and the quantity that can be purchased is restricted by the distributor (NIBSC).

Box 3.4 Cutoffs for Iron Status from a Laboratory Perspective

Evidence-based cutoffs for both deficiency and excesses have been established for iron status and are described in Chap. 4. The assays used should be reliable and valid across the full physiological range, but assay optimization should prioritize precision and accuracy of the concentration range closest to the cutoff value.

Before applying a cutoff value to categorize sample results as indicating deficiency, sufficiency, or excess, it is essential to consider the calibration of the assay being used for measuring the biomarker concentrations in the samples relative to the calibration of the assay used to establish the cutoff values. In some cases, the supplier of assay materials will provide information about expected ranges for their particular assay. This information should be included, along with specifications of the assay used, any time assay results are reported.

Laboratory Capacity Strengthening

The costs of establishing and maintaining a well-equipped and staffed laboratory to perform the range of biochemical analyses required to measure biomarkers for assessing iron status are significant limitations to the measurement of micronutrient biomarkers in LMICs. Surveys are typically carried out on an intermittent basis, making it especially difficult to meet the criteria used by global organizations for selecting an in-country lab to perform the analyses. Even in settings where clinical iron biochemical assessment is performed, this does not often translate into the ability to store, process, analyze, and capture the data results at the scale needed for a national survey. The absence of national laboratories with the demonstrated ability to analyze iron biomarkers means it is often necessary to ship specimens out of the country. Strengthening of laboratories is clearly needed and requires increased investments in human resources and training, building the necessary infrastructure, and the establishment of and participation in national and international accreditation programs [16]. Instituting regional micronutrient resource laboratories is a potential interim solution, but in the longer term, simpler iron assessment methods that meet national and international standards are necessary.

Future Directions

Variations in Hb Concentrations and the Impact on Anemia Estimates in Field Settings

The notion of differences in Hb concentrations between venous and capillary blood is not new, but further research is needed to identify cause(s) of these differences in the field context. The extent to which drop-to-drop variability impacts Hb concentrations and the extent to which recruitment of highly skilled field staff, rigorous training, and field monitoring can overcome the constraints and challenges encountered in a field environment are unclear. A potential solution is to collect capillary blood in microcontainers containing an anticoagulant, most often EDTA, but research on whether this overcomes variability issues needs to be done.

Innovations in Blood Processing

Methods that separate blood, either from capillary or venous collection, in a device that does not require centrifugation and that can stabilize field-collected samples for transport to a laboratory would be an important step toward large-scale iron assessment. Several devices have recently been offered for sale or described in experimental evaluations. These devices separate plasma either by a lateral flow across a paper substrate or by applying blood to a filter that retains the cellular components while trapping the plasma fraction in an absorbent material [44, 45]. Some of the filter devices have the advantage of allowing the use of the red blood cells for other analyses, for example, measurement of RBC folate. Barriers to wide use of these devices include limited availability, high cost, and a lack of complete vetting through field tests.

Point of Care

Noninvasive POC technologies to quantify Hb concentrations and/or diagnose anemia, such as photography of the conjunctiva and pulse oximeters, as well as POC automated analyzers that measure CBC, hold promise, but more research is needed before being put into practice [46–48]. The assessment of iron status at point of specimen collection is currently in the proof-of-concept phase. The use of these methods is especially relevant for iron because of their potential use in determining when the administration of an iron intervention would be most effective and to target iron interventions to those with diagnosed iron deficiency rather than using a blanket approach which has safety implications.

Multiplex Assays

Iron status is best assessed by the use of more than one iron biomarker in conjunction with markers of inflammation. Using conventional laboratory testing approaches requires that each specimen be tested multiple times. This makes multiplex assays, in which multiple analytes are measured simultaneously, particularly useful. Erhardt et al. described an initial step toward multiplexing in which assays for ferritin, sTfR, CRP, and AGP along with retinol-binding protein for vitamin A status assessment are combined into a system that maximizes efficiency [27] and requires a small quantity of blood (25 μL for duplicate measurement [49]). That method is in use only in the VitMin Lab (Willstaett, Germany). Since the publication of that combined approach, multiplex assays which measure all the analytes in a single well have been developed. The multiplex platforms still rely upon the principles of immunoassays, with an antibody-antigen reaction remaining at the heart of the technique, but the reaction occurs on either coated microscopic beads or planar arrays that allow the assays to detect discrete signals for multiple analytes tested in a single assay. These techniques allow measurement of multiple analytes from very small volumes of blood, such as those obtained from capillary collection, and reduce the labor costs, time, and additional laboratory consumables required [50].

Improvements in Assay Harmonization

Subtle differences in assay reactivity with protein forms in reference materials are not necessarily mirrored in endogenous forms of ferritin, sTfR, and hepcidin; thus, traceability to the WHO reference material does not guarantee comparable results between assays [51]. The past decade has seen an increasing recognition that reference materials should be commutable, meaning that

that two assays calibrated using the same reference material should provide agreement between methods in their measurement of clinical samples [52]. The ideal solution would be improvement of reference materials to ensure commutability (i.e., equal reactivity across assays), but failing that, harmonization (i.e., mathematical adjustment of the concentration values to achieve agreement between methods) using donor panels can be used as an interim measure [36, 53]. Neither approach is currently in routine use, making application of cutoff values for identifying deficiency a challenge.

Conclusion

Iron deficiency, which is the leading nutritional cause of anemia, affects billions of people globally. Despite some pre-analytical and analytical challenges, the assessment of anemia is relatively simple to conduct. Thus, both clinical diagnosis and surveillance of anemia are more common than that of iron status in LMICs. However, anemia is caused by multiple factors and is neither a specific nor sensitive measure of iron deficiency. The lack of accurate and widely available data on iron status is a major impediment to designing policies and programs to address the underlying causes of anemia. This data gap should continue to be addressed using laboratory methods that are already available while also exploring the development of and improvements in noninvasive methods, point-of-care technology, multiplex assays, and assay harmonization.

References

1. Pasricha SR, Drakesmith H, Black J, Hipgrave D, Biggs BA. Control of iron deficiency anemia in low- and middle-income countries. Blood. 2013;121(14):2607–17.
2. Lynch S, Pfeiffer CM, Georgieff MK, Brittenham G, Fairweather-Tait S, Hurrell RF, et al. Biomarkers of Nutrition for Development (BOND)-iron review. J Nutr. 2018;148(suppl_1):1001S–67S.
3. Karakochuk CD, Hess SY, Moorthy D, Namaste S, Parker ME, Rappaport AI, et al. Measurement and interpretation of hemoglobin concentration in clinical and field settings: a narrative review. Ann N Y Acad Sci. 2019;1450(1):126–46.
4. WHO. WHO guideline on use of ferritin concentrations to assess iron status in individuals and populations. Geneva: World Health Organization; 2020.
5. WHO. Haemoglobin concentrations for the diagnosis of anaemia and assessment of severity. Geneva: WHO; 2011.
6. WHO. WHO Serum transferrin receptor levels for the assessment of iron status and iron deficiency in populations. Geneva: WHO; 2014.
7. Pullum T, Kortso Collison D, Namaste S, Garrett D. Hemoglobin data in DHS surveys: intrinsic variation and measurement error. Rockville, MD: ICF; 2017.
8. Zwart A, van Assendelft OW, Bull BS, England JM, Lewis SM, Zijlstra WG. Recommendations for reference method for haemoglobinometry in human blood (ICSH standard 1995) and specifications for international haemiglobinocyanide standard (4th edition). J Clin Pathol. 1996;49(4):271–4.
9. Eurotrol. Products. https://www.eurotrol.com/en/products/.
10. Narayanan S. The preanalytic phase. An important component of laboratory medicine. Am J Clin Pathol. 2000;113(3):429–52.
11. Whitehead RD Jr, Mei Z, Mapango C, Jefferds MED. Methods and analyzers for hemoglobin measurement in clinical laboratories and field settings. Ann N Y Acad Sci. 2019;1450(1):147–71.
12. Bond MM, Richards-Kortum RR. Drop-to-drop variation in the cellular components of fingerprick blood: implications for point-of-care diagnostic development. Am J Clin Pathol. 2015;144(6):885–94.
13. Hruschka DJ, Williams AM, Mei Z, Leidman E, Suchdev PS, Young MF, et al. Comparing hemoglobin distributions between population-based surveys matched by country and time. BMC Public Health. 2020;20(1):422.
14. Whitehead RD Jr, Zhang M, Sternberg MR, Schleicher RL, Drammeh B, Mapango C, et al. Effects of preanalytical factors on hemoglobin measurement: a comparison of two HemoCue(R) point-of-care analyzers. Clin Biochem. 2017;50(9):513–20.
15. Sullivan KM, Mei Z, Grummer-Strawn L, Parvanta I. Haemoglobin adjustments to define anaemia. Tropical Med Int Health. 2008;13(10):1267–71.
16. Sayed S, Cherniak W, Lawler M, Tan SY, El Sadr W, Wolf N, et al. Improving pathology and laboratory medicine in low-income and middle-income countries: roadmap to solutions. Lancet. 2018;391(10133):1939–52.
17. Copack GmbH. Haemoglobin colour scale. www.haemoglobincolourscale.com.
18. Ingram CF, Lewis SM. Clinical use of WHO haemoglobin colour scale: validation and critique. J Clin Pathol. 2000;53(12):933–7.
19. Marn H, Critchley JA. Accuracy of the WHO Haemoglobin Colour Scale for the diagnosis of anaemia in primary health care settings in low-income

countries: a systematic review and meta-analysis. Lancet Glob Health. 2016;4(4):e251–65.
20. Chalco JP, Huicho L, Alamo C, Carreazo NY, Bada CA. Accuracy of clinical pallor in the diagnosis of anaemia in children: a meta-analysis. BMC Pediatr. 2005;5:46.
21. Punnonen K, Irjala K, Rajamaki A. Serum transferrin receptor and its ratio to serum ferritin in the diagnosis of iron deficiency. Blood. 1997;89(3):1052–7.
22. Skikne BS, Punnonen K, Caldron PH, Bennett MT, Rehu M, Gasior GH, et al. Improved differential diagnosis of anemia of chronic disease and iron deficiency anemia: a prospective multicenter evaluation of soluble transferrin receptor and the sTfR/log ferritin index. Am J Hematol. 2011;86(11):923–7.
23. Howie SR. Blood sample volumes in child health research: review of safe limits. Bull World Health Organ. 2011;89(1):46–53.
24. Peplow C, Assfalg R, Beyerlein A, Hasford J, Bonifacio E, Ziegler AG. Blood draws up to 3% of blood volume in clinical trials are safe in children. Acta Paediatr. 2019;108(5):940–4.
25. De Jongh R, Vranken J, Vundelinckx G, Bosmans E, Maes M, Heylen R. The effects of anticoagulation and processing on assays of IL-6, sIL-6R, sIL-2R and soluble transferrin receptor. Cytokine. 1997;9(9):696–701.
26. Garrett DA, Sangha JK, Kothari MT, Boyle D. Field-friendly techniques for assessment of biomarkers of nutrition for development. Am J Clin Nutr. 2011;94(2):685S–90S.
27. Erhardt JG, Estes JE, Pfeiffer CM, Biesalski HK, Craft NE. Combined measurement of ferritin, soluble transferrin receptor, retinol binding protein, and C-reactive protein by an inexpensive, sensitive, and simple sandwich enzyme-linked immunosorbent assay technique. J Nutr. 2004;134(11):3127–32.
28. Pfeiffer CM, Looker AC. Laboratory methodologies for indicators of iron status: strengths, limitations, and analytical challenges. Am J Clin Nutr. 2017;106(Suppl 6):1606S–14S.
29. Garcia-Casal MN, Pena-Rosas JP, Urrechaga E, Escanero JF, Huo J, Martinez RX, et al. Performance and comparability of laboratory methods for measuring ferritin concentrations in human serum or plasma: a systematic review and meta-analysis. PLoS One. 2018;13(5):e0196576.
30. Karakochuk CD, Whitfield KC, Rappaport AI, Barr SI, Vercauteren SM, McLean J, et al. Comparison of four immunoassays to measure serum ferritin concentrations and iron deficiency prevalence among non-pregnant Cambodian women and Congolese children. Clin Chem Lab Med. 2017;55(1):65–72.
31. Ervasti M, Kotisaari S, Romppanen J, Punnonen K. In patients who have stainable iron in the bone marrow an elevated plasma transferrin receptor value may reflect functional iron deficiency. Clin Lab Haematol. 2004;26(3):205–9.
32. Rohner F, Namaste SM, Larson LM, Addo OY, Mei Z, Suchdev PS, et al. Adjusting soluble transferrin receptor concentrations for inflammation: Biomarkers Reflecting Inflammation and Nutritional Determinants of Anemia (BRINDA) project. Am J Clin Nutr. 2017;106(Suppl 1):372S–82S.
33. Thorpe SJ, Heath A, Sharp G, Cook J, Ellis R, Worwood M. A WHO reference reagent for the Serum Transferrin Receptor (sTfR): international collaborative study to evaluate a recombinant soluble transferrin receptor preparation. Clin Chem Lab Med. 2010;48(6):815–20.
34. Pfeiffer CM, Cook JD, Mei Z, Cogswell ME, Looker AC, Lacher DA. Evaluation of an automated soluble transferrin receptor (sTfR) assay on the Roche Hitachi analyzer and its comparison to two ELISA assays. Clin Chim Acta. 2007;382(1–2, 112):–6.
35. Prentice AM, Doherty CP, Abrams SA, Cox SE, Atkinson SH, Verhoef H, et al. Hepcidin is the major predictor of erythrocyte iron incorporation in anemic African children. Blood. 2012;119(8):1922–8.
36. van der Vorm LN, Hendriks JC, Laarakkers CM, Klaver S, Armitage AE, Bamberg A, et al. Toward worldwide hepcidin assay harmonization: identification of a commutable secondary reference material. Clin Chem. 2016;62(7):993–1001.
37. Diepeveen LE, Laarakkers CMM, Martos G, Pawlak ME, Uguz FF, Verberne K, et al. Provisional standardization of hepcidin assays: creating a traceability chain with a primary reference material, candidate reference method and a commutable secondary reference material. Clin Chem Lab Med. 2019;57(6):864–72.
38. Namaste SM, Aaron GJ, Varadhan R, Peerson JM, Suchdev PS, Group BW. Methodologic approach for the Biomarkers Reflecting Inflammation and Nutritional Determinants of Anemia (BRINDA) project. Am J Clin Nutr. 2017;106(Suppl 1):333S–47S.
39. O'Callaghan KM, Roth DE. Standardization of laboratory practices and reporting of biomarker data in clinical nutrition research. Am J Clin Nutr. 2019;112(Supplement_1):453S–7S.
40. Barffour MA, Schulze KJ, Coles CL, Chileshe J, Kalungwana N, Siamusantu W, et al. Malaria exacerbates inflammation-associated elevation in ferritin and soluble transferrin receptor with only modest effects on iron deficiency and iron deficiency anaemia among rural Zambian children. Tropical Med Int Health. 2018;23(1):53–62.
41. Thorpe SJ, Walker D, Arosio P, Heath A, Cook JD, Worwood M. International collaborative study to evaluate a recombinant L ferritin preparation as an International Standard. Clin Chem. 1997;43(9):1582–7.
42. National Institute for Biological Standards and Control. Product Catalog. https://www.nibsc.org/products/brm_product_catalogue/who_standards.aspx.
43. Radboudumc. Hepcidin Reference Material. http://www.hepcidinanalysis.com/contentmenu/provided-service/reference-material/.
44. Craft N, Arredondo F, Fleshman M, Brindle E, Lillis L, Barney R, et al. Measurement of nutritional and

inflammatory biomarkers in Dry Plasma Spots (DPS) (P10-097-19). Curr Dev Nutr. 2019; 3(Suppl 1).
45. Koehler K, Marks-Nelson E, Braga CP, Beckford S, Adamec J. Validity of plasma collection cards for ferritin assessment-A proof-of-concept study. Eur J Haematol. 2020;104(6):554–61.
46. Hiscock R, Kumar D, Simmons SW. Systematic review and meta-analysis of method comparison studies of Masimo pulse co-oximeters (Radical-7 or Pronto-7) and HemoCue(R) absorption spectrometers (B-Hemoglobin or 201+) with laboratory haemoglobin estimation. Anaesth Intensive Care. 2015;43(3):341–50.
47. Collings S, Thompson O, Hirst E, Goossens L, George A, Weinkove R. Non-invasive detection of anaemia using digital photographs of the conjunctiva. PLoS One. 2016;11(4):e0153286.
48. Sireci AN. Hematology testing in urgent care and resource-poor settings: an overview of point of care and satellite testing. Clin Lab Med. 2015;35(1):197–207.
49. Measurement of the Vitamin A and iron status in blood samples. http://www.nutrisurvey.de/blood_samples/.
50. Brindle E, Lillis L, Barney R, Hess SY, Wessells KR, Ouedraogo CT, et al. Simultaneous assessment of iodine, iron, vitamin A, malarial antigenemia, and inflammation status biomarkers via a multiplex immunoassay method on a population of pregnant women from Niger. PLoS One. 2017;12(10):e0185868.
51. Kristensen GB, Rustad P, Berg JP, Aakre KM. Analytical bias exceeding desirable quality goal in 4 out of 5 common immunoassays: results of a native single serum sample external quality assessment program for cobalamin, folate, ferritin, thyroid-stimulating hormone, and free T4 analyses. Clin Chem. 2016;62(9):1255–63.
52. Miller WG, Schimmel H, Rej R, Greenberg N, Ceriotti F, Burns C, et al. IFCC Working Group recommendations for assessing commutability part 1: general experimental design. Clin Chem. 2018;64(3):447–54.
53. Hoofnagle AN. Harmonization of blood-based indicators of iron status: making the hard work matter. Am J Clin Nutr. 2017;106(Suppl 6):1615S–9S.

4 Interpretation of Biomarkers and Diagnosis of Nutritional Anaemias

Danielle Clucas and Beverley-Ann Biggs

Keywords

Anaemia · Iron deficiency · Ferritin · Vitamin B12 · Serum B12 · Holotranscobalamin Folate · Homocysteine · Methylmalonic acid

Introduction

Globally, the most common causes of anaemia are nutritional. Iron deficiency is the most prevalent, accounting for approximately 60% of cases in women and children in some areas [1]. Other causes include other nutritional deficiencies (particularly vitamin B12 and folate deficiencies), blood loss, haemolysis, haemoglobinopathies and thalassaemias, anaemia of chronic disease/inflammation and primary bone marrow pathologies. Conditions leading to anaemia vary considerably by region and are often multifactorial. Identifying the underlying cause of anaemia in a clinical setting is important to ensure the correct treatment is given. At a population level, it is vital to identify the epidemiology and pathogenesis of anaemia within countries to inform policy and guide interventions. This is achieved by the measurement of anaemia biomarkers either in clinics for individuals or in population-based surveys.

Anaemia diagnosis is based on the finding of a peripheral blood haemoglobin concentration below the recommended reference range for age and gender (Table 4.1) [2]. The aetiology of anaemia may be suggested by clinical history, examination or local prevalence data. Red blood cell (RBC) indices reported by many modern haematology analysers and RBC morphology from a blood film provide information about the underlying cause of the anaemia (Table 4.2). The most useful red cell indices include the mean cell volume (MCV), red cell count (RCC), mean cell haemoglobin (MCH), red cell distribution width (RDW) as well as the reticulocyte count and blood film report. Newer measures such as reticulocyte haemoglobin and proportion of hypochromic cells may be helpful in some cases. More specific biomarkers include measures of iron, B12 and folate status, inflammatory markers, markers of haemolysis and specialised tests, for example, for the diagnosis of specific types of haemolysis, haemoglobinopathies, thalassaemias

D. Clucas (✉)
Walter and Eliza Hall Institute of Medical Research, Parkville, Australia

Department of Medical Biology, The University of Melbourne, Parkville, Australia

Diagnostic Haematology, The Royal Melbourne Hospital, Parkville, Australia
e-mail: clucas.d@wehi.edu.au

B.-A. Biggs
Department of Medicine at the Doherty Institute, University of Melbourne, Melbourne, Australia

Victorian Infectious Diseases Service, The Royal Melbourne Hospital, Parkville, Australia
e-mail: babiggs@unimelb.edu.au

C. D. Karakochuk et al. (eds.), *Nutritional Anemia*, Nutrition and Health,
https://doi.org/10.1007/978-3-031-14521-6_4

Table 4.1 WHO recommended haemoglobin concentrations (g/L) for the diagnosis of anaemia and assessment of severity[a]. Taken from [2]

Population	Non-anaemia	Anaemia		
		Mild	Moderate	Severe
Children 6–59 months of age	110 or higher	100–109	70–99	Lower than 70
Children 5–11 years of age	115 or higher	110–114	80–109	Lower than 80
Children 12–14 years of age	120 or higher	110–119	80–109	Lower than 80
Non-pregnant women (15 years of age and above)	120 or higher	110–119	80–109	Lower than 80
Pregnant women	110 or higher	100–109	70–99	Lower than 70
Men (15 years of age and above)	130 or higher	110–129	80–109	Lower than 80

[a] At sea level

Table 4.2 Causes of anaemia—classified by mean cell volume [3, 4]

Microcytic	Normocytic	Macrocytic
Iron deficiency	Acute blood loss	B12 and/or folate deficiency
Thalassaemias	Haemolysis	Myelodysplastic syndrome
Sideroblastic anaemia	Anaemia of chronic disease	Liver disease
Anaemia of chronic disease	Bone marrow suppression/hypoplasia	Aplastic anaemia
	Primary bone marrow disorders (e.g. Leukaemia, myelofibrosis)	Pure red cell aplasia
	Early iron deficiency	Hypothyroidism
	Mixed nutritional deficiency	Associated with reticulocytosis
	Anaemia of renal disease	Chronic alcohol abuse
	Sickle cell anaemia	Medications (e.g. Hydroxyurea, methotrexate)

and bone marrow pathologies. In this chapter we will focus on biomarkers for the diagnosis of nutritional anaemias, namely, iron deficiency anaemia and the megaloblastic anaemias of vitamin B12 and folate deficiency.

Red Cell Indices and Red Blood Cell Morphology

Reticulocyte Count and Reticulocyte Haemoglobin Content

Reticulocytes are immature RBCs, containing remnants of ribosomal ribonucleic acid (RNA) [5]. The number of reticulocytes in the peripheral blood reflects erythropoietic activity and can be used to broadly classify anaemia as due to increased loss of or decreased production of RBCs. When there is anaemia with adequate substrates for erythropoiesis and normal bone marrow function, there is a compensatory increase in the reticulocyte count (reticulocytosis), for example, in acute blood loss or haemolysis. Conversely, the count is low or inappropriately "normal" for the degree of anaemia, in anaemia due to bone marrow failure or nutritional deficiency [6]. A reticulocytosis is suggested by increased polychromasia (diffusely basophilic staining red cells) on a normal blood film and is confirmed by a reticulocyte count, as determined by an automated haematology analyser or manually on a blood film after staining with a supravital stain (e.g. new methylene blue) [7].

The life span of a reticulocyte is short, approximately 4 days, compared with a mature RBC (120 days), and so reticulocyte characteristics can provide information about rapid changes in erythropoiesis that usual red cell indices cannot. Reticulocyte haemoglobin content gives an indication of the functional availability of iron for erythropoiesis [7] and is useful in the diagnosis of iron deficiency and assessing early response to iron therapy [8]. A low reticulocyte haemoglobin occurs in absolute, as well as functional, iron deficiency, and its measurement can be used to both predict and monitor response to intravenous iron therapy, where an increase can be seen as early as the second day of treatment in a responsive patient [8]. The reticulocyte haemoglobin content is also decreased in alpha- and beta-thalassaemias and some rare congenital conditions causing microcytic anaemia. Therefore, it cannot be used to assess the adequacy of iron for erythropoiesis in these conditions or to distinguish between these conditions and iron deficiency as a cause for microcytosis or microcytic anaemia [8, 9].

Mean Cell Volume

Microcytic, normocytic and macrocytic anaemias describe low haemoglobin concentrations where the red cells are small, normal in size or large, respectively, which is a common way to broadly classify anaemias. Microcytes are most commonly seen with iron deficiency and thalassaemias, while macrocytes are commonly seen in megaloblastic anaemias (from vitamin B12 and folate deficiencies). Macrocytosis may also occur with liver disease, heavy alcohol use, some myelodysplastic syndromes and the use of some medications (e.g. hydroxyurea and sulfamethoxazole/trimethoprim) and in rare congenital conditions. Another cause of an increase in MCV is a reticulocytosis, due to the larger size of these immature cells [7, 10]. While iron deficiency typically causes microcytosis and vitamin B12/folate deficiency causes macrocytosis, this may not be the case if there is a mixed nutritional deficiency. There may also be a rise or fall in MCV from the patient's baseline due to nutritional deficiency, but the MCV is still within the quoted reference range.

Mean Cell Haemoglobin

A low MCH results in hypochromic or pale RBCs on a blood film. A reduction in MCH is due to impaired haemoglobin synthesis and is seen in iron deficiency as well as thalassaemias and rarer sideroblastic anaemias [7, 10].

Red Cell Distribution Width

The RDW gives a measure of the variation in RBC volume. This is often increased in iron deficiency and may help to distinguish a mild microcytic anaemia due to iron deficiency from that due to thalassaemia trait, where the RDW is often normal. The RCC may also help in this regard, as it is increased in thalassaemia trait, due to ineffective erythropoiesis, but normal or low in anaemia due to iron deficiency. The RDW is often increased in megaloblastic anaemia and normal in other causes of a macrocytosis [7].

Percentage of Hypochromic Cells

Percentage of hypochromic cells reflects the percentage of RBCs containing less haemoglobin than normal RBCs. The percentage of hypochromic red cells is increased when erythropoiesis is iron restricted, either in absolute or functional iron deficiency [7, 11]. The percentage of hypochromic cells gives an indication of iron status over a longer period than reticulocyte haemoglobin content which changes more rapidly. Advantages of these parameters are that they can be performed on the same sample as a full blood count and have a fast turn-around time, they do not however distinguish between absolute or functional iron deficiency, or other causes of microcytic hypochromic anaemias [11].

Blood Film

Red cell morphology and other changes noted on a blood film may suggest the aetiology of anaemia. For example, the typical blood film findings in iron deficiency anaemia include microcytic hypochromic RBCs with pencil cells, or elliptocytes/elongated cells, and target cells (cells with excess cell membrane relative to the cell volume giving the appearance of a target or bull's-eye) and may be accompanied by a thrombocytosis (Fig. 4.1). The megaloblastic anaemias of vitamin B12 and folate deficiency classically show oval macrocytes and hypersegmented neutrophils. Red cells may also show tear drop cells, fragments and basophilic stippling and when severe there may be an associated thrombocytopenia and leucopenia (Fig. 4.2). Table 4.3 describes the typical blood film findings in some of the more common causes of anaemia.

To confirm the cause of anaemia suspected from red cell indices, blood film findings or clinical history or when these parameters are not

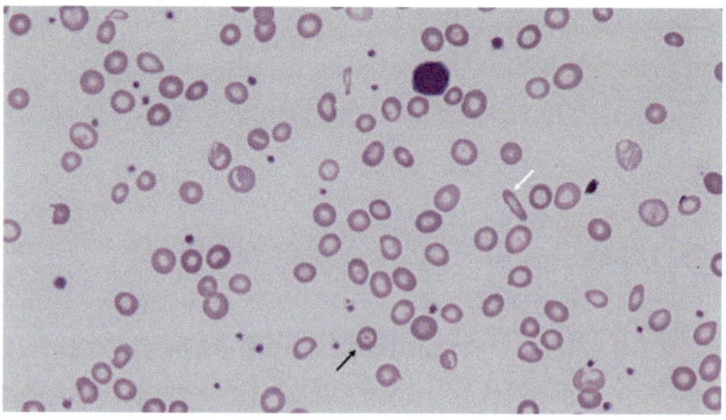

Fig. 4.1 A peripheral blood film showing typical changes of iron deficiency, with microcytic (small) hypochromic (pale) reds blood cells, pencil cells (white arrow) and target cells (black arrow)

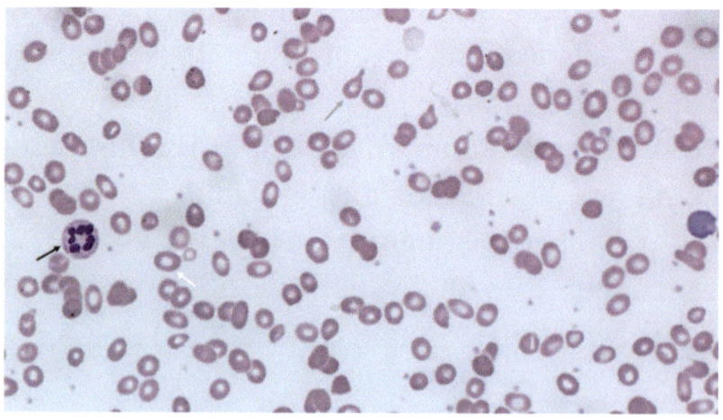

Fig. 4.2 A peripheral blood film from a patient with B12 deficiency showing oval macrocytes (large red blood cells) (white arrow), tear drop cells (grey arrow) and a hypersegmented neutrophil (black arrow)

Table 4.3 Typical blood film findings in some of the more common causes of anaemia [12–14]

Cause of anaemia	Typical blood film changes
Iron deficiency	Microcytic hypochromic red blood cells, pencil/elongated cells, target cells There may be an associated thrombocytosis
Megaloblastic anaemia (B12/folate deficiency)	Macrocytic red cells, typically macro-ovalocytes. There may also be micro tear drop cells White blood cells show hypersegmented neutrophils In severe deficiency there may be pancytopenia
Haemolysis	Increased polychromasia
Autoimmune	Spherocytes Red cell agglutination in cold agglutinin disease
Oxidative/G6PD deficiency	Bite and blister cells
Fragmentation syndromes	Schistocytes/red cell fragments There may also be keratocytes and microspherocytes Thrombocytopenia in thrombotic thrombocytopenic purpura, and to a lesser extent in haemolytic uraemic syndrome and atypical haemolytic uraemic syndrome
Anaemia of chronic disease	No specific diagnostic features on blood film. Red cells may be normocytic or microcytic
Thalassaemias	Trait—film almost normal with slight microcytosis to markedly abnormal (e.g. Hypochromia, anisopoikilocytosis, basophilic stippling, target cells) Intermedia—microcytic hypochromic red cells, anisopoikilocytosis, basophilic stippling Major—marked anisopoikilocytosis, microcytosis, hypochromia, basophilic stippling, Papenheimer bodies, target cells, tear drop cells, nucleated red blood cells

Table 4.3 (continued)

Cause of anaemia	Typical blood film changes
Haemoglobinopathies	Dependent on specific haemoglobinopathy Sickle cell anaemia: sickle cells, boat shaped cells, there may also be irregularly contracted cells and hemi-ghost cells, polychromasia, nucleated red blood cells and hyposplenic changes from 1 year of age (e.g. Howell-Jolly bodies, target cells, Pappenheimer bodies) Sickle cell/beta thalassemia: microcytosis plus changes of sickle cell anaemia Sickle cell/Hb C: Boat shaped cells, occasional cells with HbC crystals, few sickle cells, SC poikilocytes, irregularly contracted cells and target cells
Bone marrow pathology	Various changes seen depending on pathology Leucoerythroblastic (early myeloid and red blood cell precursors in the peripheral blood) and tear drop cells can signify bone marrow infiltration Abnormal cells, for example blasts in leukaemia or abnormal lymphoid cells in bone marrow infiltration with lymphoma. There may be other associated cytopenias Aplastic anaemia—cytopenias with no other specific diagnostic features on blood film Red cell aplasia—anaemia with no increase in polychromasia and no specific diagnostic features

available and only a low haemoglobin has been identified, measurement of other biomarkers for particular nutritional anaemias or other pathologies is required.

Biomarkers of Iron Status and the Diagnosis of Iron Deficiency Anaemia

Iron deficiency occurs along a spectrum. Iron depletion occurs when body iron stores have become low, but there is still enough iron for cellular purposes. This progresses to iron-deficient erythropoiesis where iron available for RBC production is limited. Haemoglobin and MCV are still within the normal range but may have fallen from the individual's baseline. Eventually, iron deficiency anaemia develops, where RBC production is reduced and haemoglobin, MCV and MCH are low [15]. Anaemia, abnormal red cell indices (as described above), dietary or medical history, or population prevalence prompts measure of more specific biomarkers of iron status.

Bone marrow aspiration with an iron, or Perls' stain, has been the gold standard for the diagnosis of iron deficiency and is diagnostic when there is no stainable particulate iron seen in an adequate sample [16]. However, this is an invasive procedure that is rarely performed solely for the diagnosis of iron deficiency given the availability of serum biomarkers, most notably serum ferritin. Bone marrow aspiration and iron stain may still be performed in complex cases of anaemia, and a diagnosis of iron deficiency may be made on a bone marrow aspirate performed for other reasons.

Readily available serum biomarkers of iron status include serum ferritin, iron, transferrin and transferrin saturation (or TIBC). Additional and emerging iron biomarkers include soluble transferrin receptor (sTfR), zinc protoporphyrin (ZPP) and hepcidin [17].

Serum Ferritin

Ferritin is the primary iron storage protein, with each ferritin molecule able to store up to 4000–

4500 iron atoms. Ferritin is found within the cytoplasm of virtually all cells of the body and is able to both safely store and release iron according to physiologic needs [18]. Serum or plasma ferritin is considered the most reliable non-invasive biomarker for the diagnosis of iron deficiency and reflects iron stores in healthy individuals when systemic inflammation is not present. Diagnostic ferritin values have been established from the few studies which have looked at ferritin concentrations in patients with microcytic anaemia who had no stainable iron in the bone marrow or who showed a therapeutic response to iron. These studies indicate a ferritin threshold of 15 μg/L to be specific (98–100%) but less sensitive (60–75%) for the diagnosis of iron deficiency. However, increasing the threshold to 30 μg/L raises the sensitivity (93–100%) at the expense of specificity (75–89%) [19–21]. The recent update of the World Health Organization (WHO) guideline on the use of ferritin concentration to assess iron status recommends a cut-off of 15 μg/L for the diagnosis of iron deficiency in children older than 5 years, adolescents and adults and 12 μg/L in infants and children under 5 years of age, in an apparently healthy population [22]. These recommendations are based largely on expert opinion, and there remain no universally accepted cut-offs. Various other specialist groups suggest other cut-offs, and reference ranges vary depending on pathology laboratory. The American Society of Haematology diagnoses iron deficiency with a ferritin of <30 μg/L in adults, with the normal range in females accepted as 20–200 μg/L and in males 40–300 μg/L [23]. The Royal College of Pathologists of Australasia (RCPA) recommends a cut-off of 30 μg/L for healthy adults and ≤20 μg/L for pre-pubescent children [24], while the Australian Iron Deficiency Expert Group suggest that ferritin <15–30 μg/L be used [25]. Despite these variations, a ferritin <15 μg/L is specific but not sensitive for the diagnosis of iron deficiency, and a ferritin concentration of <15–30 μg/L may be a reasonable compromise from the available data. A ferritin >30 μg/L, however, does not exclude iron deficiency, with higher values seen in iron deficiency when there is concurrent inflammation.

Serum ferritin is an acute phase protein, increased in the presence of inflammation, as well as in liver disease. This increase does not reflect a true increase in storage or liver iron and complicates the diagnosis of iron deficiency [26]. Failure to account for this can lead to missed diagnoses (and subsequently inadequate treatment) of iron deficiency or underestimation of population prevalence. WHO recommends that "the increase in ferritin values caused by inflammation should be accounted for in individuals and populations" [22]. It is recommended that two acute phase proteins, CRP and AGP, be measured alongside ferritin to assist with this (see Box 4.1). Many specialist groups now include a cut-off value to define iron deficiency in the presence of inflammation, such as 70 μg/L recommended by WHO for older children, adolescents and adults with inflammation and 30 μg/L for infants and children under 5 years [22]. The RCPA suggests 100 μg/L for adults in the presence of inflammation [24], while the Australian Iron Deficiency Expert Group recommends 60–100 μg/L [25]. Assessing a patient's comorbidities, inflammatory markers, RBC morphology and indices (e.g. MCV, MCH, RDW) and reticulocyte count together with the ferritin value can help to ascertain the likelihood of iron deficiency. A bone marrow biopsy in complicated cases of anaemia or assessment of response to a trial of iron therapy is also an option.

The above approach is not feasible at a population level in areas with a high prevalence of inflammation where there is a risk of underestimating the prevalence of iron deficiency if conventional ferritin ranges are used. Different approaches have been suggested for adjusting ferritin for inflammation in population studies. These include increasing the ferritin cut-off—the Biomarkers Reflecting Inflammation and Nutritional Determinants of Anemia (BRINDA) study increased the ferritin level to 30 μg/L; however, WHO guidelines now recommend a cut-off of 70 μg/L in adults with inflammation [22, 27]. This could be applied either in the entire sample or just in those with inflammation. Other approaches include excluding individuals with elevated inflammatory markers, applying arithmetic correction factors or using regression correction. The BRINDA project compared these methods and supports the use of internal regression correction, using CRP, AGP and malaria infection, in populations with elevated inflammatory markers [27]. In their analyses this led to an increase in the estimated prevalence of depleted iron stores by a median of 24.7 and 7.5 percentage points in preschool children and women of reproductive age, respectively. WHO recommends that CRP and AGP be measured along with ferritin in areas where there is widespread inflammation and that "the adjustment that best suits the country reality should be selected and used" [22].

Box 4.1 Inflammatory Markers in the Assessment of Iron Status

Measurement of inflammatory markers, although not strictly biomarkers of nutritional anaemias themselves, aids in the interpretation of other measures of nutritional anaemias. C-reactive protein (CRP) and alpha-1-acid glycoprotein (AGP) are acute phase proteins that are elevated during periods of infection and inflammation. Increases in CRP and AGP occur in different phases of the inflammatory response. CRP rises quickly but also returns to normal faster than AGP [28, 29], which rises more slowly and remains elevated for longer [30]. These markers have been used to divide the inflammatory response into phases: the 'incubation period' where CRP is elevated but AGP remains normal; 'early convalescence' when both CRP and AGP are elevated; and 'late convalescence' when CRP has returned to normal but AGP is still elevated [27].

Serum Iron and Transferrin Saturation

The vast majority of iron within the serum is bound to transferrin, the main iron transport protein [31]. Elevated or depleted serum iron levels often cause confusion when assessing iron status. Serum iron levels are labile with significant diurnal variation [32], are decreased in iron deficiency and inflammation and are affected by recent oral or intravenous iron intake [17]. Serum iron levels should not be used to diagnose iron deficiency. The only clinical situation in which a serum iron level is of value, viewed in isolation, is in a suspected case of iron poisoning [24].

The transferrin saturation gives a measure of how much transferrin is binding/transporting iron. A transferrin saturation less than 15% indicates suboptimal iron delivery for erythropoiesis [33, 34]. Transferrin saturation is often used in nutritional studies to define iron deficiency and is one of the indicators (together with serum ferritin and red cell protoporphyrin) used by the NHANES survey in their "ferritin model" which defines iron deficiency as an abnormality of at least two of the three biomarkers [35]. However, it is important to be aware that transferrin saturation is derived from serum iron. It is the ratio of serum iron to total iron binding capacity (or transferrin concentration multiplied by 25) and is therefore subject to the limitations that affect serum iron concentration [17]. A fasted morning sample may reduce variability, but due to these factors, it may not be a reliable diagnostic marker of iron status in isolation.

Soluble Transferrin Receptor

Transferrin receptor 1 (TfR1) is one of two transferrin receptors on cell membranes and is essential for iron delivery to tissues. The cells with the greatest number of TfR1 are nucleated erythroid precursors in the bone marrow. The number of TfR1 per cell is increased when iron supply is limited. Soluble transferrin receptor (sTfR) concentrations reflect the number of cellular TfR1

[36]. Increases in sTfR concentrations therefore reflect either an increase in erythropoiesis/increase in the number of nucleated erythroid cells in the bone marrow or inadequate iron stores, seen in conditions such as haemolysis, thalassaemias or polycythaemia vera and iron deficiency, respectively [37, 38]. A meta-analysis of ten studies of sTfR showed it had a sensitivity and specificity of 86% and 75%, respectively, for the diagnosis of iron deficiency [39]. Given that sTfR is also increased in states of ineffective erythropoiesis as mentioned, it is not useful for detecting iron deficiency in populations with significant rates of thalassaemia or other haemoglobinopathies [40, 41], but an advantage of this biomarker is that it is not affected by inflammation in the way that ferritin is. sTfR is increased in iron deficiency, with or without inflammation, but is normal in anaemia of chronic disease. Although it is not required for the diagnosis of uncomplicated iron deficiency, it is useful in distinguishing iron deficiency anaemia from anaemia of chronic disease [42], particularly when combined with measurement of serum ferritin in the sTfR-ferritin index (the ratio of sTfR and logarithm of serum ferritin) [43]. This index is subject to the limitations of each test, and cut-off values are assay specific and cannot be applied universally.

Zinc Protoporphyrin

Erythrocyte zinc protoporphyrin (ZPP) is used in research settings and population surveys as a biomarker of iron status. The final step in haem synthesis is the conversion of protoporphyrin IX into haem by the insertion of ferrous iron, catalysed by ferrochelatase. Erythrocyte protoporphyrin increases in RBCs when there is insufficient iron available for conversion into haem. Zinc is an alternate metal substrate for ferrochelatase, and as erythrocyte protoporphyrin increases, ZPP rises [44, 45]. ZPP is not increased in simple iron depletion, but rises when iron delivery to the bone marrow is no longer sufficient to meet the requirements for erythropoiesis, giving an indication of the severity of iron deficiency [44, 46]. In the absence of other conditions that affect ZPP, it is a sensitive measure of iron deficiency [45–47]. However, levels are also increased in lead poisoning, thalassaemia trait, some haemoglobinopathies and anaemia of inflammation [48, 49].

Hepcidin

Hepcidin is the master regulator of systemic iron homeostasis, and its production is altered, appropriately or inappropriately, in disorders of altered iron status/metabolism. Measurement of hepcidin levels may help in the diagnosis and management of these conditions [50]. In iron deficiency hepcidin is suppressed, often to undetectable levels to allow maximal iron absorption. However, hepcidin is increased in inflammatory conditions, and in patients with iron deficiency and concurrent inflammation or comorbidities, such as renal disease, hepcidin may not be suppressed to the extent expected [51]. In this setting, hepcidin levels may help to identify patients with iron deficiency who may not respond to oral iron supplementation and for whom intravenous administration may be more effective [50]. In the public health setting, it may help to identify individuals who would benefit from, and respond to, oral iron supplementation [52]. It may also be beneficial in distinguishing patients with "pure" anaemia of chronic disease from those with concomitant iron deficiency, as hepcidin levels are lower in this second group [53]. In iron loading anaemias, such as thalassaemia major and intermedia, and congenital dyserythropoietic anaemias, hepcidin levels may help to predict and monitor iron overload [54]. In the diagnostic setting, hepcidin levels would aid in the diagnosis of iron-refractory iron deficiency anaemia (IRIDA), a rare genetic condition caused by mutation in the TMPRSS6 gene and characterised by iron deficiency with inappropriately normal or high hepcidin levels [55]. Hepcidin measurement is currently limited to the research setting. Although there have been challenges in producing a reliable assay, and with worldwide standardisation, there are now both immunoassays and mass spectrometry-based assays, and there has been recent progress in the development of reference material and a proficiency testing scheme [56].

Biomarkers for the Diagnosis of Iron Deficiency Anaemia: A Summary

The classic findings in isolated iron deficiency anaemia are a microcytic hypochromic anaemia with pencil (or elongated) cells on a blood film. Red cell indices show a low MCV and MCH, low or normal RCC and reticulocyte count and a high RDW. A low ferritin is diagnostic of iron deficiency; a normal value does not however exclude it. In the presence of inflammation, the ferritin value may be within the normal range despite iron deficiency. CRP and AGP are important for diagnosing concurrent inflammation. Red cell indices, iron studies, inflammatory markers and other available iron biomarkers should be interpreted together to diagnose or exclude iron deficiency. Table 4.4 summarises the expected biomarker results in iron deficiency anaemia and how these compare to other causes of anaemia that may give some similar results.

Biomarkers of Vitamin B12 and Folate Status and the Diagnosis of Associated Anaemias

Vitamin B12 and folate deficiencies can result in a macrocytic or megaloblastic anaemia, which is due to impaired DNA synthesis. This manifests as large RBCs and hypersegmented neutrophils in the peripheral blood and megaloblastic precursors in the bone marrow (which have a characteristic nuclear chromatin pattern and asynchrony of nuclear and cytoplasmic maturation with a relatively immature nucleus). Severe megaloblastic anaemia can result in pancytopenia (a low haemoglobin, white cell and platelet count) [57]. Biomarkers of vitamin B12 and folate status include measurements of the nutrient levels themselves as well as measurement of other substances involved in their metabolism.

Vitamin B12

Vitamin B12 (or cobalamin) is transported in the plasma bound to haptocorrin or transcobalamin. Vitamin B12 bound to transcobalamin (holo-

Table 4.4 Interpreting biomarkers of iron status in iron deficiency, thalassaemia and anaemia of chronic disease. Adapted from [25]

	Haemoglobin	Mean cell volume and mean cell haemoglobin	Serum ferritin	Transferrin	Transferrin saturation[a]	Soluble transferrin receptor	Serum iron[b]
Tissue iron deficiency without anaemia	Normal	Normal or low	Low	Normal or high	Low-normal or low	High-normal or high	Low
Iron deficiency anaemia (IDA)	Low	Low (or normal in early IDA)	Low	High	Low	High	Low
IDA with inflammation	Low	Low	Low or normal	Normal or high	Low	High	Low
Thalassaemia minor	Low or normal	Low (or normal)	Normal or high	Normal	Normal or high	Normal or high	Normal
Anaemia of chronic disease	Low	Normal (may be mildly low)	Normal or high (does not imply elevated iron stores)	Normal	Low	Normal	Low

[a] Transferrin saturation should ideally be performed on a fasting morning sample

[b] Serum iron is markedly labile with significant diurnal variation. It should not be used to diagnose iron deficiency

transcobalamin, holoTC) is the active form of the vitamin, but only 20% of plasma vitamin B12 is bound to transcobalamin and in the active form [58]. Both total and active (holoTC) vitamin B12 can be measured in the serum and make up two of the four priority biomarkers of vitamin B12 status selected by the BOND Vitamin Expert Panel, together with serum methylmalonic acid (MMA) and plasma homocysteine [59]. Total vitamin B12 assays are more widely available but are less sensitive and specific for the diagnosis of vitamin B12 deficiency than holoTC [60]. Total vitamin B12 levels may be within the normal range despite low holoTC levels, and it has been recommended that holoTC also be measured if total levels are performed and are borderline or below a laboratory defined sufficiency threshold [61]. Conversely, total vitamin B12 levels may be low with normal holoTC levels such as in haptocorrin deficiency and in the third trimester of pregnancy where haptocorrin-bound vitamin B12 levels decrease by approximately 30%, but active levels are unchanged [62].

Vitamin B12 is a cofactor in two important reactions—the production of methionine from homocysteine and the conversion of methylmalonyl-CoA to succinyl-CoA. In B12 deficiency homocysteine and methylmalonic acid (MMA) (a side reaction product of methylmalonyl CoA metabolism) build up and are elevated in the serum [46, 58, 63]. MMA is the most sensitive marker of vitamin B12 deficiency and indicates whether there is adequate B12 for metabolic functions [46]. Its measurement is however not always readily available, and levels can be increased with renal impairment and bacterial overgrowth. Homocysteine also reflects adequacy of vitamin B12 for metabolic functions but is not specific for vitamin B12 deficiency. Homocysteine is also increased in folate, riboflavin and vitamin B6 deficiency, smokers, renal impairment, hypothyroidism and hyperhomocystinaemia and is ideally performed fasted (lowest in the morning, highest in the evening) [46, 63, 64].

Folate

Biomarkers of folate status include serum folate concentration, RBC folate concentration and plasma homocysteine. These were identified as priority biomarkers by the BOND Folate Expert Panel [65]. Serum folate concentration gives a measure of short-term folate status and reflects recent dietary intake [66, 67]. Improvement in diet leads to a rapid correction of serum folate levels; likewise a recent poor diet may result in low levels without necessarily indicating significantly low tissue levels [63, 67]. There is diurnal variation in folate levels and fasted samples are preferred. Red cell folate levels can be 10–20 times higher than serum, and consequently in vivo or in vitro red cell haemolysis may artefactually elevate serum folate measurements [63]. RBC folate is a sensitive marker of long-term folate status as it reflects the folate status for the life span of the RBCs, which is approximately 120 days. RBC folate is thought to correlate with liver folate concentrations and reflect tissue stores [66, 67]. RBC folate may be low and serum folate high in B12 deficiency and will respond to B12 replacement alone [68]. There is no consensus as to which of the two folate measurements is the better test for folate deficiency. Guidelines by the British Committee for Standards in Haematology recommend serum folate as the first line test for folate status [69], and serum folate appears to be more widely recommended as the most appropriate screening test [70–72]. WHO prefers red cell folate for assessing interventions aimed at improving folate status given the greater biologic variability in serum folate levels [73]. Given the issues inherent to both measures, some recommend performing both [63], and the RCPA recommends serum folate as the first line test with red cell folate reserved for when serum folate is low [61].

Plasma homocysteine is a sensitive functional biomarker of folate status, thought to reflect tissue levels [74, 75]. The major forms of intracellular folate are tetrahydrofolate (THF), 5-methyl THF and 10-formyltetrahydrofolate (10-formyl THF). 5-Methyl THF acts as the methyl group donor in the conversion of homocysteine to methionine by methionine synthase (with cobalamin as a cofactor)—producing methionine, regenerating THF and linking cobalamin to folate and 1-carbon metabolism [63, 66]. The megaloblastic anaemia in folate deficiency is thought to be caused by the decreased production of 5,10-methylene THF (due to insufficient THF) which is a cofactor in the production of dMTP, a rate-limiting step in DNA synthesis. Vitamin B12 deficiency leads to a functional folate deficiency, with a build-up of 5-methyl THF, which cannot be converted back to 5,10-methylene THF, and thus the two conditions lead to indistinguishable megaloblastic changes [63]. Folate supplementation without first excluding or treating vitamin B12 deficiency may mask the haematologic changes of vitamin B12 deficiency, allowing the neurologic changes associated with vitamin B12 deficiency to progress [76]. The role of folate in the conversion of homocysteine to methionine means that a build-up of homocysteine is also seen in folate deficiency and can be used as a biomarker in assessing an individual's folate status [63, 65]. As mentioned above, homocysteine is elevated in other conditions and so is a sensitive, but not specific, marker of folate deficiency.

Biomarkers for the Diagnosis of Nutritional Megaloblastic Anaemias: A Summary

The anaemia of vitamin B12 or folate deficiency is typically macrocytic with oval macrocytes and hypersegmented neutrophils on a blood film and an elevated MCV and RDW. Measurement of vitamin B12 (serum total or ideally active vitamin B12) or folate (serum and/or red cell) levels is usually the first step in the diagnosis of deficiency, with elevated levels of homocysteine and MMA in the case of vitamin B12 and homocysteine in the case of folate, confirming tissue deficiency (Table 4.5).

Table 4.5 Interpretation of biomarkers in the assessment of B12 and folate status. Adapted from [63]

	Normal B12 and folate status	B12 deficient	Folate deficient	Comments
Serum B12	Usually normal	Usually low, but up to 5% of patients have results within the reference range	Usually normal, but may be borderline low in severe folate deficiency, which corrects with folic acid monotherapy	May be high in liver disease, myeloproliferative neoplasms, acute inflammation, recovery from autoimmune neutropenia Low total B12 in 25% of elderly individuals. Levels also fall in normal pregnancy
Holotranscobalamin	Normal, although lower levels seen in the elderly	Low	Normal	Subject to recent dietary change within 24 h. Useful in pregnancy as levels are not affected by trimester
Serum folate	Usually normal	Usually normal. High serum folate may be seen in B12 deficiency	Usually low, but normal levels are found with recent dietary improvement	Highly influenced by recent folic acid intake. Low levels may be seen with recent deterioration in diet and are rapidly normalised by improvement in diet Haemolysis in vivo or in vitro may cause spurious elevations of serum folate

(continued)

Table 4.5 (continued)

	Normal B12 and folate status	B12 deficient	Folate deficient	Comments
Red cell folate	Usually normal	Low	Usually low, but normal in very acute deficiency state	High serum folate and low red cell folate may be seen in B12 deficiency—corrects with treatment of B12 deficiency
Plasma homocysteine	Usually normal	High in B12 deficiency and in 50% of samples from patients with low B12 consistent with metabolic B12-deficient state	High	Not specific for B12 or folate deficiency. May also be elevated in smokers, renal failure, in patients with MTHFR C677T mutation and hyperhomocystinaemia
Serum methylmalonic acid	Usually normal	High in B12 deficiency and in 50% of samples from patients with low B12 consistent with metabolic B12-deficient state	Usually normal, but high in 5% of patients who are folate deficient	Also elevated in renal impairment, with high intake of methionine and in 10% of normal subjects. Should not be used in isolation without total B12 or holotranscobalamin measurement
Urinary methylmalonic acid	Normal	High	Normal	Not affected by renal impairment

Conclusion

Nutritional deficiencies are the most common causes of anaemia worldwide, with iron deficiency accounting for the majority of cases. Red cell indices, blood film morphology and more specific biomarkers aid in identifying the underlying cause of anaemia in both populations and individuals. Despite the limitations discussed, serum ferritin remains the most reliable biomarker of iron status. Serum total or active vitamin B12 and serum or RBC folate are the recommended initial investigations for their respective deficiencies.

References

1. WHO the global prevalence of anaemia in 2011. Geneva: World Health Organisation; 2015.
2. WHO. Haemoglobin concentrations for the diagnosis of anaemia and assessment of severity. Vitamin and Mineral Nutrition Information System. Geneva: World Health Organization; 2011. Available from: https://apps.who.int/iris/bitstream/handle/10665/85839/WHO_NMH_NHD_MNM_11.1_eng.pdf.
3. Buttarello M. Laboratory diagnosis of anemia: are the old and new red cell parameters useful in classification and treatment, how? Int J Lab Hematol. 2016;38(Suppl 1):123–32.
4. Wang M. Iron deficiency and other types of anemia in infants and children. Am Fam Physician. 2016;93(4):270–8.
5. Bain BJ. Performing a blood count. In: Bain BJ, editor. Blood cells: a practical guide. 4th ed. Malden, MA: Blackwell Publishing; 2006. p. 20–60.
6. Riley RS, Ben-Ezra JM, Goel R, Tidwell A. Reticulocytes and reticulocyte enumeration. J Clin Lab Anal. 2001;15(5):267–94.
7. Briggs C, Bain BJ. Basic haematological techniques. In: Bain BJ, Bates I, Laffan MA, Mitchell Lews S, editors. Dacie and Lewis practical haematology. 11th ed. Elsevier Churchill Livingstone; 2012. p. 23–56.
8. Piva E, Brugnara C, Spolaore F, Plebani M. Clinical utility of reticulocyte parameters. Clin Lab Med. 2015;35(1):133–63.
9. Brugnara C. Reticulocyte cellular indices: a new approach in the diagnosis of anemias and monitoring of erythropoietic function. Crit Rev Clin Lab Sci. 2000;37(2):93–130.
10. Bain BJ. Morphology of blood cells. In: Bain BJ, editor. Blood cells: a practical guide. 4th ed. Malden, MA: Blackwell Publishing; 2006. p. 61–174.
11. Rehu M, Ahonen S, Punnonen K. The diagnostic accuracy of the percentage of hypochromic red blood cells (%HYPOm) and cellular hemoglobin in reticulocytes (CHr) in differentiating iron deficiency ane-

mia and anemia of chronic diseases. Clin Chim Acta. 2011;412(19–20):1809–13.

12. Bain BJ. Quantitative changes in blood cells. In: Bain BJ, editor. Blood cells: a practical guide. Fourth ed. MA, USA: Blackwell Publishing; 2006. p. 217–62.
13. Bain BJ. Disorders of red cells and platelets. In: Bain BJ, editor. Blood cells: a practical guide. Fourth ed. MA, USA: Blackwell Publishing; 2006. p. 283–397.
14. Bain BJ. Disorders of white cells. In: Bain BJ, editor. Blood cells: a practical guide. Fourth ed. MA, USA: Blackwell Publishing; 2006. p. 398–468.
15. Minck S, Jayasuriya P, Leahy M, Gallagher T. Iron deficiency: translating new evidence into practice. Healthed Expert Monogr 2017;(16):1–11.
16. Hughes DA, Stuart-Smith SE, Bain BJ. How should stainable iron in bone marrow films be assessed? J Clin Pathol. 2004;57(10):1038–40.
17. Worwood M, May A. Iron deficiency anaemia and iron overload. In: Bain BJ, Bates I, Laffan MA, Mitchell Lews S, editors. Dacie and Lewis practical haematology. 11th ed. Churchill Livingstone Elsevier; 2012. p. 175–200.
18. Harrison PM, Arosio P. The ferritins: molecular properties, iron storage function and cellular regulation. Biochim Biophys Acta. 1996;1275(3):161–203.
19. Hallberg L, Bengtsson C, Lapidus L, Lindstedt G, Lundberg PA, Hulten L. Screening for iron deficiency: an analysis based on bone-marrow examinations and serum ferritin determinations in a population sample of women. Br J Haematol. 1993;85(4):787–98.
20. Harju E, Pakarinen A, Larmi T. A comparison between serum ferritin concentration and the amount of bone marrow stainable iron. Scand J Clin Lab Invest. 1984;44(6):555–6.
21. Milman N, Bangsbøll S, Pedersen NS, Visfeldt J. Serum ferritin in non-dialysis patients with chronic renal failure: relation to bone marrow iron stores. Scand J Haematol. 1983;30(4):337–44.
22. WHO guideline on use of ferritin concentrations to assess iron status in individuals and populations. Geneva: World Health Organisation; 2020.
23. Camaschella C. Iron deficiency: new insights into diagnosis and treatment. Hematology Am Soc Hematol Educ Program. 2015;2015:8–13.
24. Iron studies standardised reporting protocol: The Royal College of Pathologists of Australasia; 2013. https://www.rcpa.edu.au/getattachment/554ba672-4d34-4e7c-b812-5741359bca78/Iron-Studies-Standardised-Reporting-Protocol.aspx.
25. Pasricha S-RS, Flecknoe-Brown SC, Allen KJ, Gibson PR, McMahon LP, Olynyk JK, et al. Diagnosis and management of iron deficiency anaemia: a clinical update. Med J Australia. 2010;193(9):525–32.
26. Koorts A, Viljoen M. Acute phase proteins: ferritin and ferritin isoforms. 2011.
27. Namaste SM, Rohner F, Huang J, Bhushan NL, Flores-Ayala R, Kupka R, et al. Adjusting ferritin concentrations for inflammation: Biomarkers Reflecting Inflammation and Nutritional Determinants of Anemia (BRINDA) project. Am J Clin Nutr. 2017;106(Suppl 1):359s–71s.
28. Vigushin DM, Pepys MB, Hawkins PN. Metabolic and scintigraphic studies of radioiodinated human C-reactive protein in health and disease. J Clin Invest. 1993;91(4):1351–7.
29. Pepys MB. C-REACTIVE PROTEIN FIFTY YEARS ON. Lancet. 1981;317(8221):653–7.
30. Aronsen KF, Ekelund G, Kindmark C, Laurell CB. Sequential changes of plasma proteins after surgical trauma. Scand J Clin Lab Inv. 1972;29(sup124):127–36.
31. Ganz T. Systemic iron homeostasis. Physiol Rev. 2013;93(4):1721–41.
32. Høyer K. Physiologic variations in the iron content of human blood serum. Acta Med Scand. 1944;119(6):562–76.
33. Bullock GC, Delehanty LL, Talbot AL, Gonias SL, Tong WH, Rouault TA, et al. Iron control of erythroid development by a novel aconitase-associated regulatory pathway. Blood. 2010;116(1):97–108.
34. Bainton DF, Finch CA. THE DIAGNOSIS OF IRON DEFICIENCY ANEMIA. Am J Med. 1964;37:62–70.
35. Cogswell ME, Looker AC, Pfeiffer CM, Cook JD, Lacher DA, Beard JL, et al. Assessment of iron deficiency in US preschool children and nonpregnant females of childbearing age: National Health and Nutrition Examination Survey 2003-2006. Am J Clin Nutr. 2009;89(5):1334–42.
36. Ponka P, Lok CN. The transferrin receptor: role in health and disease. Int J Biochem Cell Biol. 1999;31(10):1111–37.
37. Huebers HA, Beguin Y, Pootrakul P, Einspahr D, Finch CA. Intact transferrin receptors in human plasma and their relation to erythropoiesis. Blood. 1990;75(1):102–7.
38. Flowers CH, Skikne BS, Covell AM, Cook JD. The clinical measurement of serum transferrin receptor. J Lab Clin Med. 1989;114(4):368–77.
39. Infusino I, Braga F, Dolci A, Panteghini M. Soluble Transferrin Receptor (sTfR) and sTfR/log ferritin index for the diagnosis of iron-deficiency anemia a meta-analysis. Am J Clin Pathol. 2012;138(5):642–9.
40. Rees DC, Williams TN, Maitland K, Clegg JB, Weatherall DJ. Alpha thalassaemia is associated with increased soluble transferrin receptor levels. Br J Haematol. 1998;103(2):365–9.
41. George J, Yiannakis M, Main B, Devenish R, Anderson CB, An U, et al. Genetic hemoglobin disorders, infection, and deficiencies of iron and vitamin A determine anemia in young Cambodian children. J Nutr. 2012;142:781–7.
42. Cook JD, Skikne BS, Baynes RD. Serum transferrin receptor. Annu Rev Med. 1993;44:63–74.
43. Lopez A, Cacoub P, Macdougall IC, Peyrin-Biroulet L. Iron deficiency anaemia. Lancet. 2016;387(10021):907–16.
44. Labbé RF, Vreman HJ, Stevenson DK. Zinc protoporphyrin: a metabolite with a mission. Clin Chem. 1999;45(12):2060–72.

45. Magge H, Sprinz P, Adams WG, Drainoni M-L, Meyers A. Zinc protoporphyrin and iron deficiency screening: trends and therapeutic response in an urban pediatric center. JAMA Pediatr. 2013;167(4):361–7.
46. Lynch S, Pfeiffer CM, Georgieff MK, Brittenham G, Fairweather-Tait S, Hurrell RF, et al. Biomarkers of Nutrition for Development (BOND)—iron review. J Nutr. 2018;148(suppl_1):1001S–67S.
47. Yu KH. Effectiveness of zinc protoporphyrin/heme ratio for screening iron deficiency in preschool-aged children. Nutr Res Pract. 2011;5(1):40–5.
48. Hirsch RE, Pulakhandam UR, Billett HH, Nagel RL. Blood zinc protoporphyrin is elevated only in sickle cell patients with low fetal hemoglobin. Am J Hematol. 1991;36(2):147–9.
49. Tillyer ML, Tillyer CR. Zinc protoporphyrin assays in patients with alpha and beta thalassaemia trait. J Clin Pathol. 1994;47(3):205–8.
50. Girelli D, Nemeth E, Swinkels DW. Hepcidin in the diagnosis of iron disorders. Blood. 2016;127(23):2809–13.
51. Ganz T, Olbina G, Girelli D, Nemeth E, Westerman M. Immunoassay for human serum hepcidin. Blood. 2008;112(10):4292–7.
52. Pasricha SR, Atkinson SH, Armitage AE, Khandwala S, Veenemans J, Cox SE, et al. Expression of the iron hormone hepcidin distinguishes different types of anemia in African children. Sci Transl Med. 2014;6(235):235re3.
53. Theurl I, Aigner E, Theurl M, Nairz M, Seifert M, Schroll A, et al. Regulation of iron homeostasis in anemia of chronic disease and iron deficiency anemia: diagnostic and therapeutic implications. Blood. 2009;113(21):5277–86.
54. Kroot JJ, Tjalsma H, Fleming RE, Swinkels DW. Hepcidin in human iron disorders: diagnostic implications. Clin Chem. 2011;57(12):1650–69.
55. Finberg KE, Heeney MM, Campagna DR, Aydinok Y, Pearson HA, Hartman KR, et al. Mutations in TMPRSS6 cause iron-refractory iron deficiency anemia (IRIDA). Nat Genet. 2008;40(5):569–71.
56. Aune ET, Diepeveen LE, Laarakkers CM, Klaver S, Armitage AE, Bansal S, et al. Optimizing hepcidin measurement with a proficiency test framework and standardization improvement. Clin Chem Lab Med. 2020.
57. Bain BJ, Clark DM, Wilkins BS. Disorders of erythropoiesis, granulopoiesis and thrombopoiesis. In: Bain BJ, Clark DM, Wilkins BS, editors. Bone marrow pathology. 4th ed. Wiley-Blackwell; 2010.
58. Markle HV, Greenway DC. Cobalamin. Crit Rev Cl Lab Sci. 1996;33(4):247–356.
59. Allen LH, Miller JW, de Groot L, Rosenberg IH, Smith AD, Refsum H, et al. Biomarkers of Nutrition for Development (BOND): vitamin B-12 review. J Nutr. 2018;148(suppl_4):1995S–2027S.
60. Nexo E, Hoffmann-Lücke E. Holotranscobalamin, a marker of vitamin B-12 status: analytical aspects and clinical utility. Am J Clin Nutr. 2011;94(1):359s–65s.
61. Vitamin B12 and Folate testing—use and interpretation. 2015. https://www.rcpa.edu.au/getattachment/3f3667c3-34e7-47b7-93cf-e744ece8cfc7/Vitamin-and-B12-Folate-Testing-Use-and-Interpret.aspx.
62. Morkbak AL, Hvas AM, Milman N, Nexo E. Holotranscobalamin remains unchanged during pregnancy. Longitudinal changes of cobalamins and their binding proteins during pregnancy and postpartum. Haematologica. 2007;92(12):1711–2.
63. Hamilton MS, Blackmore S. Investigation of megaloblastic anaemia: cobalamin, folate and metabolite status. In: Bain BJ, Bates I, Laffan MA, Mitchell Lews S, editors. Dacie and Lewis practical haematology. 11th ed. Elsevier Churchill Livingstone; 2012. p. 201–28.
64. Haynes BM, Pfeiffer CM, Sternberg MR, Schleicher RL. Selected physiologic variables are weakly to moderately associated with 29 biomarkers of diet and nutrition, NHANES 2003-2006. J Nutr. 2013;143(6):1001s–10s.
65. Bailey LB, Stover PJ, McNulty H, Fenech MF, Gregory JF 3rd, Mills JL, et al. Biomarkers of nutrition for development-folate review. J Nutr. 2015;145(7):1636s–80s.
66. Bailey LB. Folic acid. In: Zempleni J, Rucker RB, McCormick DB, Suttie JW, editors. Handbook of vitamins. 4th ed. Boca Raton, FL: Taylor and Francis Group; 2007. p. 385–412.
67. Herbert V. Making sense of laboratory tests of folate status: folate requirements to sustain normality. Am J Hematol. 1987;26(2):199–207.
68. Perry J, Lumb M, Laundy M, Reynolds EH, CHANARIN I. Role of vitamin B12 in folate coenzyme synthesis. Brit J Haematol. 1976;32(2):243–8.
69. Devalia V, Hamilton MS, Molloy AM. Guidelines for the diagnosis and treatment of cobalamin and folate disorders. Br J Haematol. 2014;166(4):496–513.
70. Phekoo K, Williams Y, Schey SA, Andrews VE, Dudley JM, Hoffbrand AV. Folate assays: serum or red cell? J R Coll Physicians Lond. 1997;31(3):291–5.
71. Farrell CJ, Kirsch SH, Herrmann M. Red cell or serum folate: what to do in clinical practice? Clin Chem Lab Med. 2013;51(3):555–69.
72. Galloway M, Rushworth L. Red cell or serum folate? Results from the National Pathology Alliance benchmarking review. J Clin Pathol. 2003;56(12):924–6.
73. WHO. Guideline: optimal serum and red blood cell folate concentrations in women of reproductive age for prevention of neural tube defects. Geneva: World Health Organization; 2015.
74. Mason JB. Biomarkers of nutrient exposure and status in one-carbon (methyl) metabolism. J Nutr. 2003;133(Suppl 3):941s–7s.
75. Jacob RA, Gretz DM, Taylor PC, James SJ, Pogribny IP, Miller BJ, et al. Moderate folate depletion increases plasma homocysteine and decreases lymphocyte DNA methylation in postmenopausal women. J Nutr. 1998;128(7):1204–12.
76. Green R, Miller JW. Vitamin B12. In: Zempleni J, Rucker RB, McCormick DB, Suttie JW, editors. Handbook of vitamins. 4th ed. Taylor and Francis Group: Boca Raton, FL; 2007. p. 413–57.

Effects of Inflammation on Micronutrient Biomarkers Associated with Anemia

5

Melissa F. Young and Parminder S. Suchdev

Keywords

Anemia · α1-acid glycoprotein · Inflammation · BRINDA · C-reactive protein · Micronutrients

Introduction

Anemia remains an important global health problem that contributes to increased morbidity and mortality, particularly in women and children. To make progress on global goals to reduce anemia and to accurately assess nutritional status in the presence of inflammation, it is imperative to understand the role of inflammation and infection on anemia, as well as the micronutrient biomarkers associated with anemia. While iron deficiency may be a common cause of anemia in some populations, other nutritional and non-nutritional risk factors need to be considered, especially in settings with a high burden of infectious diseases. Currently, the World Health Organization is revising global guidelines for anemia assessment and has highlighted the understanding of the role of infectious and environmental factors in the etiology of anemia as an important direction for future research [1, 2]. Infection and inflammation are both known causes of non-nutritional anemia (e.g., anemia of chronic disease, hemolytic anemia from malaria, blood loss from hookworm infection) and important factors to consider for nutritional anemia (e.g., iron and other micronutrient deficiencies) due to the confounding effects of inflammation on micronutrient biomarkers [1, 3].

In this chapter we define inflammation as an innate body defense characterized by the acute-phase response (APR) [4]. The APR can be activated by a variety of stressors, including microbial invasion, tissue injury, chronic disease states, immunologic disorders, and psychological stress [5]. The APR stimulates liver hepatocytes to produce acute-phase proteins (APPs) which can be measured in blood and reflect an individual's inflammatory status. An inflammatory response can be characterized as acute (self-limiting and lasting days to weeks) or chronic (prolonged and characterized inflammatory responses that fail to regulate themselves) [3, 4]. Inflammation can also be characterized as clinical (individual has clear symptoms of the inciting cause of inflammation) or subclinical (no outward evidence of illness and detected only biochemically based on elevated APPs).

M. F. Young
Hubert Department of Global Health, Emory University, Atlanta, GA, USA
e-mail: melissa.young@emory.edu

P. S. Suchdev (✉)
Hubert Department of Global Health, Emory University, Atlanta, GA, USA

Department of Pediatrics and Emory Global Health Institute, Emory University, Atlanta, GA, USA
e-mail: psuchde@emory.edu

C. D. Karakochuk et al. (eds.), *Nutritional Anemia*, Nutrition and Health,
https://doi.org/10.1007/978-3-031-14521-6_5

This chapter is not intended to be a systematic review of the literature, but instead aims to summarize the effects of inflammation on micronutrient biomarkers associated with anemia in population-based surveys (Table 5.1), to describe approaches to adjust for these confounding effects (Table 5.2), and to identify key research gaps and priorities (Table 5.3). For the purposes of this chapter, we focus only on micronutrients that are known causes of anemia and also of public health relevance (namely, iron, vitamin A, zinc, folate, vitamin B-12, riboflavin).

Table 5.1 Summary of the effect of inflammation on micronutrient biomarkers associated with anemia

Nutrient	Commonly used biomarker	Magnitude and direction of inflammation effect
Iron	Serum or plasma ferritin	+++
	Serum of plasma sTfR	++
	Total body iron	+
Vitamin A[a]	Serum or plasma retinol	– –
	Serum or plasma RBP	– –
Zinc[a]	Serum or plasma zinc	–
Folate	Red blood cell folate	0
	Serum or plasma folate	0
Vitamin B-12	Serum or plasma vitamin B-12	0
Riboflavin	Erythrocyte glutathione reductase activation coefficient (EGRac)	Unknown

Adopted from Raiten, 20154 and BRINDA analyses [3, 10, 12–17]. *RBP* retinol binding protein; *sTfR* soluble transferrin receptor; – decrease, + increase, +++ major increase, 0 no change or inconsistent, or unknown

[a] Relationships between nutrient biomarker and inflammation are consistent for children but not for women

Table 5.2 Summary of approaches to adjust micronutrient biomarkers for inflammation

Approach	Description of the approach	Valid	Precise	Feasible	Inflammation severity	Notes/considerations
Ignore inflammation (nothing is done to account for APP)	This approach is common when APPs were not measured	✘	✔	✔	✘	Potential biased estimate of micronutrient status
Exclude individuals with inflammation	Remove individuals with elevated APPs	✘	✘	✔	✘	(1) Relies on concrete APP cutoffs, (2) may lose sample size (precision), and (3) may introduce bias since subset of population without inflammation may differ than subset with inflammation (validity)
Change nutrient biomarker cutoff	Use fixed higher or lower cutoff for micronutrient indicator for either (1) individuals with inflammation or (2) in settings of high inflammation	✘	✘	✔	✘	(1) Does not account for varying degrees of inflammation; (2) cutoff values may differ by target group or context of the survey, e.g., area with a high level of malaria; (3) may introduce bias

Table 5.2 (continued)

Approach	Description of the approach	Valid	Precise	Feasible	Inflammation severity	Notes/considerations
Four-level categorical inflammation correction factor approach (as known as Thurnham's internal correction factors)	Use CRP and AGP to create four categories (no inflammation, incubation, early convalescence and late convalescence) and apply an internal correction factor	✘	✔	✔	✘	(1) Requires both CRP and AGP, (2) does not account for potential confounders and effect modifiers, (3) produces similar estimates as exclusion approach
BRINDA regression correction approach	Use linear regression to adjust the concentrations of micronutrient biomarkers using CRP and AGP	✔	✔	✔	✔	(1) Requires data on both CRP and AGP and (2) requires statistical software and knowledge of statistics/equations to conduct the correction correctly

Adopted from Raiten, 2015 [4]. *AGP* α1-acid glycoprotein; *APP* acute-phase protein; *CF* correction factor; *CRP* C-reactive protein

Table 5.3 When to apply the BRINDA regression correction approach

Recommended	Not recommended
• Ferritin (WRA, PSC) – CRP and AGP • Retinol binding protein and retinol (PSC) – CRP and AGP • sTfR (WRA, PSC) – AGP only • Total body iron (WRA, PSC) – CRP and AGP (ferritin), AGP (sTfR) • Zinc (PSC) – CRP and AGP	• Retinol binding protein (WRA, SAC) • Zinc (WRA) • Folate (PSC, WRA) • RBC folate (PSC, WRA) • Vitamin B-12 (PSC, WRA)

PSC preschool-age children; *SAC* school-age children; *WRA* women of reproductive age (nonpregnant). Evidence is summarized from BRINDA publications [12–17, 23]. Ferritin, RBP, sTfR, zinc can be measured in serum or plasma

Effects of Inflammation on Micronutrient Biomarkers

Micronutrient biomarkers are objective measures used to estimate nutritional status or a response to a nutrition intervention. Biomarkers should ideally be precise (e.g., reproducible, limited variability), valid (e.g., accurate), cost-effective, feasible, and acceptable [6]. Confounders of biomarkers (e.g., age, sex, pre-analytic and analytic factors) need to be considered for appropriate interpretation. The APR has the potential to influence micronutrient biomarkers, as some nutrition biomarkers are also acute-phase proteins, and thus their concentrations may temporarily increase or decrease during the APR. This confounding effect is particularly problematic in settings with a high burden of inflammation, where the interpretation of micronutrient status may be inaccurate and lead to inappropriate diagnoses in individuals or improper allocation of resources to address micronutrient deficiencies [7]. The effects of inflammation on micronutrient biomarkers are complex, bidirectional, and indicator-specific [4, 8].

A review of the clinically relevant biomarkers of inflammation is outside the scope of this chapter, but they are reviewed elsewhere [4, 5]. Examples of two frequently measured APPs to assess inflammation are C-reactive protein (CRP) and α1-acid glycoprotein (AGP). CRP measures acute inflammation; it rises rapidly and remains elevated for approximately a week after symptom resolution, whereas AGP measures chronic inflammation; it rises more slowly but remains elevated for several weeks [5, 9]. In order to fully capture the APR and understand the effect of inflammation on micronutrient biomarkers across the APR continuum, measuring both CRP and AGP is recommended [10].

The *Eunice Kennedy Shriver* National Institute of Child Health and Human Development (NICHD) Biomarkers of Nutrition for Development (BOND), Inflammation and Nutrition Science for Programs and Interpretation of Research Evidence (INSPIRE), and Biomarkers Reflecting Inflammation and Nutritional Determinants of Anemia (BRINDA) projects have all explored the effects of inflammation on micronutrient biomarkers, as well approaches to account for these confounding effects [4, 8, 11].

The BOND program was formed in 2009 as a collaboration between NICHD and Bill & Melinda Gates Foundation that aimed to provide guidance on the selection and interpretation of nutrition biomarkers to be incorporated into the community's research, clinical, program, and policy-making activities [8]. The project involved expert working groups to review each of these domains, as well as the evidence base for case-study micronutrients. This project was valuable in building consensus around terminology, summarizing current knowledge, and identifying critical areas of further research. One of the key cross-cutting issues identified was the challenge of inflammation and nutrient assessment, which led to the initiation of the INSPIRE project in 2012 [4]. The goal of the INSPIRE project was to review evidence on the relationships between nutrition, immune function, and inflammatory response. The INSPIRE project provided a detailed review of evidence on what is known on the impact of acute or chronic inflammation on the selection, use, and interpretation of nutrition biomarkers.

Building on the prior work from BOND and INSPIRE, the BRINDA project was formed in 2012 including investigators from universities, government and non-governmental organizations, the private sector, as well as country representatives [11]. The goal of BRINDA is to refine approaches to estimate the prevalence of nutritional status and thus improve the targeting, design, and effectiveness of nutrition research and programs. Findings from BRINDA have informed global guidelines on the interpretation of micronutrient biomarkers in settings of inflammation and risk factors for anemia. To date, BRINDA has compiled secondary data from 43 population-based nutrition surveys from all WHO geographic regions, including data on approximately 40,000 preschool children, 56,000 women of reproductive age, 21,000 adolescents, 29,000 school-age children, and 14,000 pregnant women. The BRINDA project examines relationships between inflammation biomarkers (CRP and AGP) and micronutrient biomarkers and provides global guidance on the adjustment of micronutrient biomarkers for inflammation, as well as evaluates factors associated with anemia and their relative contribution to the prevalence of anemia.

Collectively the work of BOND, INSPIRE, and BRINDA has advanced our understanding of the complex bidirectional relationship between micronutrient biomarkers and inflammation. For the purposes of this chapter, we focus on summarizing evidence specifically on the effect of inflammation on biomarkers for six micronutrients associated with anemia, including iron, vitamin A, zinc, folate, vitamin B-12, and riboflavin (Table 5.1).

Iron

Iron deficiency is one of the most common micronutrient disorders across the globe. There are many biomarkers of iron status that have been previously reviewed [18]. Two commonly used biomarkers to assess iron status are ferritin [19] and soluble transferrin receptor (sTfR) [20]. Ferritin is an iron storage protein and sensitive biomarker of body iron stores [19]. However, ferritin is also an APP and is positively associated with inflammation [4, 10, 16]. Consistent moderate correlations between ferritin and AGP (median, 0.30; range, 0.05–0.44) and CRP (median, 0.25; range, 0.05–0.44) have been reported across multiple population-based surveys in children as part of the BRINDA project [10]. Likewise among women, ferritin is consistently associated with inflammation biomarkers. STfR is a widely used biomarker of tissue iron availability [20]. While traditionally, sTfR has been believed to be largely unaffected by infection or inflammation, this is not always the case. In the BRINDA project, relationships between sTfR and inflammation were dependent on the inflammation biomarker. Among children, there was a weak to moderate positive correlation between sTfR and AGP (median, 0.18), but a weak inconsistent relation between sTfR and CRP (median, 0.11), with similar findings observed in women [10]. Prior work has likewise proposed a biological rationale for adjusting sTfR for AGP but not CRP [10, 15, 21]. While sTfR is not an acute-phase protein, inflammation may lead to an increase in circulating sTfR through alternative mechanisms independent of the degree of erythropoiesis, the hypoxic response, or iron status.

Vitamin A

Serum retinol and retinol binding protein (RBP) are two indicators recommended by WHO for assessing the vitamin A status of populations [22]. RBP is a negative APP, and since RBP is the carrier protein for retinol, both serum retinol and RBP decrease in response to inflammation [4]. Across surveys included in the BRINDA project, there were moderate negative associations between retinol or RBP with both CRP (median, −0.26) and AGP (median, −0.20) among children. However, among women, the relationship between vitamin A biomarkers and inflammation biomarkers was inconsistent across surveys. The rationale for these differences by population group is not well understood but may be due to a lower prevalence of vitamin A deficiency and inflammation in women, immune system differences, obesity, or other unidentified effect modifiers [23]. These associations between nutrient biomarkers and inflammation biomarkers in cross-sectional surveys have also been confirmed by a recent longitudinal norovirus challenge study of 52 healthy adults in a US hospital setting where ferritin concentrations increased, and retinol and RBP concentrations decreased, in response to temporary elevations in AGP and CRP [24].

Zinc

The assessment of zinc status is complicated by the lack of a gold standard biomarker. The Zinc Expert Panel of Biomarkers of Nutrition for Development currently recommends the use of plasma or serum zinc concentrations, as well as dietary zinc intake assessment and child height-for-age [25]. Inflammation and the APR can result in redistribution of zinc from the plasma/serum to the liver, thus decreasing concentrations of this biomarker in plasma/serum [4, 26]. Among preschool children, inconsistent associations have been reported between plasma/serum zinc and inflammation biomarkers, with 6 out of 12 BRINDA datasets showing a negative correlation and the remaining were nonsignificant with the exception of 1 survey showing a significant positive assoicaiton [13]. Among women, relationships between plasma/serum zinc and AGP and CRP were weak and inconsistent.

Folate and Vitamin B-12

Vitamin B-12 and folate deficiencies in women and children remain a public health problem worldwide [27]. However, there is a lack of standardization on laboratory methods for biomarker assessment, with large differences across methodologies [12, 27–30]. Furthermore, the role of inflammation on serum/plasma vitamin B-12, serum/plasma folate, and red blood cell folate remains unclear and contradictory across the literature [4, 12]. In a recent BRINDA analysis among both women and preschool-age children, correlations between inflammation and vitamin B-12 or folate biomarkers were weak with no clear patterns of association [12].

Riboflavin

There is increasing recognition on the important role of riboflavin (vitamin B-2) for human health [31–33]. Riboflavin deficiency interferes with iron metabolism and may also cause anemia by blocking the development or maturation of erythrocyte precursors in the bone marrow [31, 33]. In addition, riboflavin deficiency also interferes with the metabolism of other B vitamins [31–33]. However, riboflavin (assessed by erythrocyte glutathione reductase activation coefficient, EGRac) is not commonly measured in population-based surveys and has not been included in prior BRINDA analyses. There remain gaps in our understanding of how riboflavin may be affected by inflammation.

Implications for Clinical Medicine and Public Health

The use of micronutrient biomarkers in individuals with inflammation can lead to incorrect diagnoses of individuals and overestimation or underestimation of the prevalence of deficiency in a population [7, 34, 35]. Figure 5.1 illustrates the theoretical impact of acute inflammation on ferritin concentrations and its impact on the classification of iron deficiency in three scenarios.

In scenario **A**, the individual is iron replete (defined here as ferritin >12 μg/L) and has a rise in serum ferritin following an acute inflammatory event, but the classification of the individual as iron replete does not change (as ferritin concentration remains above the threshold for deficiency

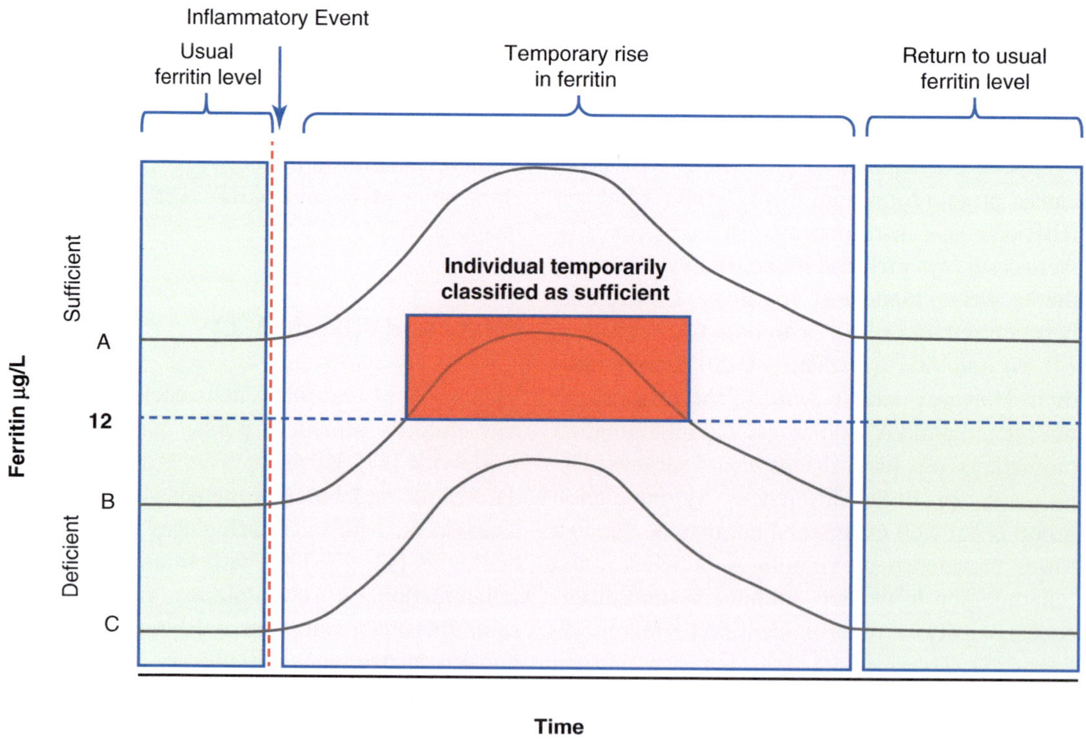

Fig. 5.1 Theoretical scenarios of serum ferritin concentrations in response to acute inflammation

before, during, and after the inflammatory event). In scenario **C**, the individual is iron deficient, and despite the rise in ferritin following an inflammatory event, the individual is still classified as iron deficient after the inflammatory event. On the other hand, in scenario **B**, we illustrate the potential misclassification of an individual. In this case, the individual is iron deficient both before and after the inflammatory event, but if iron status is assessed during the temporary rise in ferritin, we would misclassify the individual as iron replete. At the individual level, this is problematic and could lead to inappropriate clinical care. At a population level, the role of inflammation on ferritin concentrations can lead to an underestimated burden of iron deficiency for a population. This is a widespread concern as subclinical inflammation is common across the globe, affecting ~53% of preschool children and ~20% of women, based on data from household surveys of otherwise apparently healthy individuals [10]. Across BRINDA surveys in preschool children, it is reported that ignoring inflammation *underestimates* the prevalence of iron deficiency by a median 11% points (range 1–35%) and *overestimates* the prevalence of vitamin A deficiency by a median 14% points (range 3–22%) and the prevalence of zinc deficiency by a median 11% points (range 4–18%) [10, 13]. This has important implications for the public health classification of the total burden of micronutrient deficiency. The accurate measurement of the magnitude and distribution of micronutrient deficiencies is critical in planning, implementing, and evaluating interventions to improve both individual- and population-level micronutrient status, as well as for comparisons between individuals and populations.

Approaches to Adjust for the Effects of Inflammation on Micronutrient Biomarkers

There are several potential approaches for adjusting for the effects of inflammation on micronutrient biomakers [4]. Table 5.2 summarizes five statistical approaches to account for inflammation that are commonly used in the literature. The approaches vary by precision (influenced by sample size, accuracy of laboratory test), validity (influenced by selection and information bias), and feasibility (influenced by ease of use and cost). In addition to the importance of *how* to adjust micronutrient biomarkers for inflammation, another equally critical question that we review in this section is *when* to adjust. While adjustment for inflammation may be appropriate for some micronutrient biomarkers, this is not the case in all. It is important to understand the underlying biology and relationship between each micronutrient biomarker with inflammation before applying inflammation adjustment approaches.

Despite the widespread agreement on the role of inflammation on micronutrient biomarkers, many surveys simply ignore inflammation. In some cases, this is due to lack of availability of inflammation biomarker data. This is problematic given the noted prevalence of elevated CRP and AGP, even in low infection burden settings, and the established associations with some micronutrient biomarkers (e.g., serum ferritin) and thus the potential of biased estimates of nutrient deficiencies. Another approach is exclusion, where individuals with elevated CRP or AGP are excluded from the estimation of population-level deficiency prevalence rates [19, 36]. Potential concerns with this approach include that exclusion relies on concrete APP cutoffs to define inflammation, results in loss of sample size, and may introduce bias as individuals with inflammation may also be at elevated risk for nutrient deficiency but excluded from prevalence estimates. A third approach is to change the micronutrient biomarker cutoff. This approach could be used at the individual level to apply a revised cutoff among individuals with inflammation (requires measuring APP) or at a population level where the revised cutoff is applied to all individuals in suspected settings of high inflammation (does not require the measurement of APPs). For example, in the 2020 *WHO Guideline on Use of Ferritin Concentrations to Assess Iron Status in Individuals and Populations*, one recommendation is to use a higher ferritin cutoff among populations with inflammation (<30 μg/L among infants and children under 5 years and <70 μg/L among children over 5 years, adolescents, and adults) [19, 37]. While this offers a relatively easy solution, a limitation of this approach is that it does not account for varying degrees of inflammation or potential concerns of validity. Prior analyses suggest this approach may overcorrect in some settings [16]. A fourth approach is to stratify individuals into four groups based on stage of inflammation (individuals are defined by no inflammation CRP <5 mg/L and AGP <1 g/L; the incubation period CRP >5 mg/L; early convalescence CRP >5 mg/L and AGP >1 g/L; and late convalescence AGP >1 g/L) and apply an internally computed correction factor [38]. Potential limitations of this approach are that it requires collection of both CRP and AGP biomarkers, relies on clinical cutoffs of CRP and AGP (thus does not account for impact of inflammation at levels below these cutoffs), cannot control for potential confounders and effect modifiers, and produces similar estimates as the exclusion approach.

Finally, an alternative approach to adjust micronutrient biomarkers for inflammation is the BRINDA regression correction modeling approach [16, 19]. In brief, the BRINDA regression correction is a mathematical adjustment that can be used to adjust micronutrient biomarkers in settings with inflammation [10, 11]. A linear regression is used to adjust the concentrations of micronutrient biomarkers to account for the effects of inflammation (CRP and AGP) along the continuum of inflammation. This is a key advantage of the BRINDA approach as some micronutrient biomarkers (e.g., ferritin, sTfR, retinol) continue to be impacted by inflammation at levels below traditional cutoffs used to define inflammation and in settings with a low infectious disease burden [3, 10]. With this approach, linear regression analysis is conducted with the nutrient biomarker as the dependent variable and CRP, AGP, or both as the independent variables, and the slope of CRP, AGP, or both is used to adjust for the effect of inflammation. A CRP and AGP reference value (lowest decile) is applied, so that nutrient biomarker is not overadjusted at the lower values for CRP and AGP. For example, the basic adjustment equation for ferritin would be the following: Adjusted ferritin = unadjusted ferritin – $\beta 1(CRP_{obs} - CRP_{ref}) - \beta 2(AGP_{obs} - AGP_{ref})$. Further information on this approach can be found on the BRINDA website (http://www.brinda-nutrition.org/) which includes free downloadable macros and tutorials. Applying the BRINDA regression inflammation correction allows for a more accurate representation of what micronutrient concentrations would be if the inflammation resolved [3, 10].

When deciding if there is a rationale to adjust a nutrition biomarker for inflammation and apply the BRINDA regression approach, there are two important basic questions to ask as illustrated in Fig. 5.2. First, is there a clear biological rationale for the relationship between the micronutrient biomarker and inflammation? For example, as discussed earlier, serum ferritin is an APP, and there are clear, well-established mechanisms that describe why ferritin becomes elevated during inflammation [7]. For other micronutrient biomarkers, if there is no known biological mechanism for the relationship, then the BRINDA approach may not be justified. For other micronutrient biomarkers, if there is a clear biological mechanism or if the relationships between the nutrition biomarker and inflammation are unclear or unknown, the next step is to look at the data and ask the question: Is the nutrient biomarker correlated with AGP and CRP? The rationale for correction for inflammation is strengthened if there are both statistically and biologically meaningful associations between the biomarker and inflammation across multiple surveys. An important consideration is this may vary by population group, as has been reported for serum or plasma RBP and serum or plasma zinc [13, 23]. Table 5.3 provides an overview of recommendations from the BRINDA project on when adjustment of micronutrient biomarkers for inflammation may be recommended based on current evidence.

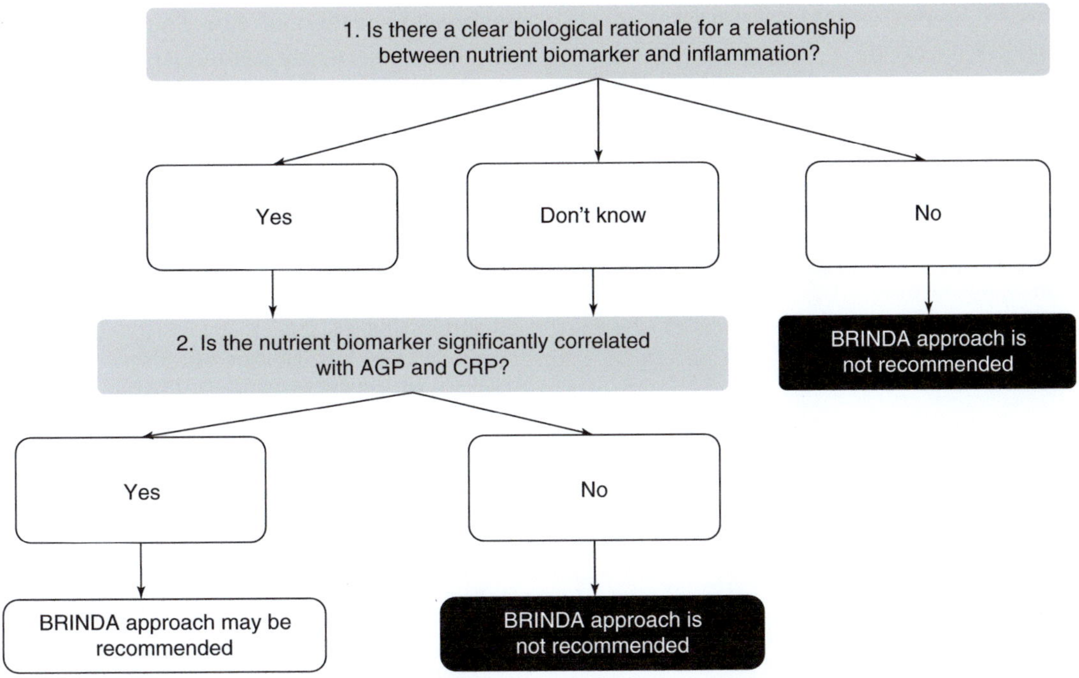

Fig. 5.2 When to apply the BRINDA regression correction approach

Research Gaps and Opportunities

Over the past decade, there have been impressive advancements in our understanding of the effects of inflammation on micronutrient biomarkers associated with anemia [4, 8, 10, 11]. In the context of nutritional anemia, there remain important research gaps in this field including understanding biological mechanisms, standardization of laboratory methods, and assessment of the validity of inflammation correction (Table 5.4).

First, there remain questions on the underlying biological mechanisms that underpin the relationships between inflammation and micronutrient biomarkers. There are many different drivers of inflammation, including malaria, COVID-19, obesity, infection, response to surgery, or trauma, among other factors, and it is unclear if the etiology of inflammation may influence the relationship between APPs and micronutrient biomarkers. Furthermore, we lack a clear understanding of why relationships between inflammation and micronutrient biomarkers vary among different population groups and study settings. For example, adjustment for inflammation is recommended for preschool-age children for RBP and serum or plasma zinc but not for women [13, 23]. This could be due to a number of different factors including etiology of inflammation, burden of inflammation or micronutrient deficiency, or other unknown mechanisms.

Lack of standardization of laboratory methods across contexts is a critical limitation of the current research on inflammation and micronutrient biomarkers. Agreement among the scientific community is needed on recommended pre- and post-analytic approaches and on the use of certified reference materials to ensure comparability of biomarker data across laboratories and over time. This was especially the case for zinc, folate, and vitamin B-12 where the lack of standardization of laboratory methods may have influenced the heterogeneity of results across contexts [12, 13]. In addition, recent research suggests different approaches for handling values below the limit of detection (LOD) or limit of quantification (LOQ) may influence the interpretation of biomarkers [39]. As a first step for making progress in this area, O'Callaghan and Roth provide recommendations for standardization of labora-

Table 5.4 Research gaps and opportunities

Biological mechanisms
• How does the etiology of inflammation (e.g., malaria, COVID-19, obesity, infection, injury) influence the relationship between acute-phase proteins and micronutrient biomarkers?
• What are the underling mechanisms driving differences in relationships between inflammation and micronutrient biomarkers across different population groups and settings?
Laboratory methods
• Can standardization of laboratory methods reduce the heterogeneity across contexts on the relationship between inflammation and micronutrient biomarkers?
• How do different approaches for handling values below the limit of detection influence interpretation of biomarkers?
• What are valid and affordable point-of-care methods to measure anemia, inflammation, and micronutrients concurrently?
Validity of inflammation correction on the assessment of nutritional anemia
• Are methods for adjusting for the effects of inflammation on micronutrient biomarkers appropriate for other population groups (e.g., pregnant women, infants, men, etc.)?
• Are there other APP biomarkers that better capture inflammation response?
• What is the effect of inflammation on other micronutrient biomarkers (EGRAC, vitamin D, choline, vitamin E, etc.)?
• How do findings from the BRINDA project conducted in large population-based surveys translate to the clinical setting?

tory practices and reporting of biomarker data [40]. In addition, further research is needed to advance our knowledge on the development and use of point-of-care methods to measure anemia, inflammation, and micronutrients.

There remain many new areas of research yet to be fully examined to better understand the validity of inflammation correction on the assessment of nutritional anemia. Much of the research to date has focused on PSC and WRA, and questions remain on the appropriateness of extending this research to other population groups, such as pregnant women, infants, or men. In addition, further research is needed to examine the potential use of other biomarkers of inflammation (such as IL-6) and to expand research to additional micronutrients (riboflavin, vitamin D, choline, vitamin E, etc.). Furthermore, more research is needed to understand how findings from the BRINDA project conducted in large population-based surveys translate to the clinical setting.

References

1. Chaparro CM, Suchdev PS. Anemia epidemiology, pathophysiology, and etiology in low- and middle-income countries. Ann N Y Acad Sci. 2019;1450(1):15–31.
2. Garcia-Casal MN, Pasricha SR, Sharma AJ, Pena-Rosas JP. Use and interpretation of hemoglobin concentrations for assessing anemia status in individuals and populations: results from a WHO technical meeting. Ann N Y Acad Sci. 2019;1450(1):5–14.
3. Suchdev PS, Williams AM, Mei Z, et al. Assessment of iron status in settings of inflammation: challenges and potential approaches. Am J Clin Nutr. 2017;106(Suppl 6):1626S–33S.
4. Raiten DJ, Sakr Ashour FA, Ross AC, et al. Inflammation and Nutritional Science for Programs/Policies and Interpretation of Research Evidence (INSPIRE). J Nutr. 2015;145(5):1039S–108S.
5. Suchdev PS, Boivin MJ, Forsyth BW, Georgieff MK, Guerrant RL, Nelson CA 3rd. Assessment of neurodevelopment, nutrition, and inflammation from fetal life to adolescence in low-resource settings. Pediatrics. 2017;139(Suppl 1):S23–37.
6. Mayeux R. Biomarkers: potential uses and limitations. NeuroRx. 2004;1(2):182–8.
7. Tomkins A. Assessing micronutrient status in the presence of inflammation. J Nutr. 2003;133(5 Suppl 2):1649S–55S.
8. Raiten DJ, Namaste S, Brabin B, et al. Executive summary—biomarkers of nutrition for development: building a consensus. Am J Clin Nutr. 2011;94(2):633S–50S.
9. Thurnham D, McCabe G. Influence of infection and infl ammation on biomarkers of nutritional status with an emphasis on vitamin A and iron. In: World Health Organization. Report: Priorities in the assessment of vitamin A and iron status in populations, Panama City, Panama, 15–September 17, 2010. Geneva, Switzerland: WHO Press; 2012.
10. Namaste SML, Ou J, Williams AM, Young MF, Yu EX, Suchdev PS. Adjusting iron and vitamin A status in settings of inflammation: a sensitivity analysis of the Biomarkers Reflecting Inflammation and Nutritional Determinants of Anemia (BRINDA) approach. Am J Clin Nutr. 2019;112(Suppl 1):458S–67S.
11. Suchdev PS, Namaste SM, Aaron GJ, et al. Overview of the Biomarkers Reflecting Inflammation and Nutritional Determinants of Anemia (BRINDA) Project. Adv Nutr. 2016;7(2):349–56.
12. Young MF, Guo J, Williams A, et al. Interpretation of vitamin B-12 and folate concentrations in population-based surveys does not require adjustment for inflam-

mation: Biomarkers Reflecting Inflammation and Nutritional Determinants of Anemia (BRINDA) project. Am J Clin Nutr. 2020;111(4):919–26.
13. McDonald CM, Suchdev PS, Krebs NF, et al. Adjusting plasma or serum zinc concentrations for inflammation: Biomarkers Reflecting Inflammation and Nutritional Determinants of Anemia (BRINDA) project. Am J Clin Nutr. 2020;111(4):927–37.
14. Larson LM, Guo J, Williams AM, et al. Approaches to assess vitamin A status in settings of inflammation: Biomarkers Reflecting Inflammation and Nutritional Determinants of Anemia (BRINDA) Project. Nutrients. 2018; 10(8).
15. Rohner F, Namaste SM, Larson LM, et al. Adjusting soluble transferrin receptor concentrations for inflammation: Biomarkers Reflecting Inflammation and Nutritional Determinants of Anemia (BRINDA) project. Am J Clin Nutr. 2017;106(Suppl 1):372S–82S.
16. Namaste SM, Rohner F, Huang J, et al. Adjusting ferritin concentrations for inflammation: Biomarkers Reflecting Inflammation and Nutritional Determinants of Anemia (BRINDA) project. Am J Clin Nutr. 2017;106(Suppl 1):359S–71S.
17. Mei Z, Namaste SM, Serdula M, et al. Adjusting total body iron for inflammation: Biomarkers Reflecting Inflammation and Nutritional Determinants of Anemia (BRINDA) project. Am J Clin Nutr. 2017;106(Suppl 1):383S–9S.
18. Lynch S, Pfeiffer CM, Georgieff MK, et al. Biomarkers of Nutrition for Development (BOND)-Iron Review. J Nutr. 2018;148(suppl_1):1001S–67S.
19. WHO guideline on use of ferritin concentrations to assess iron status in individuals and populations. Geneva: World Health Organization; 2020. Licence: CC BY-NC-SA 3.0 IGO.
20. Serum transferrin receptor levels for the assessment of iron status and iron deficiency in populations. Vitamin and Mineral Nutrition Information System. Geneva: World Health Organization; 2014 (WHO/NMH/NHD/MNM/14.6). http://apps.who.int/iris/bitstream/10665/133707/1/WHO_NMH_NHD_EPG_14.6_eng.pdf?ua=1. Accessed 17 Feb 2021.
21. Kasvosve I, Gomo ZA, Nathoo KJ, et al. Association of serum transferrin receptor concentration with markers of inflammation in Zimbabwean children. Clin Chim Acta. 2006;371(1-2):130–6.
22. WHO. Serum retinol concentrations for determining the prevalence of vitamin A deficiency in populations. Vitamin and Mineral Nutrition Information System. Geneva, World Health Organization; 2011 (WHO/NMH/NHD/MNM/11.3). http://www.who.int/vmnis/indicators/retinol.pdf. Accessed 17 Feb 2021.
23. Larson LM, Namaste SM, Williams AM, et al. Adjusting retinol-binding protein concentrations for inflammation: Biomarkers Reflecting Inflammation and Nutritional Determinants of Anemia (BRINDA) project. Am J Clin Nutr. 2017;106(Suppl 1):390S–401S.
24. Williams AM, Ladva CN, Leon JS, et al. Changes in micronutrient and inflammation serum biomarker concentrations after a norovirus human challenge. Am J Clin Nutr. 2019;110(6):1456–64.
25. King JC, Brown KH, Gibson RS, et al. Biomarkers of Nutrition for Development (BOND)-Zinc Review. J Nutr. 2015;146(4):858S–85S.
26. Cousins RJ, Leinart AS. Tissue-specific regulation of zinc metabolism and metallothionein genes by interleukin 1. FASEB J. 1988;2(13):2884–90.
27. de Benoist B. Conclusions of a WHO Technical Consultation on folate and vitamin B12 deficiencies. Food Nutr Bull. 2008;29(Suppl 2):S238–44.
28. Allen LH, Miller JW, de Groot L, et al. Biomarkers of Nutrition for Development (BOND): Vitamin B-12 Review. J Nutr. 2018;148(suppl_4):1995S–2027S.
29. Pfeiffer CM, Sternberg MR, Hamner HC, et al. Applying inappropriate cutoffs leads to misinterpretation of folate status in the US population. Am J Clin Nutr. 2016;104(6):1607–15.
30. Pfeiffer CM, Lacher DA, Schleicher RL, Johnson CL, Yetley EA. Challenges and Lessons Learned in Generating and Interpreting NHANES Nutritional Biomarker Data. Adv Nutr. 2017;8(2):290–307.
31. Powers HJ. Riboflavin (vitamin B-2) and health. Am J Clin Nutr. 2003;77(6):1352–60.
32. Saedisomeolia A, Ashoori M. Riboflavin in human health: a review of current evidences. Adv Food Nutr Res. 2018;83:57–81.
33. Thakur K, Tomar SK, Singh AK, Mandal S, Arora S. Riboflavin and health: a review of recent human research. Crit Rev Food Sci Nutr. 2017;57(17):3650–60.
34. Raiten DJ, Ashour FAS, Ross AC, et al. Inflammation and Nutritional Science for Programs/Policies and Interpretation of Research Evidence (INSPIRE). J Nutr. 2015;145(5):1039S–108S.
35. Haynes BM, Pfeiffer CM, Sternberg MR, Schleicher RL. Selected physiologic variables are weakly to moderately associated with 29 biomarkers of diet and nutrition, NHANES 2003-2006. J Nutr. 2013;143(6):1001S–10S.
36. WHO. Serum ferritin concentrations for the assessment of iron status and iron deficiency in populations. Vitamin and Mineral Nutrition Information System. Geneva: World Health Organization; 2011.
37. WHO/CDC. Assessing the iron status of populations: report of a joint World Health Organization/Centers for Disease Control and Prevention technical consultation on the assessment of iron status at the population level. Geneva, Switzerland; 2004.
38. Thurnham DI, McCabe LD, Haldar S, Wieringa FT, Northrop-Clewes CA, McCabe GP. Adjusting plasma ferritin concentrations to remove the effects of subclinical inflammation in the assessment of iron deficiency: a meta-analysis. Am J Clin Nutr. 2010;92(3):546–55.
39. Gosdin L, Sharma AJ, Suchdev PS, Jefferds ME, Young MF, Addo OY. Limits of Detection in Acute-Phase Protein Biomarkers Affect Inflammation Correction of Serum Ferritin for Quantifying Iron Status among School- Age and Preschool-Age Children and Reproductive-Age Women. J Nutr. 2022;152(5):1370–7. J Nutr. 2022;152(5):1370–7. https://doi.org/10.1093/jn/nxac035.
40. O'Callaghan KM, Roth DE. Standardization of laboratory practices and reporting of biomarker data in clinical nutrition research. Am J Clin Nutr. 2019;112(Suppl 1):453S–7S.

Part II

Special Populations

Nutritional Anemia in Infants and Children

6

Magnus Domellöf and Staffan K. Berglund

Keywords

Nutritional anemia · Infant · Child
Adolescent · Iron deficiency · Biomarkers
Neurodevelopment · Infections · Diet
Supplements

Nutritional Anemia in Children

Children are at high risk of nutritional anemia. The global anemia prevalence in children <5 years of age in 2016 was 42%, with the prevalence ranging from 60% in sub-Saharan Africa and 55% in South Asia to 16% in the European Union and 9% in North America [1]. The proportion of anemias caused by nutritional deficiencies varies substantially between populations [2].

Iron deficiency anemia (IDA) is by far the most common nutritional anemia in infants and children, commonly assumed to cause 50% of all global cases of anemia. Even though this number recently has been debated, the true proportion probably lies between 25 and 50% [3, 4]. Other nutritional deficiencies that have been associated with anemia in children include vitamin B_{12}, folate, and vitamin A deficiency. These often coexist with iron deficiency (ID), making causal attribution more difficult. Globally, non-nutritional causes of anemia in children are also common, including infectious diseases (e.g., malaria, hookworm, diarrhea, and respiratory tract infections) and genetic causes (e.g., thalassemia and sickle cell disease). Due to this diversity in etiology of anemia, it is prudent to determine the regional or national prevalence of anemia, ID, and other specific nutrient deficiencies before any measures are taken to prevent nutritional anemia in pediatric populations.

Anemia Caused by B_{12} Deficiency

Vitamin B_{12}, also known as cobalamin, is an essential vitamin that acts as a coenzyme in DNA synthesis in all cells. Lack of vitamin B_{12} causes macrocytic anemia and impaired neuronal myelination that leads to neurological symptoms. In children, vitamin B_{12} deficiency is relatively less common, due to a very low prevalence of atrophic gastritis, the most common cause of vitamin B_{12} deficiency anemia in adults.

The original version of this book was revised. An erratum to this book can be found at https://doi.org/10.1007/978-3-031-14521-6_28

M. Domellöf (✉)
Department of Clinical Sciences, Pediatrics, Umeå University, Umeå, Sweden
e-mail: magnus.domellof@umu.se

S. K. Berglund
Department of Clinical Sciences, Pediatrics, Umeå University, Umeå, Sweden

Wallenberg Centre for Molecular Medicine (WCMM), Umeå University, Umeå, Sweden

C. D. Karakochuk et al. (eds.), *Nutritional Anemia*, Nutrition and Health,
https://doi.org/10.1007/978-3-031-14521-6_6

Vegetarian mothers have a high risk of vitamin B_{12} deficiency during pregnancy, and this can lead to vitamin B_{12} deficiency in the fetus and infant. Severe macrocytic anemia due to vitamin B_{12} deficiency, as well as other micronutrient deficiencies, has been described in a few case reports of infants of vegan mothers [5]. There are also case reports of severe vitamin B_{12} deficiency in infants fed a vegan diet [6]. Mild or moderate anemia associated with vitamin B_{12} deficiency is not uncommon in populations where a majority are vegetarian, e.g., India. In a recent survey in India, anemia was attributed to vitamin B_{12} deficiency in 9–12% of cases in children of different ages [7]. However, a recent randomized controlled trial (RCT) showed no effect of supplementation of vitamin B_{12} and/or folic acid on hemoglobin concentrations among young children in India [8], and general vitamin B_{12} supplementation of populations is not recommended, except as part of multiple micronutrient supplements.

Other Nutritional Anemias

Anemia due to folate deficiency is most often observed together with ID [9], and many supplementation programs use a combination of iron and folate. Isolated folate deficiency as a cause of clinically significant anemia in children is very rare. Vitamin A deficiency is prevalent mainly among children in low-income countries, and vitamin A supplementation of children between 6 months and 5 years of age in populations at risk has been shown to significantly reduce the risk of all-cause mortality, diarrhea-specific mortality, and night blindness [10]. Vitamin A deficiency is also associated with anemia, even though the contribution of vitamin A deficiency to the global prevalence of childhood anemia is likely to be very small [4].

Deficiencies of vitamins B6, C, D, and E, riboflavin, and copper have also been associated with anemia, but these do not play any significant role in the global burden of nutritional anemia [11].

ID in Children of Different Ages

Within the pediatric population, infants and young children <5 years, especially around the age of 12–36 months, and menstruating adolescent girls are at the highest risk of ID. Risk factors for IDA in children are shown in Table 6.1.

The Newborn and the First 6 Months of Life

A healthy, term newborn infant has a high concentration of iron-rich hemoglobin (on average 170 g/L) and some additional iron stored as ferritin (Fig. 6.1). Delayed cord clamping increases the total blood volume of the newborn by about a third, substantially contributing to the newborn's iron endowment [12].

After birth, the dramatically increased systemic oxygen tension in the tissues of the newborn leads to inactivation of the hypoxia inducible factor (HIF-1α) [13], decreased production of erythropoietin (EPO) [14], and an almost com-

Table 6.1 Risk factors for IDA in children

Perinatal factors
• Severe maternal IDA
• Low birth weight (<2500 g)
• Early cord clamping
• Male sex (risk factor for IDA during early childhood)
Environmental factors
• Low socioeconomic status
• High local prevalence of IDA
• High local prevalence of infection/inflammation
• Hookworm or other intestinal parasites
• Lead exposure
Dietary factors
• Prolonged exclusive breastfeeding (>6 months)
• High intake of cow's milk
• Non-iron-fortified infant formula
• Lack of iron-rich diet (meat, iron fortified products) at 6–36 months of age
• Low iron diet after 3 years of age
• General malnutrition
Blood loss
• Occult gastrointestinal blood loss
• Large menstrual blood losses (adolescent girls)

plete suppression of erythropoiesis during the first 2 months of life. During this time, the hemoglobin concentration falls to on average about 115 g/L, and the iron is recirculated, thereby increasing ferritin-bound iron. The resulting iron stores cover the infant's requirements until the birth weight has doubled, which occurs at about 5–6 months of age, making the infant virtually independent on dietary iron during this period. IDA is thus uncommon in this age interval, with the exception of risk groups such as low birth weight or preterm infants, who will deplete their iron stores earlier due to lower iron stores at birth and a faster growth rate (Fig. 6.2).

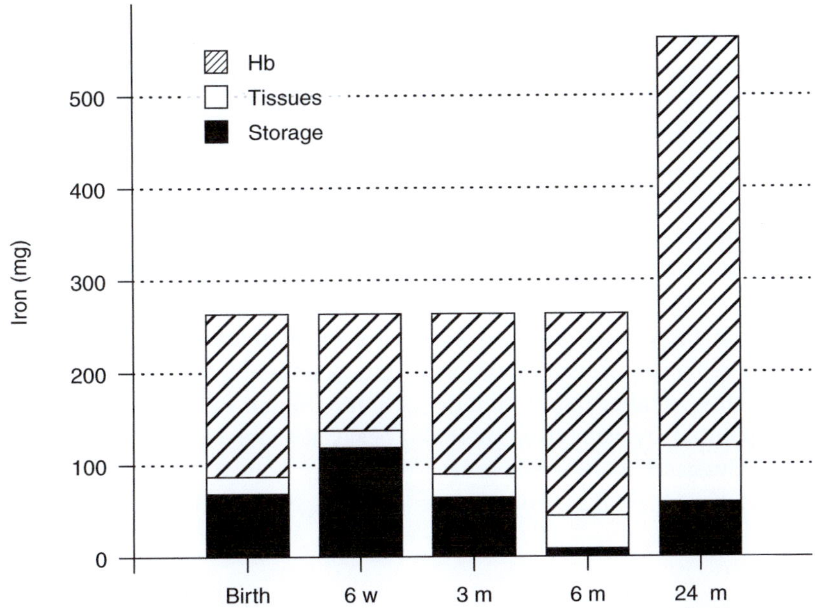

Fig. 6.1 Body iron compartments and total body iron in an normal infant with a birth weight of 3,500 g

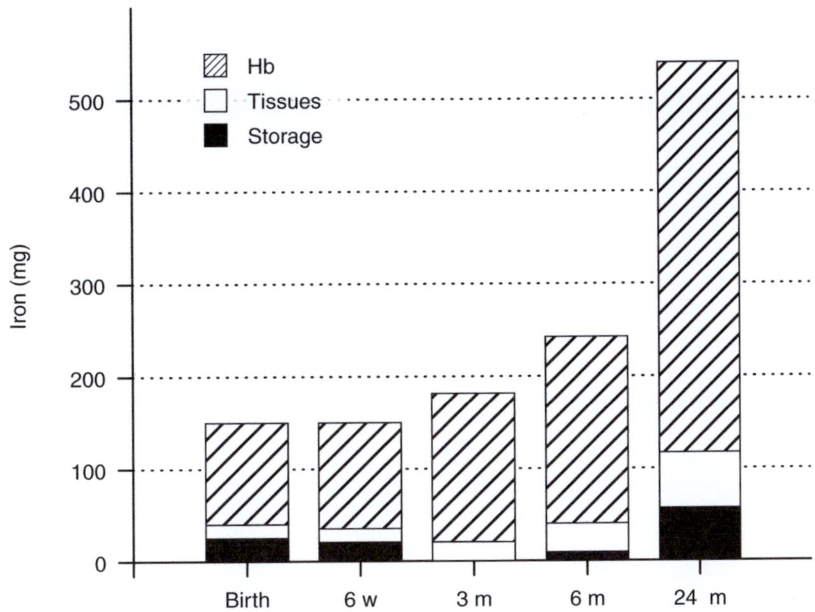

Fig. 6.2 Body iron compartments and total body iron in an infant with a low birth weight of 2,000 g

Breast milk has a very low iron concentration (0.3 mg/L), which is compatible with the newborn's low dietary iron needs and which possibly also has a preventive effect against infections due to a low iron availability for potential gastrointestinal pathogens.

Like in adults, intestinal iron absorption in newborns and infants is believed to occur mainly via the divalent metal transporter 1 (DMT1). A lactoferrin receptor is also expressed on the luminal side of the enterocyte in young infants, but it is not known whether milk lactoferrin significantly contributes to iron absorption. The membrane-bound protein ferroportin is responsible for iron transport from the enterocyte to the plasma compartment, but it is not clear whether this process is regulated in the same way as in adults. Studies have suggested that there may be a limited capacity for downregulation of iron absorption in iron-replete infants younger than 6 months, which is also supported by data from animal studies [15]. This suggests that excessive iron supplements or high iron intakes from infant formula should be avoided in young infants who are not iron deficient, in order to avoid iron overload.

The Older Infant and Toddler

At 6 months of age, iron stores from birth are depleted and the infant becomes dependent on dietary iron. The iron metabolism of the 6-month-old infant is shown in Fig. 6.3. Similarly, as in adults, basal iron losses are almost negligible, and iron from senescent erythrocytes is recirculated to the bone marrow for use in the erythropoiesis. However, in contrast to the adult situation, iron needs for erythropoiesis exceed the amount of recirculated iron, due to the continuous expansion of blood volume which occurs with body growth. Iron requirements between 6 and 24 months of life are therefore higher than during any other period of life (Figs. 6.1 and 6.3), and the risk ID and IDA peaks at about 1–3 years of age. The exact peak can vary between populations; in the USA, the peak age for ID was recently shown to be

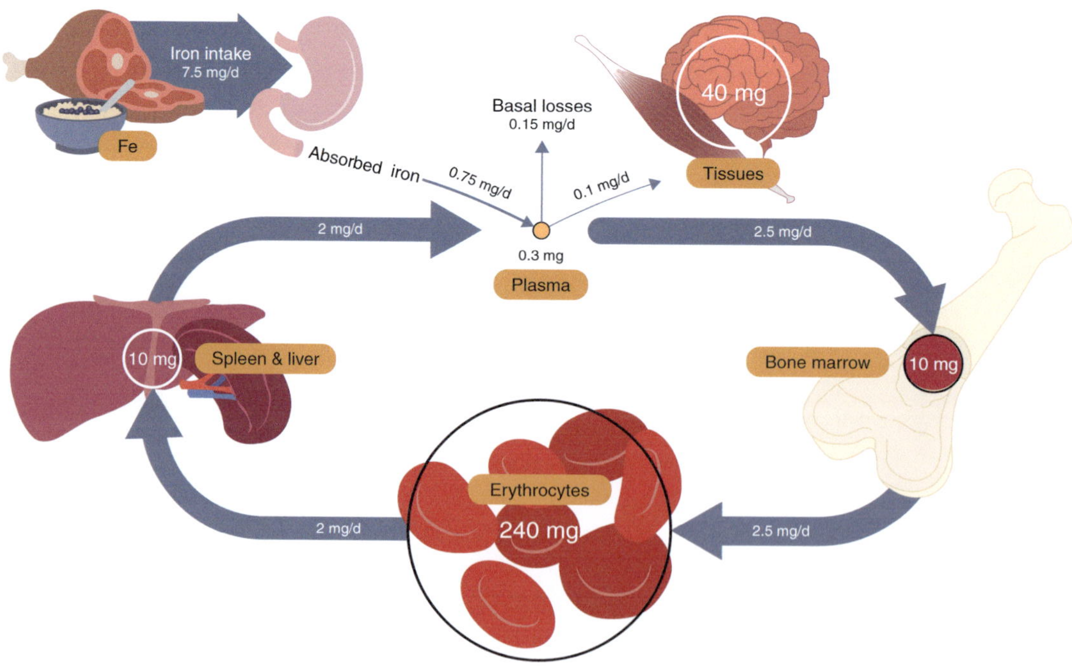

Fig. 6.3 The iron metabolism of the 6-month-old infant

15–24 months, when 16% of the population was affected [16]. A recent European study of children aged 12–23 months found that the prevalence of ID was 12% [17]. In countries with a high anemia prevalence, the peak extends up to 5 years of age [11]. Identified risk factors for ID are shown in Table 6.1. A vegan diet is likely to increase the risk for IDA in this age group, but epidemiological data are lacking.

The Preschool and School Child

At preschool and school age, especially at 3–5 years of age, IDA is globally still a major public health problem in populations with a high prevalence of general malnutrition and a high burden of infections [11]. While obesity is also associated with ID, hemoglobin concentrations generally tend to be within the normal range.

The Adolescent

In infants and toddlers, males have a higher risk of IDA than females. This is partly explained by a faster growth rate and thereby higher iron requirements in boys, but there are also inherent sex differences in, e.g., mean cell volume [18]. In preschool/school children, the risk of IDA is approximately equal between sexes. However, from puberty and onwards, females will have increased blood loss due to menstruation. Thus, adolescent girls are a risk group for IDA, with a prevalence of anemia up to 50% in high-risk regions such as India [19].

Biomarkers of Iron Status in Children

Due to the large changes in iron metabolism and iron compartments during the first months and years of life, there are considerable physiological changes in iron status biomarkers during the same period. Thus, it is of utmost importance to use adequate reference intervals for biomarkers at different ages as exemplified in Table 6.2 [20–24].

The combination of ferritin and hemoglobin is usually recommended for basic screening of IDA in children at risk [20]. For additional sensitivity and specificity, a combination of iron status biomarkers is often recommended, and mean cell volume, transferrin saturation, soluble transferrin receptors, zinc protoporphyrin, reticulocyte hemoglobin, and hepcidin are commonly used. However, their sensitivity and specificity for ID are not completely known in the pediatric population, and reference intervals for several of these biomarkers differ between laboratories and assays due to the lack of international standards.

Table 6.2 Reference intervals

Age	0–1 weeks	2 months	4 months	6–24 months	2–5 years	6–11 years	12–14 years	15–18 years	
Sex								Females	Males
Hb, g/L	135–225	90–140	105–140	105–140	110–140	115–155	120–155	120–155*	130–170
S-Ferritin, µg/L	40–500	40–400	20–300	10–200	12–200	15–200	15–200	15–150	15–200
MCV, fL	95–118	77–115	73–90	70–90	73–90	76–95	77–98	77–98	77–98

Adapted from [11, 20–24]

Iron Status and Inflammation

The load of infections is very high among preschool children in sub-Saharan Africa and moderately high in many low-income countries in Asia [4]. The difficulties of assessing iron status and the prevalence of IDA in a state of inflammation are well-known, since both acute and chronic inflammation will increase ferritin, decrease hemoglobin, and affect other iron status biomarkers [25]. In population studies, this can be partly compensated for by adjusting ferritin levels for the inflammatory markers C-reactive protein and α1-acid glycoprotein [26].

This is further complicated since infections and other states of inflammation can cause ID. A high infection load has been shown to result in chronically increased hepcidin levels, blocking iron absorption, in turn leading to ID [27]. This suggests that prevention and treatment of infections can be a useful adjunct to iron supplements in areas with a high prevalence of IDA and a high infection load.

Health Consequences of ID and Effects of Iron Supplements

IDA is the most well-known effect of ID, but the major concern in infants and children is that ID is associated with impaired neurodevelopment.

IDA

Even severe IDA in young children is mostly asymptomatic and thus difficult to diagnose. Pallor is the most common symptom, but fatigue, limited capacity for physical activity, palpitations, headache, dizziness, and insomnia are typical symptoms of severe IDA in older children as well as in adults. Severe IDA is also associated with impaired growth in children.

It is quite clear that iron supplements reduce the risk of anemia in children at risk of IDA. Meta-analyses, mostly from studies in low- and middle income countries (LMICs), show that iron supplements significantly reduce the risk of anemia in the age groups 6 months to 5 years of age [28, 29]. The reduction of IDA is substantial, with a typical risk ratio of 0.14 (95% CI 0.10–0.22) [30].

ID and Brain Development

The brain is the fastest-growing organ during the last trimester of pregnancy and during the first 2 years of life. Iron is essential for neurogenesis and the differentiation of brain cells during this sensitive period of brain development. In animal models, a clear causal relationship has been demonstrated between ID in infancy and impaired brain development and function, an effect which is depending on the timing, duration, and severity of ID [31, 32]. Several of the alterations in the brain, observed in animal models of ID, are long-lasting and do not reverse if iron therapy is provided [33]. It has also been suggested that iron is prioritized for erythropoiesis over other functions, and consequently, functional deficits in the brain may appear before IDA occurs [34]. Several domains of brain function have been shown in animal models to be affected by ID, including myelination, neurotransmitter synthesis and function, energy metabolism, and neuronal growth and branching of dendrites.

It is well-known that children with IDA have impaired neurodevelopment. It was shown already in the 1980s that toddlers with IDA have a significantly lower mental development index compared to controls [35]. Furthermore, IDA has been associated with impaired cognitive and motor development, behavioral problems, and mental health problems (anxiety, depression), effects that have been shown to be long-lasting, persisting at least up to adolescence [36, 37]. Mechanisms compatible with dopamine deficiency have been suggested [38]. However, observational studies can be confounded by socioeconomic factors and other nutrient deficiencies. Evidence from clinical trials is needed in order to determine causality and to identify effective interventions.

The Prenatal Situation

Even though supplementation of pregnant women with iron and folic acid is strongly recommended for prevention of maternal anemia and neural tube defects in the offspring, it does not directly influence the iron status of the newborn. Iron supplementation by itself has no clear effect on birth weight or other neonatal outcomes [39, 40], while multiple micronutrient supplementation of pregnant women may decrease the risk of low birth weight, which in turn is a risk factor for IDA in the offspring [41]. A recent meta-analysis showed no significant effect of antenatal iron supplementation of pregnant mothers on neurodevelopment in the offspring [42].

Infants and Preschool Children

In infants and young children <5 years, the results of meta-analyses are conflicting, mostly due to the considerably different inclusion criteria. Of three meta-analyses published in 2013, assessing the effects of iron supplementation on neurodevelopment assessed with the Bayley Scales of Infant Development, two meta-analyses showed no significant effect [30, 43], and one meta-analysis, including only trials of non-anemic infants, showed improved psychomotor development [44]. The latter suggests that early, preventive interventions may be useful since IDA may have irreversible effects on brain development. The two most recent meta-analyses of effects of iron supplementation in children <5 years both show positive effects on neurodevelopment [29, 45]. Tam et al. (2020) included five iron supplementation studies performed in low- and middle-income countries, including about 1000 children <5 years. Iron-supplemented children had significantly higher scores for motor development (effect size +0.28 SD, 95% CI 0.15–0.40, $p < 0.01$) and mental development (effect size +0.14 SD, 95% CI 0.01–0.28, $p = 0.03$). Larson et al. (2019) included 23 intervention studies of iron or multiple micronutrient supplementation, exploring different outcomes related to motor and/or mental development. The pooled analysis showed a significant positive overall effect of iron supplementation on motor development with an effect size of +0.11 SD (0.04–0.18). Taken together, these meta-analyses suggest a possible positive effect, mainly on motor development. However, there is a lack of sufficiently powered, high-quality RCTs with long-term follow-up of neurodevelopmental outcomes. In future studies, long-term effects on behavior, attention, mental health, and fine motor skills should be included, since there is increasing evidence that these functions are affected by previous or concurrent ID and/or IDA.

Low Birth Weight Infants

It is noteworthy that the above meta-analyses have generally not included studies on low birth weight (LBW < 2500 g) infants, even though this is one of the most important risk groups for IDA. The global prevalence of LBW is 15.5%, ranging from 4–9% in Europe to 28% in South Asia [46]. LBW infants include preterm infants, term infants, and small for gestational age (SGA) infants.

Even though it is well-known that LBW infants are at high risk of IDA [47], as well as for poor neurodevelopmental outcomes [48], there is a severe lack of studies investigating the effects of early iron intake on later neurodevelopmental outcomes in LBW infants.

A Cochrane review in 2012 investigated the effect of enteral iron supplementation in preterm and low birth weight infants and included 21 studies, but, even though most studies of sustained iron supplementation showed effects on hemoglobin, none evaluated neurodevelopmental outcomes [49]. Since the Cochrane review, only one new study has been published on this topic, providing the best current evidence. In that RCT, LBW infants born with a birth weight between 2000 and 2500 g were randomized to iron supplements or placebo from 6 weeks to 6 months of age, and it was demonstrated that iron supplementation not only improved short-term iron status outcomes but also reduced the risk of later behavioral problems at 3 and 7 years of age [50].

School-Age Children

Results from meta-analyses are divergent also in school-age children. In a meta-analysis of 14 RCTs of children from 6 years and adolescents, Falkingham et al. (2010) found that iron supplementation improved attention and concentration irrespective of baseline iron status (effect size +0.59 SD; 0.29–0.90) [51]. In anemic groups, supplementation improved IQ by 2.5 points (1.24–3.76) but had no effect on non-anemic participants. The studies were small and methodologically weak, and a modest publication bias was observed. In a meta-analysis of five studies of children 5–12 years, Guo et al. (2015) showed no effect on cognitive performance [52]. Lam et al. (2017) investigated iron interventions and multiple micronutrient interventions in school-age children and found a consistent improvement in cognitive performance along with improved iron status in subjects who were anemic at baseline [53].

Health Economic Aspects

Due to the long-term effects of IDA on neurodevelopment, attempts have been made to quantify the economic impact. In India, childhood IDA has been estimated to cause a loss of 8.3 million disability-adjusted life years (DALYs), and the annual production losses were estimated to be 24 billion USD, corresponding to 1.3% of the GDP [54].

Adverse Effects of Iron Supplements in Children

Since there is evidence that iron supplementation may benefit health, it might be argued that infants and children would benefit from generous iron supplementation. However, there are several reasons why excessive iron intakes can be harmful: (1) Iron is a highly reactive pro-oxidant, which will cause significant cell damage if not tightly bound to transferrin, ferritin, or other transport/storage protein; (2) iron is an essential nutrient for most pathogens and may thus increase the risk of infections; and (3) humans have no mechanism for iron excretion, which means that excessive intake and subsequent absorption of iron in an iron-replete individual will lead to iron overload.

The capacity of iron to switch between its two oxidation states Fe^{2+} (ferrous) and Fe^{3+} (ferric) underlies its essential role in oxygen transport and electron-transfer reactions, but this also renders iron a highly effective catalyst in the formation of free oxygen radicals. Normally, iron is safely sequestered in transport or storage proteins such as transferrin, lactoferrin, and ferritin. Free iron or non-transferrin-bound iron increases oxidative stress, which is associated with many diseases in children and adults, including cardiovascular, neurological, and autoimmune disorders. In preterm infants, retinopathy of prematurity and bronchopulmonary dysplasia are examples of oxidative disorders. It is generally not recommended to give any iron before 2 weeks of age to newborns since data suggests that antioxidant systems are not fully active until that age [55].

Adverse effects of iron that have been suggested to occur in children include diarrhea, gut dysbiosis, malaria, other infections, poor growth, and even poor neurodevelopment [56].

Iron and Infections

Iron is essential for the growth of many pathogens, so humans and other animals have a mechanism to deprive the pathogens of iron: Within hours of infection or other inflammatory stimulus, there is a cytokine-driven increase of hepcidin production, resulting in drastically reduced plasma iron concentrations [57]. Thus, the pivotal iron regulatory peptide hepcidin is also an important part of the immune system.

Two RCTs, both published in 2006, showed the somewhat alarming results that iron supplementation of infants and young children in malarious regions can result in increased malaria morbidity as well as increased mortality [58, 59]. However, subsequent RCTs have shown that iron supplementation of children in malarious regions is safe and effective, provided that malaria prevention and treatment are provided, which is also confirmed in the most recent Cochrane review from 2016 [60].

It has not been clearly shown that iron supplementation would increase the risk of infections other than malaria in children, even though many studies show an increased risk of diarrhea [61]. A recent meta-analysis showed that the risk of diarrhea was only significantly increased when iron was given as a part of a multiple micronutrient powder, which might be related to an interaction between iron and zinc [29].

Iron and the Microbiome

Recent studies suggest that iron supplements change the gut microbiome, resulting in more *Clostridum* spp. and pathogenic gram-negative bacteria and less lactobacilli and bifidobacteria [62, 63]. Interestingly, species of lactic acid bacteria (bifidobacteria and especially lactobacilli) are exceptional among living organisms by having extremely low iron requirements [64]. These dysbiotic effects of iron are a likely mechanism behind the association between iron supplements and diarrhea discussed above [65]. Dysbiosis may also explain the association between iron supplementation and poor growth, which has been observed in some studies, especially in iron-replete infants [56], even though there are conflicting results from recent meta-analyses regarding possible negative effects of iron supplementation on growth [29, 30, 66].

Iron and Poor Neurodevelopment

Iron accumulation in the brain has been associated with neurodegenerative disorders in adults. Thus, even though iron supplements in general improve neurodevelopment in children as described above, there is also a concern that excessive iron intakes may impair brain development. Animal experiments show that elevated iron intake in early life can have negative effects on brain morphologic and biochemical outcomes [67]. The only human study showing similar results is a RCT of an iron-fortified formula containing 12 mg/L given during 6 months to non-anemic 6-month-old Chilean infants with a low risk of ID. Infants from the original study ($n = 835$) had lower cognitive scores at follow-up at 10 ($n = 473$) and 16 ($n = 405$) years of age. The effect was mainly limited to those who had an initial higher hemoglobin level, a proxy for iron repletion [68]. No clear conclusions can be drawn from this single study, but it supports the general rule to avoid excessive iron intakes in iron-replete infants.

Interventions to Decrease the Prevalence of IDA in Children

Delayed Cord Clamping

Delayed cord clamping (DCC), i.e., waiting 1–3 min after birth to clamp and cut the umbilical cord, facilitates placental transfusion, increasing the newborn's blood volume by about 30%, with a considerable impact on total body iron. A meta-analysis from 2019, including 1799 term infants from 4 studies, shows that DCC reduces the risk of IDA at 4–12 months with a risk ratio of 0.68 (95% CI 0.49–0.94) [69]. DCC has also been shown to result in increased myelin content in the internal capsule and other early maturing brain regions associated with motor, visual, and sensory processing/function [70], and it has been shown to improve fine motor function at 4 years of age [71], indicating that this easily implemented and low-cost intervention can prevent neurodevelopmental impairment caused by ID. In addition to these effects, in preterm infants, DCC has also been shown to reduce the risk of intraventricular hemorrhage, chronic lung disease, patent ductus arteriosus, necrotizing enterocolitis, late-onset sepsis, and retinopathy of prematurity [72]. Despite overwhelming evidence and the endorsement by numerous authorities, including the WHO, the practice of DCC is only slowly adopted worldwide, suggesting the need for targeted education of stakeholders [73].

Breastfeeding

Due to the many positive health effects of breast milk, exclusive breastfeeding is recommended for all infants during the first 6 months of life [74]. Even though breast milk has a low iron content, this is fully compatible with the low iron needs of the healthy infant during this period, and a recent meta-analysis found no convincing evidence that introducing iron-containing foods before 6 months offers any advantages in terms of iron status [75]. However, prolonged exclusive breastfeeding beyond 6 months is associated with a clear risk of IDA [76] and should thus be avoided. Low birth weight infants need iron supplements in addition to breastfeeding already from 2–6 weeks of age, since they deplete their iron stores more rapidly, see section "The Newborn and the First 6 Months of Life" and Fig. 6.2 [20].

Iron Supplemented Infant Formulas and Follow-On Formulas

Iron bioavailability from breast milk is high, about 50%, while iron bioavailability from infant formula is only about 10%. Additionally, cow's milk in infant formulas may increase intestinal blood losses [77]. Thus, infant formula needs to have a higher iron concentration than breast milk. The importance of iron fortification of infant formulas for the prevention of IDA has been known for more than 50 years and has been confirmed in several RCTs [20]. However, the optimal level of iron fortification is still controversial, with most infant formulas being iron fortified to 4–8 mg/L in Europe and 12 mg/L in the USA. Even lower levels of iron fortification (2 mg/L) are being studied. Follow-on formulas, for use after 6 months of age, when iron requirements are considerably higher, are usually iron fortified at levels between 7 and 13 mg/L, but there is insufficient evidence on the effects of different levels of fortification on IDA and neurodevelopment. Adequately powered, RCTs with long-term follow-up of neurodevelopmental outcomes are urgently needed to determine optimal levels of iron fortification of infant formulas and follow-on formulas.

Iron Supplements

Iron supplements can effectively prevent or treat IDA in pediatric populations at risk, as described above. Iron supplements can be administered as mixture or syrup, which is suitable for infants and young children, or tablets, which are suitable for school children and adolescents. Multiple micronutrient supplementation can be administered as mixture/syrup, tablets, lipid-based nutrient supplements, or powder for point-of-use fortification. All of these forms of iron supplementation have been shown to be effective in children, even though isolated iron supplementation is the most studied and may have higher efficacy with regard to anemia compared to multiple micronutrient supplementation [29]. However, in settings where multiple micronutrient deficiencies are common, the latter would be preferred.

Iron-Rich Foods

During the critical period between 6 and 24 months, iron requirements are very high, and it is thus important to provide an iron-rich diet, preferably while still partially breastfeeding. Feeding solids or fluids while partially breastfeeding is called complementary feeding. There is clear evidence that iron-fortified or multiple micronutrient-fortified complementary foods, mostly cereals and milk-based drinks, improve iron status and decrease the risk of anemia in infants and toddlers [20]. Meat-based complementary foods have also been shown to be effective in preventing ID [75]. In theory, complementary foods heavily based on beans, lentils, and other iron-rich vegetables might be effective, but this has not been shown in studies [75].

In preschool and school children, point-of-use fortification of foods with micronutrient powders containing iron is effective in reducing anemia prevalence in LMIC. Even though some studies have shown promising results [78, 79], it is less clear whether other food-based interventions in school children and adolescents are similarly effective [80]. Population-level iron fortification of flour or condiments has been shown to decrease the prevalence of anemia and ID in children [81, 82].

Avoiding Cow's Milk

It is well-known that the use of unfortified cow's milk as a drink for infants and a high intake of unfortified cow's milk in toddlers considerably increase the risk of ID and IDA [20, 83]. This is due to the low iron content of cow's milk, possible increased intestinal iron losses, and the fact that it will replace iron-rich foods in the diet [77].

Conclusions

Nutritional anemia is a significant public health problem in children, associated with poor neurological function and impaired brain development. Young children (<3–5 years) and adolescent girls are at the highest risk. ID is by far the most common cause of nutritional anemia in children, but other deficiencies, such as vitamin B_{12}, can be prevalent in some settings. Iron supplements should be targeted to risk groups since unnecessary iron supplements can have adverse effects in iron-replete children. Recommended interventions for prevention and treatment of nutritional anemia in children are shown in Table 6.3.

Table 6.3 Recommended interventions

The following interventions can be recommended to reduce the prevalence of nutritional anemia in children:
In all populations
1. Universal implementation of delayed umbilical cord clamping
2. Formula-fed infants should receive formula fortified with iron, vitamin B_{12}, and other micronutrients
3. Low birth weight infants (<2500 g) should receive daily iron supplements from 2–6 weeks of age at least to 6 months of age [76]
4. Ensure iron-rich diet for infants and toddlers at 6–36 months of age, and avoid high intakes of unfortified cow's milk in this age interval [6, 76]
5. Screening of adolescent girls for ID and, if needed iron, iron supplementation
In populations with a high prevalence of anemia
1. Gather local baseline data on the most common causes of anemia in different age groups, as well as the prevalence of infections/inflammation, to guide the intervention programs
2. Iron supplements (alone or together with other micronutrients) or point-of-use fortificants (e.g., micronutrient powders or lipid-based nutrient supplements) are recommended for prevention and treatment. For prevention, it is especially important to target infants/toddlers at 6–23 months of age [11]
3. If infection/inflammation is common, public health measures should be taken to prevent and treat malaria, HIV, helminthic infections, as well as respiratory and gastrointestinal infections, especially in children under 3–5 years of age. Malaria prevention/treatment is especially important if iron supplementation is given
4. Locally adapted anemia prevention programs should include training of healthcare workers, dietary counseling, and community participation

References

1. (WHO) WHO. 2016. https://data.worldbank.org/indicator/SH.ANM.CHLD.ZS.
2. Neufeld LM, Beal T, Larson LM, Cattaneo FD. Global landscape of malnutrition in infants and young children. In: Michaelsen KF, Neufeld LM, Prentice AM, editors. Global landscape of nutrition challenges in infants and children. Basel, Switzerland: Karger AG; 2020.
3. Petry N, Olofin I, Hurrell RF, Boy E, Wirth JP, Moursi M, et al. The proportion of anemia associated with iron deficiency in low, medium, and high human development index countries: a systematic analysis of national surveys. Nutrients. 2016;8(11)
4. Engle-Stone R, Aaron GJ, Huang J, Wirth JP, Namaste SM, Williams AM, et al. Predictors of anemia in preschool children: Biomarkers Reflecting Inflammation and Nutritional Determinants of Anemia (BRINDA) project. Am J Clin Nutr. 2017.
5. Guez S, Chiarelli G, Menni F, Salera S, Principi N, Esposito S. Severe vitamin B12 deficiency in an exclusively breastfed 5-month-old Italian infant born to a mother receiving multivitamin supplementation during pregnancy. BMC Pediatr. 2012;12:85.
6. Fewtrell M, Bronsky J, Campoy C, Domellöf M, Embleton N, Fidler Mis N, et al. Complementary feeding: a position paper by the European Society for Paediatric Gastroenterology, Hepatology, and Nutrition (ESPGHAN) Committee on Nutrition. J Pediatr Gastroenterol Nutr. 2017;64(1):119–32.
7. Sarna A, Porwal A, Ramesh S, Agrawal PK, Acharya R, Johnston R, et al. Characterisation of the types of anaemia prevalent among children and adolescents aged 1-19 years in India: a population-based study. Lancet Child Adolesc Health. 2020;4(7):515–25.
8. Kumar T, Taneja S, Sachdev HPS, Refsum H, Yajnik CS, Bhandari N, et al. Supplementation of vitamin B12 or folic acid on hemoglobin concentration in children 6-36 months of age: a randomized placebo controlled trial. Clin Nutr. 2017;36(4):986–91.
9. Huang Y, Wang L, Huo J, Wu Q, Wang W, Chang S, et al. Prevalence and causes of anaemia in children aged 6-23 months in rural Qinghai, China: findings from a cross-sectional study. BMJ Open. 2019;9(9):e031021.
10. Imdad A, Mayo-Wilson E, Herzer K, Bhutta ZA. Vitamin A supplementation for preventing morbidity and mortality in children from six months to five years of age. Cochrane Database Syst Rev. 2017;3:CD008524.
11. (WHO) WHO. Nutritional anaemias: tools for effective prevention and control. Geneva, Switzerland; 2017.
12. Andersson O, Hellstrom-Westas L, Andersson D, Domellöf M. Effect of delayed versus early umbilical cord clamping on neonatal outcomes and iron status at 4 months: a randomised controlled trial. BMJ. 2011;343:d7157.
13. Park AM, Sanders TA, Maltepe E. Hypoxia-inducible factor (HIF) and HIF-stabilizing agents in neonatal care. Semin Fetal Neonatal Med. 2010;15(4):196–202.
14. Lundgren P, Hellgren G, Pivodic A, Savman K, Smith LEH, Hellstrom A. Erythropoietin serum levels, versus anaemia as risk factors for severe retinopathy of prematurity. Pediatr Res. 2019;86(2):276–82.
15. Lonnerdal B. Development of iron homeostasis in infants and young children. Am J Clin Nutr. 2017.
16. Oatley H, Borkhoff CM, Chen S, Macarthur C, Persaud N, Birken CS, et al. Screening for iron deficiency in early childhood using serum ferritin in the primary care setting. Pediatrics. 2018;142(6).
17. Akkermans MD, van der Horst-Graat JM, Eussen SR, van Goudoever JB, Brus F. Iron and vitamin D deficiency in healthy young children in western europe despite current nutritional recommendations. J Pediatr Gastroenterol Nutr. 2016;62(4):635–42.
18. Domellöf M, Lonnerdal B, Dewey KG, Cohen RJ, Rivera LL, Hernell O. Sex differences in iron status during infancy. Pediatrics. 2002;110(3):545–52.
19. Kumari R, Bharti RK, Singh K, Sinha A, Kumar S, Saran A, et al. Prevalence of iron deficiency and iron deficiency anaemia in adolescent girls in a Tertiary Care Hospital. J Clin Diagn Res. 2017;11(8):BC04–BC6.
20. Domellöf M, Braegger C, Campoy C, et al. Iron requirements of infants and toddlers. J Pediatr Gastroenterol Nutr. 2014;58(1):119–29.
21. Domellöf M, Dewey KG, Lönnerdal B, Cohen RJ, Hernell O. The diagnostic criteria for iron deficiency in infants should be reevaluated. J Nutr. 2002;132(12):3680–6.
22. Dallman PR. Blood and blood forming tissues. Rudolph AM (Ed.), Pediatrics (ed 16), Appleton-Century-Crofts, Inc., Philadelphia (1977).
23. Larsson SM, Hillarp A, Hellström-Westas L, Domellöf M, Lundahl T, Andersson O. When age really matters; ferritin reference intervals during infancy revisited. Scand J Clin Lab Invest. 2019;79(8):590–4.
24. Nelson Textbook of Pediatrics - 15th edition. Behrman RE, editor: W.B. Saunders Co; 1996.
25. Suchdev PS, Williams AM, Mei Z, Flores-Ayala R, Pasricha SR, Rogers LM, et al. Assessment of iron status in settings of inflammation: challenges and potential approaches. Am J Clin Nutr. 2017.
26. Thurnham DI, McCabe LD, Haldar S, Wieringa FT, Northrop-Clewes CA, McCabe GP. Adjusting plasma ferritin concentrations to remove the effects of subclinical inflammation in the assessment of iron deficiency: a meta-analysis. Am J Clin Nutr. 2010;92(3):546–55.
27. Prentice AM, Bah A, Jallow MW, Jallow AT, Sanyang S, Sise EA, et al. Respiratory infections drive hepcidin-mediated blockade of iron absorption leading to iron deficiency anemia in African children. Sci Adv. 2019;5(3):eaav9020.
28. Petry N, Olofin I, Boy E, Donahue Angel M, Rohner F. The effect of low dose iron and zinc intake on child

micronutrient status and development during the first 1000 days of life: a systematic review and meta-analysis. Nutrients. 2016;8(12).
29. Tam E, Keats EC, Rind F, Das JK, Bhutta AZA. Micronutrient supplementation and fortification interventions on health and development outcomes among children under-five in low- and middle-income countries: a systematic review and meta-analysis. Nutrients. 2020;12(2).
30. Pasricha SR, Hayes E, Kalumba K, Biggs BA. Effect of daily iron supplementation on health in children aged 4-23 months: a systematic review and meta-analysis of randomised controlled trials. Lancet Glob Health. 2013;1(2):e77–86.
31. Beard JL. Why iron deficiency is important in infant development. J Nutr. 2008;138(12):2534–6.
32. Georgieff MK. The role of iron in neurodevelopment: fetal iron deficiency and the developing hippocampus. Biochem Soc Trans. 2008;36(Pt 6):1267–71.
33. Lozoff B, Georgieff MK. Iron deficiency and brain development. Semin Pediatr Neurol. 2006;13(3):158–65.
34. Zamora TG, Guiang SF 3rd, Widness JA, Georgieff MK. Iron is prioritized to red blood cells over the brain in phlebotomized anemic newborn lambs. Pediatr Res. 2016;79(6):922–8.
35. Lozoff B, Brittenham GM, Wolf AW, McClish DK, Kuhnert PM, Jimenez E, et al. Iron deficiency anemia and iron therapy effects on infant developmental test performance. Pediatrics. 1987;79(6):981–95.
36. Lozoff B, Beard J, Connor J, Barbara F, Georgieff M, Schallert T. Long-lasting neural and behavioral effects of iron deficiency in infancy. Nutr Rev. 2006;64(5 Pt 2):S34–43; discussion S72–91.
37. Beard J. Recent evidence from human and animal studies regarding iron status and infant development. J Nutr. 2007;137(2):524S–30S.
38. Lozoff B. Early iron deficiency has brain and behavior effects consistent with dopaminergic dysfunction. J Nutr. 2011;141(4):740S–6S.
39. Pena-Rosas JP, De-Regil LM, Garcia-Casal MN, Dowswell T. Daily oral iron supplementation during pregnancy. Cochrane Database Syst Rev. 2015;(7):CD004736.
40. Abraha I, Bonacini MI, Montedori A, Di Renzo GC, Angelozzi P, Micheli M, et al. Oral iron-based interventions for prevention of critical outcomes in pregnancy and postnatal care: an overview and update of systematic reviews. J Evid Based Med. 2019;12(2):155–66.
41. Keats EC, Haider BA, Tam E, Bhutta ZA. Multiple-micronutrient supplementation for women during pregnancy. Cochrane Database Syst Rev. 2019;3:CD004905.
42. Jayasinghe C, Polson R, van Woerden HC, Wilson P. The effect of universal maternal antenatal iron supplementation on neurodevelopment in offspring: a systematic review and meta-analysis. BMC Pediatr. 2018;18(1):150.
43. Wang B, Zhan S, Gong T, Lee L. Iron therapy for improving psychomotor development and cognitive function in children under the age of three with iron deficiency anaemia. Cochrane Database Syst Rev. 2013(6):CD001444.
44. Szajewska H, Ruszczynski M, Chmielewska A. Effects of iron supplementation in nonanemic pregnant women, infants, and young children on the mental performance and psychomotor development of children: a systematic review of randomized controlled trials. Am J Clin Nutr. 2010;91(6):1684–90.
45. Larson LM, Kubes JN, Ramirez-Luzuriaga MJ, Khishen S, et al. Effects of increased hemoglobin on child growth, development, and disease: a systematic review and meta-analysis. Ann N Y Acad Sci. 2019;1450(1):83–104.
46. Domellöf M. Meeting the iron needs of low and very low birth weight infants. Ann Nutr Metab. 2017;71(Suppl 3):16–23.
47. Lundström U, Siimes MA, Dallman PR. At what age does iron supplementation become necessary in low-birth-weight infants? J Pediatr. 1977;91(6):878–83.
48. Oudgenoeg-Paz O, Mulder H, Jongmans MJ, van der Ham IJM, Van der Stigchel S. The link between motor and cognitive development in children born preterm and/or with low birth weight: a review of current evidence. Neurosci Biobehav Rev. 2017;80:382–93.
49. Mills RJ, Davies MW. Enteral iron supplementation in preterm and low birth weight infants. Cochrane Database Syst Rev. 2012(3):CD005095.
50. Berglund SK, Chmielewska A, Lindberg J, Westrup B, Hagglof B, Norman M, et al. Effects of iron supplementation of low birth weight infants on cognition and behavior at 7 years-a randomized controlled trial. Pediatr Res. 2017.
51. Falkingham M, Abdelhamid A, Curtis P, Fairweather-Tait S, Dye L, Hooper L. The effects of oral iron supplementation on cognition in older children and adults: a systematic review and meta-analysis. Nutr J. 2010;9:4.
52. Guo XM, Liu H, Qian J. Daily iron supplementation on cognitive performance in primary-school-aged children with and without anemia: a meta-analysis. Int J Clin Exp Med. 2015;8(9):16107–11.
53. Lam LF, Lawlis TR. Feeding the brain—the effects of micronutrient interventions on cognitive performance among school-aged children: a systematic review of randomized controlled trials. Clin Nutr. 2017;36(4):1007–14.
54. Plessow R, Arora NK, Brunner B, Tzogiou C, Eichler K, Brugger U, et al. Social costs of iron deficiency anemia in 6-59-month-old children in India. PLoS One. 2015;10(8):e0136581.
55. Berger HM, Mumby S, Gutteridge JM. Ferrous ions detected in iron-overloaded cord blood plasma from preterm and term babies: implications for oxidative stress. Free Radic Res. 1995;22(6):555–9.
56. Domellöf M. Benefits and harms of iron supplementation in iron-deficient and iron-sufficient chil-

dren. Nestle Nutr Workshop Ser Pediatr Program. 2010;65:153–62; discussion 62–5.
57. Ganz T. Iron and infection. Int J Hematol. 2018;107(1):7–15.
58. Sazawal S, Black RE, Ramsan M, Chwaya HM, Stoltzfus RJ, Dutta A, et al. Effects of routine prophylactic supplementation with iron and folic acid on admission to hospital and mortality in preschool children in a high malaria transmission setting: community-based, randomised, placebo-controlled trial. Lancet. 2006;367(9505):133–43.
59. Richard SA, Zavaleta N, Caulfield LE, Black RE, Witzig RS, Shankar AH. Zinc and iron supplementation and malaria, diarrhea, and respiratory infections in children in the Peruvian Amazon. Am J Trop Med Hyg. 2006;75(1):126–32.
60. Neuberger A, Okebe J, Yahav D, Paul M. Oral iron supplements for children in malaria-endemic areas. Cochrane Database Syst Rev. 2016;2:CD006589.
61. Ghanchi A, James PT, Cerami C. Guts, germs, and iron: a systematic review on iron supplementation, iron fortification, and diarrhea in children aged 4-59 months. Curr Dev Nutr. 2019;3(3):nzz005.
62. Jaeggi T, Kortman GA, Moretti D, Chassard C, Holding P, Dostal A, et al. Iron fortification adversely affects the gut microbiome, increases pathogen abundance and induces intestinal inflammation in Kenyan infants. Gut. 2015;64(5):731–42.
63. Simonyte Sjodin K, Domellöf M, Lagerqvist C, Hernell O, Lonnerdal B, Szymlek-Gay EA, et al. Administration of ferrous sulfate drops has significant effects on the gut microbiota of iron-sufficient infants: a randomised controlled study. Gut. 2018.
64. Weinberg ED. The Lactobacillus anomaly: total iron abstinence. Perspect Biol Med. 1997;40(4):578–83.
65. Paganini D, Uyoga MA, Kortman GAM, Cercamondi CI, Winkler HC, Boekhorst J, et al. Iron-containing micronutrient powders modify the effect of oral antibiotics on the infant gut microbiome and increase post-antibiotic diarrhoea risk: a controlled study in Kenya. Gut. 2019;68(4):645–53.
66. Cai C, Granger M, Eck P, Friel J. Effect of daily iron supplementation in healthy exclusively breastfed infants: a systematic review with meta-analysis. Breastfeed Med. 2017.
67. Agrawal S, Berggren KL, Marks E, Fox JH. Impact of high iron intake on cognition and neurodegeneration in humans and in animal models: a systematic review. Nutr Rev. 2017.
68. Gahagan S, Delker E, Blanco E, Burrows R, Lozoff B. Randomized controlled trial of iron-fortified versus low-iron infant formula: developmental outcomes at 16 years. J Pediatr. 2019;212:124–30.e1.
69. Zhao Y, Hou R, Zhu X, Ren L, Lu H. Effects of delayed cord clamping on infants after neonatal period: a systematic review and meta-analysis. Int J Nurs Stud. 2019;92:97–108.
70. Mercer JS, Erickson-Owens DA, Deoni SCL, Dean DC 3rd, Collins J, Parker AB, et al. Effects of delayed cord clamping on 4-month ferritin levels, brain myelin content, and neurodevelopment: a randomized controlled trial. J Pediatr. 2018;203(266–72):e2.
71. Andersson O, Lindquist B, Lindgren M, Stjernqvist K, Domellöf M, Hellstrom-Westas L. Effect of delayed cord clamping on neurodevelopment at 4 years of age: a randomized clinical trial. JAMA Pediatr. 2015;169(7):631–8.
72. Fogarty M, Osborn DA, Askie L, Seidler AL, Hunter K, Lui K, et al. Delayed vs early umbilical cord clamping for preterm infants: a systematic review and meta-analysis. Am J Obstet Gynecol. 2018;218(1):1–18.
73. Anton O, Jordan H, Rabe H. Strategies for implementing placental transfusion at birth: a systematic review. Birth. 2019;46(3):411–27.
74. (WHO) WHO. Infant and Young Child Nutrition (WHA55.25); 2002. http://apps.who.int/gb/archive/pdf_files/WHA55/ewha5525.pdf.
75. Obbagy JE, English LK, Psota TL, Wong YP, Butte NF, Dewey KG, et al. Complementary feeding and micronutrient status: a systematic review. Am J Clin Nutr. 2019;109(Supplement_7):852s–71s.
76. Chantry CJ, Howard CR, Auinger P. Full breastfeeding duration and risk for iron deficiency in U.S. infants. Breastfeed Med. 2007;2(2):63–73.
77. Ziegler EE. Consumption of cow's milk as a cause of iron deficiency in infants and toddlers. Nutr Rev. 2011;69(Suppl 1):S37–42.
78. Wang X, Hui Z, Dai X, Terry PD, Zhang Y, Ma M, et al. Micronutrient-fortified milk and academic performance among chinese middle school students: a cluster-randomized controlled trial. Nutrients. 2017;9(3)
79. Scott SP, Murray-Kolb LE, Wenger MJ, Udipi SA, Ghugre PS, Boy E, et al. Cognitive performance in indian school-going adolescents is positively affected by consumption of iron-biofortified pearl millet: a 6-month randomized controlled efficacy trial. J Nutr. 2018;148(9):1462–71.
80. Salam RA, Das JK, Ahmed W, Irfan O, Sheikh SS, Bhutta ZA. Effects of preventive nutrition interventions among adolescents on health and nutritional status in low- and middle-income countries: a systematic review and meta-analysis. Nutrients. 2019;12(1).
81. Sadighi J, Nedjat S, Rostami R. Systematic review and meta-analysis of the effect of iron-fortified flour on iron status of populations worldwide. Public Health Nutr. 2019;22(18):3465–84.
82. Hess S, Tecklenburg L, Eichler K. Micronutrient fortified condiments and noodles to reduce anemia in children and adults—a literature review and meta-analysis. Nutrients. 2016;8(2):88.
83. Daly A. Prevention of anaemia in inner-city toddlers by the use of a follow-on formula. Prof Care MotherChild. 1997;7(5):141–2, 6.

Nutritional Anemia in Pregnancy and Lactation

7

Anuraj H. Shankar, Rina Agustina, and Yuni Setiyawati

Background

Worldwide, maternal anemia affects over 40% of pregnant and lactating women and is considered a major public health burden [1]. During pregnancy, anemia is associated with increased maternal infections, fatigue, decreased cognitive function, preterm birth, and elevated maternal morbidity and mortality. Risks to the child due to maternal anemia include poor fetal growth and development, premature birth, still birth, increased morbidity and mortality, and poor cognitive development. Anemia during lactation adversely affects maternal postpartum health and recovery, breast milk quality, and infant health [2]. Although maternal anemia has multiple causes, the most proximal is insufficient intake of specific nutrients, especially iron, needed to meet the demands for synthesis of hemoglobin and erythrocytes [2]. However, as shown in Fig. 7.1, it must be acknowledged that maternal nutritional anemia has secondary causes which include infection, poor quality of antenatal and postnatal care, food insecurity, low socioeconomic status, poor quality implementation of maternal nutrition programs, and genetic factors. Progress on decreasing maternal anemia, and nutritional anemia, has been slow and inconsistent as seen in Fig. 7.2. The World Health Assembly (WHA) Global Nutrition Target is to reduce anemia in women of reproductive age by 50% by 2025, and current progress is lagging.

Herein, we review the assessment, epidemiology, etiology, and interventions related to maternal nutritional anemia. We present evidence for the simplest and most apparent of interventions, iron supplementation or multiple micronutrient supplementation (MMS), and highlight the gap in knowledge specifically for interventions for nutritional anemia of pregnancy and lactation in the context of nutrition-specific interventions, those directed at the immediate causes of anemia such as diet and infection, and nutrition-sensitive interventions directed at underlying determi-

A. H. Shankar (✉)
Oxford University Clinical Research Unit – Indonesia, Jakarta, Indonesia

Centre for Tropical Medicine and Global Health, Nuffield Department of Medicine, University of Oxford, Oxford, UK

Summit Institute for Development, Mataram, Indonesia
e-mail: anuraj.shankar@ndm.ox.ac.uk

R. Agustina
Department of Nutrition, Faculty of Medicine, Universitas Indonesia - Dr Cipto Mangunkusumo General Hospital, Jakarta, Indonesia

Human Nutrition Research Centre, Indonesian Medical Education and Research Institute, Faculty of Medicine, Universitas Indonesia, Jakarta, Indonesia

Y. Setiyawati
Summit Institute for Development, Mataram, Indonesia

C. D. Karakochuk et al. (eds.), *Nutritional Anemia*, Nutrition and Health,
https://doi.org/10.1007/978-3-031-14521-6_7

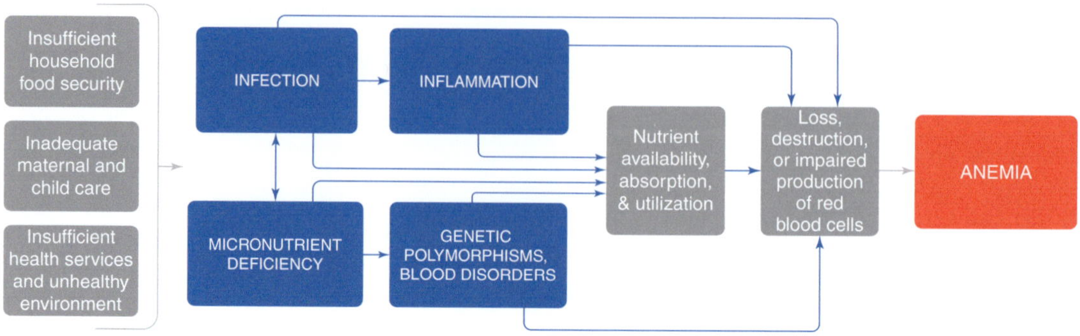

Fig. 7.1 Anemia causal framework. (Modified from Moorthy D, et al. Adv Nutr 2020;11:1631–1645)

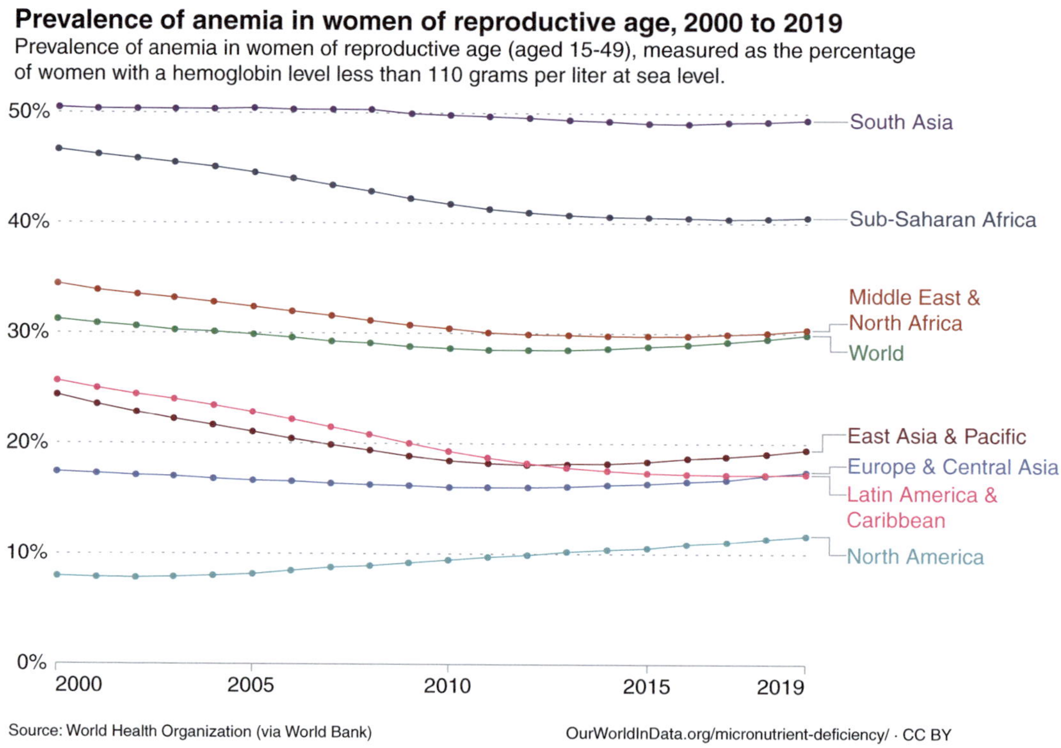

Fig. 7.2 Trends in prevalence of anemia in women of reproductive age from 2000 to 2019

nants of anemia, such as food insecurity or insufficient maternal and child healthcare services. Gaps in data persist in how to effectively deliver even the simplest of interventions to address maternal nutritional anemia, as evidenced by persistent high rates and debates around the most relevant causes. There is a need to seek solutions in the context of precision medicine and precision public health and to embrace digital health and address issues of frontline health worker performance and adopt more preventive and promotive approaches with strong community engagement. Such changes will likely require a change in how programs are designed and deployed, focusing more on local innovations, e.g., from and with communities, rather than traditional top-down approaches from global organizations that have been unable to meet the needs. The post-pandemic world is an opportunity to take stock in what has worked, and not worked, and forge innovations and novel pathways to create impact at scale.

Epidemiology

Iron deficiency is the most common cause of maternal nutritional anemia globally and contributes to approximately 50% of all anemia among pregnant and lactating women [3, 4]. It is notable that the proportion of iron deficiency anemia varies substantially depending on the region of the world and prevalence of other causes of anemia [5]. As detailed below, deficiencies of other nutrients including vitamins A, B2 (riboflavin), B6 (pyridoxine), B12 (cobalamin), C, D, and E, folate, and copper contribute to nutritional anemia. As mentioned, nearly half of all maternal anemia reflects iron deficiency anemia, with global estimates suggesting 10–20% of pregnant and lactating women are affected [6]. As such, WHO recommends universal iron and folic acid (IFA) supplementation for pregnant women containing 30–60 mg of iron, with the higher dose preferred in settings where anemia in pregnant women is ≥40%, along with 400 μg of folic acid; and intermittent use of iron and folic acid supplements by non-anemic women is a recommended alternative to prevent anemia and improve gestational outcomes in areas where the prevalence of anemia among pregnant women is lower than 20%, with the suggested dose being 120 mg elemental iron and 2800 μg folic acid weekly throughout pregnancy [7, 8]. There are no specific WHO recommendations for supplementation of lactating women.

It is clear the context for low- and middle-income countries (LMICs) versus high-income countries (HICs) differs, as illustrated in Fig. 7.3. In LMICs, maternal iron deficiency anemia has been reported as over 40%. In HICs, for example, in the United States, iron deficiency and/or iron deficiency anemia has been reported as 2–3% in pregnant and lactating women, although 15–16% among non-Hispanic Black, Mexican American, and low-income pregnant women [9]. In Europe, iron deficiency anemia varied from 3% in Switzerland to 15% in Belgium [10]. Despite the

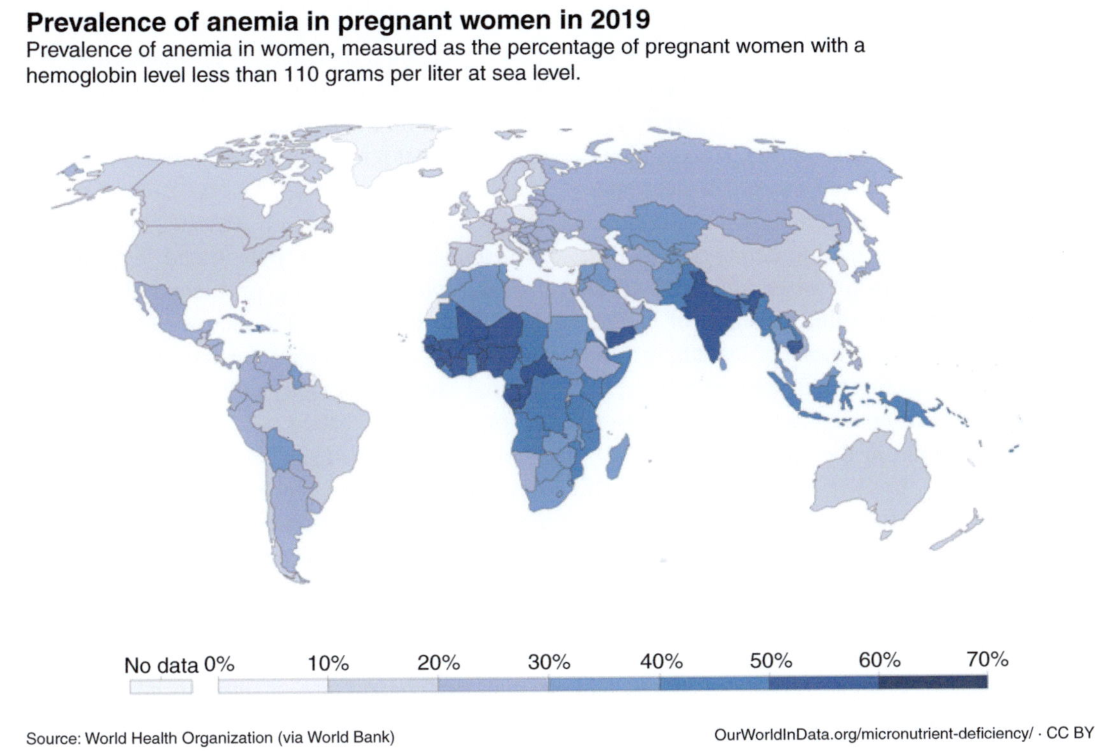

Fig. 7.3 Global prevalence of anemia in pregnant women in 2019

lack of WHO cut points for iron-replete status, the majority of these HIC populations are likely to be iron-replete [11], even among marginalized ethnic groups and low socioeconomic status individuals. Given this LMIC and HIC heterogeneity, concerns persist about the risk of adverse outcomes of high intakes of iron during pregnancy or lactation. Physiologic adaptations for iron homeostasis occur in pregnancy to meet the higher needs for iron [12], and these may potentially enhance risks from high iron intakes in iron-replete individuals, or those with hemoglobinopathies, and with potential consequences for gestational duration, gestational diabetes mellitus, and gastrointestinal health [12–16].

Biology

Anemia

Anemia is defined as a reduced absolute number of circulating erythrocytes [17] or a condition in which their number and/or oxygen-carrying capacity cannot meet physiologic needs [18]. Anemia is most often diagnosed by a low hemoglobin (Hb) concentration or a low hematocrit [17], but can also be diagnosed by erythrocyte count, mean corpuscular volume, blood reticulocyte count, blood film analysis, or Hb electrophoresis [19]. Hb concentration is the most common method and indicator used to define anemia [20]. The main role of Hb for oxygen delivery to the tissues accounts for clinical signs of anemia including fatigue, shortness of breath, palpitations, and conjunctival and palmar pallor [21]. Clinical signs and history can be used to assess the risk of anemia in the absence of laboratory data, but are of limited value [22, 23]. WHO defines anemia for pregnant women with trimester-specific cutoffs of Hb <110 g/L for the first trimester, <105 g/L for the second trimester, and <110 g/L for the third trimester, with the cutoff for severe anemia being <70 g/L. For lactating women anemia is defined as Hb <120 g/L and severe anemia as <80 g/L [18]. Severe anemia is particularly important due to risks for high-output heart failure and death and can exacerbate complications of labor and delivery [17]. Defining Hb concentration cutoffs for pregnancy and lactation has been a challenge and an ongoing process, requiring an understanding of age, gestational age of the pregnancy, genetics, and environmental factors. During pregnancy, because of the expansion of blood volume and consequent dilution effect, Hb concentration naturally declines during the first and second trimesters, rising gradually again in the third trimester [24]. Physiological factors such as hemoglobinopathies, behavior, and environmental conditions, such as altitude, diet, and smoking, all affect Hb concentrations during pregnancy and lactation [18].

Nutrient Deficiencies

Nutritional anemia in pregnancy and lactation occurs when the intake of specific nutrients is unable to meet the demands for synthesis of erythrocytes and hemoglobin, the primary oxygen-carrying molecule in the body [2]. While iron is the most common nutritional deficiency causing anemia, deficiencies of vitamins A, B6, B12, C, D, and E, folate, riboflavin, and copper can also have a role. Diets that are poor in one micronutrient tend to be poor in multiple micronutrients as shown in Fig. 7.4 and can lead to synergistic increased risk of anemia [2]. Risk for nutritional anemia is potentiated by nutrient losses, poor absorption, or increased demand. Infectious diseases tend to increase loss of nutrients due to the acute phase response, or gastrointestinal infections may directly impair gut absorption; and certain specific infections such hookworm which ingest blood, or malaria which destroys erythrocytes, increase demand for nutrients to drive erythropoiesis. Other physiologic conditions may inhibit nutrient absorption, such as the effects of atrophic gastritis on intrinsic factor to facilitate vitamin B12 absorption. And behavioral factors, such as diets high in phytate which can chelate iron or imbalanced intakes of divalent metals such as iron, zinc, copper, calcium, or manganese, which share the same trans-

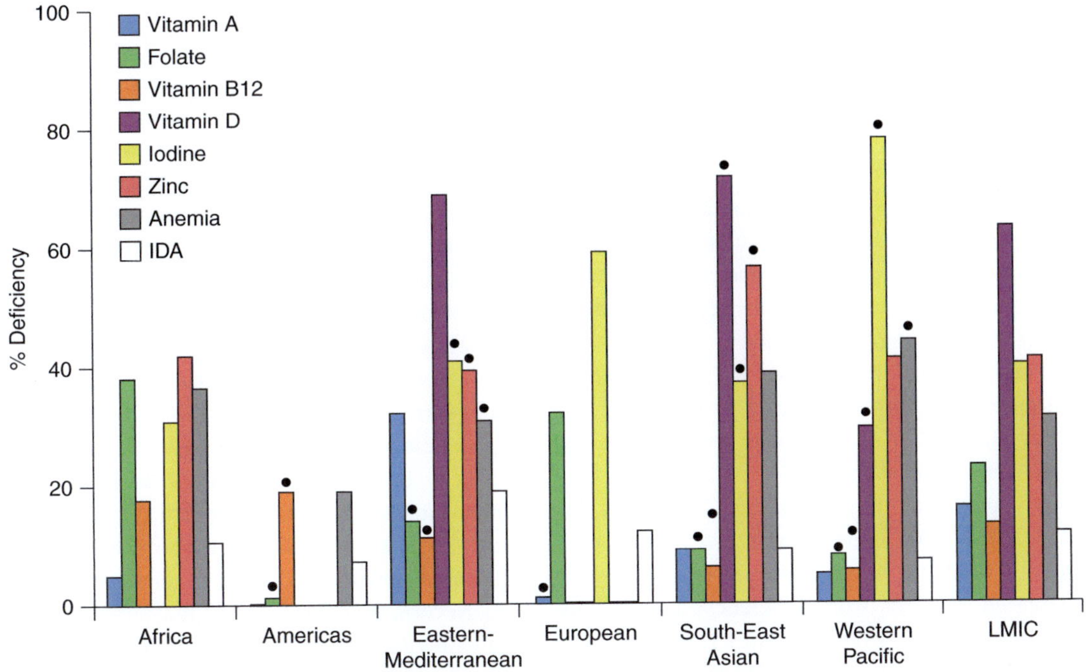

Fig. 7.4 Regional estimates of micronutrient deficiencies and anemia among women of reproductive age. Data are from 52 national and regional surveys published between 2013 and July 2017 using the World Health Organization VMNIS database. Missing bars mean no data were available for that micronutrient in the specific region. *LMIC* low- and middle-income countries; *IDA* iron deficiency anemia. Black circles indicate <3 countries contributed data. (From Bourassa MW, et al. Ann N Y Acad Sci. 2019 May; 1444(1): 6–21)

porter, can interfere with iron and copper absorption and affect anemia. In addition, genetic polymorphisms can impair iron uptake or uptake and metabolism of other nutrients that might influence anemia [25]. Pregnancy and lactation increase the demand for nutrients, thereby exacerbating the impact of the above conditions.

Iron

Iron is the most crucial nutrient required for production of well-functioning erythrocytes. This is due to its central role in synthesis of iron-protoporphyrin or heme, the core oxygen-binding moiety of hemoglobin, which is the primary oxygen-carrying protein within the erythrocyte. When dietary iron intake cannot meet needs and iron stores are depleted, then iron deficiency anemia occurs. Specifically, erythrocyte synthesis is compromised, and intra-erythrocytic hemoglobin and heme decrease, resulting in hypochromic or microcytic anemia. Expansion of maternal blood volume and fetal growth during pregnancy and blood loss during childbirth increase the need for erythrocytes and therefore iron as detailed below. Similarly, the demands of lactation increase the need for many nutrients, some of which affect erythropoiesis.

The physiological demands for elemental iron in pregnancy are high and estimated at 1000–1200 mg overall during gestation [10, 12]. Approximately two-thirds is for maternal adaptations to support the pregnancy, such as erythropoiesis, and the other one-third for placental and fetal needs [12]. Iron needs are lower in the first trimester at 0.8 mg/day, even less than pre-pregnancy, and highest in the third trimester at 3.0–7.5 mg/day [14] due to maternal metabolic and physiologic processes and fetal growth [12]; and the iron needed for fetal growth alone in the third trimester is approximately 330–400 mg. These needs may be met by mobilizing maternal iron stores in replete women, and approximately

300 mg of this total iron is recycled and available to the mother as erythrocytes and blood volume contract postpartum [26]. As such, about 750 mg of additional elemental iron is needed during pregnancy beyond that from maternal stores in replete women. For women with low iron stores, 1000 mg or more of additional iron might be required. Despite these dynamic and progressive physiologic needs, reference intakes for iron tend to average the need across all gestational ages rather than varying by trimester.

Poor maternal iron intake and status reduce the amount of iron transferred to the fetus and infant. Infants of women with iron deficiency anemia may be at increased risk for iron deficiency anemia as shown in some [27, 28] but not all studies [29]. Preterm and low birthweight infants tend to have lower iron stores and increased risk for iron deficiency anemia. As mentioned above, iron deficiency is estimated to contribute approximately 50% of all cases of anemia among pregnant women [3, 4]. However, it is noteworthy that epidemiological studies suggest the proportion of anemia due to iron deficiency was lower in countries where the prevalence of anemia was >40%, and especially in rural populations [30]. Other studies suggest the high prevalence of anemia in women cannot be explained by nutritional anemias nor hemoglobinopathies [31, 32], although severe maternal anemia tends to be more iron-dependent and responsive to supplementation [3]. Nevertheless, approximately half of all anemia cases will have causes other than iron deficiency and will not likely respond to iron supplementation.

The United States, Canada, Australia, and New Zealand recommend 50% higher intakes for pregnant than for nonpregnant women of reproductive age. However, the United Kingdom and Europe suggest no increase, and WHO does not specify intakes for pregnancy, but does recommend supplementation dose as mentioned above. The iron reference intakes therefore vary internationally, with the Recommended Nutrient Intake (RNI) that meets the needs for 97.5% of the population of pregnant women spanning from 11.5 to 27 mg/day.

Vitamin A

Vitamin A has long been recognized for its role in nutritional anemia [33]. It modulates erythropoiesis, thereby directly affecting anemia, and lymphopoiesis, thereby contributing indirectly to anemia caused by infectious diseases [33]. Vitamin A also plays a role in iron metabolism wherein deficiency decreases mobilization of iron from stores in the liver and spleen and contributes to anemia [33]. Anemia due to vitamin A deficiency is therefore accompanied by increased iron stores in the liver and spleen and increased serum ferritin concentrations [34], distinct from iron deficiency anemia with loss of iron stores and decreased serum ferritin. Vitamin A deficiency among pregnant women is prevalent in many LMICs and characterized by low serum vitamin A levels and reported night blindness [35]. Several trials have shown that supplementation with vitamin A or pro-vitamin A carotenoids, or consumption of diets adequate in these nutrients, can increase hemoglobin concentrations without iron supplementation [36].

B Vitamins

B vitamins have ubiquitous and pleiotropic roles during pregnancy and lactation, and several of them may influence anemia. Vitamin B2 (riboflavin) is crucial for iron metabolism, including iron mobilization from stores, iron absorption, and retention of iron [37], and is important for hemoglobin production [36]. Riboflavin deficiency has been documented in pregnant and lactating women and is more prevalent where meat and dairy product consumption is low [38]. Riboflavin supplements, given with iron, have a greater effect on hemoglobin than iron alone [37]. Vitamin B12 (cobalamin) and folate are crucial for DNA synthesis and cell division and therefore erythropoiesis [39]. Deficiencies in these lead to macrocytic anemia. Vitamin B12 deficiency is more prevalent where animal-source food consumption is low, but can also result from malabsorption, particularly for those suffering from gastric atrophy [40]. Estimates of the prevalence of vitamin B12 deficiency place it at approximately 5% [41]. Vitamin B9 (folate) deficiency is more prevalent where unfortified wheat or rice is consumed as a staple and where legume and green leafy vegetable consumption is low [40, 41]. Pregnant and lactating women living in malaria-endemic regions are at higher risk for folate deficiency [36]. Overall, the relative contributions of vitamin B12 or folate deficiency to nutritional anemia in pregnancy and lactating women are greater for women consuming both poor quality and vegetarian diets deficient in vitamin B12 and folate and in places where food fortification is not practiced [42]. It should be noted that vitamin B12 or folate deficiency does not necessarily or always manifest in higher prevalence of anemia [42]. Vitamin B6 (pyridoxine) is crucial for heme synthesis. Deficiency can cause the microcytic and hypochromic anemia, similar in appearance to iron deficiency, as well as normocytic or sideroblastic anemia [36]. The prevalence of vitamin B6 deficiency among pregnant and lactating women tends to be low, but its impact on anemia remains to be fully documented [36].

Vitamins C, D, and E

Vitamin C affects iron metabolism by enhancing absorption of nonheme iron in the gut and improving mobilization of iron stores [36]. Deficiency may exacerbate hemolysis by making erythrocytes more vulnerable to oxidative damage and decreasing integrity of capillaries leading to hemorrhagic blood loss [36]. Vitamin C deficiency is more prevalent in pregnant and lactating women and is exacerbated by smoking or potentially by exposure to smoke from biomass cooking stoves [43]. Supplementation can increase hemoglobin serum ferritin levels even without additional iron [36]. Vitamin D may affect calcitriol production in the bone marrow that supports erythropoiesis [44], although this and other potential mechanisms are poorly understood. Deficiency has been associated with anemia in several studies [44]. Vitamin E limits oxidation of polyunsaturated fatty acids in the erythrocyte membrane, thereby protecting against hemolytic anemia [36]. The impact of this on anemia in pregnancy and lactation is unclear, although clear effects are observed in premature and low birth weight infants or individuals with vitamin E malabsorption syndrome.

Copper

Copper is essential for enzymes needed for iron metabolism, especially for ceruloplasmin which oxidizes ferrous iron and mobilizes stored iron for synthesis of heme and hemoglobin and for erythropoiesis [45]. Copper deficiency can cause normocytic hypochromic and microcytic normochromic anemia [45, 46]. Copper deficiency is rare, but is more prevalent in preterm and low birthweight infants given milk diets, or infants recovering from malnutrition or on prolonged total parenteral nutrition, prolonged diarrhea, or persons with copper malabsorption syndromes [45]. Interestingly, because iron, zinc, and copper share the same intestinal transporter, high iron or zinc intakes can interfere with copper absorption, as can high intakes of other divalent metals such as calcium or manganese.

Overweight and Obesity

Overweight and obesity are on the rise globally, and in pregnant and lactating women, and have been linked with iron deficiency and anemia [46]. One mechanism is suggested to involve hepcidin, a peptide hormone produced primarily in the liver and regulating iron homeostasis [47, 48]. Hepcidin regulates expression of ferroportin-1, the only known iron transporter, which affects plasma iron and iron stores [46]. Higher body iron levels and inflammation increase hepcidin which in turn decreases ferroportin-1 expression, thereby decreasing iron absorption and iron bioavailability in the plasma. Conversely, anemia and hypoxia decease hepcidin which increases ferroportin-1 expression [46]. As such, in obese individuals who suffer from subclinical inflammation, hepcidin levels are elevated leading to poorer iron status despite similar iron intakes as normal-weight persons [47]. Research suggests that iron deficiency in obese or overweight individuals can be due to reduction in iron absorption and mobilization from increased hepcidin production. In addition, while obesity is associated with iron deficiency, hemoglobin concentrations may be within normal [46, 48]. Implications for nutritional anemia in obese or overweight pregnant or lactating women need further research.

Genetic Factors

In addition to the well-documented genetic contribution to anemia from hemoglobinopathies such as sickle cell trait and the thalassemias, the field of nutrigenomics has identified gene mutations and variations that may influence nutritional anemia in pregnancy and lactation. For iron, allelic variants in iron regulatory or transport proteins, such as ferroportin-1 or hepcidin, have been observed in some ethnic subpopulations and may enhance susceptibility to either high iron stores or iron deficiency [49]. Similarly, investigation of several of the nutrients contributing to nutritional anemia has led to discovery of genetic variants [35]. Vitamin A deficiency has been shown to vary between different ethnic groups, which may be causally associated with genetic variants conferring risk for low retinol levels [50]. Similarly, polymorphisms in the genes encoding the two sodium-dependent vitamin C transporter proteins (SVCT1 and SVCT2) are strongly associated with vitamin C status due to their roles in direct transport, absorption, and vitamin C accumulation in tissues. Genetic variants of proteins participating in vitamin D metabolism, its binding to receptors, and transport can impact vitamin D availability and status [51]. For vitamin E, genetic variations can influence vitamin E status by impairing metabolism, absorption and uptake, transport, and liver storage or catabolism. For the B vitamins, several polymorphisms in genes encoding enzymes and transport proteins of folate metabolism are reported to affect folate status. Moreover, vitamin B12 genes have been identified related to co-factors, regulators of vitamin transport, and membrane cobalamin transporters. Other factors have been discovered involved in enzymatic reactions of the one-carbon cycle such as methylenetetrahydrofolate reductase (MTHFR), which is also a riboflavin-dependent enzyme, and in the methionine cycle where 5-methyl-THF is used by methionine synthase (MTR) and methionine synthase reductase encoded by MTRR gene that is required for the reactivation of MTR, a process that supports vitamin B12-dependent conversion of homocysteine to methionine and the formation of tetrahydrofolate (THF). These illustrate how genetic variations may affect nutritional anemia during pregnancy and lactation [35].

Interventions

As indicated herein, the causes of maternal anemia and nutritional anemia in pregnant and lactating women are multifactorial. They arise from poor nutrition, infection, chronic diseases, and genetic etiologies. A recent synthesis and meta-review aimed to assess the impact of nutrition-specific interventions and nutrition-sensitive interventions [52]. For pregnant women, the authors concluded that daily iron-folic acid supplementation and use of insecticide-treated bednets were associated with increased Hb concentration and reduced risk of anemia, and delayed cord clamping at birth was associated with improved Hb status in the newborn. Other interventions in children indicated benefits of micronutrient powders, malaria treatment, daily and intermittent iron supplementation, and deworming. The meta-review highlighted the relative lack of evidence from multifaceted interventions in pregnant and lactating women with regard to either nutrition-specific or nutrition-sensitive approaches.

Supplementation with Iron and Other Micronutrients

Iron and other micronutrient supplements for adolescents found a 31% reduction in anemia when iron was given with or without other micronutrients (RR, 0.69; 95% CI, 0.62, 0.76) [52]. A similar result in pregnant women was seen when either multiple micronutrient supplements or iron, with or without folic acid, was provided [53]. This was echoed in the analysis of the impact of maternal multiple micronutrient supplementation (MMS), typically the UNIMMAP preparation [54], which showed it to be equivalent to iron and folic acid alone (RR = 0.98; 95% CI, 0.86, 1.11) [55]. A recent paper came to the same conclusion wherein the effects on maternal anemia of the UNIMMAP MMS containing 30 mg iron were the same as iron and folic supplements with 60 mg iron (RR = 0.99; 95% CI, 0.92–1.07), thereby highlighting the importance of other nutrients in anemia reduction [56]. Another analysis showed that vitamin A supplementation during pregnancy was associated with a reduced risk of anemia (RR = 0.64; 95% CI, 0.43, 0.94) [57]. A review of vitamin B12 supplementation [58] reported an increase in Hb concentration in women and children, and another review concluded that vitamin C supplementation increased Hb concentrations in children and nonpregnant women, but not in pregnant women [36], and another review reported no difference in Hb concentrations in pregnant women given zinc supplements [59].

Other Nutrition-Related Interventions

The meta-review addressed additional nutrition-specific and nutrition-sensitive interventions [52]. For *food fortification* overall effects were associated with increases in Hb concentration, but there were no specific data on the impact on anemia in pregnant or lactating women. For *dietary diversity*, of seven studies reviewed, there were two animal-source food interventions showing a decrease in anemia, but none were in pregnant or lactating women, and only one was in nonpregnant women in Peru. One review on consumption of animal-source foods in adults reported a positive association on Hb concentrations with intakes of 85–300 g/day. *Agriculture and food security* interventions typically evaluated the impact of home gardens, aquaculture and small fisheries, dairy development, and raising of livestock, but again no data were available for pregnant or lactating women. However, nonsignificant reductions in anemia in women were reported in one study. For *family planning* two of five studies of birth spacing on maternal anemia showed an increased risk of maternal anemia for birth intervals less than <24 months. *Conditional cash transfers* were also reviewed, and all three showed improvements in child Hb levels, but again no specific data on pregnant or lactating women was presented.

Conclusions

Nutritional anemia affecting pregnant and lactating women remains a substantial problem globally, and progress over the last decade has been slow. Although the etiologies are complex, it is clear that iron supplementation alone can have a substantial effect in most settings in LMICs, reducing anemia levels by up to 50% if adherence to supplementation is adequate. In addition, although it has long been known that other nutrients can contribute to nutritional anemia, the transition to universal MMS has been slow despite the benefits offered for anemia, and for newborn birth weight, preterm birth, and infant mortality, especially for girl babies and infants of women who are anemic [60, 61]. Other relationships also need to be explored, for example, it has recently been observed that the gut microbiome may play an important role in anemia in pregnancy by promoting hematopoiesis and modulating levels of short-chain fatty acids (SCFAs) that affect bone marrow and immune function [62]. And as mentioned, control of inflammation and infectious diseases can have an important role in nutritional modulation of anemia.

However, in regard to nutritional supplements, we note that formulating the proper composition may not be sufficient to attain impact. Indeed, the majority of iron and folic acid supplementation programs have not achieved high coverage or compliance of 80% or more. This may be due, in part, to the program designs based on one-dimensional solutions that lack person-centered design and promotion of a product, such as iron folic acid supplements or MMS, that are appealing to women. For example, it has been observed that the cheapest product may not always be the most cost-effective one and that investments to define the supplement product design, packaging, and appearance can lead to high compliance and high impact [63].

Beyond the product itself is the means of delivery and engagement with pregnant and lactating women. The current push for digital tools provides strong potential to enhance tracking and customized targeting of complex interventions that would combine a well-designed nutritional product with health promotion messages and integrate this with apps for antenatal care to optimize service delivery, such as with the WHO ANC app [64]. Further customization would be possible with frontline assessment for anemia and specific nutrient deficiencies using rapid tests linked with readers for rapid processing and point-of-care decision support to avoid potential inadequate or over-supplementation [65]. Moreover, linking these tools into a system of well-trained frontline health workers is likely to further enhance impact [66], especially if multiple frontline workers can be coordinated as teams to optimally support more complex nutrition-specific and nutrition-sensitive interventions for pregnant and lactating women. These approaches would likely also fill the substantial gaps in knowledge of what works or not to reduce nutritional anemia in pregnant and lactating women.

Currently, novel solutions are needed in the context of precision medicine and precision public health and to adopt more preventive and promotive approaches. As mentioned above, focusing more on local innovations, rather than traditional top-down approaches from global organizations, may be more likely to be successful. The post-pandemic world is an opportunity to forge new pathways with organizations at the grass roots creating local solutions with global impact.

References

1. World Health Organization. World-wide prevalence of anaemia 1993–2005: WHO global database on anaemia. Geneva, Switzerland: WHO Press; 2005.
2. Stevens GA, Finucane MM, De-Regil LM, Paciorek CJ, Flaxman SR, Branca F, et al. Global, regional, and national trends in haemoglobin concentration and prevalence of total and severe anaemia in children and pregnant and non-pregnant women for 1995–2011: a systematic analysis of population-representative data. Lancet Glob Health. 2013;1(1):e16–25. https://doi.org/10.1016/s2214-109x(13)70001-9.
3. Balarajan Y, Ramakrishnan U, Özaltin E, Shankar AH, Subramanian SV. Anaemia in low-income and middle-income countries. Lancet. 2011;378(9809):2123–35. https://doi.org/10.1016/s0140-6736(10)62304-5.
4. The global prevalence of anaemia in 2011. Geneva: World Health Organization; 2015. http://apps.who.int/iris/bitstream/10665/177094/1/9789241564960_eng.pdf?ua=1&ua=1. Accessed 21 May 2022.
5. Assessing the iron status of populations. Second edition including literature reviews. Report of a Joint World Health Organization/Centers for Disease Control and Prevention technical consultation on the assessment of iron status at the population level, Geneva, Switzerland, 6–8 April 2004. Geneva: World Health Organization; 2007. http://apps.who.int/iris/bitstream/10665/75368/1/9789241596107_eng.pdf?ua=1&ua=1. Accessed 21 May 2022.
6. Petry N, Olofin I, Hurrell RF, Boy E, Wirth JP, Moursi M, Donahue AM, Rohner F. The proportion of anemia associated with iron deficiency in low, medium, and high human development index countries: a systematic analysis of national surveys. Nutrients. 2016;8:693.
7. World Health Organization. Daily iron supplementation in children 6–23 months of age. https://apps.who.int/iris/rest/bitstreams/909299/retrieve. Accessed 21 May 2022.
8. World Health Organization. Who recommendations on antenatal care for a positive pregnancy experience. https://apps.who.int/iris/rest/bitstreams/1064182/retrieve. Accessed 21 May 2022.
9. Gupta PM, Hamner HC, Suchdev PS, Flores-Ayala R, Mei Z. Iron deficiency and adequacy in young children, non-pregnant, and pregnant women in the United States. Am J Clin Nutr. 2017;106:1640S–6S.
10. Milman N, Taylor C, Merkel J, Brannon P. Iron status in pregnant women and women of reproductive age in Europe. Am J Clin Nutr. 2017;106:1655S–62S.
11. Taylor CL, Brannon PM. Introduction to workshop on iron screening and supplementation in iron-replete pregnant women and young children. Am J Clin Nutr. 2017;106:1547S–54S.
12. Fisher AL, Nemeth E. Iron homeostasis during pregnancy. Am J Clin Nutr. 2017;106:1567S–74S.

13. Lönnerdal B. Development of iron homeostasis in infants and young children. Am J Clin Nutr. 2017;106:1575S–80S.
14. Bothwell TH. Iron requirements in pregnancy and strategies to meet them. Am J Clin Nutr. 2000;72:257S–64S.
15. Zhang C, Rawal S. Dietary iron intake, iron status and gestational diabetes. Am J Clin Nutr. 2017;106:1672S–80S.
16. Paganini D, Zimmermann MB. The effects of iron fortification and supplementation on the gut microbiome and diarrhea in infants and children: a review. Am J Clin Nutr. 2017;106:1688S–93S.
17. Schreir SL. Approach to the adult patient with anemia. In Mentzer WC, editor. Waltham, MA: UpToDate Inc.; 2018.
18. World Health Organization. Haemoglobin concentrations for the diagnosis of anaemia and assessment of severity. 2011. https://apps.who.int/iris/bitstream/handle/10665/85839/WHO_NMH_NHD_MNM_11.1_eng.pdf?sequence=22&isAllowed=y. Accessed 21 May 2022.
19. Balarajan Y, Ramakrishnan U, Özaltin E, et al. Nutritional anaemias: tools for effective prevention and control. Geneva: World Health Organization; 2017. Licence: CC BY-NC-SA 3.0 IGO.
20. Centers for Disease Control. CDC criteria for anemia n children and childbearing-aged women. MMWR Morb MortalWkly Rep. 1989;38:400–4.
21. World Health Organization. Pregnancy, childbirth, postpartum and newborn care: a guide for essential practice. Geneva: World Health Organization; 2003.
22. World Health Organization. Handbook: IMCI integrated management of childhood illness. Geneva: World Health Organization; 2005.
23. Chalco JP, Huicho L, Alamo C, et al. Accuracy of clinical pallor in the diagnosis of anaemia in children: a meta-analysis. BMC Pediatr. 2005;5:46.
24. International Nutritional Anemia Consultative Group (INACG). Adjusting hemoglobin values in program surveys. INACG/USAID; 2002.
25. Niforou A, Konstantinidou V, Naska A. Genetic variants shaping inter-individual differences in response to dietary intakes—a narrative review of the case of vitamins. Front Nutr. 2020;7:558598. https://doi.org/10.3389/fnut.2020.558598.
26. Vricella LK. Emerging understanding and measurement of plasma volume expansion in pregnancy. Am J Clin Nutr. 2017;106:1620S–5S.
27. Colomer J, Colomer C, Gutierrez D, Jubert A, Nolasco A, Donat J, et al. Anaemia during pregnancy as a risk factor for infant iron deficiency: report from the Valencia Infant Anaemia Cohort (VIAC) study. Paediatr Perinat Epidemiol. 1990;4(2):196–204.
28. Kilbride J, Baker TG, Parapia LA, Khoury SA, Shuqaidef SW, Jerwood D. Anaemia during pregnancy as a risk factor for iron deficiency anaemia in infancy: a case-control study in Jordan. Int J Epidemiol. 1999;28(3):461–8. https://doi.org/10.1093/ije/28.3.461.
29. Ziegler EE, Nelson SE, Jeter JM. Iron stores of breastfed infants during the first year of life. Nutrients. 2014;6(5):2023–34. https://doi.org/10.3390/nu6052023.
30. Petry N, Olofin I, Hurrell R, Boy E, Wirth J, Moursi M, et al. The proportion of anemia associated with iron deficiency in low, medium, and high human development index countries: a systematic analysis of national surveys. Nutrients. 2016;8(11):693–701.
31. Karakochuk C, Whitfield K, Barr S, Lamers Y, Devlin A, Vercauteren S, et al. Genetic hemoglobin disorders rather than iron deficiency are a major predictor of hemoglobin concentration in women of reproductive age in rural prey Veng, Cambodia. J Nutr. 2015;145(1):134–42. https://doi.org/10.3945/jn.114.198945.
32. Wieringa F, Dahl M, Chamnan C, Poirot E, Kuong K, Sophonneary P, et al. The high prevalence of anemia in Cambodian children and women cannot be satisfactorily explained by nutritional deficiencies or hemoglobin disorders. Nutrients. 2016;8(6):348–60. https://doi.org/10.3390/nu8060348.
33. Semba RD, Bloem MW. The anemia of vitamin A deficiency: epidemiology and pathogenesis. Eur J Clin Nutr. 2002;56(4):271–81. https://doi.org/10.1038/sj.ejcn.1601320.
34. Michelazzo FB, Oliveira JM, Stefanello J, Luzia LA, Rondo PH. The influence of vitamin A supplementation on iron status. Nutrients. 2013;5(11):4399–413. https://doi.org/10.3390/nu5114399.
35. Maia SB, Souza ASR, de Fátima Costa Caminha M, da Silva SL, de Sá Barreto Luna Callou Cruz R, Dos Santos CC, Filho MB. Vitamin A and pregnancy: a narrative review. Nutrients. 2019;11(3):681. https://doi.org/10.3390/nu11030681.
36. Fishman SM, Christian P, West KP. The role of vitamins in the prevention and control of anaemia. Public Health Nutr. 2000.
37. Rohner F, Zimmermann MB, Wegmueller R, Tschannen AB, Hurrell RF. Mild riboflavin deficiency is highly prevalent in school-age children but does not increase risk for anaemia in Cote d'Ivoire. Br J Nutr. 2007;97(5):970–6. https://doi.org/10.1017/s0007114507665180.
38. Powers HJ. Riboflavin (vitamin B-2) and health. Am J Clin Nutr. 2003;77(6):1352–60.
39. Field MS, Kamynina E, Chon J, Stover PJ. Nuclear folate metabolism. Annu Rev Nutr. 2018;38:219–43. https://doi.org/10.1146/annurev-nutr-071714-034441.
40. Allen LH. Causes of vitamin B12 and folate deficiency. Food Nutr Bull. 2008;29(2 Suppl):S20–34.
41. McLean E, de Benoist B, Allen LH. Review of the magnitude of folate and vitamin B12 deficiencies worldwide. Food Nutr Bull. 2008;29(2 Suppl):S38–51. https://doi.org/10.1177/15648265080292S107.
42. Metz J. A high prevalence of biochemical evidence of vitamin B12 or folate deficiency does not translate

into a comparable prevalence of anemia. Food Nutr Bull. 2008;29(2 Suppl):S74–85.

43. Page CM, Patel A, Hibberd PL. Does smoke from biomass fuel contribute to anemia in pregnant women in Nagpur, India? A cross-sectional study. PLoS One. 2015;10(5):e0127890. https://doi.org/10.1371/journal.pone.0127890.
44. Atkinson MA, Melamed ML, Kumar J, Roy CN, Miller ER 3rd, Furth SL, et al. Vitamin D, race, and risk for anemia in children. J Pediatr. 2014;164(1):153–8.e151. https://doi.org/10.1016/j.jpeds.2013.08.060.
45. Turnlund JR. Copper. In: Shils ME, Olson JA, Shike M, Ross AC, editors. Modern nutrition in health and disease. Philadelphia: Lippincott Williams & Wilkins; 1999. p. 241–52.
46. Tussing-Humphreys L, Pusatcioglu C, Nemeth E, Braunschweig C. Rethinking iron regulation and assessment in iron deficiency, anemia of chronic disease, and obesity: introducing hepcidin. J Acad Nutr Diet. 2012;112(3):391–400. https://doi.org/10.1016/j.jada.2011.08.038.
47. Aeberli I, Hurrell RF, Zimmermann MB. Overweight children have higher circulating hepcidin concentrations and lower iron status but have dietary iron intakes and bioavailability comparable with normal weight children. Int J Obes. 2009;33(10):1111–7. https://doi.org/10.1038/ijo.2009.146.
48. Cepeda-Lopez AC, Aeberli I, Zimmermann MB. Does obesity increase risk for iron deficiency? A review of the literature and the potential mechanisms. Int J Vit Nutr Res. 2010;80(45):263–70. https://doi.org/10.1024/0300-9831/a000033.
49. Gordeuk VR, Brannon PM. Ethnic and genetic factors of iron status in women of reproductive age. Am J Clin Nutr. 2017;106:1594S–9S.
50. Suzuki M, Wang T, Garretto D, Isasi CR, Cardoso WV, Greally JM, Quadro L. Disproportionate Vitamin A deficiency in women of specific ethnicities linked to differences in allele frequencies of vitamin A-related polymorphisms. Nutrients. 2021;13:1743. https://doi.org/10.3390/nu13061743.
51. Szili B, Szabó B, Horváth P, Bakos B, Kirschner G, Kósa JP, Toldy E, Putz Z, Lakatos P, Tabák A, Takács A. Impact of genetic influence on serum total- and free 25-hydroxyvitamin-D in humans. J Steroid Biochem Mol Biol. 2018;183:62–7. https://doi.org/10.1016/j.jsbmb.2018.05.007.
52. Moorthy D, Merrill R, Namaste S. Iannotti L The impact of nutrition-specific and nutrition-sensitive interventions on hemoglobin concentrations and anemia: a meta-review of systematic reviews. Adv Nutr. 2020;11:1631–45.
53. Allen LH, Peerson JM, Olney DK. Provision of multiple rather than two or fewer micronutrients more effectively improves growth and other outcomes in micronutrient deficient children and adults. J Nutr. 2009;139:1022–30.
54. Bourassa MW, Osendarp SJM, Adu-Afarwuah S, Ahmed S, Ajello C, Bergeron G, et al. Review of the evidence regarding the use of antenatal multiple micronutrient supplementation in low- and middle-income countries. Ann N Y Acad Sci. 2019;1444(1):6–21.
55. Oh C, Keats EC, Bhutta ZA. Vitamin and mineral supplementation during pregnancy on maternal, birth, child health and development outcomes in low- and middle-income countries: a systematic review and meta-analysis. Nutrients. 2020;12(2):491. https://doi.org/10.3390/nu12020491.
56. Gomes F, Agustina R, Black RE, Christian P, Dewey KG, Kraemer K, Shankar AH, Smith ER, Thorne-Lyman A, Tumilowicz A, Bourassa MW. (2022). Multiple micronutrient supplements versus iron-folic acid supplements and maternal anemia outcomes: an iron dose analysis. Ann N Y Acad Sci. 2022. https://doi.org/10.1111/nyas.14756.
57. McCauley ME, van den Broek N, Dou L, Othman M. Vitamin A supplementation during pregnancy for maternal and newborn outcomes. Cochrane Database Syst Rev. 2015;(10):CD008666.
58. Swaminathan S, Thomas T, Kurpad AV. B-vitamin interventions for women and children in low-income populations. Curr Opin Clin Nutr Metab Care. 2015;18:295–306.
59. Villar J, Merialdi M, Gulmezoglu AM, Abalos E, Carroli G, Kulier R, de Onis M. Nutritional interventions during pregnancy for the prevention or treatment of maternal morbidity and preterm delivery: an overview of randomized controlled trials. J Nutr. 2003;133(5 Suppl 2):1606S–25S.
60. Supplementation with Multiple Micronutrients Intervention Trial (SUMMIT) Study Group, Shankar AH, Jahari AB, Sebayang SK, Aditiawarman, Apriatni M, Harefa B, Muadz H, Soesbandoro SD, Tjiong R, Fachry A, Shankar AV, Atmarita, Prihatini S, Sofia G. Effect of maternal multiple micronutrient supplementation on fetal loss and infant death in Indonesia: a double-blind cluster-randomised trial. Lancet. 2008;371:215–27.
61. Smith ER, Shankar AH, Wu LS, Aboud S, Adu-Afarwuah S, Ali H, et al. Modifiers of the effect of maternal multiple micronutrient supplementation on stillbirth, birth outcomes, and infant mortality: a meta-analysis of individual patient data from 17 randomised trials in low-income and middle-income countries. Lancet Glob Health. 2017;5(11):e1090–100.
62. Long Y, Liang F, Guo R, Zhu C, Zhao X, Wang X, Liu F, Jiang M, Liang Q, Zeng S, Han M, Qin J, Li S, Li S, Yang H. Gut microbiota signatures in gestational anemia. Front Cell Infect Microbiol. 2021;11:549678. https://doi.org/10.3389/fcimb.2021.549678.
63. Permatasari IK, Syah IF, Guntjoro R, Sadhu S, Odipatra R, Satria A, Widowati F, Nurjannah, Ramdhani NI, Shankar AH. Better quality for better impact: optimized packaging and appearance of maternal multiple micronutrient supplements for pregnant women in Indonesia. 2020. https://sightandlife.org/wp-content/uploads/2020/04/SightandLife_SpecialReport_MMS_2020_Better-Quality-for-Better-Impact.pdf. Accessed 22 May 2022.

64. Haddad SM, Souza RT, Cecatti JG, Barreix M, Tamrat T, Gulas C, Mehl G, Syah IF, Shankar AH, Tuncalp O. Building a mobile application of the WHO antenatal care recommendations: methodological intersection between evidence, clinical logic and digital technology. J Med Internet Res. 2020;22:e16355.
65. Lubell-Doughtie P, Bhatt S, Wong R, Shankar AH. Transforming rapid diagnostic tests for precision public health: open guidelines for manufacturers and users. JMIR Biomed Eng. 2022;7(2):e26800. https://doi.org/10.2196/26800.
66. Shankar AV, Zaitu A, Kadha JK, Sebayang SK, Apriatni M, Sulastri A, Sunarsih E, Shankar AH. Programmatic effects of a large scale multiple micronutrient supplementation trial in Indonesia: using community facilitators as intermediaries for behavior change. Food Nutr Bull. 2009;30:S207–14.

8 Nutritional Anemia in the Elderly

Susan J. Fairweather-Tait

Keywords

Anemia · Hemoglobin · Elderly · Iron · Folate
Vitamin B_{12}

Definition of Elderly

The term "elderly" refers to chronological age, and most developed countries categorize elderly people as aged 60 or 65 years and over [1]. However, the ageing process is not uniform both between and within populations due to differences in genetics, lifestyle, and overall health [2]. At the biological level, ageing results from the impact of accumulated molecular and cellular damage over time, but these changes are not linear or consistent and not closely associated with chronological age. During the process of ageing, there is a gradual decrease in physical and mental capacity and a growing risk of disease, and this leads, eventually, to death. In 2020, the global number of people aged 65 years or over was 727 million, and this is expected to double by 2050 [3]. Currently, elderly people account for 9.3% of the global population, but by 2050, this figure is expected to increase to 16% [3]. Healthy ageing is defined by WHO as "the process of developing and maintaining the functional ability that enables wellbeing in older age" [4]. There is growing recognition of the importance of healthy ageing, and, coupled with the current demographic changes, this may lead to a revised definition of "elderly," taking account of different health characteristics as well as number of years since birth.

Diagnosis of Anemia

The World Health Organization (WHO) defines anemia for people living at sea level as mild, moderate, or severe [5], according to the Hb concentration (g/L):

- Men (15 years of age and above): mild 110–129 g/L, moderate 80–109 g/L, severe <80 g/L.
- Women (15 years and above): mild 110–119 g/L, moderate 80–109 g/L, severe <80 g/L.

However, the appropriateness of these values, which were developed more than 40 years ago, has been questioned. Data from the 1999–2012 National Health and Nutrition Examination Survey (NHANES) show that Hb reference intervals decrease with age in men aged 20–79 years, whereas female reference intervals are essentially stable, but with a slight increase after the meno-

S. J. Fairweather-Tait (✉)
Norwich Medical School, University of East Anglia, Norwich, UK
e-mail: s.fairweather-tait@uea.ac.uk

C. D. Karakochuk et al. (eds.), *Nutritional Anemia*, Nutrition and Health,
https://doi.org/10.1007/978-3-031-14521-6_8

Table 8.1 Examples of the effects of age, sex, and ethnicity on Hb concentration

(a) Age- and sex-specific reference limits for Hb concentration (g/L) (adapted from [7])

	Male Percentiles				Female Percentiles			
Age (years)	*n*	2.5th	50th	97.5th	*n*	2.5th	50th	97.5th
60–70	44,403	130	149	169	52,374	120	137	155
70–80	35,735	123	145	167	43,718	117	135	154
80–90	12,095	115	141	166	17,191	112	133	154
90–100	932	110	134	164	2442	107	130	153

(b) Hb concentrations (g/L) of healthy adult women: data from NHANES and NDNS stratified by race (adapted from [9])

	n	Mean ± SD	Derived cut-off
White	5231	135.9 ± 10.1	119.2
Black	2707	126.0 ± 12.1	106.0
Mexican and Hispanic	3356	132.7 ± 11.0	114.2
Asian	575	129.9 ± 10.7	112.2

pause [6]. Recently, Zierk et al. (2020) applied a data mining approach to a large dataset of 3,029,904 clinical samples collected for routine blood counts in Germany between 2012 and 2017. After exclusion of abnormal samples (e.g., raised CRP), reference intervals were calculated from an indirect algorithm described and validated previously. The strength of this approach is that it uses data from a "real world" population to which the reference intervals are ultimately applied, while still excluding outliers. There was a significant fall in Hb concentration every decade for men ($p < 0.001$) and women ($p < 0.05$) as shown in Table 8.1. They concluded that men's Hb, hematocrit, and red cell count reference intervals decline continuously with age, whereas changes in women start later and are less pronounced. Milman et al. (2007) also reported a significant age-related decline in Hb concentration in both men and women [8].

In addition, separate cut-offs for diagnosing anemia, based on ethnicity/race, have been proposed. Individuals of African descent have lower Hb concentrations than Caucasian populations, partially due to the greater prevalence of genetic Hb disorders in persons of African descent. Varghese et al. [9] examined the Hb distributions in nine rounds of the National Health and Nutrition Examination Survey (NHANES) and two rounds of the UK National Diet and Nutrition Survey (NDNS), and the mean Hb concentrations of Blacks, Mexicans and Hispanics, and Asians were lower than concentrations in Whites (Table 8.1). The WHO cut-off for anemia, defined as the value corresponding to the 4.95th percentile of a healthy reference population, was estimated separately for each ethnic group. Based on the pooled analysis, the derived Hb cut-off was lower for Mexican/Hispanic, Blacks, and Asians, whereas the cut-off for Whites was comparable to the WHO-recommended cut point of 120 g/L. For men aged 60 years and over, Beutler and Waalen (2006) proposed a Hb cut-off value of 132 g/L for white men and 127 g/L for black men [10]. However, the WHO cut-off values are still the gold standard because there is, as yet, no official recommendation to change them for older people.

Prevalence and Pathogenesis of Anemia in the Elderly

Anemia affects one third of the world's population [11] and is particularly common in young children and women of reproductive age. In adults, the prevalence increases with age and is affected by health status and environmental factors, primarily the diet [12]. Sub-Saharan Africa, South Asia, the Caribbean, and Oceania had the highest anemia prevalence across all age groups and both sexes in 2010 [13]. Large prospective registry studies observe mild anemia in 10–24% of people aged 65 years and over [14]. Elderly patients admitted to hospital are more frequently affected by anemia, and the prevalence is even higher in nursing home residents [14]. Assuming a global prevalence of 17%, it is likely that 15 million older people suffer from anemia in Europe with a similar level in the USA [14]. In people older than 80 years, it is estimated that approximately 50% are anemic [15] (Table 8.2).

Anemia in the elderly is often multifactorial due to the presence of multiple concomitant morbidities which increase with advancing age. At least one third of anemias are the result of iron deficiency, and folate and vitamin B12 deficiencies are not uncommon [16]. Other etiologies include CKD insufficiency and chronic inflammation, but around one third of cases are unexplained [16]. The mean corpuscular volume is an essential diagnostic tool as it distinguishes between nutritional anemias (microcytic or macrocytic red cells) and those resulting from chronic inflammation, renal failure, and unknown causes (normocytic red cells).

Table 8.2 Conditions that may lead to nutritional anemia in the elderly

Factors	
Dietary	
Nutrient deficiencies	Consequence
Iron	IDA (iron deficiency anemia) [12]
Folate	Folate deficiency (megaloblastic anemia) [18]
Vitamin B12	B_{12} deficiency (megaloblastic anemia) [19]
Riboflavin	EGRac ≥1.4 weakly associated with presence of anemia [20]
Copper	Copper deficiency anemia [21, 22]
Vitamin C	Scurvy (normocytic anemia) [23]
Physiological	
Loss of appetite, malnutrition	IDA, folate, and B_{12} deficiency [24]
Achlorhydria, *Helicobacter pylori*, gastritis	IDA and B_{12} deficiency [25]
Blood loss	IDA [26]
Regular intake of medications, e.g., aspirin, ibuprofen	IDA [27]
Prescribed drugs, e.g., antimetabolites and anticoagulants	Folate deficiency [14]

Serum ferritin concentrations below 19 μg/L are highly suggestive of iron deficiency anemia [17]. However, serum ferritin concentrations are elevated in the presence of infection and inflammation, conditions that are quite common in the elderly population. Raised C-reactive protein (>5 mg/L) or α-1-acid glycoprotein concentrations (>1 g/L) are used to diagnose infection or inflammation, and there are methods proposed for adjusting for this to estimate iron stores (see Chap. 5). The soluble transferrin receptor-ferritin index can be used to distinguish between iron deficiency anemia and other types of anemia; an index of more than 1.5 supports the diagnosis of iron deficiency anemia [17]. Fecal occult blood tests will detect GI blood loss. In the absence of iron deficiency anemia, the most likely cause of microcytic or normocytic anemia is anemia of chronic disease, which is unrelated to nutritional deficiencies.

Vitamin B deficiencies are more pronounced in the elderly, and a peripheral blood smear and reticulocyte count are the initial steps in evaluating the cause of macrocytic anemia (see Chap. 13). Serum vitamin B_{12} and folate concentrations should then be measured. When these are borderline, elevated methylmalonic acid signifies vitamin B_{12} deficiency, and high homocysteine indicates folate deficiency.

Iron deficiency is the most common [12], followed by folate [18] and vitamin B_{12} [19] deficiencies. Clinical riboflavin deficiency occurs mainly in low-income countries, where it is associated with anemia, but suboptimal riboflavin status is also associated with lower hemoglobin and higher rates of anemia [20]. Riboflavin deficiency impairs red blood cell synthesis by altering flavin-dependent release of iron from stores, decreasing iron absorption, and increasing the rate of iron loss from the gastrointestinal tract. Additionally, riboflavin deficiency can affect Hb production through impaired flavin-dependent synthesis of 5′-phosphate, which is required for the first step in heme biosynthesis. Copper deficiency is rare [21] but can result in microcytic, normocytic, or macrocytic anemia. Zinc supplements or high intakes, e.g., from denture adhesives that contain zinc, exacerbate copper deficiency and cause zinc-induced copper deficiency anemia [22]. Vitamin C deficiency can also cause anemia [23].

A summary of physiological causes of anemia includes factors that affect the supply of key nutrients and the functioning of the GI tract, including loss of appetite and malnutrition [24], achlorhydria, *H. pylori* infection and gastritis [25], and blood loss [26]. The regular ingestion of nonsteroidal anti-inflammatory medications is another cause [27], and prescribed antimetabolite/anticoagulant drugs can cause folate deficiency [14].

Iron Deficiency

One of the most common causes of iron deficiency anemia in low- and middle-income countries is low iron bioavailability [12, 28]. This is not the case for older adults in high-income countries as Western diets generally contain iron of higher bioavailability. An example of supporting evidence is a study in 80-year-old Danish men and women whose iron intake and/or bioavailability of dietary iron was adequate to maintain a "favorable" iron status. There was a low prevalence of iron deficiency and a moderate prevalence of iron overload, and the use of vitamin-mineral supplements containing iron had no influence on iron status [29].

Intakes of iron vary widely between individuals and countries, but there is a consistent downward trend with age, most noticeably in the very old (≥85 years), which mirrors falling energy expenditure. Appetite may decrease, and types of food eaten may change as people age, in association with social change such as reduced mobility (which affects shopping and cooking), dental and digestive problems, financial constraints, mental health (e.g., depression and dementia), and bereavement. In the UK, mean daily iron intakes of 11.5, 10.6, and 10.1 mg were reported for 65–74-, 75–84-, and ≥ 85-year-old elderly people, respectively; in Denmark, intakes were 11.8 and 9.7 mg/day for 65–74- and 75–80-year-olds, respectively [30]. When energy requirements are lower, unless the micronutrient density of the diet is increased, micronutrient intakes will also fall. The major sources of bioavailable iron in the diet are meat, fish, poultry, and green vegetables. If elderly people consume less of these and rely more on ultra-processed foods that do not contain much iron, and cereal foods, especially wholegrain products that contain phytate (which reduces iron bioavailability), then they will be at risk of becoming iron deficient.

There is very little information regarding the effects of ageing on iron absorption from the GI tract. One investigation carried out many years ago proposed that malabsorption was the most significant cause of low serum iron and Hb levels [31]. Another more recent study reported that iron malabsorption diseases (atrophic body gastritis, Hp-related pangastritis, and celiac disease) affect almost 60% of early (65–74 years) and late (>75 years) elderly groups [32].

The widespread age-related decline in kidney function is accompanied by reduced secretion of erythropoietin (a signalling molecule that stimulates the production of red blood cells, decreases hepcidin expression, and enhances iron absorption), and this will eventually lead to anemia. Treatment includes iron supplements and erythropoietin-stimulating agents. In the USA, data from the NHANES showed that 14% of adults had chronic kidney disease (CKD) and that anemia was twice as common in this group (15.4%) than in the general population (7.6%). The prevalence of anemia increased with stage of CKD, from 8.4% at stage 1 to 53.4% at stage 5 [33].

Folate Deficiency

Anemia due to folate deficiency is less common than iron deficiency, but, like iron, it increases with age [34]. Deficiency in elderly people usually arises because of inadequate levels of intake and a restricted diet. Foods fortified with folic acid provide an important supply of folate because, unlike food folate, the absorption of folic acid is not reduced when there is gastric atrophy until it is very severe.

Folate deficiency is common in chronic alcoholics consuming >80 g ethanol/day. Multiple factors contribute to its progression, including low folate intake, poor absorption due to impaired transcription of the intestinal folate carrier, reduced liver uptake and storage, and increased urinary excretion [35].

Vitamin B_{12} (Cobalamin) Deficiency

The two most common causes of vitamin B_{12} deficiency in the elderly are inadequate dietary intake and gastric atrophy, which impairs the release of B_{12} from food for subsequent absorption. The prevalence of vitamin B_{12} deficiency increases with age. Reported values vary from 11 to 90%, depending on the definition of B_{12} deficiency and the population: elderly vegans [36] and institutionalized elderly having the highest prevalence [37]. For example, among residents aged over 65 years living in an institution, 53.7% had anemia and 34.9% had vitamin B_{12} deficiency [37]. The majority (86.6%) of the residents were ≥75 years old.

Malabsorption causes vitamin B_{12} depletion over time, depending on the size of the body stores. Fortified foods are therefore recommended for the elderly. Furthermore, since about 1% of it is absorbed by passive transport, even when intrinsic factor is lacking, high-dose supplementation can be used to treat deficiency.

Vitamin B_{12} is only found in animal food products and fortified foods; therefore, elderly vegans may be at high risk of vitamin B_{12} deficiency. In a sub-study of 785 older men and women (mean age 58.6 ± 13.3 years, range 29–94 years) from the Adventist Health Study [38], the intake of low vitamin B_{12} (<2.0 μg/day) was 15.2% in vegans, 10.6% in lacto-ovo-vegetarians, and 6.5% in nonvegetarians. However, there were no differences in biomarkers of vitamin B_{12} status between the groups, which the authors suggest is due to intake from fortified food and supplements, and in their conclusion they stress the importance of regular supplemental vitamin B_{12} intake in elderly individuals.

The Impact of Anemia on Health

Anemia is usually a consequence of underlying disease (Table 8.3). For example, there is a high probability that the hypoalbuminemia observed in thin elderly people is associated with anemia [39–41], but no evidence for a causal relationship exists. Clarifying the etiology is critical

Table 8.3 Conditions associated with anemia and potential health consequences. (Adapted from [12])

Condition	Possible explanation
Ageing	Inflammageing [57]
Frailty	Hypoalbuminemia [39, 40]
Thinness	Malnutrition [41]
Hemorrhoids	Blood loss
Inflammatory bowel disease (ulcerative colitis and Crohn's disease)	Blood loss and inflammation (↑ hepcidin)
Gastritis and GI ulcers	B_{12} deficiency, blood loss
Helicobacter pylori infection	Iron deficiency [50, 51]
Erythrocyte disorders (autoimmune hemolytic anemia, hemolysis)	Impaired Hb synthesis
Chronic inflammatory diseases (rheumatoid and osteoarthritis, hepatitis)	Inflammation (↑ hepcidin)
Cancer (GI tumors, breast and prostate cancer)	Multiple etiologies
Obesity	Inflammation (↑ hepcidin)
Renal disease (CKD)	Erythropoietin deficiency [33]
Metabolic disorders (hypo- or hyperthyroidism, diabetes)	Iron or erythropoietin deficiency
Alzheimer's disease	Perturbed Hb synthesis [42]
Health consequences	
Cardiovascular disease [52]	
Dementia [47]	
Depression [46]	
Decline in physical performance [43]	
Reduced muscle strength and increased risk of falling [44]	
Restless legs syndrome [48]	
Mortality [52]	

both to establish the most appropriate treatment and to undertake follow-up investigations to identify possible diseases. Non-nutritional anemia may result from blood loss (IBD, hemorrhoids), elevated hepcidin resulting from systemic inflammation (chronic inflammatory disorders such as arthritis, obesity), erythropoietin deficiency (CKD), high serum ferritin (tumor-derived in some cancers), and impaired Hb synthesis (erythrocyte disorders) [12]. There is a strong association between low Hb and Alzheimer's disease (AD), with a 3.41-fold increase in anemia in AD being reported [42]. Although the etiology is unknown, it has been suggested that it involves the oxidation of red cell Hb by amyloid beta (Aβ) protein; Aβ is enriched in red cell membranes in AD compared to healthy controls [42].

Various adverse health outcomes are attributed to anemia, including decline in physical performance, cognitive impairment, depression, dementia, susceptibility to falling, frailty, restless legs syndrome, and mortality (Table 8.3). Most of these are associations, and the underlying mechanisms are yet to be identified. Anemia results in diminished muscular oxygenation, which could explain fatigue, decline in physical performance [43], and reduced muscle strength [44].

Iron deficiency anemia commonly co-occurs with depressive symptoms in older people, but it is unclear whether the anemia is nutritional in origin or due to chronic disease. There is a plausible underlying pathway as iron plays an important role in the oxygenation of the brain and the synthesis of many neurotransmitters, and, specifically, dopamine function, which may explain mood disorders [45]. The InCHIANTI study of 986 Italian men and women, with a mean age of 75 years, reported that the risk of anemia progressively and significantly increases with severity of depression [46]. There is growing evidence for a link between iron deficiency anemia and dementia. A population-based cohort study in Taiwan (all newly diagnosed anemia patients, $n = 26,343$) concluded that newly diagnosed anemia is a risk factor for dementia; the adjusted subdistribution hazard ratio (SHR) of dementia risk in anemic patients was 1.14 (95% confidence interval [CI], 1.08~1.21, $p < 0.001$). Patients with iron supplements tended to exhibit a lower dementia risk (adjusted SHR, 0.84; 95% CI, 0.75, 0.94, $p = 0.002$) compared to patients without iron supplement [47].

Iron deficiency is also associated with restless legs syndrome (RLS), a neurologic disorder characterized by peculiar symptoms typically occurring in the evening and at night. The prevalence is between 5 and 10% in Caucasian populations, and it is twice as common in women as men. Elderly people are more affected than children and adults, with the prevalence increasing up to 60–70 years of age. In elderly patients with RLS, the two main problems are cognitive impairment, causing a difficult identification of the symptoms, and comorbidities, which are far more common in this patient population, thus complicating diagnosis and treatment [48]. Iron deficiency and dopamine metabolism are the two main pathophysiological mechanisms underlying RLS symptoms [48]. A recent systematic review concluded that treatment for 4 weeks with iron (oral or IV) was associated with a significant improvement in the International Restless Legs Syndrome score [49]. A link between RLS and *Helicobacter pylori* infection has been reported [50], and eradication of *Helicobacter pylori* was found to prevent subclinical iron deficiency anemia in older patients [51].

In a prospective study in Taiwan examining the association between iron deficiency and cardiovascular disease (CVD) and mortality, the severity of deficiency was found to be positively associated with both CVD and all-cause mortality [52]. In relation to mortality, anemia and hypoalbuminemia are important markers for older adults at risk of death within 5 years. It was demonstrated that one of these biomarkers gave a twofold increased risk for mortality, but when both were present, the risk was fourfold [39]. The presence of anemia is therefore a useful indicator for health professionals when undertaking geriatric screening, such as in primary care.

Management

The type of anemia and underlying cause(s) determine the most appropriate treatment. In addition, any comorbidities should be taken into account.

For microcytic anemia, oral iron therapy should be considered first, provided there is no evidence of malabsorption. Conventional treatment involves two to three oral doses per day of ferrous sulfate, which provides 100–200 mg iron. However, there are a number of commonly reported adverse side effects, including abdominal discomfort, nausea, vomiting, diarrhea, constipation, and black stools. Alternative forms and lower doses of iron are proposed to improve tolerance, for example, ferric citrate. The efficacy of 210 mg iron per day (minimum) was tested in patients with chronic kidney disease without the need for hemodialysis (NDD-CKD) [53]. Gastrointestinal disorders were the most common adverse events, with diarrhea reported in 24% and 19% and constipation in 19% and 13% of patients treated with ferric citrate and placebo, respectively. The authors concluded that oral ferric citrate was a safe and efficacious treatment for iron deficiency anemia in patients with NDD-CKD.

Low-dose oral iron supplements (15 mg iron/day) are reported to be as effective as higher doses of iron (50 mg iron/day) in anemic octogenarians [54]. After 2-month treatment, Hb and serum ferritin values increased from 100 to 113 g/L in the low iron group and from 102 to 116 g/L in the high iron group. Adverse side effects were significantly more common in the high iron group. Alternate day dosing with iron is another recommended strategy that reduces adverse side effects of oral iron supplements. Iron absorption is greater with alternate day than with consecutive day dosing in iron-deficient anemic women [55]. If oral iron therapy is ineffective, parenteral iron should be given, usually as one to five infusions, followed 6–8 weeks later by blood tests to check that the treatment has been successful [17].

Anemia caused by folate or vitamin B_{12} deficiency can be treated with oral supplements. Patients with folate deficiency should have concomitant vitamin B_{12} deficiency corrected first because repletion of folate can mask concurrent vitamin B_{12} deficiency. Early recognition and treatment of vitamin B_{12} deficiency are crucial since a proportion of patients develop severe complications, such as bone marrow failure and irreversible neurological impairment [19].

Public Health Nutrition

As with all diet-related chronic diseases, prevention is the optimal goal, but the difficulties of mitigating anemia on a global basis are well-recognized [56]. There are particular problems in countries in which the diets contain iron of low bioavailability and where there is a high prevalence of diseases and disorders such as thalassemia, sickle cell anemia, malaria, and hookworm infestation. Low-grade inflammation, often referred to as inflammageing [57], is commonly found in older people as a consequence of osteoarthritis and other age-related conditions (Table 8.3). Inflammation is associated with increased hepcidin expression (which reduces iron absorption) and may be one of the explanations for the high prevalence of IDA in this population group.

Various public health strategies are employed to address anemia, in particular iron deficiency anemia, with varying degrees of success. These include food-based dietary recommendations, food fortification, nutrient supplements, and biofortification. In order to reduce the risk of anemia in older people, it is important to ensure that iron, folate, and vitamin B_{12} requirements are met under conditions of falling energy expenditure. Consuming micronutrient dense foods is one option, although introducing dietary change is always a challenge. The development of biofortified plant foods is a promising way forward [58]. A recent meta-analysis of studies examining the efficacy of iron-biofortified (compared with conventional) staple crops on iron status and functional outcomes showed that cognitive performance in attention and memory domains significantly improved, although there were no effects on outcomes such as iron deficiency or anemia [59].

Conclusion

The elderly are a nutritionally vulnerable group, and anemia is a widespread problem which increases substantially with age. Iron deficiency is the most common cause of nutritional anemia. A wide range of conditions found in the elderly are associated with anemia, such as frailty, bowel disorders, chronic inflammatory diseases, certain cancers, metabolic disorders, and renal disease. Anemia has a major impact on the health of elderly people, including decline in physical performance, reduced muscle strength, risk of falling, depression, cognitive decline, and dementia, but the mechanisms for many of these associations still need to be elucidated.

References

1. United Nations, Department of Economic and Social Affairs, Population Division. World population ageing 2019: highlights (ST/ESA/SER.A/430). 2019.
2. Levine ME. Modeling the rate of senescence: can estimated biological age predict mortality more accurately than chronological age? J Gerontol A Biol Sci Med Sci. 2013;68:667–74. https://doi.org/10.1093/gerona/gls233.
3. United Nations Department of Economic and Social Affairs, Population Division. World population ageing 2020 highlights: living arrangements of older persons (ST/ESA/SER.A/451). 2020.
4. WHO. 2018. https://www.who.int/news-room/fact-sheets/detail/ageing-and-health. Accessed 30 Nov 2020.
5. World Health Organization. Nutritional anaemias. Report of a WHO Scientific Group. World Health Organ Tech Rep Ser. 1968;405:5–37.
6. Fulgoni VL, Agarwal S, Kellogg MD, Lieberman HR. Establishing pediatric and adult RBC reference intervals with NHANES data using piecewise regression. Am J Clin Pathol. 2019;151:128–42. https://doi.org/10.1093/ajcp/aqy116.
7. Zierk J, Krebs A, Rauh M, Metzler M, Löscher A, Strasser E, Krause SW. Blood counts in adult and elderly individuals: defining the norms over eight decades of life. Br J Haematol. 2020. https://doi.org/10.1111/bjh.16430.
8. Milman N, Pedersen AN, Ovesen L, Schroll M. Hemoglobin concentrations in 358 apparently healthy 80-year-old Danish men and women. Should the reference interval be adjusted for age? Aging Clin Exp Res. 2008;20:8–14.
9. Varghese JS, Thomas T, Kurpad AV. Evaluation of haemoglobin cut-off for mild anaemia in Asians—analysis of multiple rounds of two national nutrition surveys. Indian J Med Res. 2019;150:385–9.
10. Beutler E, Waalen J. The definition of anemia: what is the lower limit of normal of the blood hemoglobin concentration? Blood. 2006;107(5):1747–50. Epub 2005 Sep 27.
11. Chaparro CM, Suchdev PS. Anemia epidemiology, pathophysiology, and etiology in low- and middle-income countries. Ann N Y Acad Sci. 2019;1450:15–31. https://doi.org/10.1111/nyas.14092. Epub 2019 Apr 22.
12. Wawer AA, Jennings A, Fairweather-Tait SJ. Iron status in the elderly: a review of recent evidence. Mech Ageing Dev. 2018;175:55–73. https://doi.org/10.1016/j.mad.2018.07.003. Epub 2018 Jul 21.
13. Kassebaum NJ, Jasrasaria R, Naghavi M, Wulf SK, Johns N, Lozano R, Regan M, Weatherall D, Chou DP, Eisele TP, Flaxman SR, Pullan RL, Brooker SJ, Murray CJ. A systematic analysis of global anemia burden from 1990 to 2010. Blood. 2014;123:615–24.
14. Stauder R, Valent P, Theur I. Anemia at older age: etiologies, clinical implications, and management. Blood. 2018;131:505–14.
15. Tettamanti M, Lucca U, Gandini F, Recchia A, Mosconi P, Apolone G, Nobili A, Tallone MV, Detoma P, Giacomin A, Clerico M, Tempia P, Savoia L, Fasolo G, Ponchio L, Della Porta MG, Riva E. Prevalence, incidence and types of mild anemia in the elderly: the "Health and Anemia" population-based study. Haematologica. 2010;95(11):1849–56.
16. Girelli D, Marchi G, Camaschella C. Anemia in the elderly. HemaSphere. 2018;2:3. https://doi.org/10.1097/HS9.0000000000000040.
17. Lanier JB, Park JJ, Callahan RC. Anemia in older adults. Am Fam Physician. 2018;98:437–42.
18. Socha DS, DeSouza SI, Flagg A, Sekeres M, Rogers HJ. Severe megaloblastic anemia: vitamin deficiency and other causes. Cleve Clin J Med. 2020;87(3):153–64. https://doi.org/10.3949/ccjm.87a.19072.
19. Marchi G, Busti F, Zidanes AL, Vianello A, Girelli D. Cobalamin deficiency in the elderly. Mediterr J Hematol Infect Dis. 2020;12(1):e2020043. https://doi.org/10.4084/MJHID.2020.043. eCollection 2020.
20. Aljaadi AM, How RE, Loh SP, Hunt SE, Karakochuk CD, Barr SI, McAnena L, Ward M, McNulty H, Khor GL, Devlin AM, Green TJ. Suboptimal biochemical riboflavin status is associated with lower hemoglobin and higher rates of anemia in a sample of Canadian and Malaysian women of reproductive age. J Nutr. 2019;149:1952–9. https://doi.org/10.1093/jn/nxz151.

21. Altarelli M, Ben-Hamouda N, Schneider A, Berger MM. Copper deficiency: causes, manifestations, and treatment. Nutr Clin Pract. 2019;34:504–13. https://doi.org/10.1002/ncp.10328. Epub 2019 Jun 17.
22. Myint ZW, Oo TH, Thein KZ, Tun AM, Saeed H. Copper deficiency anemia: review article. Ann Hematol. 2018;97:1527–34. https://doi.org/10.1007/s00277-018-3407-5.
23. Na IS, Nguyen K, Potenzi B, Cheah M. Now you C me: a case of scurvy presenting as depression and anaemia. BMJ Case Rep. 2020;13(3):e233645. https://doi.org/10.1136/bcr-2019-233645.
24. Bianchi VE. Role of nutrition on anemia in elderly. Clin Nutr ESPEN. 2016;11:e1–e11. https://doi.org/10.1016/j.clnesp.2015.09.003. Epub 2015 Dec 9.
25. Annibale B, Esposito G, Lahner E. A current clinical overview of atrophic gastritis. Expert Rev Gastroenterol Hepatol. 2020;14(2):93–102. https://doi.org/10.1080/17474124.2020.1718491. Epub 2020 Jan 24.
26. Lopez-Contreras MJ, Zamora-Portero S, Lopez MA, Marin JF, Zamora S, Perez-Llamas F. Dietary intake and iron status of institutionalized elderly people: relationship with different factors. J Nutr Health Aging. 2010;14:816–21.
27. Fleming DJ, Jacques PF, Massaro JM, D'Agostino RB Sr, Wilson PW, Wood RJ. Aspirin intake and the use of serum ferritin as a measure of iron status. Am J Clin Nutr. 2001;74:219–26.
28. Fairweather-Tait S, Speich C, Mitchikpè CES, Dainty JR. Dietary iron bioavailability: a simple model that can be used to derive country-specific values for adult men and women. Food Nutr Bull. 2020;41(1):121–30. https://doi.org/10.1177/0379572119885482. Epub 2019 Nov 20.
29. Milman N, Pedersen AN, Ovesen L, Schroll M. Iron status in 358 apparently healthy 80-year old Danish men and women: relation to food composition and dietary and supplemental iron intake. Ann Hematol. 2004;83:423–9.
30. Fabian E, Elmadfa I. Nutritional situation of the elderly in the European Union: data of the European Nutrition and Health Report (2004). Ann Nutr Metab. 2008;52(suppl 1):57–61.
31. Montgomery RD, Haeney MR, Ross IN, Sammons HG, Barford AV, Balakrishnan S, Mayer PP, Culank LS, Field J, Gosling P. The ageing gut: a study of intestinal absorption in relation to nutrition in the elderly. Q J Med. 1978;47:187–24.
32. Vannella L, Aloe Spiriti MA, Di Giulio E, Lahner E, Corleto VD, Monarca B, Delle Fave G, Annibale B. Upper and lower gastrointestinal causes of iron deficiency anemia in elderly compared with adult outpatients. Minerva Gastroenterol Dietol. 2010.
33. Stauffer ME, Fan T. Prevalence of anemia in chronic kidney disease in the United States. PLoS One. 2014;9(1):e84943. https://doi.org/10.1371/journal.ponw.0084943.
34. Clarke R, Grimley Evans J, Schneede J, Nexo E, Bates C, Fletcher A, Prentice A, Johnston C, Ueland PM, Refsum H, Sherliker P, Birks J, Whitlock G, Breeze E, Scott JM. Vitamin B12 and folate deficiency in later life. Age Ageing. 2004;33:34–41.
35. Allen LH. Causes of vitamin B12 and folate deficiency. Food Nutr Bull. 2008;29(2 Suppl):S20–34.
36. Pawlak R, Parrott SJ, Raj S, Cullum-Dugan D, Lucus D. How prevalent is vitamin B12 among vegetarians? Nutr Rev. 2013;71:110–7.
37. Wong CW, Ip CY, Leung CP, Leung CS, Cheng JN, Siu CY. Vitamin B12 deficiency in the institutionalized elderly: a regional study. Exp Geront. 2015;69:221–5.
38. Haddad EH, Jaceldo-Siegl K, Oda K, Fraser GE. Associations of circulating methylmalonic acid and vitamin B-12 biomarkers are modified by vegan dietary pattern in adult and elderly participants of the Adventist Health Study 2 Calibration Study. Curr Dev Nutr. 2020;4(2):nzaa008. https://doi.org/10.1093/cdn/nzaa008. eCollection 2020 Feb.
39. Corona LP, de Oliveira Duarte YA, Lebrão ML. Markers of nutritional status and mortality in older adults: the role of anemia and hypoalbuminemia. Geriatr Gerontol Int. 2018;18:177–82.
40. Röhrig G, Becker I, Polidori MC, Schulz RJ, Noreik M. Association of anemia and hypoalbuminemia in German geriatric inpatients. Z Gerontol Geriat. 2015;48:619–24.
41. Silva EC, Roriz AK, Eickemberg M, Mello AL, Côrtes EB, Feitosa CA, Medeiros JM, Ramos LB. Factors associated with anemia in the institutionalized elderly. PLoS One. 2016;11(9):e0162240. https://doi.org/10.1371/journal.pone.0162240. eCollection 2016.
42. Faux NG, Rembach A, Wiley J, Ellis KA, Ames D, Fowler CJ, Martins RN, Pertile KK, Rumble RL, Trounson B, Masters CL, AIBL Research Group, Bush AI. An anemia of Alzheimer's disease. Mol Psychiatry. 2014;19(11):1227–34. https://doi.org/10.1038/mp.2013.178. Epub 2014 Jan 14.
43. Penninx BW, Guralnik JM, Onder G, Ferrucci L, Wallace RB, Pahor M. Anemia and decline in physical performance among older persons. Am J Med. 2003;115:104–10.
44. Penninx BWJH, Pahor M, Ceasri M, Corsi AM, Woodman RC, Bandinelli S, Guralnick JM, Ferrucci L. Anemia is associated with disability and decreased physical performance and muscle strength in the elderly. J Am Geriatr Soc. 2004;52:719–24.
45. Stewart R, Hirani V. Relationship between depressive symptoms, anemia, and iron status in older residents from a National Survey population. Psychosom Med. 2012;74:208–13.
46. Onder G, Penninx BW, Cesari M, Bandinelli S, Lauretani F, Bartali B, Gori AM, Pahor M, Ferrucci L. Anemia is associated with depression in older adults: results from the InCHIANTI study. J Gerontol A Biol Sci Med Sci. 2005;60:1168–72.
47. Hong CT, Hsieh YC, Liu HY, Chiou HY, Chien LN. Association between anemia and dementia—a nationwide, population-based cohort study in Taiwan. Curr Alzheimer Res. 2020. https://doi.org/10.2174/1567205017666200317101516.

48. Didato G, Di Giacomo R, Rosa GJ, Dominese A, de Curtis M, Lanteri P. Restless legs syndrome across the lifespan: symptoms, pathophysiology, management and daily life impact of the different patterns of disease presentation. Int J Environ Res Public Health. 2020;17(10):3658. https://doi.org/10.3390/ijerph17103658.
49. Avni T, Reich S, Lev N, Gafter-Gvili A. Iron supplementation for restless legs syndrome—a systematic review and meta-analysis. Eur J Intern Med. 2019;63:34–41.
50. Rezvani F, Sayadnasiri M, Rezaei O. Restless legs syndrome in patients infected with Helicobacter pylori. Neurol Res. 2018;40:581–5. https://doi.org/10.1080/01616412.2018.1454704. Epub 2018 Apr 6.
51. Maruyama M, Kamimura K, Hoshiyama A, Hoshiyama K, Hoshiyama M, Hoshiyama Y, Terai S. Effect of Helicobacter pylori eradication on elder cases: observational study in community-based medicine. World J Clin Cases. 2017;5:412–8. https://doi.org/10.12998/wjcc.v5.i12.412.
52. Hsu HS, Li CI, Liu CS, Lin CC, Huang KC, Li TC, Huang HY, Lin WY. Iron deficiency is associated with increased risk for cardiovascular disease and all-cause mortality in the elderly living in long-term care facilities. Nutrition. 2013;29:737–43.
53. Fishbane S, Block GA, Loram L, Neylan J, Pergola PE, Uhlig K, Chertow GM. Effects of ferric citrate in patients with nondialysis-dependent CKD and iron deficiency anemia. J Am Soc Nephrol. 2017;28:1851–8. https://doi.org/10.1681/ASN.2016101053. Epub 2017 Jan 12.
54. Rimon E, Kagansky N, Kagansky M, Mechnick L, Mashiah T, Namir M, Levy S. Are we giving too much iron? Low-dose iron therapy is effective in octogenarians. Am J Med. 2005;118:1142–7.
55. Stoffel NU, Zeder C, Brittenham GM, Moretti D, Zimmermann MB. Iron absorption from supplements is greater with alternate day than with consecutive day dosing in iron-deficient anemic women. Haematologica. 2019. https://doi.org/10.3324/haematol.2019.220830. [Epub ahead of print].
56. Schümann K, Solomons NW. Perspective: what makes it so difficult to mitigate worldwide anemia prevalence? Adv Nutr. 2017;8:401–8.
57. Ferrucci L, Fabbri E. Inflammageing: chronic inflammation in ageing, cardiovascular disease, and frailty. Nat Rev Cardiol. 2018;15(9):505–22. https://doi.org/10.1038/s41569-018-0064-2.
58. Vasconcelos MW, Gruissem W, Bhullar NK. Iron biofortification in the 21st century: setting realistic targets, overcoming obstacles, and new strategies for healthy nutrition. Curr Opin Biotechnol. 2017;44:8–15. https://doi.org/10.1016/j.copbio.2016.10.001. Epub 2016 Oct 22.
59. Finkelstein JL, Fothergill A, Hackl LS, Haas JD, Mehta S. Iron biofortification interventions to improve iron status and functional outcomes. Proc Nutr Soc. 2019;78(2):197–207. https://doi.org/10.1017/S0029665118002847.

Iron Deficiency and Anaemia in Athletes

9

Peter Peeling, Alannah McKay, and Marc Sim

Keywords

Iron · Athlete · Exercise · Training Adaptation · Physical capacity · Supplement Performance · Diet

Introduction

Iron is a fundamental component of numerous processes that lend themselves to sports performance and physical capacity. For instance, iron is imperative for oxygen transport and mitochondrial energy production, both of which have significant implications to aerobic capacity. Furthermore, the links between iron and cognitive processing could be important to sport where rapid decision-making is necessary. Finally, the association between iron and the immune system is pertinent, since maintaining an overall healthy athlete is essential in reducing the number of days of training lost to illness. Accordingly, it is for these four reasons (oxygen transport, energy production, cognitive processing and immune function) that iron is an essential mineral relevant to athletic performance.

Despite the clear importance of iron to human function, numerous exercise-relevant avenues are apparent for increased iron use (i.e. haematological adaptation increasing red blood cell volume) and iron loss (i.e. sweating, gastrointestinal bleeding, haematuria and haemolysis), which need to be replaced on a daily basis. However, no innate process of endogenously producing iron exists to fulfil our daily needs, making the diet (or supplementation) our only means of replenishing these losses. Accordingly, iron deficiency (ID) is a common condition in athlete populations, with a particularly high prevalence in four core groups: (1) female athletes, due to a combination of exercise-induced iron losses and (periodically) menstrual bleeding; (2) vegetarians, due to a lack of haem iron in the diet; (3) individuals competing in endurance-based sports, due to the accumulation of numerous exercise-induced iron loss mechanisms; and (4) energy restricted athletes, likely a result of diet restriction, poor nutrition, or lack of time between training sessions. Although

P. Peeling (✉)
School of Human Sciences (Exercise and Sport Science), The University of Western Australia, Crawley, WA, Australia

The Western Australian Institute of Sport, Mount Claremont, WA, Australia
e-mail: peter.peeling@uwa.edu.au

A. McKay
Mary MacKillop Institute for Health Research, Australian Catholic University, North Sydney, NSW, Australia

M. Sim
School of Medical and Health Sciences, Edith Cowan University, Joondalup, WA, Australia

School of Medicine, Royal Perth Hospital Unit, The University of Western Australia, Crawley, WA, Australia

C. D. Karakochuk et al. (eds.), *Nutritional Anemia*, Nutrition and Health,
https://doi.org/10.1007/978-3-031-14521-6_9

these four groups are identified as 'greater risk' populations, it is still important to recognise that both intermittent sport and male athletes are also susceptible to ID. Accordingly, athletes of both sexes (up to ~15% of male and ~50% of female athlete cohorts) across a range of sport types (e.g. endurance, team sports) have been shown to present with compromised iron stores [1, 2], an issue that can impact physical performance capacity if not corrected in the early stages of depletion.

On this basis, the following chapter will define the various stages of ID reported in sports medicine literature, before progressing to highlight the impact of such mineral deficit on physical performance outcomes. Next, we will take a mechanistic look at the various avenues of iron loss and malabsorption in relation to exercise, before culminating with the various methods of treatment to correct ID in athlete populations.

What Constitutes an Iron Deficiency in Athlete Populations?

A negative iron balance in athletes may result from a range of factors including inadequate dietary intake, exercise-induced iron losses and inflammation [3, 4]. For female athletes, iron losses are exacerbated by menses [5]. Over time, such events can compromise iron stores and increase an athlete's susceptibility to ID. Debate currently exists as to the most appropriate haematological variables (and their cut-off values) that should be considered when assessing an athlete's iron status. For a list of iron-related biomarkers, their respective thresholds and the associated limitations, readers are directed to a comprehensive summary by Clenin and colleagues [6]. Regardless, we propose that the minimum routine clinical assessment of ID in athletes includes analysis of the iron indices: serum ferritin, haemoglobin concentration and transferrin saturation [3]. These indices are essential for adopting a three-stage approach when categorising ID in athlete populations (Table 9.1).

Table 9.1 Common iron indices thresholds required to categorise the severity of iron deficiency in athletes

Progressive stages of iron deficiency in athletes	Serum ferritin (μg/L)	Total haemoglobin (g/L)	Transferrin saturation (%)
Stage 1—Iron deficiency (ID)	<35	>115	>16
Stage 2—Iron-deficient non-anaemia (IDNA)	<20	>115	<16
Stage 3—Iron-deficient anaemia (IDA)[a]	<12	<115	<16

[a] Serum soluble transferrin receptor levels of 2.5 mg/L may also be considered a reasonable threshold for identification of IDA [7]

Stage 1 ID is characterised by an initial reduction in serum ferritin, highlighting a depletion in total iron stores [8, 9]. Notably, haemoglobin and other markers of iron status remain relatively unaffected in this stage. Once ferritin stores are compromised, Stage 2 ID inevitably follows if no remedial action is taken. This stage is characterised by low circulating iron levels, including a reduction in iron supply to erythroid marrow. Such events are distinguished by a decrease in transferrin saturation and may include an increased total iron binding capacity. Both Stage 1 and 2 ID are collectively referred to as iron-deficiency non-anaemia (IDNA), as healthy haemoglobin levels are maintained, despite the presence of potentially insufficient iron stores. As previously highlighted, due to the lack of clinical consensus, a serum ferritin range of <12 to 40 μg/L has been used in various literature to categorise IDNA in athletes. Subsequently, once iron transport and storage are limited, haemoglobin synthesis can no longer be maintained. Such events represent Stage 3 ID, where serum ferritin, haemoglobin and transferrin saturation are all compromised, reflecting a state of iron deficiency anaemia (IDA); of note, others have proposed that IDA manifests when haemoglobin falls below 115–120 g/L [6, 9–17]. Nevertheless, caution must be exercised when assessing iron status from single indices. For example, in active populations, a training-induced adaptation of expanded plasma volume can dilute red blood cells, making haemoglobin levels appear reduced when measured in blood, which, in isolation, could lead to a misdiagnosis of iron deficiency, known as pseudo-anaemia [18] or sports anaemia [19]. Additionally, we know that serum ferritin can increase as an acute phase reactant after completing moderate-intensity exercise [20, 21], and therefore, several factors should be considered when standardising blood collection procedures for athlete populations.

With this in mind, a framework to standardise the conditions and frequency of blood screening for iron status in athletes is proposed by Sim et al. [22]. When deciding the appropriate frequency of blood screening (e.g. annually, biannually, quarterly), factors such as gender, type of sport, any history of ID, dietary preferences, energy availability and unexplained poor performance need to be considered. Blood collection should also occur under standardised conditions, including (1) samples obtained in the morning, (2) the individual presenting in a well-hydrated state (waking urinary specific gravity <1.025), (3) low to moderate activity conducted in the preceding 24 h and (iv) no signs of infection or illness.

Impact of Iron Deficiency on Physical Capacity and Performance

Performance implications of sub-optimal iron stores likely depend on the severity of ID. Compromised performance as a result of ID can be attributed to the role of iron in metabolic pathways, which include (1) haemoglobin and myoglobin for oxygen transport and (2) the production of non-haem iron sulphur enzymes and haem-containing cytochromes heavily involved in the oxidative production of energy in the form of adenosine triphosphate [4]. Unsurprisingly during IDA (Stage 3), aerobic performance is severely impacted [23]. Nevertheless, during IDNA (Stages 1 and 2), compromised tissue oxidative capacity can also impair aerobic performance [10, 24]. Such outcomes may place a higher demand on anaerobic metabolism, which can negatively impact endurance performance by increasing lactate production (lowering blood pH) and muscle glycogen use.

Despite the key role iron plays in energy production, the effects of iron supplementation to improve performance in IDNA individuals remain equivocal [9, 11, 25–29]. For example, a systematic review (18 trials and 2 companion papers, n = 1170 individuals) of both trained and untrained IDNA individuals (serum ferritin ≤20 μg/L and haemoglobin >120 g/L) reported no effect of iron supplementation on maximal oxygen uptake (VO_{2max}) or time-trial methods of testing exercise performance [30]. Additionally, a second systematic review specific to IDNA athletes (12 studies, n = 283 participants, 91% female) reported that half of all studies found no performance benefits were found across a range of performance-based physical tests (e.g. shuttle run, 3000 m run, time-to-fatigue) after iron supplementation was provided to improve iron stores [31].

Similar findings have been reported by several well-designed randomised, double-blind, placebo-controlled trials [9, 15, 17, 26, 29]. For example, despite improving iron status through intramuscular iron injections (5 × 2 mL of 100 mg elemental iron over 10 days) in eight iron-deplete female athletes (serum ferritin = 19 μg/L, serum soluble transferrin receptor = 5.9 mg/L), no changes in running VO_{2max}, exercise economy (@70% VO_{2max}) or time to exhaustion were observed [9]. Similarly, in IDNA female netballers (serum ferritin <40 μg/L and haemoglobin >125 g/L), this same intramuscular iron injection protocol (as above) did not enhance performance across a suite of physiological tests (vertical jump, 10 s power, 5 × 6 s repeat sprint test and a 20 m multi-stage shuttle run) [25]. Comparable findings have also been reported in 18 IDNA female runners (serum ferritin <20 μg/L and haemoglobin ≥120 g/L) after 8 weeks of oral iron supplements (100 mg iron as ferrous sulphate per day), where endurance performance (VO_{2max} and time-to-exhaustion) remained unchanged [17].

Contrary to the aforementioned work, a meta-analysis (12 studies, n = 443, 82% female) reported that iron supplementation can improve

VO_{2max} in IDNA individuals (serum ferritin ≤35 μg/L and haemoglobin >120 g/L) [10]. Notably, the greatest effects on aerobic power were recorded in individuals with low VO_{2max} (<40 mL/kg/min), typically associated with untrained populations. Such observations limit the generalisability of these results to well-trained athletes. In support of this concept, when considering untrained IDNA active women (*n* = 42, serum ferritin <16 μg/L, haemoglobin >120 g/L), 6 weeks of oral iron supplements (2 x 50 mg ferrous sulphate per day, each containing 10 mg of elemental iron, in conjunction with a training programme) improved 15 km cycling time-trial performance by ~6.5% [15]. As oxygen-carrying capacity generally remains unaffected by IDNA, these positive results were attributed to an increase in tissue iron status, which was proposed to enhance muscle oxidative capacity and the efficiency of oxygen utilisation at the tissue level [15]. Conversely, in a separate study of 37 untrained IDNA women (serum ferritin <16 μg/L, haemoglobin >120 g/L), no improvements in 15 km cycling time-trial performance were recorded, despite receiving a higher dose of iron supplementation (135 mg/day ferrous sulphate containing 45 mg elemental iron or placebo) for 8 weeks [26]. However, the iron-supplemented group in this study did demonstrate an improved exercise efficiency, as indicated by 2.0 kJ/min lower energy expenditure and a 5.1% lower fractional utilisation of peak oxygen consumption. Observational work in 165 IDNA female rowers (Hb >120 g/L) also reports that lower ferritin stores (<20 μg/L vs. ≥20 μg/L) were retrospectively associated (2–3 months prior) with slower (~21 s) 2 km rowing TT ergometer performances [32]. However, in a follow-up RCT, oral iron supplements consumed for 6 weeks (100 mg/day ferrous sulphate) did not improve 4 km rowing time-trial performance, regardless of the favourable effects on energy expenditure and efficiency [29].

Despite ambiguity regarding the effect of iron supplements provided to IDNA populations, the negative impacts of IDA on performance are well established. This has been attributed to a range of factors including compromised aerobic endurance, work capacity and energy efficiency. Specifically, once erythropoiesis and oxygen transport are impaired, a reduction in VO_{2max} inevitably occurs. Other serious health consequences of IDA that can affect performance may include extreme lethargy, disturbances in immunity, poor thermoregulation as well as impaired brain and muscle metabolism [33]. Considering the health and performance implications of IDA, commencing iron supplements in the early stages of the condition should be a priority to prevent these significant impairments from occurring. From an athletic perspective, a case study reported that iron supplements (both oral and parenteral) provided over 15 weeks to an elite anaemic female runner not only improved her iron status (serum ferritin 9.9–27 μg/L and haemoglobin 88–130 g/L) but also enabled a gradual increase in training load, which, in combination, likely facilitated a 3000 m personal best run performance in the following weeks post-supplementation [34].

Collectively, the interpretation of this work, especially for IDNA populations, is complicated by a range of factors. These include the varied methods by which performance has been assessed (e.g. VO_{2max}, time to exhaustion, submaximal exercise economy), the different iron supplementation protocols employed (oral vs. parenteral administration), the various cut-points of iron indices used to categorise ID, the training status of the population measured (untrained vs. well-trained athletes) and the time differential between a supplement-induced increases in iron status and the time required for positive training adaptations to occur. However, in general, any positive effects of iron supplements on performance capacity are likely dependent on the severity of ID and the treatment strategy used to correct it. Specifically, individuals presenting with IDA may experience the largest performance benefits after iron supplementation; however, for individuals with IDNA, where aerobic capacity is typically unchanged, the negative impacts of iron-deficient erythropoiesis (Stage 2), due to its role in the pathway to energy production, cannot be excluded.

Mechanisms of Iron Deficiency in Athlete Populations

While iron is clearly important for athletic performance, there are numerous exercise-associated mechanisms capable of compromising iron stores in athletes. Key adaptive processes that occur in response to exercise such as erythropoiesis, DNA synthesis and oxidative enzyme production are all iron-dependent processes that draw upon an athlete's available iron stores [35]. Consequently, these stores may be compromised if dietary iron intake is not adequate to support the increases in iron demand.

In addition to iron for adaptive response, there are also multiple exercise-associated avenues of iron loss suggested to contribute to ID in athletes. For instance, iron can be lost through sweat, an important physiological mechanism that is upregulated to assist thermoregulation during exercise. While the amount of iron lost in sweat is considered small (~0.14 mg/L) [36], these losses may become substantial in athletes who exercise multiple times per day or in those training in hot environments. In addition to sweat, haemolysis is another exercise-induced avenue of iron loss, primarily occurring in response to the high impact forces from foot strike [37] and from the circulatory system compression associated with vigorous muscle contraction [38]. This trauma results in the destruction of red blood cells, resulting in the haemoglobin and associated iron content to spill into the surrounding plasma. While there are inherent recycling mechanisms in place to clear the haemolysed red blood cell and free iron from circulation via macrophage activity [39], the efficacy of this process may be impaired by exercise-induced increases in hepcidin, which acts to degrade the ferroportin export channels on the cell surface of the macrophage. Finally, haematuria and gastrointestinal (GI) bleeding are also reported as potential avenues by which iron can be lost [3], both of which are commonly reported processes that can occur in response to high-intensity or prolonged exercise. Collectively, accumulation of exercise-induced iron loss mechanisms may have negative implications for an athlete's iron stores, which may contribute to the high prevalence of ID reported in athletic populations.

In the last 15 years, the iron regulatory hormone, hepcidin, has been implicated as an exercise-induced mechanism that can alter iron metabolism in athletes. Exercise-induced increases in the inflammatory cytokine, interleukin-6 (IL-6), directly upregulate hepcidin activity, likely through the signalling processes that increase hepatocyte hepcidin production [40]. The resultant hepcidin-ferroportin interactions act to limit iron absorption from enterocytes in the gut, in addition to reducing the iron recycling potential of macrophages [41]. Although this process is a necessary homeostatic mechanism of iron balance, this exercise-induced increase in IL-6 is followed ~3–6 h later by a subsequent peak in circulating hepcidin levels [42]. Accordingly, iron absorption during this time is likely to be transiently impaired, potentially curtailing an athlete's opportunity to appropriately replenish their iron stores. Consequently, the timing of dietary iron (or supplement) intake becomes important and, where possible, should occur at a time away from this post-exercise period of hormone elevation, to maximise the prospects for absorption. In athletes that are training multiple times per day, this may be particularly challenging due to the prospect of chronically elevated hepcidin levels. In such instances, it is important to consider the diurnal variation of hepcidin, which is lowest in the morning and gradually increases throughout the day [43]. The magnitude of the post-exercise hepcidin response also appears influenced by its diurnal variation, with greater levels reported when exercise is performed in the afternoon, as compared to the morning [44]. With this in mind, iron absorption is likely to be greatest in the morning (with or without exercise) and should be considered by athletes and sports dieticians when developing strategies to optimise iron absorption around exercise.

Manipulating the IL-6 response magnitude to exercise has been explored as a potential strategy to minimise post-exercise hepcidin expression and improve iron absorption. Exercise duration is one of the strongest determinants of the post-exercise IL-6 response, which increases exponentially as exercise duration progresses [45]. Its influence also impacts post-exercise hepcidin levels, with longer training sessions also exacerbating the post-exercise concentrations [46]. Conversely, exercise intensity and modality (i.e. running vs. cycling) are shown to have a lesser impact on this post-exercise response [21].

Interestingly, the release of IL-6 is accelerated by muscle glycogen depletion [47], which means it is possible for carbohydrate ingestion to preserve muscle glycogen stores and attenuate the signal for increased IL-6 production. This prospect *could* have subsequent positive effects for curtailing elevated post-exercise hepcidin levels. However, research to date exploring the use of short-term dietary carbohydrate intake, both prior to [48, 49] and during exercise [50], in addition to chronic dietary carbohydrate manipulations (>7 days) [51, 52], have largely been unable to attenuate the post-exercise hepcidin response via increases in carbohydrate consumption. Rather, it seems more evident that exercising in a state of low glycogen availability is responsible for augmenting post-exercise hepcidin levels [48, 49], and therefore, appropriate carbohydrate feeding around exercise is likely good practice to minimise (but not attenuate) this response.

Treatment of Iron Deficiency in Athletes

Decisions relevant to the treatment approach taken to rectify an iron deficiency in athletes are generally made on the basis of condition severity. Currently, there are three well-accepted approaches to treatment: (1) increasing the intake of iron-rich foods in the diet; (2) oral iron supplementation; or (3) parenteral iron administration.

Increasing Dietary Iron Intake

The most conservative treatment for ID is dietary intervention, which is a common initial consideration when athletes present with iron stores close to the 'healthy' lower limit (i.e. serum ferritin 30–35 μg/L). The recommended dietary iron intake is 8 mg/day for males and 18 mg/day for females of menstruating age [53]. Accordingly, an appropriate initial response to any form of dietary correction should involve counsel with a trained sports dietician to evaluate if the required needs are able to be met simply through a 'food first' approach. The best food choices for obtaining dietary iron come in the form of animal meat sources, primarily due to the fact that haem iron is better absorbed at the gut than the less efficient non-haem form found in plant-based foods [4]. Regardless, vegetarian athletes can find iron-rich options in foods such as leafy green vegetables (e.g. spinach, cabbage, bok choy), fortified or whole grain cereals, oats and various noodles and rices. Of note, dietary assessment and advice should include the co-consumption of iron absorption enhancers, such as vitamin C, while avoiding the intake of iron absorption inhibitors, such as phytates, calcium and tannins (found in tea and coffee), when eating foods with the intent of optimising iron absorption from the meal [54].

Although a dietary assessment and optimisation of iron intake from 'food first' choices should be the initial approach to correcting an ID, it must be noted that it is generally hard to significantly improve iron stores through food intake alone, and therefore, in instances of compromised iron status, oral iron supplementation is commonly considered.

Oral Iron Supplementation

Persistent subjective feelings of lethargy, fatigue and general malaise, in association with a blood panel showing (at minimum) compromised iron stores, may provide indication for the sports physician and dietician to consider recommending a period of oral iron supplementation. Oral iron supplements are usually provided in the ferrous form as either ferrous fumarate, ferrous sulphate or ferrous gluconate preparations. Currently, ferrous sulphate preparations are the established standard treatment for depleted iron stores, with the literature showing strong efficacy of effect when consumed in doses of 60–120 mg of elemental iron per day, for 8–12 weeks [11, 22, 55]. However, a significant limitation in the commitment to such supplementation protocols exists on the basis of commonly reported GI distress symptoms that manifest from regular oral iron intake [56].

In order to reduce the GI disturbance incurred from oral iron supplements, alternative slow-release preparations, such as polysaccharide-iron complexes, have been developed, which appear to be efficacious with promising rates of gut tolerability [57]. Alternatively, it is also possible that the frequency of supplement intake could be altered to reduce the incidence of GI distress, without impacting the efficacy of response. For instance, Stoffel et al. [58] reported a greater fractional and cumulative iron absorption in non-athletic females who supplemented with 60 mg of iron as ferrous sulphate on alternate days for 28 days, as compared with women who supplemented with 60 mg of iron as ferrous sulphate daily for a 14-day period. These positive outcomes were based on the proposition that intermittent-day supplementation avoids a hepcidin-related suppression of intestinal iron uptake following the initial high iron dose—i.e. alternate-day supplementation protocols give the body's hepcidin response time to recover. When applied to an athlete cohort in training, McCormick et al. [59] showed that 8 weeks of alternate-day iron supplementation (105 mg elemental iron per tablet) increased iron stores to the same magnitude as daily supplementation, despite 50% less iron being consumed over the 8-week period. Importantly, such outcomes were concurrent with a lower incidence of GI upset in the alternate-day supplement group. Accordingly, it appears that an effective oral iron supplement strategy for athletes considered to have compromised iron stores is to consume ~100 mg of iron from an oral polysaccharide-iron complex source, on alternate days, for up to 12 weeks.

Parenteral Iron Administration

Although the outcomes from oral iron supplementation are positive, the process is slow (i.e. weeks), and the magnitude of effect may be underwhelming or persistently unresponsive in severe cases. Accordingly, when an athlete's blood profile indicates an anaemic state (i.e. Stage 3 ID) and their haemoglobin mass appears compromised, parenteral iron administration might be considered by the sports physician. Parenteral iron administration has the benefit of bypassing the gut, where key limitations in absorption exist. The response to an intravenous iron source is rapid, with literature reporting a 200–400% increase in serum ferritin after follow-up assessment conducted between 1 and 56 days post-administration [11, 28]. Although rapid, McKay et al. [60] report a high variability between athletes subsequent to an intravenous iron infusion and recommend an individualised approach to follow-up testing, with efficacy checks at 1 and 6 months post-infusion to track the rate of ferritin decay. Furthermore, it should also be noted that both Woods et al. [61] and Burden et al. [28] reported significant and rapid increases in serum ferritin subsequent to intravenous iron administration in IDNA athletes; however, neither study showed any impact on athletic performance outcomes. Conversely, Garvican et al. [11] showed benefits to endurance capacity in IDA athletes (i.e. haemoglobin mass compromised) after an infusion-derived increase in serum ferritin, likely a result of facilitated erythropoiesis, suggesting this form of treatment is best applied in more severe cases of ID. Finally, it should be considered that parenteral iron administration comes with some, albeit low, risks of negative side effects, which may be as mild as skin staining at the site of injection, through to (very rare) anaphylaxis [62]. Accordingly, the decision to follow this treatment strategy should be made in consultation with a trained sports physician.

Conclusion

It is clear from the evidence presented in this chapter that iron is a fundamental mineral of imperative importance to an athlete's health, physical capacity and performance potential. The various roles that iron plays within the body appear to have many interactions with the processes that contribute to optimal physical output. Therefore, it is essential that athletes maintain healthy iron stores to ensure their haematological adaptation, oxygen transport and energy production potential are realised. Despite such importance, ID is a common diagnosis in athlete populations, likely due to the myriad of exercise-related mechanisms (e.g. haemolysis, GI bleeding, inflammation and hepcidin elevations) that concurrently act to tax iron stores. Although the existing panel of blood markers to measure an athlete's iron status are lacking true consensus, inferences can be made via the reporting of (at a minimum) subjective symptoms of persistent fatigue, in association with low serum ferritin stores and, in more severe cases, compromised haemoglobin levels. Although the impact on physical capacity appears to manifest only in the later stages of ID, early treatment (i.e. at Stage 1 or 2) is likely to prevent the late-stage negative outcomes. Accordingly, the treatment options include an increase in dietary iron intake, the use of oral iron supplements or, in more severe cases, the use of parenteral iron administration. Of course, the direction taken with respect to the treatment strategy used should be decided upon in consultation with a trained sports dietician and sports physician.

References

1. Milic R, Martinovic J, Dopsaj M, Dopsaj V. Haematological and iron-related parameters in male and female athletes according to different metabolic energy demands. Eur J App Physiol. 2011;111(3):449–58.
2. Nabhan D, Bielko S, Sinex JA, Surhoff K, Moreau WJ, Schumacher YO, et al. Serum ferritin distribution in elite athletes. J Science Med Sport. 2020;23(6):554–8.
3. Peeling P, Dawson B, Goodman C, Landers G, Trinder D. Athletic induced iron deficiency: new insights into the role of inflammation, cytokines and hormones. Eur J App Physiol. 2008;103(4):381–91.
4. Beard J, Tobin B. Iron status and exercise. Am J Clin Nutr. 2000;72(2):594S–7S.
5. Sim M, Dawson B, Landers G, Trinder D, Peeling P. Iron regulation in athletes: exploring the menstrual cycle and effects of different exercise modalities on hepcidin production. Int J Sport Nutr Exerc Metab. 2014;24(2):177–87.
6. Clénin G, Cordes M, Huber A, Schumacher YO, Noack P, Scales J, et al. Iron deficiency in sports-definition, influence on performance and therapy. Swiss Med Weekly. 2015;145:w14196.
7. Koulaouzidis A, Said E, Cottier R, Saeed A. Soluble transferrin receptors and iron deficiency, a step beyond ferritin. A systematic review. J Gastrointestin Liver Dis. 2009;18(3):345–52.
8. Garza D, Shrier I, Ford P, Brown M, Matheson G. The clinical value of serum ferritin tests in endurance athletes. Clin J Sports Med. 1997;7(1):46–53.
9. Peeling P, Blee T, Goodman C, Dawson B, Claydon G, Beilby J, et al. Effect of iron injections on aerobic-exercise performance of iron-depleted female athletes. Int J Sport Nutr Exer Metab. 2007;17(3):221–31.
10. Burden RJ, Morton K, Richards T, Whyte GP, Pedlar CR. Is iron treatment beneficial in, iron-deficient but non-anaemic (IDNA) endurance athletes? A systematic review and meta-analysis. Br J Sports Med. 2015;49(21):1389–97.
11. Garvican LA, Saunders PU, Cardoso T, Macdougall IC, Lobigs LM, Fazakerley R, et al. Intravenous iron supplementation in distance runners with low or suboptimal ferritin. Med Sci Sport Exer. 2014;46(2):376–85.
12. DellaValle DM, Haas JD. Iron status is associated with endurance performance and training in female rowers. Med Sci Sport Exer. 2012;44(8):1552–9.
13. Fogelholm M, Jaakkola L, Lampisjärvi T. Effects of iron supplementation in female athletes with low serum ferritin concentration. Int J Sports Med. 1992;13(02):158–62.
14. Friedmann B, Weller E, Mairbaurl H, Bärtsch P. Effects of iron repletion on blood volume and performance capacity in young athletes. Med Sci Sport Exer. 2001;33(5):741–6.
15. Hinton PS, Giordano C, Brownlie T, Haas JD. Iron supplementation improves endurance after training in iron-depleted, nonanemic women. J Appl Physiol. 2000;88(3):1103–11.
16. Lamanca JJ, Haymes EM. Effects of iron repletion on VO_{2max}, endurance, and blood lactate in women. Med Sci Sport Exer. 1993;25(12):1386–92.
17. Klingshirn L, Pate R, Bourque S, Davis J, Sargent R. Effect of iron supplementation on endurance capacity in iron-depleted female runners. Med Sci Sport Exer. 1992;24(7):819–24.

18. Bärtsch P, Mairbäurl H, Friedmann B. Pseudo-anemia caused by sports. Ther Umsch Rev Ther. 1998;55(4):251–5.
19. Sim M, Peeling P, Dawson B, Trinder D. Exercise-induced anemia, in the Encyclopedia of Exercise Medicine in Health and Disease edited by FC Mooren. New York: Springer; 2013. p. 330.
20. Sim M, Dawson B, Landers G, Swinkels DW, Tjalsma H, Yeap BB, et al. Oral contraception does not alter typical post-exercise interleukin-6 and hepcidin levels in females. J Sci Med Sport. 2015;18(1):8–12.
21. Sim M, Dawson B, Landers G, Swinkels DW, Tjalsma H, Trinder D, et al. Effect of exercise modality and intensity on post-exercise interleukin-6 and hepcidin levels. Int J Sport Nutr Exerc Metab. 2013;23(2):178–86.
22. Sim M, Garvican-Lewis LA, Cox GR, Govus A, McKay AK, Stellingwerff T, et al. Iron considerations for the athlete: a narrative review. Eur J App Physiol. 2019;119(7):1463–78.
23. Myhre KE, Webber BJ, Cropper TL, Tchandja JN, Ahrendt DM, Dillon CA, et al. Prevalence and impact of anemia on basic trainees in the US air force. Sports Med-Open. 2016;2(1):23.
24. Haas JD, Brownlie T. Iron deficiency and reduced work capacity: a critical review of the research to determine a causal relationship. J Nutr. 2001;131(2):676S–90S.
25. Blee T, Goodman C, Dawson B, Stapff A. The effect of intramuscular iron injections on serum ferritin levels and physical performance in elite netballers. J Sci Med Sport. 1999;2(4):311–21.
26. Zhu YI, Haas JD. Altered metabolic response of iron-depleted nonanemic women during a 15-km time trial. J Appl Physiol. 1998;84(5):1768–75.
27. Hinton P, Sinclair L. Iron supplementation maintains ventilatory threshold and improves energetic efficiency in iron-deficient nonanemic athletes. Eur J Clin Nutr. 2007;61(1):30.
28. Burden R, Pollock N, Whyte G, Richards T, Moore B, Busbridge M, et al. Effect of intravenous iron on aerobic capacity and iron metabolism in elite athletes. Med Sci Sport Exer. 2015;47(7):1399–407.
29. Dellavalle DM, Haas JD. Iron supplementation improves energetic efficiency in iron-depleted female rowers. Med Sci Sport Exer. 2014;46(6):1204–15.
30. Houston BL, Hurrie D, Graham J, Perija B, Rimmer E, Rabbani R, et al. Efficacy of iron supplementation on fatigue and physical capacity in non-anaemic iron-deficient adults: a systematic review of randomised controlled trials. BMJ Open. 2018;8(4).
31. Rubeor A, Goojha C, Manning J, White J. Does iron supplementation improve performance in iron-deficient nonanemic athletes? Sports Health. 2018;10(5):400–5.
32. DellaValle DM, Haas JD. Impact of iron depletion without anemia on performance in trained endurance athletes at the beginning of a training season: a study of female collegiate rowers. Int J Sport Nutr Exer Metab. 2011;21(6):501–6.
33. Bothwell TH, Charlton R, Cook J, Finch CA. Iron metabolism in man. Exp Physiol. 1980;65(3):255–6.
34. Garvican LA, Lobigs L, Telford R, Fallon K, Gore CJ. Haemoglobin mass in an anaemic female endurance runner before and after iron supplementation. Int J Sport Physiol Perform. 2011;6(1):137–40.
35. Beard JL. Iron biology in immune function, muscle metabolism and neuronal functioning. J Nutr. 2001;131(2):568S–80S.
36. Waller MF, Haymes EM. The effects of heat and exercise on sweat iron loss. Med Sci Sport Exer. 1996;28(2):197–203.
37. Telford RD, Sly GJ, Hahn AG, Cunningham RB, Bryant C, Smith JA. Footstrike is the major cause of hemolysis during running. J Appl Physiol. 2003;94(1):38–42.
38. Selby GB, Eichner ER. Endurance swimming, intravascular hemolysis, anemia, and iron depletion: new perspective on athlete's anemia. Am J Med. 1986;81(5):791–4.
39. Kristiansen M, Graversen JH, Jacobsen C, Sonne O, Hoffman H-J, Law SA, et al. Identification of the haemoglobin scavenger receptor. Nature. 2001;409(6817):198–201.
40. Wrighting DM, Andrews NC. Interleukin-6 induces hepcidin expression through STAT3. Blood. 2006;108(9):3204–9.
41. Nemeth E, Tuttle MS, Powelson J, Vaughn MB, Donovan A, Ward DM, et al. Hepcidin regulates cellular iron efflux by binding to ferroportin and inducing its internalization. Science. 2004;306(5704):2090–3.
42. Peeling P, Dawson B, Goodman C, Landers G, Wiegerinck ET, Swinkels DW, et al. Effects of exercise on hepcidin response and iron metabolism during recovery. Int J Sport Nutr Exer Metab. 2009;19(6):583–97.
43. Troutt JS, Rudling M, Persson L, Ståhle L, Angelin B, Butterfield AM, et al. Circulating human hepcidin-25 concentrations display a diurnal rhythm, increase with prolonged fasting, and are reduced by growth hormone administration. Clin Chem. 2012;58(8):1225–32.
44. McCormick R, Moretti D, McKay AK, Laarakkers CM, Vanswelm R, Trinder D, et al. The Impact of morning versus afternoon exercise on iron absorption in athletes. Med Sci Sport Exer. 2019;51(10):2147–55.
45. Fischer CP. Interleukin-6 in acute exercise and training: what is the biological relevance. Exerc Immunol Rev. 2006;12(6–33):41.
46. Newlin MK, Williams S, McNamara T, Tjalsma H, Swinkels DW, Haymes EM. The effects of acute exercise bouts on hepcidin in women. Int J Sport Nutr Exer Metab. 2012;22(2):79–88.
47. Steensberg A, Febbraio MA, Osada T, Schjerling P, Van Hall G, Saltin B, et al. Interleukin-6 production in contracting human skeletal muscle is influenced by pre-exercise muscle glycogen content. J Physiol. 2001;537(2):633–9.
48. Badenhorst CE, Dawson B, Cox GR, Laarakkers CM, Swinkels DW, Peeling P. Acute dietary carbohydrate manipulation and the subsequent inflammatory and

hepcidin responses to exercise. Eur J App Physiol. 2015;115(12):2521–30.
49. McKay AK, Heikura IA, Burke LM, Peeling P, Pyne DB, van Swelm RP, et al. Influence of periodizing dietary carbohydrate on iron regulation and immune function in elite triathletes. Int J Sport Nutr Exer Metab. 2020;30(1):34–41.
50. Sim M, Dawson B, Landers G, Wiegerinck ET, Swinkels DW, Townsend M-A, et al. The effects of carbohydrate ingestion during endurance running on post-exercise inflammation and hepcidin levels. Eur J App Physiol. 2012;112(5):1889–98.
51. Badenhorst CE, Dawson B, Cox GR, Sim M, Laarakkers CM, Swinkels DW, et al. Seven days of high carbohydrate ingestion does not attenuate post-exercise IL-6 and hepcidin levels. Eur J App Physiol. 2016;116(9):1715–24.
52. McKay AK, Peeling P, Pyne DB, Welvaert M, Tee N, Leckey JJ, et al. Acute carbohydrate ingestion does not influence the post-exercise iron-regulatory response in elite keto-adapted race walkers. J Sci Med Sport. 2019;22(6):635–40.
53. Trumbo P, Yates AA, Schlicker S, Poos M. Dietary reference intakes: vitamin A, vitamin K, arsenic, boron, chromium, copper, iodine, iron, manganese, molybdenum, nickel, silicon, vanadium, and zinc. J Acad Nutr Dietetics. 2001;101(3):294.
54. Deakin V, Peeling P. Prevention, detection and treatment of iron depletion and deficiency in athletes. In Clinical sports nutrition. McGrow-Hill Education; 2015. p. 266–309.
55. Dawson B, Goodman C, Blee T, Claydon G, Peeling P, Beilby J, et al. Iron supplementation: oral tablets versus intramuscular injection. Int J Sport Nutr Exer Metab. 2006;16(2):180–6.
56. Tolkien Z, Stecher L, Mander AP, Pereira DI, Powell JJ. Ferrous sulfate supplementation causes significant gastrointestinal side-effects in adults: a systematic review and meta-analysis. PLoS One. 2015;10(2):e0117383.
57. Yasa B, Agaoglu L, Unuvar E. Efficacy, tolerability, and acceptability of iron hydroxide polymaltose complex versus ferrous sulfate: a randomized trial in pediatric patients with iron deficiency anemia. Int J Pediatric. 2011;2011.
58. Stoffel NU, Cercamondi CI, Brittenham G, Zeder C, Geurts-Moespot AJ, Swinkels DW, et al. Iron absorption from oral iron supplements given on consecutive versus alternate days and as single morning doses versus twice-daily split dosing in iron-depleted women: two open-label, randomised controlled trials. Lancet Haematol. 2017;4(11):e524–e33.
59. McCormick R, Dreyer A, Dawson B, Sim M, Lester L, Goodman C, et al. The effectiveness of daily and alternate day oral iron supplementation in athletes with suboptimal iron status (Part 2). Int J Sport Nutr Exer Metab. 2020;30(3):191.
60. McKay AK, Goods P, Binnie MJ, Goodman C, Peeling P. Examining the decay in serum ferritin following intravenous iron infusion: a retrospective cohort analysis of olympic sport female athletes. App Physiol Nutr Metab. 2020 (in-press).
61. Woods A, Garvican-Lewis LA, Saunders PU, Lovell G, Hughes D, Fazakerley R, et al. Four weeks of IV iron supplementation reduces perceived fatigue and mood disturbance in distance runners. PLoS One. 2014;9(9):e108042.
62. Rampton D, Folkersen J, Fishbane S, Hedenus M, Howaldt S, Locatelli F, et al. Hypersensitivity reactions to intravenous iron: guidance for risk minimization and management. Haematologica. 2014;99(11):1671–6.

Part III

Sources of Iron and Bioavailability

10 Sources of Iron: Diet, Supplemental, and Environmental

Frank T. Wieringa, Marjoleine A. Dijkhuizen, and Jacques Berger

Keywords

Hemoglobin · Anemia · Iron deficiency · Iron fortification · Animal-based foods · Dietary diversification

Animal-based foods have traditionally played an important role in combating iron deficiency, because of the high bioavailability of heme iron. However, with the urgent need to change to more sustainable and durable diets, greatly increasing meat consumption to reach recommended daily intakes of iron is not desirable in the present context. Therefore, alternative, more sustainable sources of dietary iron need to be identified, such as fish or insects. Also, plant-based foods can be good sources of dietary iron, such as soybeans and lentils. Algae, seaweeds, and mushrooms are other foods that can provide important amounts of iron, but are often underutilized.

Iron fortification and supplementation are interventions aimed at either specific population groups (pregnant and lactating women, children between 6 and 24 months) or at the general population (e.g., iron fortification of staple foods). These interventions are often implemented in combination with other micronutrients (e.g., folic acid). Bio-fortification aims to increase iron content of foods by breeding techniques and even genetic modification approaches.

Non-intentional increases of iron in the diet can arise from contamination, either during the processing (e.g., milling) or during the preparation (e.g., brewing) of foods or drinks. Also drinking water can contain high amounts of iron, and even though having a low bioavailability, this iron can contribute to overall iron status of populations, resulting in iron nutrition being better than expected based on dietary assessment in some populations.

To improve iron status of populations vulnerable for iron deficiency, it is not only important to identify potential iron-rich food sources, but also take into account acceptability and cultural habits. In many countries, food taboos play an important role in the etiology of iron deficiency and anemia. Finally, affordability and iron bioavailability of the foods identified need to be considered too. Designing sustainable, acceptable, affordable, and durable diets that provide enough

F. T. Wieringa (✉) · J. Berger
Alimentation, Nutrition, Santé (ANS), UMR 267 – QualiSud, Institut de Recherche pour le Développement (IRD), Montpellier, France

QualiSud, Université de Montpellier, CIRAD, Institut Agro, IRD, Avignon Université, Université de La Réunion, Montpellier, France
e-mail: franck.wieringa@ird.fr

M. A. Dijkhuizen
Department of Nutrition, Exercise and Sports, Faculty of Science, University of Copenhagen, Frederiksberg C, Denmark

C. D. Karakochuk et al. (eds.), *Nutritional Anemia*, Nutrition and Health,
https://doi.org/10.1007/978-3-031-14521-6_10

iron (and other vitamins and minerals) for populations, especially those with a high demand for iron such as pregnant and lactating women and young children, will be a major challenge the coming years.

Introduction

The paradox of iron deficiency in humans is well-known: While iron is one of the most abundant minerals on earth, an estimated two billion people are iron deficient [1]. But most forms of iron present in the earth's crust, such as hematite (Fe_2O_3), are not bioavailable for humans and, hence, cannot serve as source of iron for human metabolism. Thus, for centuries, humans have depended on relatively costly or rare iron-rich foods and more or less bioavailable iron compounds in efforts to improve health. Hippocrates, in the fourth century B.C., has been credited of using watercress, a vegetable rich in iron, as part of his treatments [2]. But it would take almost six centuries before the nutritional importance of iron itself for human health was described by Boussingault [1]. Amazingly, Jean-Baptiste Boussingault was not medically trained but a geologist, who also, for example, reported on the role of minerals in soil in plant growth or nitrogen balance in animals [1]. And it took a further 50 years, until 1928, before the role of iron in treating nutritional anemia was clearly demonstrated by Mackay [2]. And even though the role of iron in treating nutritional anemia is known for almost a century now and iron deficiency is probably the most prevalent micronutrient deficiency globally, most efforts in the last decades to reduce the prevalence of anemia and iron deficiency have not been altogether successful, and thus the prevalence of anemia and iron deficiency continues to remain high.

Before discussing in more detail different potential dietary and non-dietary sources of iron, it should be made clear in advance that there is a huge difference in the bioavailability of different iron compounds. Dietary iron occurs mainly in three forms: elemental iron, either as ferrous iron ($Fe2+$) or as ferric iron ($Fe3+$), and heme iron, that is, $Fe2+$ chelated into a heme complex as found in hemoglobin or myoglobin. Heme iron (with dietary sources obviously coming from animal-source foods) has a much higher bioavailability (in the range of 10–40%) than ferric iron (bioavailability in the range of 5–15%) coming from plant-based foods, as ferric iron first needs to be reduced to its ferrous state before it can be absorbed [3]. Hence, whether iron, ingested through the mouth, ends up being absorbed in the duodenum and becomes part of human metabolism or, as is the case for most of the iron consumed, leaves the gut with the stools is for an important part determined by its chemical form. When iron comes from foods and diets, it is obvious that in addition to iron, other (micro)nutrients are also ingested and these can induce, depending on their interactions (see Chap. 20), promoting or inhibiting effects on the absorption and bioavailability of iron. Furthermore, specific conditions in the gut itself such as acidity, enzymatic activity, microbiome composition, and parasite infestation are not constant and can vary according to age, health, and populations and affect iron bioavailability directly or indirectly (such as through inflammation and microbial metabolism). As iron bioavailability is covered extensively in Chap. 10, the current chapter will focus mainly on the potential sources of iron available to humans, rather than the intricate details of absorption itself for each compound or food. However, where needed, the bioavailability and wider context of certain iron formulations will be discussed.

Iron Sources

Iron can come from many different sources, and these sources can be consumed unwittingly of the iron content or specifically sought out to increase iron intake. In this chapter, we have divided iron sources into three different categories:

I. Common dietary sources of iron: iron in everyday foods and diets.
II. Intentionally increased iron intake (dietary and non-dietary).
III. Non-intentionally increased iron intake.

In the first category, the common dietary sources, iron intake is discussed in the context of typical examples of regular foods and ordinary diets worldwide, as well as the impact of dietary restrictions on iron intake is covered. Furthermore, the increased iron requirements in pregnancy and lactation in relation to dietary iron sources are examined. Under intentionally enhanced intake of iron, we discuss fortification and bio-fortification of staple foods and specific food items with iron as well as iron supplementation. In addition, iron-specific dietary diversification and food-based interventions are also considered, including interventions targeting food processing and cooking techniques. Finally, under the non-intentional sources of iron, contamination of foods with environmental iron including iron-rich drinking water is discussed.

Common Dietary Iron Sources

Dietary patterns around the world differ widely, and as the iron content of foods consumed also ranges widely, the contribution of diet to overall iron intake ranges from negligible to excessive intakes. Surprisingly perhaps, there is no clear consensus on the amount of iron that needs to be consumed on a daily basis. Different recommendations, with different physiological bases, are in common use. For example, the estimated average requirement (EAR), set by the Institute of Medicine (IOM, USA), estimates the average intake needed in a given population, whereas the recommended dietary allowance (RDA) or recommended dietary intake (RDI) gives the amount of iron needed to assure that 97.5% of a population achieves the requirements for that nutrient. The IOM assumes a bioavailability of iron of 18%, whereas the FAO/WHO have made recommendations based on diets with different bioavailability, some of them as low as 5% (Table 10.1). As a result, recommended dietary intakes of iron range from 3 mg/day to >50 mg/day, and perhaps even more perplexing to non-nutritionists is that some recommended intakes from FAO/WHO are higher than the upper limits set by the IOM.

Table 10.1 FAO/WHO and IOM recommended daily intake recommendations for iron (mg/day), by age group

	FAO/WHO recommended nutrient intakes[b]			Institute of Medicine[c] Dietary reference Intakes		
	Estimated bioavailability					
Age (years)[a]	5%	10%	15%	EAR	RDA	UL[d]
0.5–1	18.6	9.3	6.2	6.9	11	40
1–3	11.6	5.8	3.9	3.0	7.0	40
4–6	12.6	6.3	4.2	4.1	10	40
7–8	17.8	8.9	5.9	4.1	10	40
9–10	17.8	8.9	5.9	5.7–5.9	8	40
11–13 male	29.2	14.6	9.7	5.9	8	40
11–13 female (pre-menarche)	28.0	14.0	9.3	5.7	8	40
11–13 female (post-menarche)	65.4	32.7	21.8	–	–	40
14–17 male	37.6	18.8	12.5	7.7	11	45
14–17 female	62.0	31.0	20.7	7.9	15	45
Male (>18 years)	27.4	18.8	9.1	6	8.0	45
Female (18–50 years)	58.8	29.4	19.6	8.1	18	45
Female lactating (>18 years)	30	15	10	6.5	9	45
Pregnant women (>18 years)[e]	–	–	–	22	27	45
Female post-menopausal	22.6	11.3	7.5	5	8	45

[a] The age categories of the FAO/WHO and Institute of Medicine recommendations differ slightly

[b] Vitamin and mineral requirements in human nutrition: 2nd edition. WHO/FAO. 2004

[c] Dietary references intakes for vitamin A, vitamin K, arsenic, boron, chromium, copper, iodine, iron, manganese, molybdenum, nickel, silicon, vanadium, and zinc. Institute of Medicine, 2001. *EAR* estimated average requirement; *FAO* Food and Agricultural Organization of the United Nations; *IOM* Institute of Medicine; *RDA* Recommended Dietary Allowance; *UL* tolerable upper intake levels; *WHO* World Health Organization

[d] UL or tolerable upper intake levels were determined on appearance of gastrointestinal side effects when iron was consumed on an empty stomach

[e] WHO recommends supplementation of 30–60 mg elemental iron per day for pregnant women

It is estimated that today >40% of the world population has an inadequate intake of iron, with diets in Asia and sub-Saharan Africa especially lacking in iron [23]. Milman, using data from 49 dietary intake surveys in 29 European countries, reported median intakes in Europe varying from 7.6 mg of total iron/day (Bosnia) to 18.5 mg total iron/day (Lithuania and Slovakia) [4]. Interestingly, 19 out of these 29 countries reported daily iron intakes for nonpregnant women of reproductive age (WRA) of <11 mg/day, and in almost all countries, >50% of women had a daily intake of <15 mg/day, the most commonly used RDA for WRA. Dietary iron intake in several African countries was even more variable, ranging from 3.8 mg/day in South Africa to >50 mg/day in Ethiopia [5]. Iron intakes in WRA were inadequate in 34% of women in Kenya, to 100% of women in South Africa. In contrast, dietary iron intake in WRA in Ethiopia was inadequate in <12% of the women [5]. Ferguson et al. used linear programming to identify for which nutrients the recommended nutrient intakes (RNIs) were likely not to be met in five Southeast Asian countries [6]. They found that realistic ordinary diets were unlikely to provide the RNI for iron in infants in Cambodia, Indonesia, Laos, Thailand, and Vietnam and for WRA in Cambodia and Vietnam, even when including two servings of chicken liver/week.

Iron in Animal-Based Foods

Increasing intake of iron-rich foods to allow individuals to meet daily iron requirements is often considered synonymous to increasing intake of animal-source foods. Common foods associated with a high iron content are often also animal-source foods, such as liver and blood-containing products. As animal-source foods contain heme iron, the bioavailability of the iron is also high. Chicken liver, for example, contains ~10 mg of iron/100 g [7], while sausages containing blood are reported to have from ~7 mg of iron/100 g (Scottish black pudding) to up to 30–50 mg iron/100 g (Spanish and Peruvian blood sausages) [3]. In several Asian countries, so-called blood curd is popular either as a snack or added to soups. Blood curd contains ~25 mg iron/100 g [8]. However, these products are almost never consumed daily and more often restricted to special occasions. Contrary to popular belief, other forms of animal products contain considerably less iron, even though highly bioavailable, with chicken or beef meat containing only ~1.0–4.0 mg iron/100 g. Eggs are also not a good source of iron, containing on average 1.8 mg iron/100 g, which is mainly concentrated in the egg yolk. Moreover, egg white appears to inhibit the absorption of non-heme iron [9]. Cow's milk is a disappointingly poor iron source (0.5 mg iron/L), and cow's milk consumption in early childhood is even associated with iron deficiency [10].

However, at the same time, the EAT-Lancet commission report on sustainable and healthy diets promotes a sharp shift towards eating less animal-source foods derived from animal husbandry. Indeed, this report acknowledges the delicate balance between increasing nutrient intake and decreasing the impact on climate change in many low- and middle-income countries while estimating that, by 2050, only 13 g of protein from animal-source foods per day is available for sub-Saharan Africa [11]. Hence, alternative dietary sources of iron with a lower carbon footprint need to be identified (e.g., fish, shellfish) and preferentially introduced into local diets. Several species of fish are rich in micronutrients, including iron that is mainly in the form of heme iron and high molecular complex-bound non-heme iron, both of which have a higher bioavailability than non-heme iron from plant sources [12]. Studies from Bangladesh and Cambodia report iron content of small freshwater fish ranging from 0.6 to 14.4 mg total iron/100 g raw edible freshwater fish and from 0.3 to 3.3 mg total iron/100 g for marine fish [13–15]. In Bangladesh, 3 out of 25 species of fish had a high iron content (>5.0 mg/100 g), with heme iron ranging from 0.4 to 4.9 mg. In Cambodia, over 50% (9 out of 16) of the fish species analyzed had a high iron content, with heme iron ranging from 1.3 to 5.4 mg/100 g [16]. Interestingly, the fish *Esomus longimanus*, which is found in rice fields in Cambodia, contained 45.1 mg iron per 100 g edible parts, of which 36.0 mg was heme iron. One serving of traditional Cambodian sour soup made with this species of fish would supply ~45% and ~ 42% of the daily requirement of iron in WRA and children, respectively. Shrimp and prawns were reported to have total iron concentrations ranging from 0.6 to 14.3 mg/100 g, with the percentage of heme iron ranging from 18% to 93% of total iron (0.4–4.9 mg/100 g). Adding small dried fish to plant-based diets can substantially enhance the content (and bioavailability) of iron in the diet, as well as increase the amount of other minerals, such as zinc and calcium. Consumption of fish in the world has quadrupled in the last 40 years, and in many countries, especially in South and Southeast Asia, fish represents ~28–75% of animal protein consumption, with the lowest-income households spending more money on fish than on other animal-source products [12]. This underscores the potential value of fish as a source of dietary iron among vulnerable groups [17] and the relevance of initiatives such as improving aquaculture and marine practices to safeguard and increase their potential as a sustainable food source. This would thereby contribute to more sustainable diets and could reduce the impact of food systems on climate change [18].

Insects are drawing increased attention as a potentially nutrient-rich food source in human diets. More than 2000 insect species are edible and are consumed frequently in tropical regions. Several insect species (e.g., crickets, palm weevils, termites, and caterpillars) are especially rich in zinc and iron [19]. In Thailand, the iron content of edible parts from four different insects obtained from supermarkets of street hawkers ranged from 2.8 mg iron/100 g for the mulberry silkworm (*Bombyx mori L.*) to 9.1 mg iron/100 for the scarab beetle (*Holotrichia* sp.) [20]. A study comparing four commonly consumed insects with sirloin beef showed that cricket and sirloin beef had comparable high levels of iron, higher than grasshopper or buffalo worms. However, iron solubility was higher from insects than beef, and the in vitro iron bioavailability in buffalo worms and sirloin was comparable to that of ferrous sulfate ($FeSO_4$) [21]. However, there are also some disadvantages to insect consumption, as they contain anti-nutrient components (e.g., chitin and chitosan) and also may contain allergens and toxic bioactive compounds, host parasites, and pathogenic bacteria. Lastly, insects may potentially be contaminated with pesticides and heavy metals from the environment [20, 22].

Iron in Plant-Based Foods

Plant-based foods have the potential to be iron-rich, even more than animal-source foods, but iron bioavailability is much lower. However, the largest component of most diets is generally plant-based foods, rather than animal-source foods, as they are more affordable, more accessible, and, in some cases, more acceptable, than animal-source foods. For example, legumes, including beans, peas, and lentils, are good sources of iron. Soybeans contain around 7.8 mg iron/100 g, and fermented soybean products can provide from 1.8–2.1 mg iron/100 g of tofu or tempeh up to 12 mg iron/100 g for Japanese natto. Lentils are another iron-rich food, providing 7 mg iron/100 g. White, lima, red kidney and navy beans, chickpeas, and black-eyed peas provide 3.5–5.2 mg iron per 100 g of cooked product. Nuts and seeds are also iron-rich plant-based foods. Seeds that are richest in iron include pumpkin, sesame, hemp, and flaxseeds, containing ~12–42 mg iron/100 g. Nuts, including almond, cashews, pine, and macadamia nuts, contain ~3.5–5.6 mg iron/100 g. Some types of vegetables also contain high concentrations of iron and are often also rich in vitamin C, a nutrient that can enhance iron absorption. Leafy greens, such as spinach, kale, swiss chard, collard, and beet greens, contain ~2–5 mg iron/100 g of cooked product. Other vegetables, such as broccoli, cabbage, and brussels sprouts, contain ~0.6–1.4 mg iron/100 g of cooked product. Whole grains, such as amaranth, spelt, oats, and quinoa, contain ~2.2–4.1 mg iron/100 g of cooked product. However, phytates, fibers, and plant matrix effects may significantly reduce iron bioavailability in these foods as well as, albeit often to a lesser extent, in all plant-based foods.

Algae and seaweed are also micronutrient-rich (including iron), although the nutritional composition of brown, red, and green seaweeds varies between species, season, and ecology of the harvesting location [23]. In Venezuela, four species of marine algae (*Ulva* sp., *Sargassum* sp., *Porphyra* sp., *and Gracilariopsis* sp.) were shown to be good sources of ascorbic acid and (bioavailable) iron, with iron concentrations ranging from 15.5 mg (*Prophyra* sp.) to 196 mg/100 g of dry weight (*Gracilariopsis* sp.) [24]. All algae, added as a dose between ~10 and 20 g to a rice-based meal, significantly increased iron absorption, up to fivefold of the absorption value of the rice-based meal alone, probably due to both the high vitamin C concentration and a low or non-existent phytate content (an antinutrient that can reduce iron absorption). Samples of edible algae *Porphyra vietnamensis* growing along different localities of the West Coast of India had iron concentrations in a range of ~33–298 mg iron/100 g of dry weight [25]. However, edible seaweed can also contain significant heavy metal concentrations, even though intake is generally below toxic levels, unless there is regular and sizeable consumption of seaweed. Bioaccumulation of arsenic is a risk, and more studies of heavy metal toxicokinetics are needed before any recommendations can be made [23]. For *P. vietnamensis*, the recommended daily intake was 1.3 g/day to avoid any risk of arsenic toxicity. Spirulina, a cyanobacteria or blue-green algae that has received a lot of attention in the last 20 years, could also be a good source of iron and other micronutrients, as iron content ranges between 58 and 180 mg/100 g of dry weight [26]. Finally, a potential source of iron is mushrooms. A study on the iron content of 30 edible mushrooms in Turkey found an average content of 36 mg iron/100 g of edible parts (ranging from 5 to 84 mg iron/100 g) [27]. However, in general, mushrooms are not normally consumed on a daily basis, and more research is warranted in this area.

Iron Intake in Specific Cases: Dietary Restrictions and Increased Requirements

Certain individuals or population groups abstain from consuming certain food groups because of religious beliefs or cultural taboos. For examples, some individuals follow vegan or vegetarian diets, which lack animal-source foods. These diets are often associated with an increased risk for both iron deficiency and anemia [28]. However, Clarys et al. showed that the overall dietary iron intakes of vegans in Belgium were at least as high as those of their peers who were consuming an omnivorous diet (23 vs. 17 mg iron/day); hence, differences in iron status are most likely due to the lower bioavailability of iron from plant-based diets [29]. Food taboos are another factor that can influence iron intakes, but are often ignored or not well-documented. In many cultures, food taboos exist—especially for pregnant and lactating women—often resulting in a lower intake of essential nutrients. For example, in North Laos, up to 80% of women adhered to postpartum food restrictions, which included eating only rice in the postpartum month(s). In a study in Addis Ababa, Ethiopia, almost 20% of pregnant women avoided certain foods during pregnancy, including organ meat and dark green leafy vegetables. Women avoiding these food groups had a significant higher risk for anemia [30]. Dietary restrictions can also arise from traditional and social hierarchic food distribution patterns within the household, often allocating expensive, animal-source foods to the adult men, resulting in restricted access to high-iron foods by women and children. Many traditional beliefs and practices also restrict infant diets, often withholding animal-source foods during the first year or beyond. In Thailand, a common belief is that a child should not be given fish, before she/he can say "Pla" (meaning fish in Thai), to avoid the risk of choking on the bones.

Nutritional status of the mother during pregnancy and lactation is an important determinant of the nutritional status of the newborn, but most iron is already transferred to the infant during the last trimester of pregnancy and during delivery, with maternal iron preferentially being transferred to the fetus, as long as maternal iron status permits [31]. Indeed, the amount of iron in human breastmilk is low, ~0.6 mg/L during the first month of lactation and declining to around 0.2–0.3 mg/L at 6 months postpartum, with apparently no correlation between maternal iron status and breastmilk iron concentration [32]. Iron in human breastmilk is present as lactoferrin, which has a very high bioavailability (~50%) [33]. Lactoferrin serves both as an iron-carrier and chelator, thereby potentially having bacteriostatic activities. Yet, despite the high bioavailability of lactoferrin, concern exists over the iron intake of fully breastfed infants after 4 months, with iron deficiency being more prevalent in infants exclusively breastmilk for 6 months [34]. Iron intake in the second half of infancy should come mainly from complementary foods, with recommended intakes of iron ranging from 6 to 18 mg/day depending on the bioavailability of iron in the diet (Table 10.1). Unfortunately, most traditional complementary foods, especially in low- and middle-income countries (LMIC), have a low nutrient density, and when they contain iron, this is often found in combination with fiber and phytic acid, which may reduce nutrient absorption [35]. Concomitantly, infants and young children require high nutrient intakes and absorption to support their high growth velocity. As a result, many infants and young children in LMIC become iron deficient during the first 2 years of life, as dietary iron intakes are low and bioavailability of ingested iron is low as well. Moreover, boy infants appear to be at an even higher risk for anemia and iron deficiency than girls [36, 37]. One possible explanation for these sex-specific differences may be the higher growth rate of male infants, as compared to females, leading to increased iron requirements in males. We estimated that daily iron intake of male infants should be almost 1 mg/day higher than that of female infants to achieve similar iron body stores [36].

General Considerations on Dietary Sources of Iron

Unfortunately, data on the iron status of a population or data on the iron content of foods is not always available, and many iron-rich foods are underutilized. In many cases, iron deficiency prevalence is estimated from anemia prevalence, which is inaccurate as anemia is caused by a myriad of causes, which may comprise of both nutritional and non-nutritional causes. It is also important to evaluate diets that are actually and realistically consumed, especially in the most at-risk populations. In LMICs, where nutritional anemia is often a serious public health problem, the risk of iron deficiency is often higher in young children and in WRA, especially in pregnant and lactating women. And as prevalence of iron deficiency is higher in lower socioeconomic status groups, the dietary iron sources that are affordable and available are often limited. It is thus crucial for approaches that aim to improve dietary diversity to consider specific situations and constraints to assess how the local food basket can realistically contribute to covering nutrient requirements, especially iron requirements in this case.

Intentionally Increased Iron Intake (Dietary and Non-dietary)

The intentional enhancement of iron intakes can be roughly divided into dietary strategies and non-dietary strategies. Dietary strategies encompass dietary diversification, bio-fortification, and fortification of staple foods, whereas non-dietary strategies include supplementation, as well adaptation of food processing techniques. Dietary strategies and supplementation are covered under other chapters in this book (see Chaps. 26 and 27). Therefore, only a brief summary is provided and some examples are given in Table 10.2.

Supplementation is regarded as the most straightforward intervention to improve dietary iron intakes, although it is often considered as a short- to medium-term solution to fight iron deficiency. However, supplementation programs, such as iron and folic acid (IFA) supplements for pregnant and lactating women, have been in place for decades. The World Health Organization recommends IFA supplements for pregnant women at risk for iron deficiency, with supplements providing 30–60 mg of elemental iron/tablet, and women typically receive 90–180 tablets, to be taken during pregnancy and during the first months of lactation. Recommended iron intake in

Table 10.2 Examples of interventions to intentionally increase dietary iron intake

	Intervention strategies to increase dietary iron intake			
Target group	Supplementation	Fortification	Bio-fortification	Dietary diversification
Pregnant and lactating women	IFA supplements, containing 30–60 mg of iron	Iron-fortified drinks [48] Iron-fortified foods [48]		
Women of reproductive age	Weekly IFA supplements [49]	Iron-fortified drinks [48]		
Adolescent girls (10–19 years)	Intermittent IFA supplements	Fortified drinks [50]		
Young children (6–23 months)	Home fortification with micronutrient powders [51]			
Whole population	–	(Mandatory) fortification of rice, wheat, or maize flour, condiments [52]	Rice (genetically modified or conventional breeding), sweet potato, cassava root, wheat [53]	Increased intake of legumes [54]

IFA iron and folic acid

pregnancy is high (>20 mg/day, Table 10.1), whereas the tolerable upper intake level (UL) set by the IOM is 45 mg/d, giving a narrow window, and indeed complaints on gastrointestinal side effects are not uncommon. A Cochrane review on daily IFA supplements showed that this strategy is effective, with iron deficiency at term reduced by 57% [38]. Moreover, limited evidence suggests that improving iron status of women before conception through weekly IFA supplements can have a positive impact on birth weight [39]. However, the long-term sustainability of providing iron supplements is questionable, as well as that there is a potential negative interaction with infectious diseases, with, for example, a study from Tanzania showing an increase in morbidity and mortality in children receiving iron and folic acid supplements, not only due to malaria but also to other infectious diseases [40]. A specialized type of supplementation is home fortification with micronutrient powders (MNPs), which could be regarded as a method of delivery "in-between" supplementation and fortification. The purpose of home fortification with MNPs is to increase micronutrient intake of children between 6 months and 2 years of age, by adding the MNP to the meal of a child, thereby providing ~12.5 mg of elemental iron. The use of MNP reduces the risk for anemia and iron deficiency by an estimated 18% and 53%, respectively [41]. However, some studies have reported an increase in diarrheal disease with the use MNPs, and there is also a concern for increased gut inflammation and negative effects on the child's intestinal microbiome due to the high iron content [42]. In view of the serious potential drawbacks and the many implementation and uptake challenges of the existing supplementation strategies, new iron supplementation approaches are needed, with new formulations that provide a lower overall dose of iron, but with a higher bioavailability, as extensively described in Chap. 26.

Food-based approaches include a wide range of different strategies such as dietary diversification, food fortification, and bio-fortification. Food-based approaches aim to deliver micronutrients through the diet, and these interventions are considered appropriate as medium- and long-term strategies, with good acceptability and sustainability. Dietary diversification aims to increase the number of food groups being consumed, thereby providing a wider variety and higher concentrations of nutrients in the diet. These interventions are discussed in detail in Chap. 27.

If the iron content of diets is low, bio-fortification or iron fortification of staple foods can be used to increase iron intakes, either as a parallel approach or as a transitional supportive approach until behavioral changes in dietary diversity come into effect. Indeed, iron fortification is feasible for a wide range of food vehicles, including rice, fish and soy sauce, salt, or bouillon cubes [43]. However, some strategies appear to be more effective than others [44, 45]. Also, there is concern about monitoring fortification programs, as many LMIC countries lack the resources for certifying appropriate levels of iron fortification. A recent estimate from four African countries showed that iron-fortified foods contributed to <15% of the RDI for WRA, mainly because iron fortification levels were below standard. If standards were met, iron-fortified foods could contribute up to 65% of the RNI for WRA [46]. Bio-fortification aims at increasing iron content of crops through breeding techniques or genetic engineering. However, pure conventional breeding techniques might sometimes be insufficient, for example, for rice, while genetic engineering of rice could potentially increase iron content of the rice kernel up to four times [47]. Food fortification and bio-fortification are described in detail in Chaps. 24 and 27.

Indirect Methods to Increase Dietary Iron Intake: Food Processing and Preparation

Food processing in its simplest forms includes milling, grinding, and cooking and has the potential to markedly increase the bioavailability of iron. The development of interventions to optimize food processing techniques to improve iron content and bioavailability may provide sustainable tools to improve dietary iron uptake at minimal cost. Examples are parboiling of rice, germination, limited washing of rice, absorption cooking, or the promotion of whole grain or partially milled grains. Parboiling is the process of heat treatment of rice after soaking. For example, by using iron-fortified water during the soaking process, the parboiled rice can obtain significantly higher iron concentrations than rice soaked with regular water. However, other processes are less straightforward, such as the germination of white sorghum, which not only reduced phytate content but also iron content; hence, overall effects on iron status remain to be investigated [55].

Another approach is using food processing techniques to improve the bioavailability of iron. For example, fermentation is one of the oldest food processing techniques known to mankind [56]. Fermentation of maize and of black-eyed peas (Vigna *unguiculata*) significantly increased iron uptake in Caco-2 cells [57, 58]. While most fermentation processes do not significantly increase the iron content of foods, they may have a positive impact on iron bioavailability by reducing the phytate content, breaking down the plant matrix, and sometimes increasing the content of iron absorption enhancing substances, such as vitamin C. A special case is the fermentation of complementary foods, mainly maize- or sorghum-based porridges in East and West Africa, either spontaneously with lactic acid bacilli or added yeast. Although most studies show increases in iron solubility after fermentation, the question remains whether there is a real impact on iron bioavailability as phytic acid-iron ratios remained high [59].

Over the last decades, other non-dietary interventions have been developed with the aim to increase the iron intake of populations. For example, the practice of cooking in iron pots, rather than in aluminum pots, was introduced as potential intervention to increase iron intake, as iron leaches into the food during cooking. A study conducted in Ethiopia showed a positive impact of the use of iron pots on iron status in young children. The authors estimated that cooking in iron pots resulted in 0.24 mg available elemental iron/100 g cooked food, compared to 0.05 mg available elemental iron/100 g cooked food from aluminum pots [60]. However, given the low amount of iron in the cooked food in relation to the RDA of iron and the low bioavailability of iron, whether this increase on iron status was clinically important is questionable. Harvey et al. reviewed the impact of non-food sources of iron, including iron of cooking pots, and concluded that any impact on iron status is highly uncertain [61], while a more recent review is relatively more positive on the potential impact of cooking in iron pots [62]. But in a well-conducted study in Benin, serum ferritin concentrations were lower, rather than higher, in children and women using iron pots for 6 months [63].

The consumption of traditional beers in Southern Africa has also been associated with higher iron status and has even been associated with iron overload [64]. Beer brewed in iron pots in South Africa contained between ~15 and 68 mg iron/L, and ~ 10% of the beer consumers had evidence of iron overload [65]. The long brewing process and the relative acidity of the home brew were factors that likely promoted the increased iron content and bioavailability.

The impact of the more recent, and excessively promoted, "Lucky Iron Fish" on iron status is in contrast highly questionable. These small iron ingots in the form of a fish are added to the water while cooking food, and iron is purportedly leached into the water (and into the cooked food). Depending on acidity, 3–80 mg iron/L is reported to be released [66]. But the surface of cast-iron cooking pots is much larger than of the ingot; hence, the biological plausibility of these small ingots leaching so much iron is questionable. Indeed, a randomized controlled trial in Cambodia did not find any impact of the Lucky Iron Fish on iron status [67], and furthermore, there are also concerns that heavy metals such as arsenic and lead could leach out of the iron ingot. More research on these products is needed to establish their safety and efficacy.

Non-intentionally Increased Iron Intake (Dietary and Non-dietary)

Finally, dietary iron intakes can be increased non-intentionally by inadvertent high iron concentrations in foods, or even non-foods, as a result of external or environmental factors.

Environmental Contaminants

Non-intentional enhancement of iron intake is most often the result of contamination of foods or drinks. A well-known example is the Ethiopian cereal teff, which when processed traditionally in small-scale iron grinding mills can lead to daily iron intakes of >200 mg [61]. However, studies report wide variations in the amount of iron that can be absorbed due to iron contamination of foods. In Senegal, the amount of iron in millet that came from contamination varied between 10 and 80% of the total iron content [68], and Greffeuille et al. reported that traditional milling of maize in Benin doubled or even tripled iron content [69]. An important question is how much of the contaminating iron is freely available for absorption. An extreme example of non-intentional non-dietary iron intake is pica. Pica is often defined as the craving for eating abnormal substances, such as earth, clay, or solid ice (in large amounts). Data from studies on pica suggests that most iron coming from soil is not bioavailable. Pica is often associated with iron deficiency, and one hypothesis on the etiology of geophagy (eating of earth) is that iron deficiency triggers geophagy, as a way to replenish iron stores [70]. However, even though soils and clays often contain large amounts of iron, in the order of 2–3 mg/g, bioavailability of the iron is very low. Indeed, addition of soils or clay to cooked white beans reduced iron uptake in Caco-2 cells, suggesting an inhibitory effect [71].

Iron in the Environment

Another non-intentional source of dietary iron intake can occur when drinking water or soil content is also high in iron. Karakochuk et al. analyzed groundwater from wells in Prey Veng province in Cambodia and reported that ~70% of samples exceeded the recommended maximum level for iron, with a mean concentration of 1.4 mg iron/L [72]. Indeed, iron coming from groundwater could explain the discrepancy between dietary iron content of foods in Cambodia [6] and biochemical data showing very low levels of iron deficiency in the population [73]. In a study in Bangladesh, iron in drinking water ranged from 0 to 79 mg iron/L, with iron content in some areas up to ~4 mg iron/L, contributing to a daily intake of ~11 mg/day. Pregnant women living in the high-iron areas had significant lower risk for iron deficiency and iron deficiency anemia [74]. Finally, iron soil content is associated with plant growth, and iron-deficient soils can lead to retarded plant growth and chlorosis. Increasing the iron content of soil can be done through application of ferrous sulfate (FeSO4) or organic fertilizers. The higher iron content of the cultivated plant can help to increase dietary iron intakes and thereby reduce the risk for iron deficiency populations consuming those plants [75].

To conclude, the first step to identify strategies to increase iron status in humans is to assess dietary iron intakes and sources. Dietary iron can come from many different food sources or can be consumed as a result of food contamination, food processing, or the environment. In addition, non-dietary strategies, such as oral supplementation with iron tablets, are commonly used to increase iron intakes in individuals. But a high dietary iron intake is not equivalent to a high iron status, as iron bioavailability is a critical determinant of iron uptake and is affected by many factors. Furthermore, a fine balance is needed between improving iron status when needed, without unnecessary exposure to high amounts of (poorly absorbable) iron with potentially negative health effects, not even mentioning the potential toxicity of iron overload. Ultimately, a single golden bullet to solve the problem of iron deficiency does not exist. This is the lesson that needs to be drawn from all public health interventions in the last few decades aimed at reducing the prevalence of anemia and iron deficiency. Therefore, a wider perspective is needed, starting with comprehensive measurement of the prevalence of iron deficiency and/or anemia in a population; an extensive examination of the potential causes, underlying risk factors, and the groups most affected; and, finally, the determination of optimal approaches to address iron deficiency and/or anemia in the target population.

References

1. Carpenter KJ. A short history of nutritional science: Part 1 (1785–1885). J Nutr. 2003;133:638–45.
2. Mackay HM. Anaemia in infancy: its prevalence and prevention. Arch Dis Child. 1928;3:117.
3. Gulec S, Anderson GJ, Collins JF. Mechanistic and regulatory aspects of intestinal iron absorption. American Journal of Physiology-Gastrointestinal and Liver. Physiology. 2014;307:G397–409.
4. Milman NT. Dietary iron intake in women of reproductive age in Europe: a review of 49 studies from 29 countries in the period 1993–2015. J Nutr Metab. 2019;2019:7631306.
5. Harika R, Faber M, Samuel F, Kimiywe J, Mulugeta A, Eilander A. Micronutrient status and dietary intake of iron, vitamin A, iodine, folate and zinc in women of reproductive age and pregnant women in Ethiopia, Kenya, Nigeria and South Africa: a systematic review of data from 2005 to 2015. Nutrients. 2017;9:1096.
6. Ferguson EL, Watson L, Berger J, Chea M, Chittchang U, Fahmida U, Khov K, Kounnavong S, Le BM, Rojroongwasinkul N. Realistic food-based approaches alone may not ensure dietary adequacy for women and young children in South-East Asia. Matern Child Health J. 2019;23:55–66.
7. Kongkachuichai R, Napatthalung P, Charoensiri R. Heme and nonheme iron content of animal products commonly consumed in Thailand. J Food Compos Anal. 2002;15:389–98.
8. Wang FS, Lin CW. The effects of heating and chemical treatment on the haem and non-haem iron content of heat-induced porcine blood curd. J Sci Food Agric. 1994;65:209–13.
9. Hurrell RF, Lynch SR, Trinidad TP, Dassenko SA, Cook JD. Iron absorption in humans: bovine serum albumin compared with beef muscle and egg white. Am J Clin Nutr. 1988;47(1):102–7.
10. Ziegler EE. Consumption of cow's milk as a cause of iron deficiency in infants and toddlers. Nutr Rev. 2011;69(Suppl 1):S37–42.
11. Willett W, Rockström J, Loken B, Springmann M, Lang T, Vermeulen S, Garnett T, Tilman D, DeClerck F, Wood A, et al. Food in the Anthropocene: the EAT-Lancet Commission on healthy diets from sustainable food systems. Lancet (London, England). 2019;393:447–92.
12. Kawarazuka N, Béné C. Linking small-scale fisheries and aquaculture to household nutritional security: an overview. Food Security. 2010;2:343–57.
13. Roos N, Thorseng H, Chamnan C, Larsen T, Gondolf UH, Bukhave K, Thilsted SH. Iron content in common Cambodian fish species: perspectives for dietary iron intake in poor, rural households. Food Chem. 2007;104:1226–35.
14. Roos N, Wahab MA, Hossain MAR, Thilsted SH. Linking human nutrition and fisheries: incorporating micronutrient-dense, small indigenous fish species in carp polyculture production in Bangladesh. Food Nutr Bull. 2007;28:S280–S93.
15. Wheal MS, DeCourcy-Ireland E, Bogard JR, Thilsted SH, Stangoulis JC. Measurement of haem and total iron in fish, shrimp and prawn using ICP-MS: implications for dietary iron intake calculations. Food Chem. 2016;201:222–9.
16. Roos N, Islam MM, Thilsted SH. Small indigenous fish species in Bangladesh: contribution to vitamin A, calcium and iron intakes. J Nutr. 2003;133:4021S–6S.
17. Hicks CC, Cohen PJ, Graham NAJ, Nash KL, Allison EH, D'Lima C, Mills DJ, Roscher M, Thilsted SH, Thorne-Lyman AL, et al. Harnessing global fish-

eries to tackle micronutrient deficiencies. Nature. 2019;574:95–8.
18. Costello C, Cao L, Gelcich S, Cisneros-Mata MÁ, Free CM, Froehlich HE, Golden CD, Ishimura G, Maier J, Macadam-Somer I, et al. The future of food from the sea. Nature. 2020;588:95–100.
19. van Huis A. Edible insects are the future? Proc Nutr Soc. 2016;75:294–305.
20. Köhler R, Kariuki L, Lambert C, Biesalski H. Protein, amino acid and mineral composition of some edible insects from Thailand. J Asia Pac Entomol. 2019;22:372–8.
21. Latunde-Dada GO, Yang W, Vera Aviles M. In vitro iron availability from insects and sirloin beef. J Agric Food Chem. 2016;64:8420–4.
22. Imathiu S. Benefits and food safety concerns associated with consumption of edible insects. NFS J. 2020;18:1–11.
23. Cherry P, O'Hara C, Magee PJ, McSorley EM, Allsopp PJ. Risks and benefits of consuming edible seaweeds. Nutr Rev. 2019;77:307–29.
24. García-Casal MN, Pereira AC, Leets I, Ramírez J, Quiroga MF. High iron content and bioavailability in humans from four species of marine algae. J Nutr. 2007;137:2691–5.
25. Rao PS, Mantri VA, Ganesan K. Mineral composition of edible seaweed Porphyra vietnamensis. Food Chem. 2007;102:215–8.
26. Gutiérrez-Salmeán G, Fabila-Castillo L, Chamorro-Cevallos G. Aspectos nutricionales y toxicológicos de Spirulina (arthrospira). Nutr Hosp. 2015;32:34–40.
27. Gençcelep H, Uzun Y, Tunçtürk Y, Demirel K. Determination of mineral contents of wild-grown edible mushrooms. Food Chem. 2009;113:1033–6.
28. Haider LM, Schwingshackl L, Hoffmann G, Ekmekcioglu C. The effect of vegetarian diets on iron status in adults: a systematic review and meta-analysis. Crit Rev Food Sci Nutr. 2018;58:1359–74.
29. Clarys P, Deliens T, Huybrechts I, Deriemaeker P, Vanaelst B, De Keyzer W, Hebbelinck M, Mullie P. Comparison of nutritional quality of the vegan, vegetarian, semi-vegetarian, pesco-vegetarian and omnivorous diet. Nutrients. 2014;6(3):1318–32.
30. Mohammed SH, Taye H, Larijani B, Esmaillzadeh A. Food taboo among pregnant Ethiopian women: magnitude, drivers, and association with anemia. Nutr J. 2019;18(1):19.
31. Cao C, Fleming MD. The placenta: the forgotten essential organ of iron transport. Nutr Rev. 2016;74(7):421–31.
32. Domellöf M, Lönnerdal B, Dewey KG, Cohen RJ, Hernell O. Iron, zinc, and copper concentrations in breast milk are independent of maternal mineral status. Am J Clin Nutr. 2004;79(1):111–5.
33. Cerami C. Iron nutriture of the fetus, neonate, infant, and child. Ann Nutr Metab. 2017;71(Suppl 3):8–14.
34. Chantry CJ, Howard CR, Auinger P. Full breastfeeding duration and risk for iron deficiency in U.S. infants. Breastfeed Med. 2007;2(2):63–73.
35. Dewey KG, Brown KH. Update on technical issues concerning complementary feeding of young children in developing countries and implications for intervention programs. Food Nutr Bull. 2003;24(1):5–28.
36. Wieringa FT, Berger J, Dijkhuizen MA, Hidayat A, Ninh NX, Utomo B, Wasantwisut E, Winichagoon P. Sex differences in prevalence of anaemia and iron deficiency in infancy in a large multi-country trial in South-East Asia. Br J Nutr. 2007;98:1070–6.
37. Domellöf M, Lönnerdal B, Dewey KG, Cohen RJ, Rivera LL, Hernell O. Sex differences in iron status during infancy. Pediatrics. 2002;110:545–52.
38. Peña-Rosas JP, De-Regil LM, Garcia-Casal MN, Dowswell T. Daily oral iron supplementation during pregnancy. Cochrane Database Syst Rev. 2015;2015(7):CD004736.
39. Viteri FE, Berger J. Importance of pre-pregnancy and pregnancy iron status: can long-term weekly preventive iron and folic acid supplementation achieve desirable and safe status? Nutr Rev. 2005;63:S65–76.
40. Sazawal S, Black RE, Ramsan M, Chwaya HM, Stoltzfus RJ, Dutta A, Dhingra U, Kabole I, Deb S, Othman MK, et al. Effects of routine prophylactic supplementation with iron and folic acid on admission to hospital and mortality in preschool children in a high malaria transmission setting: community-based, randomised, placebo-controlled trial. Lancet (London, England). 2006;367:133–43.
41. Suchdev PS, Jefferds MED, Ota E, da Silva LK, De-Regil LM. Home fortification of foods with multiple micronutrient powders for health and nutrition in children under two years of age. Cochrane Database Syst Rev. 2020;2(2):CD008959.
42. Paganini D, Zimmermann MB. The effects of iron fortification and supplementation on the gut microbiome and diarrhea in infants and children: a review. Am J Clin Nutr. 2017;106(Suppl 6):1688S–93S.
43. Dijkhuizen MA, Greffeille V, Roos N, Berger J, Wieringa FT. Interventions to improve micronutrient status of women of reproductive age in Southeast Asia: a narrative review on what works, what might work, and what doesn't work. Matern Child Health J. 2019;23(Suppl 1):18–28.
44. Van Thuy P, Berger J, Nakanishi Y, Khan NC, Lynch S, Dixon P. The use of NaFeEDTA-fortified fish sauce is an effective tool for controlling iron deficiency in women of childbearing age in rural Vietnam. Nutrition. 2005;135(11):2596–601.
45. Peña-Rosas JP, Mithra P, Unnikrishnan B, Kumar N, De-Regil LM, Nair NS, Garcia-Casal MN, Solon JA. Fortification of rice with vitamins and minerals for addressing micronutrient malnutrition. Cochrane Database Syst Rev. 2019;2019:CD009902. https://doi.org/10.1002/14651858.CD009902.pub2.
46. Friesen VM, Mbuya MN, Aaron GJ, Pachón H, Adegoke O, Noor RA, Swart R, Kaaya A, Wieringa FT, Neufeld LM. Fortified foods are major contributors to apparent intakes of vitamin A and iodine, but not iron, in diets of women of reproductive age in 4 African countries. J Nutr. 2020;150(8):2183–90.

47. Majumder S, Datta K, Datta SK. Rice biofortification: high iron, zinc, and vitamin-A to fight against "hidden hunger". Agronomy. 2019;9:803.
48. Athe R, Dwivedi R, Pati S, Mazumder A, Banset U. Meta-analysis approach on iron fortification and its effect on pregnancy and its outcome through randomized, controlled trials. J Family Med Primary Care. 2020;9:513–9.
49. WHO. WHO guidelines approved by the guidelines review committee. guideline: intermittent iron and folic acid supplementation in menstruating women. Geneva: World Health Organization; 2011.
50. Ziauddin Hyder SM, Haseen F, Khan M, Schaetzel T, Jalal CSB, Rahman M, Lönnerdal B, Mannar V, Mehansho H. A multiple-micronutrient-fortified beverage affects hemoglobin, iron, and vitamin A status and growth in adolescent girls in Rural Bangladesh. J Nutr. 2007;137:2147–53.
51. Tam E, Keats EC, Rind F, Das JK, Bhutta AZA. Micronutrient supplementation and fortification interventions on health and development outcomes among children under-five in low- and middle-income countries: a systematic review and meta-analysis. Nutrients. 2020;12:289.
52. Waller AW, Andrade JE, Mejia LA. Performance factors influencing efficacy and effectiveness of iron fortification programs of condiments for improving anemia prevalence and iron status in populations: a systematic review. Nutrients. 2020;12:275.
53. Connorton JM, Balk J. Iron biofortification of staple crops: lessons and challenges in plant genetics. Plant Cell Physiol. 2019;60:1447–56.
54. Mutwiri LN, Kyallo F, Kiage B, Van der Schueren B, Matthys C. Can improved legume varieties optimize iron status in low- and middle-income countries? A systematic review. Adv Nutr. 2020;11:1315–24.
55. Afify AE-MM, El-Beltagi HS, Abd El-Salam SM, Omran AA. Bioavailability of iron, zinc, phytate and phytase activity during soaking and germination of white sorghum varieties. PLoS One. 2011;6:e25512.
56. Baye K, Mouquet-Rivier C, Icard-Vernière C, Picq C, Guyot J-P. Changes in mineral absorption inhibitors consequent to fermentation of Ethiopian injera: implications for predicted iron bioavailability and bioaccessibility. Int J Food Sci Technol. 2014;49:174–80.
57. Proulx AK, Reddy MB. Fermentation and lactic acid addition enhance iron bioavailability of maize. J Agric Food Chem. 2007;55:2749–54.
58. Chawla P, Bhandari L, Sadh PK, Kaushik R. Impact of solid-state fermentation (Aspergillus oryzae) on functional properties and mineral bioavailability of black-eyed pea (Vigna unguiculata) seed flour. Cereal Chem. 2017;94:437–42.
59. Gabaza M, Muchuweti M, Vandamme P, Raes K. Can fermentation be used as a sustainable strategy to reduce iron and zinc binders in traditional African fermented cereal porridges or gruels? Food Rev Intl. 2017;33:561–86.
60. Adish AA, Esrey SA, Gyorkos TW, Jean-Baptiste J, Rojhani A. Effect of consumption of food cooked in iron pots on iron status and growth of young children: a randomised trial. Lancet. 1999;353(9154):712–6.
61. Harvey PW, Dexter PB, Darnton-Hill I. The impact of consuming iron from non-food sources on iron status in developing countries. Public Health Nutr. 2000;3(4):375–83.
62. Alves CA-O, Saleh A, Alaofè H. Iron-containing cookware for the reduction of iron deficiency anemia among children and females of reproductive age in low- and middle-income countries: a systematic review. PLoS One. 2019;14(9):e0221094.
63. Sharieff W, Dofonsou J, Zlotkin S. Is cooking food in iron pots an appropriate solution for the control of anaemia in developing countries? A randomised clinical trial in Benin. Public Health Nutr. 2008;11(9):971–7.
64. Bothwell T, Seftel H, Jacobs P, Torrance J, Baumslag N. Iron overload in Bantu subjects: studies on the availability of iron in Bantu beer. Am J Clin Nutr. 1964;14:47–51.
65. Choma S, Alberts M, Urdal P. Effect of traditional beer consumption on the iron status of a rural South African population. South Afr J Clin Nutr. 2007;20:62–8.
66. Charles CV, Summerlee AJ, Dewey CE. Iron content of Cambodian foods when prepared in cooking pots containing an iron ingot. Tropical Med Int Health. 2011;16(12):1518–24.
67. Rappaport AA-O, Whitfield KC, Chapman GE, Yada RY, Kheang KM, Louise J, Summerlee AJ, Armstrong GR, Green TJ. Randomized controlled trial assessing the efficacy of a reusable fish-shaped iron ingot to increase hemoglobin concentration in anemic, rural Cambodian women. Am J Clin Nutr. 2017;106(2):667–74.
68. Galan P, Cherouvrier F, Zohoun I, Zohoun T, Chauliac M, Hercberg S. Iron absorption from typical West African meals containing contaminating Fe. Br J Nutr. 1990;64:541–6.
69. Greffeuille V, Polycarpe Kayodé AP, Icard-Vernière C, Gnimadi M, Rochette I, Mouquet-Rivier C. Changes in iron, zinc and chelating agents during traditional African processing of maize: effect of iron contamination on bioaccessibility. Food Chem. 2011;126:1800–7.
70. Young SL. Pica in pregnancy: new ideas about an old condition. Annu Rev Nutr. 2010;30:403–22.
71. Seim GL, Ahn CI, Bodis MS, Luwedde F, Miller DD, Hillier S, Tako E, Glahn RP, Young SL. Bioavailability of iron in geophagic earths and clay minerals, and their effect on dietary iron absorption using an in vitro digestion/Caco-2 cell model. Food Funct. 2013;4:1263–70.
72. Karakochuk CD, Murphy HM, Whitfield KC, Barr SI, Vercauteren SM, Talukder A, Porter K, Kroeun H, Eath M, McLean J, et al. Elevated levels of iron in groundwater in Prey Veng province in Cambodia: a possible factor contributing to high iron stores in women. J Water Health. 2014;13:575–86.

73. Wieringa FT, Dahl M, Chamnan C, Poirot E, Kuong K, Sophonneary P, Sinuon M, Greuffeille V, Hong R, Berger J. The high prevalence of anemia in Cambodian children and women cannot be satisfactorily explained by nutritional deficiencies or hemoglobin disorders. Nutrients. 2016;8:348.
74. Ahmed F, Khan MR, Shaheen N, Ahmed KMU, Hasan A, Chowdhury IA, Chowdhury R. Anemia and iron deficiency in rural Bangladeshi pregnant women living in areas of high and low iron in groundwater. Nutrition. 2018;51:46–52.
75. Palanog AD, Calayugan MIC, Descalsota-Empleo GI, Amparado A, Inabangan-Asilo MA, Arocena EC, Cruz PC, Borromeo TH, Lalusin A, Hernandez JE, et al. Zinc and iron nutrition status in the Philippines population and local soils. Front Nutr. 2019;6:81.

Iron Bioavailability: Enhancers and Inhibitors

11

Manju B. Reddy, Isaac Agbemafle, and Seth Armah

Introduction

Iron bioavailability (IBA) refers to the amount of absorbed iron that is available for normal physiological functions and storage. Dietary iron absorption is influenced by the physicochemical form of iron and the dietary factors that influence their absorption in the gastrointestinal tract. Dietary iron exists in two distinct forms, heme and nonheme iron, and their relative proportions determine food IBA. Heme iron, which comes from hemoglobin and myoglobin, is mainly found in animal-source foods, and nonheme iron is present in both plant and animal foods. Although ~10–15% of total dietary iron originates from heme iron in meat-containing diets, it contributes to ~40% of the daily iron requirement because of its higher absorption of ~25% [1]. Dietary sources of nonheme iron include nuts, legumes, vegetables, and grain products. Absorption of nonheme iron is known to be much lower (<10%) than heme iron. The entire of nonheme iron forms a common iron pool in the digestive tract, and iron absorption from this pool is affected by factors in the diet, as well as physiological factors specific to the individual, such as iron status. The total IBA is ~14–18% from mixed diets that include both heme and nonheme iron as was estimated recently [2].

Extensive reviews were published recently on iron absorption and IBA [3–5]. Heme iron is absorbed as an intact porphyrin molecule by what is assumed to be a different mechanism than nonheme iron. The intact metaloporphyrin enters the mucosal cell using a receptor at the brush border after the globin is separated by intestinal proteolytic enzymes. Dietary heme iron absorption is relatively unaffected by dietary factors, except by calcium, but inversely influenced by the individual iron status, similar to nonheme iron. Once heme enters the enterocyte, iron is released from heme by heme oxygenase before entering the common cellular iron pool and being transferred to the plasma.

Similar to heme iron absorption, nonheme iron absorption is also inversely influenced by iron status. Nonheme iron uptake in the gut epithelium is much better characterized than for heme iron. It is transported by enterocytes through divalent metal transporter (DMT-1). Although absorption from the nonheme iron pool constitutes a major fraction of daily iron intake, unlike heme iron, its absorption depends on the

M. B. Reddy (✉)
Food Science and Human Nutrition, Iowa State University, Ames, IA, USA
e-mail: mbreddy@iastate.edu

I. Agbemafle
Fred N. Binka School of Public Health, University of Health and Allied Sciences, Ho, Ghana
e-mail: iagbemafle@uhas.edu.gh

S. Armah
Nutrition, University of North Carolina at Greensboro, Greensboro, NC, USA
e-mail: s_armah@uncg.edu

C. D. Karakochuk et al. (eds.), *Nutritional Anemia*, Nutrition and Health,
https://doi.org/10.1007/978-3-031-14521-6_11

presence of a variety of dietary components ingested simultaneously. In general, the factors that solubilize iron in the lumen dictate its bioavailability. Several dietary components, such as ascorbic acid and animal products like meat, fish, and poultry (MFP), are important in increasing IBA. Inhibitors such as phytate from bran and seeds and polyphenols from coffee, tea, and legumes could bind iron tightly and cause the inhibition of its absorption. Although it is not clear, calcium may inhibit nonheme iron absorption [6]. Vitamin A, carotenoids, oxalic acid, and inulin (non-digestible carbohydrate) have also been shown to affect iron absorption, but the data is inconclusive [1, 4]. Ferritin iron is taken up by an endocytic mechanism [7], but results from another group show that ferritin is degraded during digestion releasing nonheme iron [8]. Ferritin iron absorption is similar to ferrous sulphate in human subjects [9] and does not suggest that it is absorbed differently from nonheme iron.

While individual effects of each factor are well-studied in single meal human absorption studies, understanding the interplay of nutrients and non-nutrients and their effects in a mixed meal is complex. Nonetheless, mixed diets have generally shown smaller effect of enhancers and inhibitors on iron bioavailability compared to single meal absorption studies [10–12]. The effect of individual enhancers and inhibitors of IBA is described below.

Muscle Tissue (MFP)

Animal tissue not only offers highly absorbable heme iron but is also known to enhance nonheme iron absorption. The positive influence of animal tissue on nonheme iron absorption in humans has been reported by several researchers using single meal absorption studies. A dose-response increase in iron absorption was reported when pork meat was added to high phytate, low-ascorbic acid-containing meal suggesting the positive effect of meat even from an inhibiting meal [13].

The effect of animal tissue on nonheme iron absorption was found not to be due to differences in the quality and quantity of the proteins, and all animal tissues, such as pork, beef, chicken, liver, lamb, and fish, had similar enhancing effects on iron absorption, whereas egg, milk, cheese, and ovalbumin protein had no enhancing effect [14–16]. It is well-known that animal tissue enhances nonheme iron absorption, but the mechanism is not clear. The positive influence of animal tissue has been attributed to an unknown "factor" hypothesized to prevent iron from polymerizing and maintain iron in a stable soluble form suitable for absorption [17]. A clear understanding of the positive effect of meat has not yet been achieved, but the data suggest that proteins and/or their constituents in meat interact with nonheme iron and maintain its solubility. Meat proteins may possess nonheme iron absorption-enhancing capabilities because of certain amino acids and intermediary products, likely produced during gastrointestinal digestion. These substituents may chelate and solubilize iron, thereby facilitating nonheme iron absorption by the gut mucosa.

Researchers have also suggested that the amino acid profile of proteins was responsible for the differences observed in iron absorption. Initially, evidence suggested that the enhancing effect of cysteine-containing peptides released from digestion of meat was responsible for reducing and chelating iron [18]. Histidine and lysine were also found to increase iron absorption when given concurrently with ferric iron in rat intestinal segments [19]. Extrapolating the results from rat studies to humans is however questionable due to the limited sensitivity of rats to enhancing and inhibiting dietary factors [20]. A further study suggested that the "meat factor" may not be due to a single peptide fraction but more likely to be a multitude of small peptides [21].

In a human study, the protein fraction of chicken and beef were shown to be responsible for increasing iron absorption, even though the authors did not clearly rule out the potential enhancing effect of other fractions in the meat [22]. Histidine content of low-molecular-weight beef proteins produced following in vitro digestion was shown to be responsible for increased

IBA in a cell culture model [23]. However, using a similar cell culture model, another research group [24] showed that the low-molecular-weight carbohydrates of fish muscle tissue were responsible for increasing nonheme iron uptake in caco-2 cells. These carbohydrates are suggested as oligosaccharides, possibly glycosaminoglycans, which are part of the muscle tissue matrix.

In a pilot study with a food supplement that contained fish cartilage glycosaminoglycans containing no iron, researchers reported an improvement in iron status in 4 months [25], which supports the enhancing effects of glycosaminoglycans on IBA. However, it does not rule out the confounding effect of other components present in the cartilage. On the contrary, no enhancing effect of commercial glycosamines was found in humans when iron absorption was measured with stable isotopes [26], but authors suggested that differences between naturally occurring glycosamines and the commercial product may be attributed to these disagreements. Using a combination of biochemical methods to identify and purify the components in beef coupled with testing in humans showed that purified L-a-glycerophosphocholine can also enhance iron absorption from a meal containing low amounts of inhibitors [27]. However, based on the information available to date, no clear evidence exists to clearly identify the nature of the "meat factor."

The enhancing effect of meat from whole diets is not clear. In a controlled feeding study, researchers showed that adding 60 g pork meat to the high phytate Polish and Danish diet for 5-day increased iron absorption significantly [28]. On the contrary, only a marginal increase was observed when the subjects increased their animal tissue intake to 300 g/day for 5-day compared to their habitual diet [12]. Nonetheless, a recent meta-analysis indicates that there is a positive association of animal flesh foods and iron status in adults within the developed countries, but it is not clear on the optimum quantity or frequency of flesh intake required to maintain or achieve a healthy iron status [29].

Ascorbic Acid

Ascorbic acid (AA), mainly found in fruits and vegetables, is well-known for its reducing and antioxidant properties and, most importantly, as a powerful enhancer of iron absorption. AA acts by forming a soluble chelate with iron at the low pH of the stomach, which is maintained in the intestine, thus preventing the formation of insoluble and unabsorbable iron compounds with other ligands (i.e., phytates) [30]. Investigations by other researchers suggest that the AA-iron complex is absorbed intact in the duodenum, and others indicate that the binding mechanism predominates over the ferrireductase activity of AA [31]. Interestingly, AA is a cofactor of duodenal cytochrome b (Dcytb), the main enzyme that reduces iron from ferric to ferrous form at the luminal membrane of the enterocyte [32]. Thus, AA increases iron absorption by reduction mechanisms involving ferric to ferrous conversions, allowing its effective transport.

There is ample evidence from many single-meal radioisotope studies in humans on the dose-dependent enhancing effect of native or added AA on iron absorption. When tested with added AA, the increase in iron absorption from a semi-synthetic meal was directly proportional to the amount of AA added over a range of 25–1000 mg [33]. Similarly, Ballot et al. [34] showed that iron absorption with different fruit juices was closely correlated with the AA content of the juices. The addition of 15 mg synthetic AA also improved the nonheme iron absorption from a basic rice meal by 98% [35].

Even in the presence of inhibitors such as phytate, polyphenols, calcium and the proteins in milk products [30, 36], AA can counteract their inhibitory effects to increase the absorption of both native and fortification iron. For example, the inhibitory effects of phytic acid from cereals were overcome by AA to increase iron absorption up to 84% in maize and 48% in wheat [37]. Evidence from other studies suggest that adding 50 mg or more AA prevented the dose-dependent inhibitory effects of polyphenols and phytates on nonheme iron absorption from meals [30, 36].

However, comparing single meal to whole meal studies, AA enhancing effect on iron absorption is modest in whole meal studies [11]. This is probably the reason why a systematic review by Hunt et al. [38] did not show a significant effect on iron status after prolonged supplementation with AA.

Other authors have argued that the AA/Fe molar ratio is an important determinant for the final effect on iron absorption. Available evidence point to a 2:1 ratio for low phytate content foods and up to 4:1 for high phytate content food [31, 39]. However, it should be noted AA is sensitive to temperature and air exposure and that food processing techniques may decrease its concentration and oxidize it to decrease its enhancing effect on iron absorption [31].

Phytic Acid

Phytic acid (myo-inositol hexakisphosphate, or IP6) is the primary inhibitor of iron absorption in plant-based diets. When phytic acid is bound with minerals such as calcium or magnesium, it is refred as phytate. Phytate is present in generous amounts in nuts, legumes, and seeds, reaching up to ~5% by weight [40]. In these foods, it is the predominant storage form of phosphorus, storing close to 80% of phosphorus in some foods [40]. Phytate intake is also very high in developing countries due to the frequent consumption of plant-based foods and is of major concern mostly because of its contribution to mineral deficiencies, particularly iron and zinc. For example, daily phytate intake in Nigeria is about 3× the daily intake in the UK [41]. Phytate is an ester of inositol with up to six phosphate groups that are partially ionized at physiological pH [40]. The negatively charged phosphate groups provide strong affinity for metallic cations including iron. Phytate binds to these metals to produce complexes that are insoluble, hence rendering them almost unabsorbable [42]. The inhibitory effect of phytate is mostly attributed to the higher inositol phosphates with five or six phosphate groups (myo-inositol hexaphosphate-IP6 and myo-inositol pentaphosphate IP5), with little or no effect of the lower inositol phosphates on iron solubility [43].

Phytate inhibits iron absorption in a dose-dependent manner, hence reducing phytate content of the meal leads to improved absorption. For example, Hurrell et al. [44] demonstrated that reducing the phytate content of soy protein isolates from 4.9–8.4 mg/g to ≤0.01 mg/g resulted in 4–5× improvement in iron absorption. It is recommended that, to improve iron absorption from phytate-rich foods, the phytate to iron molar ratio should be reduced to less than 1:1 in cereal or legume-based meals that do not contain any iron absorption enhancers or less than 6:1 in meals that contain meat or ascorbic acid [1]. This recommendation is particularly necessary in countries or populations where iron deficiency is prevalent. The inhibitory effect of phytic acid can be reversed by the addition of ascorbic acid suggesting that it has lesser affinity for iron than ascorbic acid [30]. Reducing the phytate content of meals can be achieved by several methods including milling, heat treatment, soaking, germination, fermentation, and addition of exogenous phytase enzyme [45]. Many of these food processing techniques are used commonly in low-resource countries.

Phytases are enzymes that catalyze the phosphate monoester hydrolysis of phytate to produce intermediate and lower forms of inositol phosphates (IP-1, IP-2, IP-3, IP-4, and IP-5) which have lower binding capacities for iron, zinc, and other metallic cations [43]. Increased phytase activity in germination occurs through de novo synthesis of the enzyme or endogenous phytase activation or both [46]. Germination has been reported to decrease phytate content by as much as 40% [46]. In fermentation, microflora on the surface of cereal grains produce phytase that breaks down phytate. The fermentation process also provides a suitable pH for the enzymatic breakdown of phytate [47]. Soaking helps to reduce phytate content in foods which have phytates stored in water-soluble forms, such as sodium or potassium phytates [47].

Despite the overwhelming data on the significant inhibitory effect of phytate on nonheme iron absorption, it has also been shown that the inhibitory effect is less pronounced when a mixed meal is considered, as compared to what is observed in single-meal studies. For example, the inhibitory effect of a mixed diet that was high in phytate, calcium, and polyphenols consumed over a 2-week period was statistically significantly lower (3.2% absorption) compared to the inhibitory effect observed when absorption was measured from a single meal (2.3% absorption) [48]. In a more recent study [49], decreased inhibitory effect of phytate on nonheme IBA was shown when persons regularly consumed high phytate diets. We have also demonstrated in a regression model using complete diet data that while among the dietary factors, phytate contributed the most significantly in determining nonheme iron absorption, it explained <1% of the variability in iron absorption, compared to ~35% for serum ferritin [50]. This supports the assertion that the inhibitory effect of phytates on nonheme iron absorption is decreased in a mixed and varied diet. These efforts to reduce the phytate content of foods, especially in the more monotonous diets in low-resource countries where iron and zinc deficiencies are rife, are still necessary to address these micronutrient deficiencies.

Polyphenols

Polyphenols are naturally occurring secondary metabolites of plants. They are known major dietary inhibitors of iron absorption because of their ability to form insoluble complexes or co-precipitates under neutral to alkaline conditions during digestion [51]. Other studies have reported polyphenols could inhibit the activity of digestive enzymes [52, 53]. It is likely that polyphenols bind to digestive enzymes to inactivate them; thus, iron may remain complexed within the non-digested starch and protein molecules. The inhibitory effect of polyphenols from vegetables, legumes, spices, red wine, different teas, cocoa, and coffee on iron uptake is dose-dependent and has been attributed to the galloyl groups in its structure [52–54].

This inhibitory nature of polyphenols present in different plant foods has been investigated in many human isotopic absorption studies. Short-term human studies suggest that all major types of food polyphenols are potential inhibitors of nonheme iron absorption, but the degree of inhibition might vary with the type of polyphenols present in the foods. For example, polyphenols from black tea are more potent inhibitors than herbal teas, while polyphenols in coffee are comparatively less inhibitory [52]. Polyphenols are also found in beans, and its removal from beans has been shown to significantly increase iron absorption by 2.6-fold [51].

Available evidence from long-term in vivo, rodent, and in vitro studies show conflicting results of the reputed inhibitory effects of polyphenols on iron absorption [55]. In one long-term in vivo study, the authors found no correlation between polyphenol (i.e., tannin) supplementation and iron absorption or status [55], while in another study, authors found a negative correlation between body iron status and coffee or tea consumption [56]. In vitro studies have recognized these conflicting results among heterogeneous classes of polyphenols due to their inherent propensity of forming mineral complexes of varying solubility, as well as their prospective reducing properties on ferric iron [57]. Considering the iron/polyphenol molar ratio, one can conclude that some polyphenols are conditionally promotive at certain molar ratios (e.g., luteolin-7-glucoside, cyanidin-3-glucoside), while others are inhibitory to iron uptake (e.g., malvidin) [57].

The inhibitory effect of polyphenols is decreased when they are consumed ~1 h after the meal [58]. Given the diverse chemical properties of polyphenols, further studies are required to elucidate if certain polyphenols can increase IBA. This is particularly important given that polyphenol bioavailability can differ according to their structural changes (i.e., deconjugation of the glycosylated moiety) that occur during passage through the gastrointestinal tract [58]. Polyphenols have also been identified to cross-link intestinal mucins, which modulates barrier properties, thus affecting nutrient absorption [58]. This may have implications in facilitating iron uptake, as mucin binding plays an imperative role. Other factors, such as gender and baseline iron status, may also influence the impact of polyphenols on iron parameters. For example, green and black tea consumption had no effect on iron status in males but significantly decreased iron status in females and furthermore in females with low baseline ferritin levels [59].

Calcium

Calcium is unique in the sense that it has been shown to inhibit both heme [6] and nonheme iron absorption [6, 60]. Initially, the inhibitory effect was suggested to occur during the transport of iron across the basolateral membrane from the enterocyte to the plasma because absorption of both forms of iron is equally inhibited. However, it was also suggested that the inhibition takes place during the initial uptake into the enterocytes [61]. It is possible that calcium might internalize the DMT1 receptor, limiting the transfer of luminal iron into enterocytes, or it might interfere with transfer of iron across the enterocyte though ferroportin (FPN). Using a cell culture model, it has been shown that FPN abundance was decreased with calcium treatment, thereby decreasing iron efflux only temporarily [62]. The authors suggested this adaptation may explain the discrepancy between long-term supplementation in single-meal studies as discussed below.

The evidence is convincing from single-meal absorption studies that some forms of supplemental calcium (e.g., calcium carbonate, calcium citrate, and calcium phosphate) inhibit nonheme iron absorption when they are consumed simultaneously with the food and the degree of inhibition varied if they were given with the high (28%) or low bioavailability (55%) meals [60]. Providing milk to a breakfast meal affected iron absorption, but the inhibitory effect of calcium was dampened when provided with orange juice, suggesting the importance of meal composition on calcium inhibition [63]. A stronger inhibition on iron absorption was reported in another study from a bread roll meal whether inorganic or dietary calcium was added in a dose-dependent manner [6]. The majority of the information on calcium inhibition came from single-meal studies fed to fasting subjects, but the magnitude of effect was diminished in the context of mixed diets that contained various enhancers and inhibitors. The effect of increasing average dietary calcium intake to 1280 mg/d from 680 mg/day for 5 days was not shown to inhibit iron absorption [10, 64]. A later study by another group supported these results showing consumption of a glass of milk with the three main meals or of an equivalent amount of calcium from fortified foods did not decrease nonheme-iron absorption from a 4-day diet [64].

It is unclear whether dietary or supplemental calcium affects iron status. In a 6-month supplementation study, calcium supplements (1200 mg/day) given with meals did not reduce plasma ferritin concentrations in iron-replete adults consuming a Western-style diet containing moderate to high amounts of calcium [65]. In a randomized controlled trial, consumption of a milk product fortified with iron that provided 100% of the recommended daily iron intake did not improve iron status over 4 months in iron-deficient women, which can be attributed to calcium but does not rule out the effect of casein in the product [66].

Conclusion

Although nonheme iron contributes a higher proportion of dietary iron intake compared to heme iron, its poor bioavailability results in lower contribution to absorbed iron. The effect of enhancers such as AA and animal tissue and inhibitors such as phytic acid, polyphenols, and calcium on nonheme iron absorption is particularly strong in single meals. In complete diets, the effects of these dietary factors are modest. Efforts to improve iron bioavailability are necessary especially in developing countries where iron deficiency is rife, and attention needs to be directed mostly on reducing phytic acid which plays a major role in iron deficiency due to its abundance in plant-source foods from these countries. Encouraging the consumption of animal-source foods would also improve iron status through both its highly bioavailable heme iron content and its enhancing effect on nonheme iron absorption.

References

1. Hurrell R, Egli I. Iron bioavailability and dietary reference values. Am J Clin Nutr. 2010;91(5):1461S–7S.
2. Armah SM, Carriquiry AL, Reddy MB. Total Iron Bioavailability From the US diet is lower than the current estimate. J Nutr. 2015;145(11):2617–21.
3. Abbaspour N, Hurrell R, Kelishadi R. Review on iron and its importance for human health. J Res Med Sci Off J Isfahan Univ Med Sci. 2014;19(2):164–74.
4. Milman NT. A review of nutrients and compounds, which promote or inhibit intestinal iron absorption: making a platform for dietary measures that can reduce iron uptake in patients with genetic haemochromatosis. J Nutr Metab. 2020;2020:7373498.
5. Blanco-Rojo RVP. Iron bioavailability from food fortification to precision nutrition. A review. Innov Food Sci Emerg Technol. 2019;51:126–38.
6. Hallberg L, Rossander-Hultén L, Brune M, Gleerup A. Calcium and iron absorption: mechanism of action and nutritional importance. Eur J Clin Nutr. 1992;46(5):317–27.
7. San Martin CD, Garri C, Pizarro F, Walter T, Theil EC, Núñez MT. Caco-2 intestinal epithelial cells absorb soybean ferritin by mu2 (AP2)-dependent endocytosis. J Nutr. 2008;138(4):659–66.
8. Hoppler M, Schönbächler A, Meile L, Hurrell RF, Walczyk T. Ferritin-iron is released during boiling and in vitro gastric digestion. J Nutr. 2008;138(5):878–84.
9. Lönnerdal B, Bryant A, Liu X, Theil EC. Iron absorption from soybean ferritin in nonanemic women. Am J Clin Nutr. 2006;83(1):103–7.
10. Reddy MB, Cook JD. Effect of calcium intake on nonheme-iron absorption from a complete diet. Am J Clin Nutr. 1997;65(6):1820–5.
11. Cook JD, Reddy MB. Effect of ascorbic acid intake on nonheme-iron absorption from a complete diet. Am J Clin Nutr. 2001;73(1):93–8.
12. Reddy MB, Hurrell RF, Cook JD. Meat consumption in a varied diet marginally influences nonheme iron absorption in normal individuals. J Nutr. 2006;136(3):576–81.
13. Bœch SB, Hansen M, Bukhave K, Jensen M, Sørensen SS, Kristensen L, et al. Nonheme-iron absorption from a phytate-rich meal is increased by the addition of small amounts of pork meat. Am J Clin Nutr. 2003;77(1):173–9.
14. Cook JD, Monsen ER. Food iron absorption in human subjects. III. Comparison of the effect of animal proteins on nonheme iron absorption. Am J Clin Nutr. 1976;29(8):859–67.
15. Björn-Rasmussen E, Hallberg L. Effect of animal proteins on the absorption of food iron in man. Nutr Metab. 1979;23(3):192–202.
16. Cook JD, Monsen ER, Food iron absorption. I. Use of semisynthetic diet to study absorption of nonheme iron. Am J Clin Nutr. 1975;28(11):1289–95.
17. Carpenter CE, Mahoney AW. Contributions of heme and nonheme iron to human nutrition. Crit Rev Food Sci Nutr. 1992;31(4):333–67.
18. Glahn RP, Van Campen DR. Iron uptake is enhanced in Caco-2 cell monolayers by cysteine and reduced cysteinyl glycine. J Nutr. 1997;127(4):642–7.
19. Van Campen D, Gross E. Effect of histidine and certain other amino acids on the absorption of iron-59 by rats. J Nutr. 1969;99(1):68–74.
20. Reddy MB, Cook JD. Assessment of dietary determinants of nonheme-iron absorption in humans and rats. Am J Clin Nutr. 1991;54(4):723–8.
21. Storcksdieck genannt Bonsmann S, Hurrell RF. Iron-binding properties, amino acid composition, and structure of muscle tissue peptides from in vitro digestion of different meat sources. J Food Sci. 2007;72(1):S019–29.
22. Hurrell RF, Reddy MB, Juillerat M, Cook JD. Meat protein fractions enhance nonheme iron absorption in humans. J Nutr. 2006;136(11):2808–12.
23. Swain JH, Tabatabai LB, Reddy MB. Histidine content of low-molecular-weight beef proteins influences nonheme iron bioavailability in Caco-2 cells. J Nutr. 2002;132(2):245–51.
24. Huh EC, Hotchkiss A, Brouillette J, Glahn RP. Carbohydrate fractions from cooked fish promote iron uptake by Caco-2 cells. J Nutr. 2004;134(7):1681–9.
25. Belluzzi A, Roda G, Tonon F, Soleti A, Caponi A, Tuci A, et al. A new iron free treatment with oral fish cartilage polysaccharide for iron deficiency chronic anemia in inflammatory bowel diseases: a pilot study. World J Gastroenterol. 2007;13(10):1575–8.
26. Storcksdieck genannt Bonsmann S, Walczyk T, Renggli S, Hurrell RF. Nonheme iron absorption in young women is not influenced by purified sulfated and unsulfated glycosaminoglycans. J Nutr. 2007;137(5):1161–4.
27. Armah CN, Sharp P, Mellon FA, Pariagh S, Lund EK, Dainty JR, et al. L-alpha-glycerophosphocholine contributes to meat's enhancement of nonheme iron absorption. J Nutr. 2008;138(5):873–7.
28. Kristensen MB, Hels O, Morberg C, Marving J, Bügel S, Tetens I. Pork meat increases iron absorption from a 5-day fully controlled diet when compared to a vegetarian diet with similar vitamin C and phytic acid content. Br J Nutr. 2005;94(1):78–83.
29. Jackson J, Williams R, McEvoy M, MacDonald-Wicks L, Patterson A. Is higher consumption of animal flesh foods associated with better iron status

among adults in developed countries? A systematic review. Nutrients. 2016;8(2):89.
30. Siegenberg D, Baynes RD, Bothwell TH, Macfarlane BJ, Lamparelli RD, Car NG, et al. Ascorbic acid prevents the dose-dependent inhibitory effects of polyphenols and phytates on nonheme-iron absorption. Am J Clin Nutr. 1991;53(2):537–41.
31. Teucher B, Olivares M, Cori H. Enhancers of iron absorption: ascorbic acid and other organic acids. Int J Vitam Nutr Res. 2004;74:403–19.
32. Latunde-Dada GO, van der Westhuizen J, Vulpe CD, Anderson GJ, Simpson RJ, McKie AT. Molecular and functional roles of duodenal cytochrome B (Dcytb) in iron metabolism. Blood Cells Mol Dis. 2002;29(3):356–60.
33. Cook JD, Monsen ER. Vitamin C, the common cold, and iron absorption. Am J Clin Nutr. 1977;30(2):235–41.
34. Ballot D, Baynes RD, Bothwell TH, Gillooly M, MacFarlane BJ, MacPhail AP, et al. The effects of fruit juices and fruits on the absorption of iron from a rice meal. Br J Nutr. 1987;57(3):331–43.
35. Gillooly M, Bothwell TH, Torrance JD, MacPhail AP, Derman DP, Bezwoda WR, et al. The effects of organic acids, phytates and polyphenols on the absorption of iron from vegetables. Br J Nutr. 1983;49(3):331–42.
36. Hallberg L, Brune M, Rossander L. The role of vitamin C in iron absorption. Int J Vitam Nutr Res Suppl. 1989;30:103–8.
37. Serna-Saldivar SO, Carrillo EP. Food uses of whole corn and dry-milled fractions. In: Corn: chemistry and technology. 3rd ed. Elsevier; 2018. p. 435–67.
38. Hunt JR, Gallagher SK, Johnson LAK. Effect of ascorbic acid on apparent iron absorption by women with low iron stores. Am J Clin Nutr. 1994;59(6):1381–5.
39. Hurrell R, Bothwell T, Cook JD, Dary O, Davidsson L, Fairweather-Tait S, et al. The usefulness of elemental iron for cereal flour fortification: a SUSTAIN Task Force report. Sharing United States Technology to Aid in the Improvement of Nutrition. Nutr Rev. 2002;60(12):391–406.
40. Abdulwaliyu I, Arekemase SO, Adudu JA, Batari ML, Egbule MN, Okoduwa SIR. Investigation of the medicinal significance of phytic acid as an indispensable anti-nutrient in diseases. Clin Nutr Exp. 2019;28:42–61.
41. International Zinc Nutrition Consultative Group (IZiNCG), Brown KH, Rivera JA, Bhutta Z, Gibson RS, King JC, et al. Assessment of the risk of zinc deficiency in populations and options for its control. Food Nutr Bull. 2004;25(1 SUPPL 2):S99–203.
42. Marie Minihane A, Rimbach G. Iron absorption and the iron binding and anti-oxidant properties of phytic acid. Int J Food Sci Technol. 2002;37(7):741–8.
43. Sandberg A-S, Brune M, Carlsson N-G, Hallberg L, Skoglund E, Rossander-Hulthén L. Inositol phosphates with different numbers of phosphate groups influence iron absorption in humans. Am J Clin Nutr. 1999;70(2):240–6.
44. Hurrell RF, Juillerat MA, Reddy MB, Lynch SR, Dassenko SA, Cook JD. Soy protein, phytate, and iron absorption in humans. Am J Clin Nutr. 1992;56(3):573–8.
45. Hurrell RF. Phytic acid degradation as a means of improving iron absorption. J Int Vitaminol Nutr. 2004;74(6):445–52.
46. Masud T, Mahmood T, Latif A, Sammi S, Hameed T. Influence of processing and cooking methodologies for reduction of Phytic acid content in Wheat (Triticum aestivum) varieties. J Food Process Preserv. 2007;31(5):583–94.
47. Gupta RK, Gangoliya SS, Singh NK. Reduction of phytic acid and enhancement of bioavailable micronutrients in food grains. J Food Sci Technol. 2015;52:676–84.
48. Cook JD, Dassenko SA, Lynch SR. Assessment of the role of nonheme-iron availability in iron balance. Am J Clin Nutr. 1991;54(4):717–22.
49. Armah SM, Boy E, Chen D, Candal P, Reddy MB. Regular consumption of a high-phytate diet reduces the inhibitory effect of phytate on nonheme-iron absorption in women with suboptimal iron stores. J Nutr. 2015;145(8):1735–9.
50. Armah SM, Carriquiry A, Sullivan D, Cook JD, Reddy MB. A complete diet-based algorithm for predicting nonheme iron absorption in adults. J Nutr. 2013;143(7):1136–40.
51. Petry N, Egli I, Zeder C, Walczyk T, Hurrell R. Polyphenols and phytic acid contribute to the low iron bioavailability from common beans in young women. J Nutr. 2010;140(11):1977–82.
52. Hurrell RF, Reddy M, Cook JD. Inhibition of non-haem iron absorption in man by polyphenolic-containing beverages. Br J Nutr. 1999;81(4):289–95.
53. Brune M, Rossander L, Hallberg L. Iron absorption and phenolic compounds: importance of different phenolic structures. Eur J Clin Nutr. 1989;43(8):547–57.
54. Disler PB, Lynch SR, Charlton RW, Torrance JD, Bothwell TH, Walker RB, et al. The effect of tea on iron absorption. Gut. 1975;16(3):193–200.
55. Delimont NM, Fiorentino NM, Kimmel KA, Haub MD, Rosenkranz SK, Lindshield BL. Long-term dose-response condensed tannin supplementation does not affect iron status or bioavailability. Curr Dev Nutr. 2017;1(10).
56. Milman N, Byg KE, Ovesen L, Kirchhoff M, Jürgensen KSL. Iron status in Danish women, 1984-1994: a cohort comparison of changes in iron stores and the prevalence of iron deficiency and iron overload. Eur J Haematol. 2003;71(1):51–61.
57. Hart JJ, Tako E, Wiesinger J, Glahn RP. Polyphenolic profiles of yellow bean seed coats and their relationship with iron bioavailability. J Agric Food Chem. 2020;68(3):769–78.
58. Georgiades P, Pudney PDA, Rogers S, Thornton DJ, Waigh TA. Tea derived galloylated polyphenols cross-link purified gastrointestinal mucins. PLoS One. 2014;9(8):e105302.

59. Schlesier K, Kühn B, Kiehntopf M, Winnefeld K, Roskos M, Bitsch R, et al. Comparative evaluation of green and black tea consumption on the iron status of omnivorous and vegetarian people. Food Res Int. 2012;46(2):522–7.
60. Cook JD, Dassenko SA, Whittaker P. Calcium supplementation: effect on iron absorption. Am J Clin Nutr. 1991;53(1):106–11.
61. Roughead ZKF, Zito CA, Hunt JR. Inhibitory effects of dietary calcium on the initial uptake and subsequent retention of heme and nonheme iron in humans: comparisons using an intestinal lavage method. Am J Clin Nutr. 2005;82(3):589–97.
62. Lönnerdal B. Calcium and iron absorption—mechanisms and public health relevance. Int J Vitam Nutr Res. 2010;80(4–5):293–9.
63. Deehr MS, Dallal GE, Smith KT, Taulbee JD, Dawson-Hughes B. Effects of different calcium sources on iron absorption in postmenopausal women. Am J Clin Nutr. 1990;51(1):95–9.
64. Grinder-Pedersen L, Bukhave K, Jensen M, Højgaard L, Hansen M. Calcium from milk or calcium-fortified foods does not inhibit nonheme-iron absorption from a whole diet consumed over a 4-d period. Am J Clin Nutr. 2004;80(2):404–9.
65. Minihane AM, Fairweather-Tait SJ. Effect of calcium supplementation on daily nonheme-iron absorption and long-term iron status. Am J Clin Nutr. 1998;68(1):96–102.
66. Toxqui L, Pérez-Granados AM, Blanco-Rojo R, Wright I, González-Vizcayno C, Vaquero MP. Effects of an iron or iron and vitamin D-fortified flavored skim milk on iron metabolism: a randomized controlled double-blind trial in iron-deficient women. J Am Coll Nutr. 2013;32(5):312–20.

Part IV

The Role of Nutrition in Anemia

Vitamin A in Nutritional Anemia

12

Alison D. Gernand, Xiaodi Xu, and Keith P. West Jr

Keywords

Vitamin A deficiency (VAD) · Anemia · β-carotene · β-cryptoxanthin · Hematinic nutrients · Erythropoiesis

Introduction

There are many nutrition-related causes of anemia beyond iron, and deficiencies such as folate, vitamin B_{12}, and vitamin A can also adversely affect hematopoiesis and lead to anemia [1]. In particular, vitamin A deficiency (VAD) may increase the risk of iron-deficient erythropoiesis and anemia as a result of altering the absorption, storage, release, or transport of iron to the marrow [2]. Because vitamin A is essential for an adequate innate and acquired immune response, VAD may also contribute to inflammation-induced sequestration of iron and other responses to infection that increase risk of anemia [3, 4]. Interventions that prevent or treat VAD therefore have the potential to help reduce risk of anemia induced by undernutrition, infection, or other inflammatory processes, especially where both VAD and anemia are highly prevalent.

While low- and middle-income countries provide context for a modern public health focus on VAD as a cause of anemia, historically its association with anemia has been observed when and where nutritional and disease stresses have been apparent [5]. Nearly a 100 years ago, Danish orphans with xerophthalmia were noted to be "weak, thin and markedly anemic" [6]. In China, Berglund and Yang described an anemia that responded to treatment with cod liver oil [7]. Nearly all infants in a case series reported from the United States in the 1930s who had died with histopathologic evidence of vitamin A deficiency had, on autopsy, sequestered deposits of iron in the liver and spleen [8]. In rat experiments, progressive vitamin A deficiency was noted to cause a fall in hemoglobin prior to developing xerophthalmia [9], degenerative changes in the bone marrow [10], and heavy deposits of hemosiderin [8]. Animal experiments were followed by early clinical studies suggesting that anemia could also be a consequence of VAD in humans [11, 12].

In the late 70s, a biphasic hematologic response also became apparent in human studies, with hemoglobin concentration initially falling, followed by a polycythemia in the presence of severe VAD [13]. The finding of hemoconcentration in late-stage VAD, attributed to a disturbance

A. D. Gernand
Department of Nutritional Sciences, College of Health and Human Development, Pennsylvania State University, State College, PA, USA

X. Xu · K. P. West Jr (✉)
Program in Human Nutrition, Department of International Health, Johns Hopkins Bloomberg School of Public Health, Baltimore, MD, USA
e-mail: kwest1@jhu.edu

C. D. Karakochuk et al. (eds.), *Nutritional Anemia*, Nutrition and Health,
https://doi.org/10.1007/978-3-031-14521-6_12

in fluid balance and reduced water intake, has since been repeatedly observed in different species [9, 10, 14].

From the mid-1950s onward, multiple population-based surveys among children and adults consistently noted an interdependence between serum retinol and blood hemoglobin levels, serving to strengthen evidence of this biologic linkage [2]. In the 1970s, Hodges and colleagues carried out a small but detailed and seminal study in which the hemoglobin concentration of 5 male volunteers on a chronic, vitamin A deficient diet dropped 30% (from a mean of 161–114 g/L), despite receiving adequate dietary iron and later, therapeutic iron supplementation [13]. Their hemoglobin returned to normal following either daily vitamin A or β-carotene supplementation, suggesting that vitamin A is required for an adequate hematologic response to iron. Subsequent studies have revealed blunted responses to supplemental iron in children marginal-to-deficient in vitamin A (assessed by plasma retinol) [15] and improved responses to iron in anemic children [16, 17], adolescents [18], and pregnant women [19] when provided with vitamin A. Over the years the metabolic interactions of vitamin A and iron deficiencies in affecting risk of anemia, and the potential of vitamin A to enhance effects of iron to attenuate risk of anemia have been of continued research, review, and program interest [1, 2, 5, 20].

After briefly reviewing vitamin A and health consequences of VAD, we focus on anemia as a disorder of VAD [21], the hematologic response to vitamin A, and plausible iron metabolic pathways that may respond to shifts in vitamin A nutriture. As childhood and pregnancy represent life stages of greatest risk for vitamin A deficiency [20, 22–24], iron deficiency, and anemia [5, 25, 26], the chapter focuses on evidence in these vulnerable groups.

Vitamin A

Vitamin A, an essential micronutrient for humans, refers to a group of fat-soluble compounds including retinol, retinal, and retinyl esters. Vitamin A is needed for vision, immune cell function, growth, and reproduction [20]. Dietary requirements are high in the first year of life to support growth and development, and are slightly higher in pregnancy and almost double in lactation compared to non-pregnant, non-lactating [27]. Dietary sources of vitamin A include preformed vitamin A (retinol and retinyl ester) in animal source foods and provitamin A carotenoids (β-carotene, α-carotene, and β-cryptoxanthin) in dark green leaves, yellow-orange vegetables and fruit, egg yolk and, increasingly, in biofortified crops and tubers [28, 29]. These sources are converted to retinal and retinoic acid and stored as retinyl esters [30]. Vitamin A status is most commonly assessed via serum or plasma retinol concentrations [31], distributions of which differ between vitamin A-sufficient and deficient populations and, among the latter, shifts in response to food-based vitamin A interventions [32]. For simplicity, we will refer to serum or plasma retinol as serum retinol.

Vitamin A Deficiency Disorders (VADD)

Vitamin A deficiency causes a wide range of health consequences, or disorders (Fig. 12.1), including poor growth, impaired host immunity, and epithelial defenses that can increase severity of infection and risk of hearing loss and death. With increased severity, VAD causes xerophthalmia, involving progressively severe stages of eye disease that include night blindness, conjunctival xerosis leading to an appearance of Bitot's spots, corneal xerosis, and potentially blinding keratomalacia. Less appreciated and recognized, VAD also causes a nutritional anemia [20]. With the exception of night blindness, consequent to a lack of retinaldehyde within the visual cycle, most lesions are likely mediated by roles of retinoic acids on nuclear receptor-mediated gene expression, transcription, translation, and further protein modifications in the absence of sufficient nutrient that modify cellular, extracellular, and systemic metabolism [30]. The prevalence of

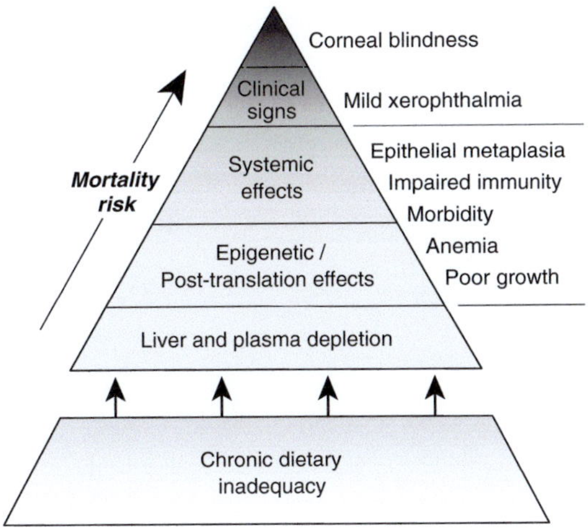

Fig. 12.1 Vitamin A deficiency disorders

VAD (serum retinol <0.70 μmol/L) among preschool children has remained at ~30% in developing regions of the world [22, 33]. However, severity and thus also consequent xerophthalmia and child mortality have likely declined in response to vitamin A supplementation programs and food fortification efforts over the past 3–4 decades [34]. Mild-to-moderate vitamin A deficiency appears to be a problem in school-aged children and adolescents, although its extent and health consequences at these ages remain poorly estimated [23]. The World Health Organization (WHO) has estimated 15% of pregnant women, or ~19 million, to be vitamin A deficient, among whom half develop night blindness [22], the most common symptom of deficiency [24] and a condition that has, in one large South Asian study, been associated with a threefold higher odds ratio (95% CI: 1.5–7.23) of anemia [35].

Anemia as a VADD

While iron deficiency is the leading cause of nutritional anemia, vitamin A joins several hematinic nutrients, including vitamins C, E, B_6, and B_{12} and folate that, when deficient, can adversely affect iron-dependent erythropoiesis and contribute to anemia [1]. Vitamin A deficiency, for example, may compromise iron absorption, storage, transport, and delivery to bone marrow [1, 2, 5], reduce erythrocytosis by lowering erythropoietin production [36–38], or may induce iron sequestration due to increased severity of infection [4]. The classic study by Hodges et al. was likely reflecting some of these blunted effects of vitamin A deficiency on iron metabolism [13] as have other studies. For example, in South Africa vitamin A deficiency appeared to blunt serum iron and transferrin saturation responses in school children who were given a soup fortified with iron (20 mg) and vitamin C (100 mg) [15]. Increased serum ferritin concentrations suggested that iron had been absorbed and stored, but not released in children whose plasma retinol concentrations were <0.70 μmol/L. In the evidence that follows, from studies of association, treatment trials, animal experiments, and in vitro studies, it seems apparent that a fraction of anemia in undernourished populations may be a consequence of VAD and thus reparable following vitamin A intervention.

Evidence of Association: Vitamin A Deficiency and Anemia

Vitamin A and hematologic status covary, as do risks of vitamin A deficiency and anemia in undernourished populations. In many settings serum retinol and hemoglobin concentrations are correlated, whether expressed on an ecological basis, as reported by Hodges et al. from eight country surveys of non-pregnant, non-lactating women in 1978 ($r = 0.77$, $n = 8$, $p < 0.05$) [13] or as seen in populations of children, adolescents, and pregnant women among which correlation coefficients have ranged from $r = 0.08$–0.90 [39–50]. A number of studies have quantified the association between serum retinol or, its surrogate retinol binding protein (RBP) and blood hemoglobin concentrations in different populations [40, 44, 50–57]. From some of these studies, it is possible to calculate the change in hemoglobin that might be expected if vitamin A status (i.e. serum retinol) was to increase in a population, as presented in Table 12.1. Estimates of changes in hemoglobin range from 0.01 to 0.77 g/L for each μg/dL increase in serum retinol.

Table 12.1 Differences in blood hemoglobin per unit increment in serum/plasma retinol from surveys and observational studies

Region	Country [reference]	Age (year)/ sex	Sample size	Increment in Hb (△g/L) per μg/dL (μmol/L) in serum retinol	Prevalence (%)	
					VAD[a]	Anemia[b]
Multiple regions	Eight countries[c] [13]	15–45/F (NPNL)[d]	NR	0.70 (20.5)	Varied	Varied
North America	Mexico [50]	0.5–11/M&F	1770	0.01 (0.3)	NR[e]	17
South America	Brazil [52]	0.5–10/M&F	1111	0.06 (1.7)	14	14
Central Asia	Kazakhstan [44]	8–17/M&F	159	0.19 (5.5)	1	27
Southeast Asia	Thailand [51]	6–12/M&F	567	0.15 (4.3)	3	31
	Thailand [53]	1–8/M&F	1060	0.54 (15.5)	44	100
South Asia	Bangladesh [40]	11–16/M	381	0.14 (3.9)	2	7
	Bangladesh [54]	5–12/M&F	242	0.17 (4.9)	<3	NR
	Pakistan [46]	4–8/M&F	120	0.77 (22.0)	17	100
	Bangladesh [55]	5–15/F	225	0.34 (9.9)	11	22
	Nepal [56][f]	15–44/F Placebo β-Carotene Vitamin A	349 479 405	0.38 (11.0) 0.29 (8.4) 0.18 (5.2)	19 14 3	73 67 68

[a] VAD = vitamin A deficiency defined as plasma/serum retinol <0.70 μmol/L (20 μg/dL)

[b] Anemia defined as Hb <110 g/L for children aged 6–59 months, Hb <115 g/L for children aged 5–11 years, Hb <115 g/L for children aged 12–14 years and non-pregnant women, and Hb <130 g/L for men aged ≥15 years

[c] Paraguay, Chile, Brazil, Uruguay, Ecuador, Venezuela, Guatemala, and Ethiopia

[d] *NPNL* non-pregnant, non-lactating women

[e] *NR* not reported; *F* female; *M* male

[f] Unpublished data among mid-gestation, pregnant women participating in a placebo-controlled maternal vitamin A or β-carotene supplement trial [56]. Anemia prevalence by treatment group in last column as observed in a population with 74% hookworm infection [57]

Studies in populations with a lower prevalence of VAD and anemia, in general, found a lower increment in hemoglobin associated with improved vitamin A status. The highest end of this range in hemoglobin increments would predict that an intervention that increases serum retinol by 5 μg/dL in a vitamin A deficient population may raise hemoglobin by 4 g/L.

The extent to which vitamin A deficiency and anemia co-occur or cluster is of interest as it reflects biologic interdependence that may exist in different population contexts [2]. Surveys reveal frequent overlap that varies, however, in extent between VAD and anemia. For example, in Nigeria, where 44% of adolescents were vitamin A deficient and 64% were anemic (Hb <120 g/L), 40% had both conditions [58]. A similar pattern has been observed among preschoolers. In the Marshall Islands where 60% of preschoolers were vitamin A deficient and 36% anemic, one-third had both conditions. The relative odds of anemia given VAD was 1.45 ($p < 0.01$) [59]. Virtually the same conditions were observed in Micronesian children [60]. In Honduras, where 48% and 40% of children aged 1–2 years were marginal-to-deficient in vitamin A and anemic, respectively, 22% had both conditions [61], whereas in lower VAD risk Venezuelan preschoolers the overlap was less, at 22%, 38%, and 8% [62]. In Vietnam, where 8% and 54% of surveyed preschoolers were vitamin A deficient and anemic, respectively, both deficient retinol and low provitamin A carotenoids were associated with anemia, represented by odds ratios of 2.06 (95% CI: 1.10–3.86) and 1.52 (95% CI: 1.01–2.28), respectively (both $p < 0.05$) [63]. Employing serum RBP as a proxy for retinol at the same cutoff (<0.70 μmol/L), deficient preschoolers in northern Cambodia exhibited an odds ratio of 3.6 (95% CI: 2.2–5.9) of being anemic relative to children above this cutoff ($p < 0.001$) [55].

In Nepal, where 54% of gravida were marginal-to-deficient in vitamin A (serum retinol <1.05 μmol/L) and 73% anemic, 43% exhibited both conditions [57], but in nearby Bangladesh, where 21% of gravida were vitamin A deficient (<0.70 μmol/L, and thus comparable to Nepal), 19% had anemia, and only 2% had both conditions [49]. Notably, in Nepal anemia was exacerbated by a high prevalence of hookworm (74%) and P. vivax malaria [57], whereas in Bangladesh, there was no hookworm, malaria or iron deficiency due to high iron content of drinking water wells, and where thalassemia was a major cause of maternal anemia [64], underscoring importance of knowing the etiology of anemia.

Effects of Vitamin A Supplementation on Hematologic Status

Clinical trials carried out in populations of children and women of reproductive age have tended to show improvement in indices of iron metabolism and erythropoiesis in response to vitamin A interventions, despite variation in nutritional risk and the dosage, frequency, duration, and form of supplementation.

Children

Initial studies in Southeast Asia in the 1970s through the 90s were directed toward discerning effects of vitamin A delivered via fortification. In Indonesia, preschool consumption of vitamin A-fortified monosodium glutamate (MSG) that provided ~240 μg of vitamin A per day (or ~33% of the current Recommended Dietary Allowance for women [27]) led to a mean hemoglobin increase of a 10 g/L vs. 2 g/L change in controls after almost a year of intervention (Table 12.2) [65]. These findings supported earlier work in Guatemala where iron indicators favorably shifted and stabilized, reflecting apparently improved iron stores and mobilization from tissues for erythropoiesis, following a national sugar fortification program that provided children with ~350 μg retinol equivalents (RE) per day [66].

Several randomized trials have been conducted in Africa, Asia, and Latin America testing effects of daily, semi-weekly, or weekly small-dose vitamin A supplementation, alone and with iron or zinc, in preventing childhood anemia for periods up to 9 months (Table 12.2). In Tanzania, a factorial trial among children (aged 9–12 years) tested the effects of 1.5 mg (5000 IU) of vitamin A alone and with 60 mg of iron given 3 days per week. After 3 months, vitamin A increased mean hemoglobin concentration by ~10 g/L over the change in controls, with a further significant increment of 8.6 g/L obtained with vitamin A plus iron, vs. a 4.0 g/L increment when iron was given alone [17]. In Guatemala, a daily supplement of 3 mg of vitamin A per day given to children 1–8 years of age for 2 months increased hemoglobin by ~6 g/L over controls. Iron alone (3 mg/kg/day) raised hemoglobin by ~10 g/L; however, providing vitamin A with iron led to no further effect [16]. In Belize, a weekly oral dose of vitamin A increased hemoglobin, while adding a weekly dose of zinc had no additional hematologic effect [67]. The comparability of these trials in their design suggests that vitamin A supplementation may facilitate absorption or mobilization of iron for erythropoiesis, although its efficacy in raising hemoglobin can be expected to be lower than supplemental iron.

In China, two randomized trials have tested effects of daily or weekly small-dose vitamin A supplementation, alone and with zinc, for periods of up to 9 months (Table 12.2). In one, a daily supplement of 500 IU vitamin A as fortified bis-

Table 12.2 Randomized trials on effects of vitamin A on anemia in children

Description of study					Baseline prevalence[a]		Changes in:[b]		
Region	Country [reference]	Subjects' age (*n*)	Length of trial	Treatment groups and regimen	Anemia (%)	VAD (%)	Hb[c] (g/L)	Serum retinol (μmol/L)	Serum ferritin (μg/L)
Africa	Morocco [38]	5-13 yr (81)	10 mo	Placebo at baseline & 5 mo 200,000 IU VA at baseline & 5 mo	54 54	20 15	1 7*,**	0.06 0.21*,**	1 −7*,**
	Tanzania [17]	9–12 yr (136)	3 mo	Placebo 3 d/wk 1.5 mg VA 3 d/wk 60 mg iron 3 d/wk 1.5 mg VA 3 d/wk + 60 mg iron 3 d/wk	100	NR	3.6* 13.5*,** 17.5*,** 22.1*,**	NR	NR
Central America	Guatemala [14]	1–8 yr (115)	2 mo	Placebo 3 mg VA/d 3 mg/kg iron/d 3 mg VA/d + 3 mg/kg iron/d	80 80 83 71	NR	3.2 9.3* 13.8*,** 14.2*,**	0.10 0.35*,** 0.13 0.36*,**	−4.9 0.1 5.5* 5.4*
	Belize [67]	2–6 yr (43)	6 mo	Placebo 70 mg zinc/wk 3030 RAE VA/wk 70 mg zinc/wk + 3030 RAE VA/wk	NR	NR	4.0 8.0*,** 12.0*,** 11.0*,**	0.05 0.16 0.18 0.12	NR
South America	Venezuela [71]	2–6 yr (80)	30 d	No supplementation 200,000 IU VA at baseline	17.6	25	0 3*	0.01 0.1*	−2.3 −0.6
	Peru [72]	6–35 mo (323)	18wk	3 mg/kg iron/d 3 mg/kg iron/d + 3 mg/kg zinc/d 3 mg/kg iron/d + 3 mg/kg zinc/d + 100,000 IU VA (single dose)	100	NR	19.5* 24.0*,** 23.8*,**	NR	24.5* 33.0*,** 30.8*,**
East Asia	China [68]	3-6 yr (580)	9 mo 3 mo 3 mo	500 IU VA/d fortified biscuits 5d/wk 1666 IU VA/d fortified biscuits 5d/wk 20,000 IU VA/wk fortified biscuits 200,000 IU VA at baseline	21.5 29.2 24.7 21.5	6.7 8.6 8.3 6.7	6.98* 5.70* 5.23* 12.54*	0.13* 0.23* 0.12* 0.08*	NR
	China [69]	<3 mo to >3 yr (127[d])	14 d	No supplement 1500 IU VA/d 10 mg zinc/d for children <6 months old or 20 mg zinc/d for children ≥6 months old 1500 IU VA/d + 10 or 20 mg zinc/d	32.28	81.89	2.23 5.11 2.43 7.43 **	0.05 0.24 0.06 0.28**	NR
South Asia	India [20]	36–66 mo (516)	24 wk	Placebo/d, 6d/wk 14 mg iron fumarate+500 IU VA + 0.05 mg folic acid/d, 6d/wk	32.6 19.1	13.0 17.5	4 4	0.0007 0.0011	−2.8* 10.4 *,**

Table 12.2 (continued)

Description of study					Baseline prevalence[a]		Changes in:[b]		
Region	Country [reference]	Subjects' age (*n*)	Length of trial	Treatment groups and regimen	Anemia (%)	VAD (%)	Hb[c] (g/L)	Serum retinol (µmol/L)	Serum ferritin (µg/L)
Southeast Asia	Indonesia [65]	0–5 yr (445)	5 mo	Unfortified MSG MSG fortified with ~240 µg RAE VA/d	NR	39 38	−2.0 10.0*,**	−0.70 0.11	NR
	Indonesia [70]	3–6 mo (800)	6 mo	100,000 IU VA at baseline + placebo 100,000 IU VA at baseline +10 mg zinc/d 100,000 IU VA at baseline +10 mg zinc/d + 10 mg iron/d 100,000 IU VA at baseline +10 mg zinc/d + 10 mg iron/d + 1000 IU VA/d	79.3 83.0 82.6 84.2	NR	−0.5* −0.64* −0.03 0.16	0.05 0.03 −0.01 0.11*	−22.2* −18.0* −10.4 −2.9
	Malaysia [74]	7–12 yr (250)	3 mo	Placebo 200,000 IU VA + 10 ug VE at baseline	48.3 48.8	NR	0.21 0.51**	NR	0.9 −1.5**
	Indonesia [75]	3–6 yr (236)	5 wk	Xerophthalmic children: Placebo 60 mg VA (single dose) Clinically normal children: Placebo 60,000 ug RAE VA (single dose) All children with HB < 11.0 g/L: Placebo 60 mg VA (single dose)	NR	100 100 50 37	7.0 5.0 5.0 5.0 14.0* 21.0*,**	0.1 1.1*,** 0.1 0.9*,** NR	4.0 16.8*,** 3.1 12.9*,** NR
	Thailand [73]	3–9 yr (134)	2 wk	No supplement 60 mg VA (single dose)	100	NR	−0.8 2.2**	−0.07* 0.15*,**	6.1 5.0
	Thailand [53]	1–8 yr (166)	4 mo	No supplement 60 mg VA+ 40 mg VE (single dose)	100	NR	2.4* 2.0*	0.13* 0.15*	12.5* 6.6*

[a] VAD = vitamin A deficiency defined as plasma/serum retinol <0.70 µmol/L (20 µg/dL); anemia defined per Hb cutoff used in study

[b] Superscripts: * denotes significantly different from baseline, $P < 0.05$; ** denotes significantly different from control at follow-up, $P < 0.05$

[c] Abbreviations: *Hb* hemoglobin; *yr* year; *mo* month; *wk* week; *d* day; *NR* not reported; *VA* vitamin A; *IU* international units; *VE* vitamin E

[d] Pediatric patients with persistent diarrhea

cuits to preschoolers led to a significant increment of 7 g/L in hemoglobin over baseline after 9 months [68]. Adding either another 1666 IU of vitamin A per day or 20,000 IU per week led to no further effect although a single dose of 200,000 IU vitamin A at the outset induced a further increment of 5.6 g/L. The second tested effects of supplementing children 3 months to ~3 years of age daily with 1500 IU of vitamin A alone and with either 10 or 20 mg zinc (based on age) [69]. After 14 days, vitamin A supplementation had increased hemoglobin concentration by 2.9 g/L over the change in controls, while no effect was observed with zinc. In Indonesia, giving anemic infants a 1000 IU vitamin A added to zinc or zinc+iron per day obtained no further beneficial effect on hemoglobin concentration [70].

Several other trials in South America, Southeast Asia, and Africa have focused on discerning effects of a single, high-potency vitamin A supplement on anemia in anemic and/or vitamin A deficient children (Table 12.2). These tests are relevant where periodic vitamin A supplementation remains a major prophylactic strategy. In Venezuela, giving a 200,000 IU oral dose of vitamin A to children conferred, after 30 days, a 3 g/L increase in hemoglobin concentration over the change observed in controls [71]. In Peru, in a 2-month trial, hemoglobin concentrations of infants and toddlers administered a single 30 mg (100,000 IU) oral dose of vitamin A at the outset, followed by daily iron, were comparable to levels of children given daily zinc with iron [72]. In an early preschooler trial in Thailand, within 2 weeks of receiving a 60 mg (200,000 IU) dose of vitamin A, serum iron, percent transferrin saturation, hemoglobin, and hematocrit significantly increased compared to controls [73] although in a second, longer follow-up trial, while serum iron and percent transferrin saturation were higher in supplemented children after 2 months, effects had disappeared after 4 months [53]. On the other hand, in a recent randomized trial among aboriginal school-aged children in Malaysia, a 200,000 IU dose of vitamin A, by 3 months, had significantly raised hemoglobin, decreased the prevalence of iron deficiency anemia, and decreased plasma ferritin compared to controls [41], the last effect possibly reflecting a reduction in infection or mobilization of iron stores. In mildly xerophthalmic and biochemically VAD preschoolers in Indonesia, a 60 mg oral dose of vitamin A increased hemoglobin by 7 g/L, but in contrast to the Malay study, also raised serum ferritin after 5 weeks [74], suggesting different mechanisms at least in the short run.

A placebo-controlled trial in Morocco (Table 12.2) compared the efficacy of two, consecutive 5-monthly rounds of vitamin A (60 mg) in mildly vitamin A deficient and anemic school-aged children [38], providing a longer term, comprehensive assessment of the hematologic response to periodic vitamin A supplementation in a population relatively unaffected by endemic infectious disease. Compared to controls whose status remained unchanged, sequential doses of vitamin A cumulatively increased serum retinol and its carrier proteins as percentages of vitamin A deficient children decreased, reflecting the intended nutritional effect. Hemoglobin gradually increased, reaching a difference of 7 g/L from controls after 10 months, and the prevalence of anemia decreased to 38% vs 59% in controls. Plasma erythropoietin (EPO) concentration increased (by 3.7 mIU/mL over controls) by 10 months, accompanied by a decrease in the regression slope of EPO on hemoglobin, interpreted to reflect a physiologic adjustment in hemoglobin (hypoxia)-induced regulation of EPO production [75] and, thus, vitamin A-mediated hematopoiesis [76]. Concentrations of transferrin receptor and serum ferritin both steadily declined while their ratio remained unchanged, suggesting that while total body iron remained unchanged, hepatic iron had been mobilized to support erythropoiesis. Given a lack of detectable change in estimated body iron stores, these findings suggest there was not an increase in iron absorption.

High-potency vitamin A appears to stimulate iron metabolism, reduce iron-deficient erythropoiesis, and improve hemoglobin homeostasis. Overall, these results are fairly consistent across time and regions, suggesting that a ~3–10 g/L increase in hemoglobin may be expected when dosing anemic and, at least mildly vitamin A deficient children [5]. The duration of effect of a single large dose may be a few months, although in populations less stressed by infectious diseases, the duration may be longer and extended by repeated, periodic dosing, as seen in Morocco.

Women of Reproductive Age

Attention to effects of vitamin A on anemia has also focused on the reproductive years, given that an estimated 25–56% of women in low-middle income countries have anemia, half of which is attributed to iron deficiency [77] and, in moderately undernourished populations, ~10% may become night blind attributable to VAD [24, 35]. Two trials in Malawi supplemented pregnant women daily with 5000 and 10,000 IU vitamin A with iron and folic acid and did not observe differences in hemoglobin response over the length of pregnancy between gravida receiving vitamin A and controls administered only iron and folic acid (Table 12.3) [78, 79]. Neither trial, however, also found a serum retinol response compared to controls against average baseline prevalences of VAD of ~29% and ~9%, respectively. In China, three controlled trials supplemented pregnant women with daily 2 mg retinol equivalents (6666 IU) in addition to daily iron and folic acid, and observed a 4–24 g/L increase in hemoglobin concentration, as well as increased serum retinol concentrations, over control responses to iron and folic acid alone (with/without also riboflavin) after 2 months of intervention [80–82]. These findings suggest that vitamin A intervened effects on erythropoiesis during pregnancy, in mild-to-moderately deficient populations, may be expected to occur when there are effects on indicators of vitamin A status.

Ahmed and colleagues in Bangladesh addressed the hematinic effects of vitamin A in a trial of non-pregnant, anemic teenagers randomized to receive weekly vitamin A, iron + folic acid, or both versus placebo receipt for 3 months [18]. Consistent with other studies, vitamin A alone increased serum retinol, hemoglobin, iron, total iron binding capacity (TIBC), and percent transferrin saturation, with a concomitant decrease in serum ferritin. A second trial among non-pregnant, anemic (Hb <100 g/L) Bangladeshi women found that a single large dose of vitamin A (60 mg) with daily iron failed to significantly improve hemoglobin concentration after 2 months beyond iron alone [84]. Only 6% of women were vitamin A deficient and serum retinol did not respond to the supplement. In India, non-pregnant, anemic 17–18-year-old adolescents were randomized to receive a dose of 200,000 IU vitamin A followed by daily iron, folic acid, and vitamin C for 100 days [83]. Consistent with other studies, vitamin A supplement use significantly increased hemoglobin, by 18 g/L, over the control group receiving only iron.

In Nepal, women were supplemented weekly with placebo, [β-carotene (42 mg) or vitamin A (7000 μg retinol equivalents)] for at least several months prior to a mid-gestational blood draw [56]. Serum retinol was lowest among placebo recipients and highest in those receiving preformed vitamin A [56, 86] (Table 12.1). Under these population experimental conditions, a larger hemoglobin difference per unit increase in serum retinol was observed in the placebo group (0.39 g/L) while the shallowest slope (0.18 g/L) was observed among mothers whose vitamin A status had become adequate, and possibly homeostatically controlled, following months of weekly preformed vitamin A receipt.

Finally, in Indonesia, two trials supplemented pregnant women with daily or weekly vitamin A in addition to daily iron and folic acid. In a factorial trial among 251 pregnant women, Suharno and colleagues observed that daily vitamin A supplementation (2.4 mg retinol) for 8 weeks significantly raised hemoglobin concentration by ~4 g/L over that of placebo recipients, an effect that explained 35% of pregnancy-related anemia [19]. Several other status indicators improved including packed cell volume, total iron binding capacity, percent transferrin saturation, and serum retinol and iron concentrations, suggestive of iron mobilization into circulation. The maximal effect (+13 g/L) was observed in women receiving both vitamin A and iron, among whom virtually all (97%) anemia had resolved. The second trial among pregnant Indonesian women that added 4800 retinol activity equivalents of vitamin A to iron (120 mg) + folic acid (500 μg) on a weekly dose schedule observed, relative to supplemental iron alone, a slight improvement in hemoglobin (by 1.6 g/L) and a reduction of 4.1 μg/dL in serum ferritin, suggestive of greater mobilization of iron stores [85].

Table 12.3 Randomized trials on the effects of vitamin A on anemia in adolescent girls/women of reproductive age (pregnant or non-pregnant)

Description of study					Baseline prevalence[a]		Changes in:[b]		
Region	Country [reference]	Subjects' age pregnancy status (n)	Length of trial	Treatment groups and regimen	Anemia (%)	VAD (%)	Hb[c] (g/L)	Serum retinol (μmol/L)	Serum ferritin (μg/L)
Africa	Malawi [78]	Pregnant (203)	Enrollment to delivery	30 mg iron/d + 400 μg folic acid/d	49	25	7.3*	−0.11*	NR
				30 mg iron/d + 400 μg folic acid/d + 3000 μg RE VA/d	51	35	4.7*	0.07	
	Malawi [79]	Pregnant (700[d])	Enrollment to delivery	Placebo/d + 60 mg iron/d + 0.25 mg folic acid/d	78.9	7.4	9	−0.03	NR
				5000 IU VA/d + 60 mg iron/d + 0.25 mg folic acid/d	80.3	7.1	8	0.025	
				10,000 IU VA/d + + 60 mg iron/d + 0.25 mg folic acid/d	81.6	11.2	10	0.05	
East Asia	China [80]	20–30 yr Pregnant (186)	2 mo	Placebo	100	NR	−1.98	−0.0671	−1.61
				60 mg iron/d			17.9*,**	−0.0114	2.11*,**
				60 mg iron/d + 0.4 mg folic acid/d			14.7*,**	0.0036	3.38*,**
				60 mg iron/d + 0.4 mg folic acid/d + 2.0 mg retinol/d			16.5*,**	0.7964 *,**	8.12*,**
	China [81]	20–35 yr Pregnant (366)	2 mo	60 mg iron/d + 400 μg folic acid	100	NR	17.2*	NR	5.6*
				60 mg iron/d + 400 μg folic acid +2 mg retinol/d			21.2*,**		9.4*
				60 mg iron/d + 400 μg folic acid +1 mg riboflavin/d			19.3*		8.1*
				60 mg iron/d + 400 μg folic acid +2 mg retinol/d + 1 mg riboflavin/d			22.6*,**		11.0*,**
	China [82]	20–35 yr Pregnant (164)	2 mo	Placebo	100	NR	−2.7	−0.059	−1.2
				60 mg ferrous sulfate/d			15.3**	0.042	1.4**
				60 mg ferrous sulfate/d + 400 μg folic acid/d			17.3**	0.061	3.1**
				60 mg ferrous sulfate/d + 400 μg folic acid/d + 2 mg retinol/d + 1 mg riboflavin/d			22.0**	0.995**	11.5**

Description of study					Baseline prevalence[a]		Changes in:[b]		
Region	Country [reference]	Subjects' age pregnancy status (n)	Length of trial	Treatment groups and regimen	Anemia (%)	VAD (%)	Hb[c] (g/L)	Serum retinol (μmol/L)	Serum ferritin (μg/L)
South Asia	India [83]	17–18 yr Non-pregnant (40)	100 d	100 mg iron/d + 500 μg folic acid/d + 60 mg VC/d 100 mg iron/d + 500 mg folic acid/d + 60 mg VC/d + 200,000 IU VA	NR	NR	13 18**	NR	NR
	Bangladesh [18]	14–19 yr Non-pregnant (480)	12 wk	Placebo 2.42 mg retinyl palmitate/wk 120 mg iron/wk + 3.5 mg folic acid/wk 120 mg iron/wk + 3.5 mg folic acid/wk + 2.42 mg retinol palmate/wk	96 82 82 92	27	1.2 3.3*,** 9.1*,** 12.2*,**	−0.01 0.15″ −0.01 0.13**	−2.9 −3.9 2.3** 5.0**
	Bangladesh [84]	15–45 yr Non-pregnant (216)	60 d	60 mg iron/d 60 mg iron/d + 200,000 IU VA (single dose) 60 mg iron/d + 15 mg zinc/d + 200,000 IU VA (single dose)	100	6	13.4 15.9* 17.9*,**	−0.03 0.09 0.04	20.0* 13.8* 16.0*
Southeast Asia	Indonesia [19]	17–35 yr Pregnant (251)	8 wk	Placebo 2.4 mg VA/d 60 mg iron/d 2.4 mg VA/d + 60 mg iron/d	100	10	2.0 6.0** 10.0** 15.0**	−0.01 0.18** 0.00 0.23**	−0.2 0.0 0.6** 0.4**
	Indonesia [85]	17–35 yr Pregnant (366)	Enrollment to delivery	120 mg iron/wk + 500 μg folic acid/wk 120 mg iron/wk + 500 μg folic acid/wk + 4800 RAE/wk	44 50	17 13	2.1 3.7*	−0.12* 0.01	−3.0 −7.1*

[a] VAD = vitamin A deficiency defined as plasma/serum retinol <0.70 μmol/L (20 μg/dL); anemia defined per Hb cutoff used in study

[b] Superscripts: * denotes significantly different from baseline, $P < 0.05$; ** denotes significantly different from control at follow-up, $P < 0.05$

[c] Abbreviations: *Hb* hemoglobin; *yr* year; *mo* month; *wk* week; *d* day; *MSG* monosodium glutamate; *NR* not reported; *RE* retinol equivalents; *RAE* retinol activity equivalents; *VA* vitamin A; *IU* international units; *VE* vitamin E; *VC* vitamin C; *NP* non-pregnant women

[d] Prevalence of HIV across treatment groups was 32.3% HIV

Mechanisms and Pathways of Interaction

The weight of evidence indicates that VAD compromises hemoglobin homeostasis through pathways responsive to vitamin A repletion. Variations in vitamin A nutriture appear to mediate iron metabolism along the internal iron and reticuloendothelial circuitry, as depicted in Fig. 12.2. Four mechanisms can be posited for how vitamin A might affect hematopoiesis and hematologic status, related to (a) influencing dynamics of tissue storage and release of iron into circulation, (b) regulating erythropoiesis, (c) modifying the sequestration and release of tissue iron associated with responses to infection, and (d) affecting iron absorption.

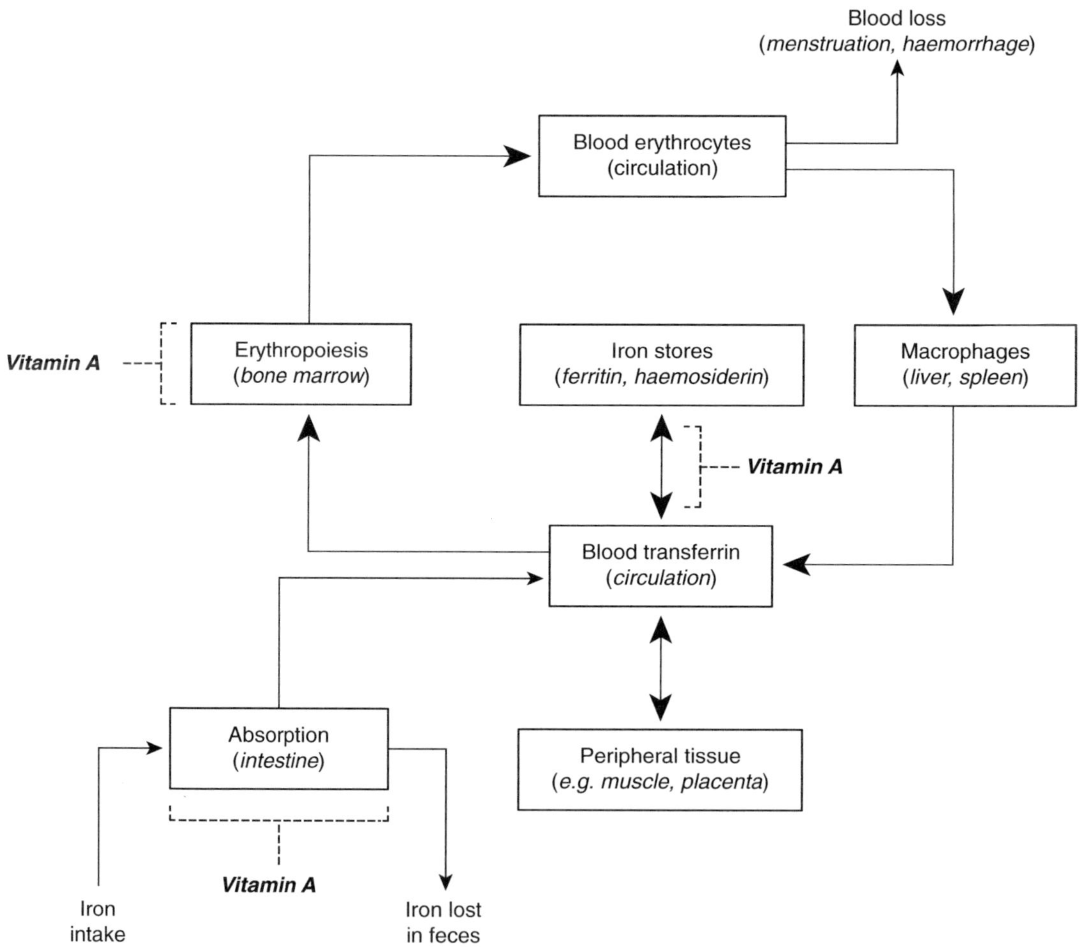

Fig. 12.2 Four mechanisms can be posited for how vitamin A might affect hematopoiesis and hematologic status

Mobilization of Tissue Iron Stores

Under normal conditions, iron not required for erythropoiesis or other iron-dependent functions is delivered by circulating transferrin to iron storage (as ferritin or hemosiderin). Mobilization is achieved when iron is released from ferritin into the circulation. As a general rule, an 8–10 mg change in ferritin storage can be inferred for each 1 μg/L change in serum ferritin concentration [87]. When measured, supplementation with vitamin A alone has usually, though not always [74], led to a modest fall in serum ferritin [38, 73, 85]. This could reflect, in part, a reduction in the acute phase reaction of serum ferritin to infection [87] mediated by vitamin A [3, 4]. However, in the absence of reported infections (e.g. elevated acute phase proteins or other clinical morbidity), a decrease in serum ferritin more likely reflects the release of utilizable iron into the bloodstream. An increase in percent transferrin saturation or decrease in total iron binding capacity further supports increased entry of iron into the circulation for delivery to the bone marrow [87]. The response of serum ferritin in these studies generally finds support from animal studies that show increased storage iron and lower femur or tibial iron in progressive vitamin A depletion [10, 88] that responds to vitamin A supplementation with lower hepatic or spleen iron concentrations. However, such responses have not been as clear in animals with marginal-to-mild vitamin A deficient states [89].

Erythropoiesis

In bone marrow, the formation of red blood cells requires differentiation and commitment of stem cells toward erythroblast development, a process requiring erythropoietin (EPO) in the latter stages of red cell development [36]. EPO is a regulatory glycoprotein hormone that is produced in the peritubular cells of the adult kidney in response to hypoxia to stimulate red cell production and longevity. In cell culture, EPO has increased in response to retinoic acid, independently of oxygen tension [90]. Few human studies have to date examined effects of vitamin A supplementation on EPO production. One, in pregnant women, failed to change circulating EPO levels with a vitamin A supplement regimen; however, vitamin A status was also not changed [79]. Also, as vitamin A was added to supplemental iron and folic acid, independent effects of vitamin A could not be examined. Among severely anemic Zanzibari preschool children high-potency vitamin A intake (30 mg < 12 months and 60 mg ≥12 months of age) induced an unexpected, precipitous decline in serum EPO levels, along with marked reductions in C-reactive protein and serum ferritin within 72 h [91]. EPO production tends to be sharply diminished in individuals with falciparum malaria, which may exacerbate anemia and make short-term treatment responses difficult to interpret [92]. In marginally vitamin A deficient and anemic Moroccan school-aged children, supplementation with vitamin A stimulated a sustained increase in EPO synthesis and erythropoiesis [38]. Although data remain incomplete, they appear sufficient to implicate a role for vitamin A in stimulating erythropoiesis via a regulatory influence on EPO [76].

Anemia of Infection

The anemia of infection is characterized by a set of cytokine-induced mechanisms that lead to shortened red blood cell survival, impaired red blood cell production, and decreased mobilization and utilization of iron. This form of iron-deficient erythropoiesis is also accompanied by up-regulation of ferritin and serum transferrin receptor [93] and down-regulation of transferrin as part of the acute phase response [2]. Vitamin A status can influence mechanisms of host resistance and severity of infection [3, 94], which in turn can have a depressive effect on serum retinol [95], factors that can lead to obscured or altered effects of a vitamin A intervention on biomarkers of erythropoiesis and anemia risk during infections, illustrated below with malaria, human immunodeficiency virus (HIV), and tuberculosis.

Malaria: Anemia of malaria can be frequent and severe, especially during pregnancy and early childhood [96–98]. Vitamin A deficiency is also common during malaria but its association with anemia may be complicated by factors beyond the inflammatory response, such risks that associated with age and seasonality, and host-parasite competition for iron and vitamin A [99, 100]. For example, iron stores may increase risk of incident malaria in endemic, as implicated in studies in Kenya [100] and Zambia [101]. Further, hemoglobin and risk of anemia may not respond to vitamin A that still reduces the severity of malaria episodes, as was seen in vitamin A trials among preschool children in Papua New Guinea [102] and in Tanzanian children with pneumonia, malaria, and HIV infection [103].

HIV: In poorly nourished populations affected by viral infections such as HIV, both VAD [104] and anemia can be common and associated with more severe disease [5]. In pregnant HIV-infected women, a positive association has been demonstrated between serum retinol and blood hemoglobin levels, as it does in non-HIV-infected populations [105]. However, few studies have tested effects of vitamin A supplementation on anemia among individuals with HIV infection. For example, 6-week-old infants of Malawian HIV-infected pregnant women supplemented daily with vitamin A (3 mg) from mid-pregnancy onward had a mean hemoglobin that was 4 g/L higher [106]. In Zimbabwe, however, neither postpartum maternal nor infant receipt of high-potency vitamin A affected infant hemoglobin or risk of anemia [107]. In Tanzania, a factorial trial that provided vitamin A (5000 IU) + β-carotene (30 mg) supplements versus other multivitamins and provided 200,000 IU or placebo to HIV-infected mothers shortly after birth reported a slightly increased hemoglobin concentrations (by 2–3 g/L) but no effects on risk of anemia or offspring during the first two postpartum years [108]. In a South African trial, HIV+/- children 6–24 months of age born to HIV-/+ mothers given daily 1250 IU of vitamin A alone versus vitamin A with zinc or with other micronutrients showed 11–24% reductions in the prevalence of anemia after 12 months [109]. Lack of a placebo renders the findings inconclusive with respect to vitamin A.

Tuberculosis: While patients with pulmonary tuberculosis are likely to be anemic, vitamin A and zinc deficient [110], a placebo-controlled trial in Indonesian adult cases reported positive effects of combined vitamin A + zinc on clinical indicators of disease recovery over a 6-month period, but no differential effect on hemoglobin [111].

Vitamin A deficiency is known to increase risk of severe infection [3, 94], consequent child mortality [20] and is contributory cause of nutritional anemia. However, effects of vitamin A on reducing anemia of infection remain sparsely researched and poorly understood across diverse infectious diseases, including SARS-CoV2 which is associated with an in-hospital anemia prevalence of ~26% [112]. The continuum from VAD to adequacy is a plausible determinant of COVID-19 severity and health consequence in undernourished populations, including risk of anemia [94], representing a research priority.

Iron Absorption

It is plausible that vitamin A or β-carotene intake or status in the gut might influence iron absorption, although the data on this pathway are presently conflicting and mechanisms unclear. Several, but not all [10], studies in rats fed vitamin A deficient diets have reported increased iron absorption with vitamin A depletion [88, 113, 114]. Human studies in Venezuela, Côte d'Ivoire, and Switzerland have evaluated iron absorption by level of dietary vitamin A intake based on erythrocyte incorporation of labeled iron as a surrogate for absorption. Among Venezuelan subjects (some of whom were anemic), low dose vitamin A (0.37–2.78 μmol) or β-carotene (0.58–2.06 μmol) supplementation of a rice, wheat, or cornmeal meal containing 2–5 mg of iron increased non-heme iron uptake by up to three-fold [115]. The studies among healthy Swiss adults [116] and school-aged children with poor iron status in Côte d'Ivoire [117], employing different methods than in Venezuela, observed a slight decrease in iron absorption with increased vitamin A intake that could not be explained.

Although a postulated mechanism includes a chelating effect of vitamin A to protect iron from the inhibitory effects of phytates, polyphenols, and tannic acid in the gut, there is not sufficient evidence in vivo for this effect [118].

Conclusions

In areas where VAD poses a substantial public health threat, it is likely to contribute to iron-deficient erythropoiesis and therefore contribute to a mild-to-moderate anemia that is responsive to vitamin A intake. The effect is clearest when both VAD and anemia are uncomplicated by infectious disease. Important to note, most studies have been undertaken in groups selected for anemia, VAD, or both. In such groups, vitamin A supplementation can be expected to raise hemoglobin concentrations by ~2–10 g/L over a period of 2 weeks to months. The range of impact of vitamin A on hemoglobin from trials generally agrees with predictions from observational studies. Effects of vitamin A may be achieved by (1) enhancing hepatic tissue mobilization and delivery of iron to bone marrow, (2) improving erythropoiesis, possibly by upregulating erythropoietin production and extending red blood cell longevity, (3) reducing sequestration of tissue iron by reducing the severity infection, and (4) facilitating iron absorption. Most evidence to date supports the first two mechanisms. The nutritional influence of vitamin A, however, on the internal iron circuit may be modulated by the type and severity of an infection, which may alter distributions of both vitamin A and iron independently, or act directly on vitamin A-iron metabolic pathways. While VAD may be a cause of anemia, its role can be expected to be modest compared to effects of iron deficiency, hookworm or malaria, where they are endemic.

References

1. Fishman SM, Christian P, West KP. The role of vitamins in the prevention and control of anaemia. Public Health Nutr. 2000;3(2):125–50.
2. Bloem MW. Interdependence of vitamin A and iron: an important association for programmes of anaemia control. Proc Nutr Soc. 1995;54(2):501–8.
3. Ross AC. The relationship between immunocompetence and vitamin A status. In: Sommer A, West Jr KP, editors. Vitamin A deficiency: health, survival, and vision. Oxford: Oxford University Press; 1996. p. 251–73.
4. Beisel WR, West KP Jr, Sommer A. Micronutrients in infection. In: Guerrant RL, Walker DH, Weller PF, editors. Tropical infectious diseases: principles, pathogens, & practice. Philadelphia: Churchill Livingstone; 1999. p. 76–87.
5. Semba RD, Bloem MW. The anemia of vitamin A deficiency: epidemiology and pathogenesis. Eur J Clin Nutr. 2002;56(4):271–81.
6. Bloch CE. Clinical investigation of Xerophthalmia and Dystrophy in Infants and Young Children (Xerophthalmia et Dystrophia Alipogenetica). J Hyg (Lond). 1921;19(3):283–304.5.
7. Berglund H, Keefer KC, Yang CS. Deficiency anemia in Chinese, responding to cod liver oil. Proc Soc Exper Biol Med. 1929;26:418–21.
8. Wolbach SB, Howe PR. Tissue changes following deprivation of fat-soluble A vitamin. J Exp Med. 1925;42(6):753–77.
9. McLaren DS, Tchalian M, Ajans ZA. Biochemical and hematologic changes in the vitamin A-deficient rat. Am J Clin Nutr. 1965;17(3):131–8.
10. Mejia LA, Hodges RE, Rucker RB. Role of vitamin A in the absorption, retention and distribution of iron in the rat. J Nutr. 1979;109(1):129–37.
11. Abbott OD, Ahmann CF, Overstreet MR. Effect of avitaminosis A on the human blood picture. Am J Physiol Legacy Content. 1939;126(2):254–60.
12. Wagner KH. Die experimentelle Avitaminose A beim Menschen. Hoppe Syelers Z Physiol Chem. 1940;264:153–89.
13. Hodges RE, et al. Hematopoietic studies in vitamin A deficiency. Am J Clin Nutr. 1978;31(5):876–85.
14. Pedersen S, et al. Haemoconcentration associated with low vitamin A status can mask anaemia. Acta Trop. 2002;84(1):55–8.
15. van Stuijvenberg ME, et al. Response to an iron fortification programme in relation to vitamin A status in 6-12-year-old school children. Int J Food Sci Nutr. 1997;48(1):41–9.
16. Mejía LA, Chew F. Hematological effect of supplementing anemic children with vitamin A alone and in combination with iron. Am J Clin Nutr. 1988;48(3):595–600.
17. Mwanri L, et al. Supplemental vitamin A improves anemia and growth in anemic school children in Tanzania. J Nutr. 2000;130(11):2691–6.
18. Ahmed F, Khan MR, Jackson AA. Concomitant supplemental vitamin A enhances the response to weekly supplemental iron and folic acid in anemic teenagers in urban Bangladesh. Am J Clin Nutr. 2001;74(1):108–15.

19. Suharno D, et al. Supplementation with vitamin A and iron for nutritional anaemia in pregnant women in West Java, Indonesia. Lancet. 1993;342(8883):1325–8.
20. Sommer A, West KP Jr. Vitamin A deficiency: health, survival, and vision. New York: Oxford University Press; 1996.
21. Sommer A, Davidson FR. Assessment and control of vitamin A deficiency: the Annecy Accords. J Nutr. 2002;132(9 Suppl):2845s–50s.
22. World Health Organization (WHO). Global prevalence of vitamin A deficiency in populations at risk 1995–2005. WHO Global Database on Vitamin A Deficiency, Geneva, Switzerland, 2009.
23. Singh V, West KP Jr. Vitamin A deficiency and xerophthalmia among school-aged children in Southeastern Asia. Eur J Clin Nutr. 2004;58(10):1342–9.
24. Christian P. Recommendations for indicators: night blindness during pregnancy—a simple tool to assess vitamin A deficiency in a population. J Nutr. 2002;132(9 Suppl):2884s–8s.
25. Gernand AD, Schulze KJ, Stewart CP, West KP Jr, Christian P. Micronutrient deficiencies in pregnancy worldwide: health effects and prevention. Nat Rev Endocrinol. 2016:1–16. https://doi.org/10.1038/nrendo.2016.37.
26. Bailey R, West KP Jr, Black RE. The epidemiology of global micronutrient deficiencies. Ann Nutr Metab. 2015;66(suppl 2):22–33.
27. Stewart CP, Fanzo J, West KP Jr, Black RE. Chapter 4: Nutrition. In: Merson MH, Black RE, Mills AJ, editors. Global health: diseases, programs, systems, and policies. 4th ed. Burlington, VT: Jones & Bartlett Learning; 2020. p. 259–333.
28. Semba RD, Askari S, Gibson S, Bloem MW, Kraemer K. The potential impact of climate change on the micronutrient-rich food supply. Adv Nutr. 2021;00:1–21.
29. Garg M, Sharma A, Vats S, Tiwari V, Kumari V, Mishra V, Krishania M. Vitamins in cereals: a critical review of content, health effects, processing losses, bioaccessibility, fortification, and biofortification strategies for their improvement. Front Hum Nutr. 2021;8:586815. https://doi.org/10.3389/fnut.2021.586815.
30. Blaner WS, Li Y. Vitamin A metabolism, storage and tissue delivery mechanisms. In: Dolle P, Niederreither K, editors. The retinoids: biology, biochemistry, and disease. 1st ed. Hoboken, NJ: Wiley-Blackwell; 2015. p. 3–34.
31. Tanumihardjo S. Biomarkers of nutrition for development. Am J Clin Nutr. 2011;94(2):658S–65S.
32. Palmer A, West KP Jr, Dalmiya N, Schultink. The use and interpretation of serum retinol distributions in evaluating the public health impact of vitamin A programmes. Public Health Nutr. 2012;15(7):1201–15.
33. Stevens GA, Bennett JE, Hennocq Q, Lu Y, De-Regil LM, Rogers L, Danaei G, Li G, White RA, Flaxman SR, Oehrle S-P, Finucane MM, Guerrero R, Bhutta ZA, Then-Paulino A, Fawzi W, Black RE, Ezzati M. Trends and mortality effects of vitamin A deficiency in children in 138 low-income and middle-income countries between 1991 and 2013: a pooled analysis of population-based surveys. Lancet Global Health. 2015;3:e528–36.
34. Wirth JP, Petry N, Tanumihardjo SA, Rogers LM, McLean E, Greig A, Garrett GS, Klemm RD, Rohner F. Vitamin A supplementation programs and country-level evidence of vitamin A deficiency. Nutrients. 2017;9(190):1–18. https://doi.org/10.3390/nu9030190.
35. Christian P, West KP Jr, Khatry SK, Katz J, Shrestha SR, Pradhan EK, Le Clerq SC, Pokhrel RP. Night blindness of pregnancy in rural Nepal—nutritional and health risks. Intl J Epidemiol. 1998;27:231–7.
36. Fisher JW. Erythropoietin: physiology and pharmacology update. Exp Biol Med (Maywood). 2003;228(1):1–14.
37. Jelkmann W, et al. Effects of antioxidant vitamins on renal and hepatic erythropoietin production. Kidney Int. 1997;51(2):497–501.
38. Zimmermann MB, et al. Vitamin A supplementation in children with poor vitamin A and iron status increases erythropoietin and hemoglobin concentrations without changing total body iron. Am J Clin Nutr. 2006;84(3):580–6.
39. Ahmed F, et al. The coexistence of other micronutrient deficiencies in anaemic adolescent schoolgirls in rural Bangladesh. Eur J Clin Nutr. 2008;62(3):365–72.
40. Ahmed F, et al. Anaemia and vitamin A status among adolescent schoolboys in Dhaka City, Bangladesh. Public Health Nutr. 2006;9(3):345–50.
41. Al-Mekhlafi HM, et al. Effects of vitamin A supplementation on iron status indices and iron deficiency anaemia: a randomized controlled trial. Nutrients. 2013;6(1):190–206.
42. Chen K, et al. Co-assessment of iron, vitamin A and growth status to investigate anemia in preschool children in suburb Chongqing, China. World J Pediatr. 2009;5(4):275–81.
43. Hamdy AM, Abdel Aleem MM, El-Shazly AA. Maternal vitamin A deficiency during pregnancy and its relation with maternal and neonatal hemoglobin concentrations among poor Egyptian families. ISRN Pediatr. 2013;2013:652148.
44. Hashizume M, et al. Anaemia, iron deficiency and vitamin A status among school-aged children in rural Kazakhstan. Public Health Nutr. 2005;8(6):564–71.
45. Jafari SM, et al. Serum retinol levels are positively correlated with hemoglobin concentrations, independent of iron homeostasis: a population-based study. Nutr Res. 2013;33(4):279–85.
46. Khan NC, et al. Sub clinical vitamin A deficiency and anemia among Vietnamese children less than five years of age. Asia Pac J Clin Nutr. 2007;16(1):152–7.
47. Khatib IM, Elmadfa I. Poor nutritional health of Bedouin preschool children in Jordan: the irony of urbanization. Ann Nutr Metab. 2009;54(4):301–9.
48. Saraiva BC, et al. Iron deficiency and anemia are associated with low retinol levels in children aged 1 to 5 years. J Pediatr. 2014;90(6):593–9.

49. Shamim AA, et al. Plasma zinc, vitamin B(12) and α-tocopherol are positively and plasma γ-tocopherol is negatively associated with Hb concentration in early pregnancy in north-west Bangladesh. Public Health Nutr. 2013;16(8):1354–61.
50. Villalpando S, et al. Distribution of anemia associated with micronutrient deficiencies other than iron in a probabilistic sample of Mexican children. Ann Nutr Metab. 2006;50(6):506–11.
51. Thurlow RA, et al. Only a small proportion of anemia in northeast Thai schoolchildren is associated with iron deficiency. Am J Clin Nutr. 2005;82(2):380–7.
52. Cardoso MA, et al. Underlying factors associated with anemia in Amazonian children: a population-based, cross-sectional study. PLoS One. 2012;7(5):e36341.
53. Bloem MW, et al. Iron metabolism and vitamin A deficiency in children in northeast Thailand. Am J Clin Nutr. 1989;50(2):332–8.
54. Ahmed F, et al. Interactions between growth and nutrient status in school-age children of urban Bangladesh. Am J Clin Nutr. 1993;58(3):334–8.
55. George J, Yiannakis M, Main B, Devenish R, Anderson C, An US, Williams SM, Gibson RS. Genetic hemoglobin disorders, infection, and deficiencies of iron and vitamin A determine anemia in young Cambodian children. J Nutr. 2012;142:781–7.
56. West KP Jr, et al. Double blind, cluster randomised trial of low dose supplementation with vitamin A or beta carotene on mortality related to pregnancy in Nepal. The NNIPS-2 Study Group. BMJ. 1999;318(7183):570–5.
57. Dreyfuss ML, et al. Hookworms, malaria and vitamin A deficiency contribute to anemia and iron deficiency among pregnant women in the plains of Nepal. J Nutr. 2000;130(10):2527–36.
58. Ayogu RN, et al. Prevalence and factors associated with anthropometric failure, vitamin A and iron deficiency among adolescents in a Nigerian urban community. Afr Health Sci. 2016;16(2):389–98.
59. Palafox NA, et al. Vitamin A deficiency, iron deficiency, and anemia among preschool children in the Republic of the Marshall Islands. Nutrition. 2003;19(5):405–8.
60. Lloyd-Puryear M, et al. Vitamin A deficiency and anemia among micronesian children. Nutr Res. 1989;9(9):1007–16.
61. Albalak R, et al. Co-occurrence of nutrition problems in Honduran children. J Nutr. 2000;130(9):2271–3.
62. Castejon HV, et al. Co-existence of anemia, vitamin A deficiency and growth retardation among children 24-84 months old in Maracaibo, Venezuela. Nutr Neuroscience. 2004;7(2):113–9.
63. Khan NC, Huan PV, Nhien NV, Tuyen LD, de Pee S, Semba RD. Relationship of serum carotenoids and retinol with anaemia among pre-school children in the northern mountainous region of Vietnam. Public Health Nutr. 2010;13(11):1863–9.
64. Merrill RD, Shamim AA, Ali H, Jahan N, Labrique AB, Schulze K, Christian P, West KP Jr. Iron status of women Is associated with the iron concentration of potable groundwater in rural Bangladesh. J Nutr. 2011;141:944–9.
65. Muhilal, et al. Vitamin A-fortified monosodium glutamate and health, growth, and survival of children: a controlled field trial. Am J Clin Nutr. 1988;48(5):1271–6.
66. Mejia LA, Arroyave G. The effect of vitamin A fortification of sugar on iron metabolism in preschool children in Guatemala. Am J Clin Nutr. 1982;36:87–93.
67. Smith JC, et al. Vitamin A and zinc supplementation of preschool children. J Am Coll Nutr. 1999;18(3):213–22.
68. Zhang X, et al. Effect of biscuits fortified with different doses of vitamin A on indices of vitamin A status, haemoglobin and physical growth levels of pre-school children in Chongqing. Public Health Nutr. 2010;13(9):1462–71.
69. Wang Y, et al. Effect of vitamin A and Zn supplementation on indices of vitamin A status, haemoglobin level and defecation of children with persistent diarrhea. J Clin Biochem Nutr. 2016;59(1):58–64.
70. Fahmida U, et al. Zinc-iron, but not zinc-alone supplementation, increased linear growth of stunted infants with low haemoglobin. Asia Pac J Clin Nutr. 2007;16(2):301–9.
71. Jimenez C, et al. A single dose of vitamin A improves haemoglobin concentration, retinol status and phagocytic function of neutrophils in preschool children. Br J Nutr. 2010;103(6):798–802.
72. Alarcon K, et al. Effects of separate delivery of zinc or zinc and vitamin A on hemoglobin response, growth, and diarrhea in young Peruvian children receiving iron therapy for anemia. Am J Clin Nutr. 2004;80(5):1276–82.
73. Bloem MW, et al. Vitamin A intervention: short-term effects of a single, oral, massive dose on iron metabolism. Am J Clin Nutr. 1990;51(1):76–9.
74. Semba RD, et al. Impact of vitamin a supplementation on hematological indicators of iron metabolism and protein status in children. Nutr Res. 1992;12(4):469–78.
75. Barosi G. Inadequate erythropoietin response to anemia: definition and clinical relevance. Ann Hemato. 1994;68(5):215–23.
76. Evans T. Regulation of hematopoiesis by retinoid signaling. Exp Hematol. 2005;33(9):1055–61.
77. Stevens GA, Finucane MM, De-Regil LM, Paciorek CJ, Flaxman SR, Branca F, Peña-Rosas JP, Bhutta ZA, Ezzati M. on behalf of Nutrition Impact Model Study Group (Anaemia). Global, regional, and national trends in haemoglobin concentration and prevalence of total and severe anaemia in children and pregnant and non-pregnant women for 1995–2011: a systematic analysis of population-representative data. Lancet Global Health. 2013;1(1):E16–25.
78. Semba RD, et al. Impact of vitamin A supplementation on anaemia and plasma erythropoietin concentrations in pregnant women: a controlled clinical trial. Eur J Haematol. 2001;66(6):389–95.

79. van den Broek NR, et al. Randomised trial of vitamin A supplementation in pregnant women in rural Malawi found to be anaemic on screening by HemoCue. BJOG. 2006;113(5):569–76.
80. Sun YY, et al. A combination of iron and retinol supplementation benefits iron status, IL-2 level and lymphocyte proliferation in anemic pregnant women. Asia Pac J Clin Nutr. 2010;19(4):513–9.
81. Ma AG, et al. Retinol and riboflavin supplementation decreases the prevalence of anemia in Chinese pregnant women taking iron and folic Acid supplements. J Nutr. 2008;138(10):1946–50.
82. Ma AG, et al. Supplementation of iron alone and combined with vitamins improves haematological status, erythrocyte membrane fluidity and oxidative stress in anaemic pregnant women. Br J Nutr. 2010;104(11):1655–61.
83. Kapil U, et al. The impact of a package of single mega dose of vitamin A and daily supplementation of iron, folic acid and vitamin C in improving hemoglobin levels. J Trop Pediatr. 2005;51(4):257–8.
84. Kolsteren P, et al. Treatment for iron deficiency anaemia with a combined supplementation of iron, vitamin A and zinc in women of Dinajpur, Bangladesh. Eur J Clin Nutr. 1999;53(2):102–6.
85. Yamini S, et al. Circulating levels of retinol, tocopherol and carotenoid in Nepali pregnant and postpartum women following long-term beta-carotene and vitamin A supplementation. Eur J Clin Nutr. 2001;55(4):252–9.
86. Muslimatun S, et al. Weekly supplementation with iron and vitamin A during pregnancy increases hemoglobin concentration but decreases serum ferritin concentration in Indonesian pregnant women. J Nutr. 2001;131(1):85–90.
87. Cook JD. Diagnosis and management of iron-deficiency anaemia. Best Pract Res Clin Haematol. 2005;18(2):319–32.
88. Strube YN, Beard JL, Ross AC. Iron deficiency and marginal vitamin A deficiency affect growth, hematological indices and the regulation of iron metabolism genes in rats. J Nutr. 2002;132(12):3607–15.
89. Beynen AC, et al. Iron status in rats fed a purified diet without vitamin A. Biol Trace Elem Res. 1992;35(1):81–4.
90. Neumcke I, et al. Effects of pro- and antioxidative compounds on renal production of erythropoietin. Endocrinology. 1999;140(2):641–5.
91. Cusick SE, et al. Short-term effects of vitamin A and antimalarial treatment on erythropoiesis in severely anemic Zanzibari preschool children. Am J Clin Nutr. 2005;82(2):406–12.
92. Burgmann H, et al. Serum levels of erythropoietin in acute Plasmodium falciparum malaria. Am J Trop Med Hygiene. 1996;54(3):280–3.
93. Rohner F, Namaste SML, Larson LM, Addo OY, Mei Z, Suchdev PS, Williams AM, Ashour FAS, Rawat R, Raiten DR, Northrop-Clewes CA. Adjusting soluble transferrin receptor concentrations for inflammation: biomarkers reflecting inflammation and nutritional determinants of anemia (BRINDA) project. Am J Clin Nutr. 2017;106(Suppl):372S–282S.
94. Stephensen CB, Leitz G. Vitamin A in resistance to and recovery from infection: relevance to SARS-CoV2. Brit J Nutr. 2021:1–10. https://doi.org/10.1017/S0007114521000246.
95. Larson LM, Guo J, Williams AM, Young MF, Ismally S, Addo OY, Thurnham D, Tanumihardjo SA, Suchdev PS, Northrop-Clewes CA. Approaches to assess vitamin A status in settings of inflammation: biomarkers reflecting inflammation and nutritional determinants of anemia (BRINDA) project. Nutrients. 2018;10:1100. https://doi.org/10.3390/nu10081100.
96. Acheampong CO, Barffour MA, Schulze KJ, Chileshe J, Kalungwana N, Saimusantu W, West KP Jr, Palmer AC. Age-specific differences in magnitude of malaria-related anemia during low and high malaria seasons in rural Zambian children. eHaem. 2021;2:349–56.
97. Nussenblatt V, Semba RD. Micronutrient malnutrition and the pathogenesis of malarial anemia. Acta Trop. 2002;82(3):321–37.
98. Ekvall H. Malaria and anemia. Curr Opin Hematol. 2003;10(2):108–14.
99. Shankar AH. Nutritional modulation of malaria morbidity and mortality. J Infect Dis. 2000;182(Suppl 1):S37–53.
100. Nabakwe EC, et al. Vitamin a deficiency and anaemia in young children living in a malaria endemic district of western Kenya. East Afr Med J. 2005;82(6):300–6.
101. Barffour MA, Schulze KJ, Coles CL, Chileshe J, Kalungwana N, Arguello M, Siamusantu W, Moss WJ, West KP Jr, Palmer AC. High iron stores I low malaria season increase malaria risk in high transmission season in a prospective cohort of rural Zambian children. J Nutr. 2017;147:1531–6.
102. Shankar AH, et al. Effect of vitamin A supplementation on morbidity due to Plasmodium falciparum in young children in Papua New Guinea: a randomised trial. Lancet. 1999;354(9174):203–9.
103. Villamor E, et al. Vitamin A supplementation and other predictors of anemia among children from Dar Es Salaam, Tanzania. Am J Trop Med Hyg. 2000;62(5):590–7.
104. Semba RD, Tang AM. Micronutrients and the pathogenesis of human immunodeficiency virus infection. Br J Nutr. 1999;81(3):181–9.

105. Friis H, et al. HIV and other predictors of serum folate, serum ferritin, and hemoglobin in pregnancy: a cross-sectional study in Zimbabwe. Am J Clin Nutr. 2001;73(6):1066–73.
106. Kumwenda N, et al. Antenatal vitamin A supplementation increases birth weight and decreases anemia among infants born to human immunodeficiency virus-infected women in Malawi. Clin Infect Dis. 2002;35(5):618–24.
107. Miller MF, et al. Effect of maternal and neonatal vitamin A supplementation and other postnatal factors on anemia in Zimbabwean infants: a prospective, randomized study. Am J Clin Nutr. 2006;(1):212–22.
108. Fawzi WW, et al. Multivitamin supplementation improves hematologic status in HIV-infected women and their children in Tanzania. Am J Clin Nutr. 2007;85(5):1335–43.
109. Chhagan MK, et al. Effect on longitudinal growth and anemia of zinc or multiple micronutrients added to vitamin A: a randomized controlled trial in children aged 6-24 months. BMC Public Health. 2010;10:145.
110. Karyadi E, Schultink W, Nelwan RHH, Gross R, Amin Z, Dolmans WMV, van der Meer JWM, Hautvast JGAJ, West CE. Poor micronutrient status of active pulmonary tuberculosis patients in Indonesia. J Nutr. 2000;130:2953–8.
111. Karyadi E, et al. A double-blind, placebo-controlled study of vitamin A and zinc supplementation in persons with tuberculosis in Indonesia: effects on clinical response and nutritional status. Am J Clin Nutr. 2002;75(4):720–7.
112. Zuin M, Rigatelli G, Quadretti L, Fogato L, Zuliani G, Roncon L. Prognostic role of anemia in COPVID-19 patients: a meta-analysis. Infect Dis Rep. 2021;13:930–7.
113. Amine EK, et al. Comparative hematology during deficiencies of iron and vitamin A in the rat. J Nutr. 1970;100(9):1033–40.
114. Roodenburg AJ, et al. Comparison between time-dependent changes in iron metabolism of rats as induced by marginal deficiency of either vitamin A or iron. Br J Nutr. 1994;71(5):687–99.
115. García-Casal MN, et al. Vitamin A and beta-carotene can improve nonheme iron absorption from rice, wheat and corn by humans. J Nutr. 1998;128(3):646–50.
116. Walczyk T, et al. No enhancing effect of vitamin A on iron absorption in humans. Am J Clin Nutr. 2003;77(1):144–9.
117. Davidsson L, et al. The effect of retinyl palmitate added to iron-fortified maize porridge on erythrocyte incorporation of iron in African children with vitamin A deficiency. Br J Nutr. 2003;2:337–43.
118. Layrisse M, et al. New property of vitamin A and beta-carotene on human iron absorption: effect on phytate and polyphenols as inhibitors of iron absorption. Arch Latinoam Nutr. 2000;50(3):243–8.

13 The Role of B-Vitamins in Nutritional Anemia

Helene McNulty

Keywords

Anemia · B-vitamin deficiency · Folate · Folic acid · Vitamin B12 · Cobalamin · Riboflavin · Food fortification · Health outcomes · Disease burden

Introduction

Reduction of anemia is one of the World Health Organization Global Nutrition Targets for 2025 [1]. Megaloblastic anemia is the major clinical manifestation of overt folate or B12 deficiency. Although the anemia arising from a deficiency of either vitamin is clinically indistinguishable, the causes are very different and differential diagnosis is essential in order to provide effective treatment. Furthermore, the absence of anemia does not imply that status of these vitamins is sufficient. Less obvious "nonanemic" manifestations can arise with low nutrient status through the lifecycle, with adverse health impacts from early life to older age. An understanding of the causes, detection, and consequences of insufficient B-vitamin status is necessary, so that appropriate public health strategies for prevention can be implemented.

H. McNulty (✉)
Nutrition Innovation Centre for Food and Health (NICHE), Ulster University, Coleraine, Northern Ireland, UK
e-mail: h.mcnulty@ulster.ac.uk

Folate Deficiency

Metabolic Role of Folate

Folate is essential for one-carbon metabolism (Fig. 13.1). This involves the transfer and utilization of one-carbon units in a network of pathways required for DNA and RNA biosynthesis, amino acid metabolism, and methylation processes via the production of S-adenosylmethionine. The generation of S-adenosylmethionine in tissues is dependent on an adequate supply of folate and vitamin B12 and is used for a great number of methylation reactions by donating its methyl group to over 100 methyltransferases for a range of substrates such as DNA, hormones, proteins, neurotransmitters, and membrane phospholipids, all of which are regulators of important biological processes [2]. Of note, in order to function effectively within one-carbon metabolism, folate needs to interact closely with related B-vitamins, namely, vitamin B12, vitamin B6, and riboflavin. This means that deficient status of one or more of these B-vitamins, or polymorphisms in folate genes, can impair one-carbon metabolism, even if folate intakes are adequate.

Causes of Folate Deficiency

The discovery of folate as an essential nutrient dates back to the 1930s when a fatal anemia of

C. D. Karakochuk et al. (eds.), *Nutritional Anemia*, Nutrition and Health,
https://doi.org/10.1007/978-3-031-14521-6_13

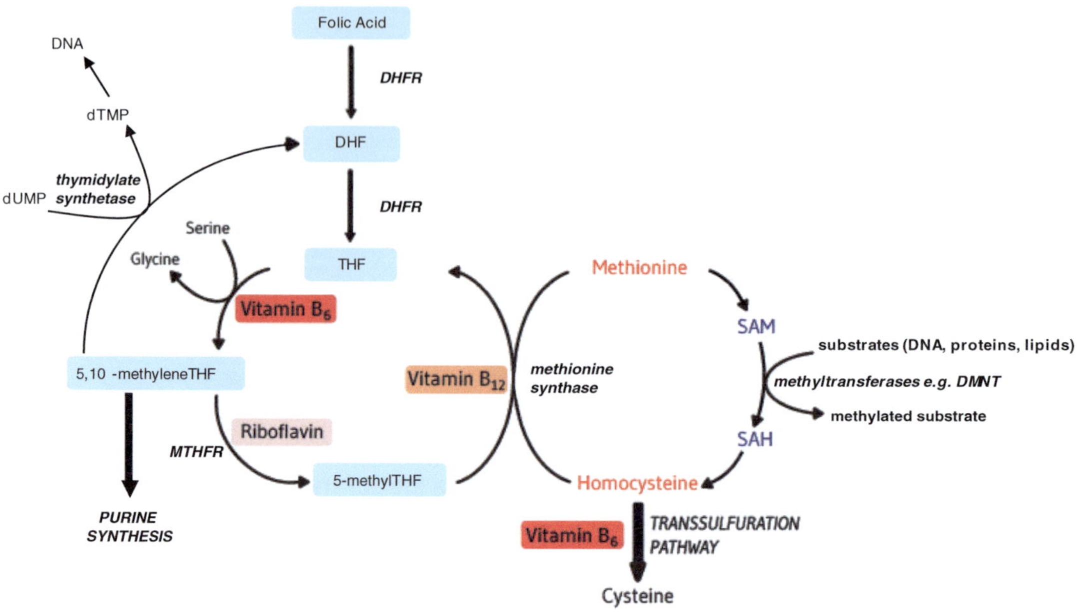

Fig. 13.1 Overview of B vitamins in one-carbon metabolism. Abbreviations: *DHF* dihydrofolate; *DHFR* dihydrofolate reductase; *DMNT* DNA methyltransferase; *dTMP* deoxythymidine monophosphate; *dUMP* deoxyuridine monophosphate; *MTHFR* methylenetetrahydrofolate reductase; *SAH* S-adenosylhomocysteine; *SAM* S-adenosylmethionine; *THF* tetrahydrofolate. (Adapted from Linus Pauling Institute at https://lpi.oregonstate.edu/mic/vitamins/folate)

pregnancy was first described in India which was subsequently proven to be responsive to treatment with food sources of the vitamin [3]. There are various causes of folate deficiency, arising from increased requirements and/or reduced availability [2]. Pregnancy is a time when folate requirement is greatly increased to sustain the demand for rapid cell replication and growth of fetal, placental, and maternal tissue. Certain gastrointestinal conditions, most notably celiac disease, can also lead to deficient folate status through chronic malabsorption. Heavy alcohol consumption and certain drugs, e.g., phenytoin and primidone (anticonvulsants) and sulfasalazine (used in inflammatory bowel disease), are also linked with folate deficiency.

Dietary folate intakes can be considered suboptimal in the diets of many people worldwide in that, although adequate in preventing megaloblastic anemia, they are often found to be insufficient in achieving biomarker concentrations of folate associated with the lowest risk of neural tube defects or other disease linked with low folate status. This widespread under-provision of folate is generally attributed to the poor stability and incomplete bioavailability of natural food folates when compared with the synthetic vitamin, folic acid. Food folates occur naturally in richest supply in green leafy vegetables, beans, liver and yeast, whereas folic acid is found in the human diet only in fortified foods and supplements. Because of their chemical structure, natural food folates are inherently unstable outside living cells and tend to have poor bioavailability [4]. In addition to their limited bioavailability, food folates (particularly green vegetables) can undergo losses during cooking, and this will substantially reduce the folate content of the food before it is even ingested.

As a result of the poor stability and limited bioavailability of folate from natural food sources, achieving optimal folate status can be challenging in practice [3]. Folate intakes and recommendations in the US and certain other countries are expressed as Dietary Folate Equivalents (DFEs), a calculation that was devised to take into account the greater bioavailability of folic acid from fortified foods compared to naturally occurring dietary folates [4, 5].

Detection of Deficient Folate Status

Biomarker status of folate is routinely assessed by measurement of folate concentrations in serum/plasma or in red blood cells as determined by either microbiological assay, or more typically in clinical laboratories, by protein binding assays. Serum folate is the earliest and most sensitive indicator of altered folate exposure and will reflect recent dietary intake [6]. Red blood cell folate parallels liver concentrations (accounting for about 50% of total body folate) and is thus considered to reflect tissue folate stores. It responds slowly to changes in dietary folate intake but is a good indicator of longer-term status in that it reflects folate intake/status over the previous 3–4 months when circulating folate is incorporated into the maturating red cells [6]. The measurement of plasma homocysteine concentration provides a functional indicator of folate status, on the basis that normal homocysteine metabolism requires an adequate supply of folate. When the status of folate is deficient or low, plasma homocysteine is invariably found to be elevated. Homocysteine is not specific for folate status, however, as it will also be elevated with B12 or other B-vitamin deficiency, certain lifestyle factors, and renal insufficiency [7].

Consequences of Deficient Folate Status

Severe Deficiency: Anemia

Clinical folate deficiency is manifested as megaloblastic anemia, a condition characterized by immature, enlarged red blood cells (reflecting impaired DNA synthesis), which is reversible with folic acid treatment. Folate-related anemia was recently reported to occur in >20% of women of reproductive age in many low- and middle-income countries, but was typically <5% in higher income economies [8]. Estimates of folate deficiency can however vary considerably depending on the method used and cut-points applied, but the microbiologic assay is recommended by the WHO and widely considered to be superior to other assays for measurement of folate status. Red blood cell and serum folate concentrations typically decrease throughout pregnancy; however, supplementation with folic acid prevents this decline [9] and can thus prevent the occurrence of megaloblastic anemia of pregnancy [10].

Other Manifestations of Insufficient Folate Status

Emerging scientific evidence supports a number of roles for folate through the lifecycle in maintaining health and preventing disease (Fig. 13.2). Because homocysteine is elevated with low folate status, it is possible that some of the reported manifestations of folate insufficiency are mediated via increased homocysteine concentrations,

Known and emerging roles of optimal status in human health

	Strength of Evidence
Early life	
Maternal health in pregnancy	Conclusive
Fetal development	Conclusive
Folate in pregnancy and Offspring health	New
Later life	
Cardiovascular health	Conclusive
Cancer prevention	Promising
Cognitive function in ageing	Promising
Bone health	Possible role

Fig. 13.2 Folate and related B vitamins throughout the lifecycle. Known and emerging roles of optimal status in human health

but it remains unclear whether homocysteine *per se* is a true risk factor for cardiovascular and other disease outcomes. In any case, homocysteine is a sensitive indicator of functional folate deficiency; in human studies, plasma homocysteine is inversely correlated with folate and shows marked lowering in response to folic acid intervention.

Neural tube defects (NTD): Maternal folate status has a major impact on early development of the embryo up to the first 4 weeks of pregnancy. Conclusive evidence has existed for over 25 years of the benefits at this time of folic acid in preventing both first occurrence [11] and recurrence [12] of NTD. These are major birth defects occurring as a result of failure of the neural tube to close properly in the first few weeks of pregnancy, leading to death of the fetus or newborn, or to various disabilities involving the spinal cord, the most common form of which is spina bifida. This conclusive evidence has led to clear folic acid recommendations for women of reproductive age which are in place worldwide.

The proposed mechanisms to explain the beneficial effects of periconceptional folic acid against NTD have focussed on the factors that could potentially impair normal folate metabolism, including polymorphisms in folate genes. Of these, an increased risk of NTD is strongly associated with the 677C → T variant in the gene coding for the folate metabolizing enzyme methylenetetrahydrofolate reductase (MTHFR) [13]. Autoantibodies against folate receptors have also been implicated in pregnancies affected by NTD [14].

Of note, although folate insufficiency is considered the major contributing factor, there is convincing evidence that low maternal vitamin B12 is an independent risk factor for an NTD-affected pregnancy [15]. Thus, future public health efforts to reduce NTD may need to target the status of not only folate but also B12 in women entering pregnancy. In addition, apart from preventing NTD, there is good evidence that periconceptional folic acid use may prevent congenital heart defects in infants [16], and possibly orofacial clefts, although the latter evidence is somewhat controversial.

Other adverse pregnancy outcomes: As pregnancy progresses, folate continues to play an important role in maternal, fetal, and neonatal health (Fig. 13.2). Deficient maternal folate status (and/or elevated homocysteine) is associated with an increased risk of a number of adverse pregnancy outcomes including gestational hypertension, preeclampsia, placental abruption, pregnancy loss, low birth weight, and intrauterine growth restriction [17]. Although there is some evidence that folic acid supplementation in pregnancy can reduce the risk of gestational hypertension and preeclampsia [18], this is conflicting. One recent RCT reported that high dose folic acid beyond the first trimester of pregnancy had no beneficial effect on preeclampsia in women at high risk for this condition [19].

In addition to protecting against the development of anemia in the mother and NTD in the offspring, there is emerging evidence linking maternal folate during pregnancy with neurodevelopment and cognitive function in the child. The biological mechanism linking maternal folate with the offspring brain is unclear, but likely involves folate-mediated epigenetic changes related to brain development and function [20]. Indeed, a wealth of literature supports the fetal origins of human disease throughout the lifecycle and emerging evidence implicates epigenetic modifications as the likely mechanism. DNA methylation, the most widely studied epigenetic mechanism for gene regulation, is dependent upon the supply of methyl donors provided by folate and related B-vitamins via S-adenosylmethionine [2]. Folate deficiency could thus lead to aberrant gene expression with consequential adverse health outcomes [21].

Cardiovascular disease (CVD): There is considerable evidence to link low status of folate and related B-vitamins (B12 and B6) with an increased risk of CVD and stroke in particular [22]. Although much of this evidence focuses specifically on plasma homocysteine (high concentrations of which are associated with endothelial dysfunction, atherosclerosis, and thrombosis), it is possible that the link with CVD is through mechanisms that are independent of homocysteine, including a role for folate and related one-carbon metabolism in blood pressure and prevention of hypertension, an important risk factor for CVD [3].

Randomized controlled trials (RCTs) show that folic acid intervention may decrease the risk of stroke by as much as 18%, and higher (over 25%) in trials with a treatment duration of >36 months, in participants with poorer baseline folate status or in those with no previous history of stroke [23]. Also, population data from the USA and Canada show an improvement in stroke mortality corresponding to the time that mandatory folic acid food fortification was introduced [24]. Thus, optimizing folate status through population-based folic acid intervention (i.e., food fortification) aimed at reducing NTD may also be beneficial in reducing CVD. Although a number of secondary prevention trials in at-risk patients failed to show a benefit of folic acid (typically in combination with vitamins B12 and B6) for CVD events generally [22], all such trials were aimed at preventing further cardiovascular events in patients with well-established pathology. A reasonable conclusion from the evidence therefore is that the administration of high dose B-vitamins to CVD patients is of no benefit in preventing another event. The same cannot be said for primary prevention, however, because the aforementioned trials did not investigate this question. Also, in one trial testing B-vitamin intervention in CVD risk, the HOPE-2 trial, a clear benefit in reducing the risk of stroke was detected but for some reason this result was overlooked in the original report [25], although subsequently reported separately [26].

Cognitive dysfunction and other neurological manifestations: Folate has a fundamental role in the nervous system throughout the lifecycle, from neural development in early life through to the maintenance of mental health and cognitive function in later life. A number of inherited disorders of folate transport and metabolism have been described [27]. These rare disorders are associated with variable neurological manifestations that can present any time from the neonatal period to adult life, including developmental delay, cognitive impairment, motor and gait abnormalities, behavioral or psychiatric symptoms, seizures, neuropathy, and vascular changes on magnetic resonance imaging (MRI).

A growing body of evidence indicates that folate and related B-vitamins may be important for maintaining cognitive health in aging, with lower B-vitamin status and/or elevated homocysteine concentrations associated with dysfunction [28]. Cognitive dysfunction refers to a spectrum ranging from mild memory loss to dementia, the latter referring to a state where the decline in memory and thinking are sufficient to impair functioning in daily living. Observational studies in this area are however complicated by the fact that poor diet can be both a cause and a consequence of impaired cognitive function and should be interpreted with caution. Only randomized trials can confirm whether low B-vitamin status is causatively linked with cognitive dysfunction. Research in this area has been very substantially underpinned by the VITACOG trial which showed that B-vitamin intervention not only improved cognitive performance in patients with mild cognitive impairment, but also slowed the rate of global and regional brain atrophy as determined using MRI [29, 30]. The totality of trial evidence suggests that any benefit of intervention with folic acid (alone or combined with vitamins B12 and B6) on cognitive function arises through correction of deficient/low status, whereas providing additional folic acid to those with optimal status likely has little effect on cognition.

Apart from memory deficits and cognitive dysfunction, depressive symptoms are well described in folate deficiency [31]. Furthermore, folate deficiency can affect the duration and clinical severity of depression and is associated with poorer response to antidepressant medication [31]. In a meta-analysis of observational studies, low folate was associated with a greater risk of depression [32]. A large cohort study of older Irish adults recently reported an incremental increase in the risk of depression as red blood cell folate declined, with an 80% higher rate of depression found among participants with the 20% lowest folate status [33]. The same study demonstrated that regular consumption of fortified foods increased dietary intakes of folate and related B-vitamins, substantially improved corresponding biomarker status, and was associated with a reduced risk of depression (by 50%) in those who consumed fortified foods on a daily basis compared to non-consumers.

Osteoporosis: Evidence implicating a role for folate and related B-vitamins in osteoporosis is typically focussed on hyperhomocysteinemia, arising from historical case reports on patients with homocystinuria, a rare autosomal recessive disease characterized by very high concentrations of plasma homocysteine (>100 μmol/L). Among the clinical features described in these patients were skeletal abnormalities, lower bone mineral density (BMD), and early onset osteoporosis.

The moderately elevated homocysteine concentrations found within the general population (and characteristic of low folate status) is also associated with an increased risk of osteoporosis, a crippling bone disease with major health and economic consequences. Potential mechanisms to explain this relationship link elevated homocysteine with increased bone resorption and bone fragility or a disturbance in collagen cross-linking. Thus, large cohort studies from various high-income countries report strong positive associations between homocysteine concentrations and risk of osteoporotic fracture or lower BMD [34, 35]. Correspondingly, a higher risk of hip fracture was reported in Norwegian women with lower (<2.9 nmol/L) compared to higher (>6.6 nmol/L) serum folate concentrations [35].

Cancer: Human and animal studies link deficient folate status with the development of various cancers, most notably of the colorectum [36]. The proposed mechanisms by which folate deficiency may promote malignant transformation are based on folate's role in one-carbon metabolism, and specifically DNA methylation and the de novo synthesis of pyrimidines and purines, nucleotides required for DNA replication and repair. Low folate status may thus alter gene expression through defective cytosine methylation, or lead to catastrophic cycles of aberrant DNA repair [37]. Controversially, however, there is also evidence that folic acid at high doses may have adverse effects on carcinogenesis. Historical evidence of the potential for such effects lies in the fact that drugs such as methotrexate, whose mechanism of action is to block folate metabolism, are effective chemotherapeutic agents. Clinical studies have more recently raised the concern that high dose folic acid may promote colorectal tumorigenesis in patients with pre-existing lesions [38].

Thus, whereas higher folate status within the dietary range is considered to be protective against certain cancers, some remain concerned that exposure to excessively high folic acid intakes could increase the growth of pre-existing neoplasms. Such concerns in relation to cancer risk have impacted public health policy in countries worldwide, with many governments delaying decisions to implement population-wide folic acid fortification, despite the widespread recognition of the benefits of such policy in preventing NTD.

Vitamin B12 Deficiency

Metabolic Role of Vitamin B12

Vitamin B12, also known as cobalamin, plays important roles in one-carbon metabolism and in mitochondrial metabolism.

In the form of methylcobalamin, vitamin B12 interacts closely with folate by acting as a cofactor for the folate-dependent enzyme, methionine synthase, which is required in the synthesis of methionine from homocysteine. Methionine, once formed, is activated by ATP to form S-adenosylmethionine, a methyl group donor used in many biological methylation reactions, including the methylation of a number of sites within DNA, RNA, and proteins [39].

In the form 5-deoxyadenosylcobalamin, vitamin B12 is required as a cofactor for the mitochondrial enzyme, methylmalonyl CoA mutase. This enzyme catalyzes the conversion of methylmalonyl CoA to succinyl-CoA, an intermediate step in the conversion of propionate to succinate, which in turn plays an important role in the metabolism of odd-chain fatty acids and ketogenic amino acids.

Causes of B12 Deficiency

Pernicious anemia is the clinical condition of severe deficiency of vitamin B12. This arises from an autoimmune gastritis characterized by B12 malabsorption owing to loss of intrinsic factor [40]. Much more commonly, however, a less severe depletion of vitamin B12 can arise from food-bound B12 malabsorption as a result of mild atrophic gastritis leading to reduced gastric acid production (hypochlorhydria), thereby diminishing B12 absorption from food because of the essential role of gastric acid in the release of B12 from food proteins during digestion. Food-bound B12 malabsorption commonly occurs in older adults and can lead to sub-clinical deficiency, where there is metabolic evidence of deficient status but without the classical hematological or neurological deficiency signs [41].

Vitamin B12 is present only in animal foods, including meat, poultry, fish and to a lesser extent eggs, milk, and dairy products. The deficient B12 status commonly found in older adults in high-income countries is rarely attributable to low dietary intakes, which are typically found to exceed dietary recommendations, but rather is the result of malabsorption related to atrophic gastritis as outlined above, and/or the use of proton pump inhibitors (e.g., omeprazole) and other gastric acid suppressant drugs, commonly prescribed for conditions such as simple heartburn or gastroesophageal reflux disease. Notably, one large community study in the US (of over 25,000 B12 deficient cases and nearly 200,000 controls) found that the long-term use of PPIs was associated with a 25–65% greater risk of vitamin B12 deficiency [42]. In addition, metformin usage in Type 2 Diabetes can also result in vitamin B12 deficiency and in turn a greater risk of cognitive dysfunction [43].

In low-income countries, however, B12 deficiency is largely the result of low dietary intakes, typically in regions where vegan diets or limited animal foods are consumed, but gastrointestinal infections and infestations, along with host–microbiota interactions, may also be contributory factors [44].

Detection of Deficient B12 Status

Vitamin B12 status can be assessed using up to four biomarkers, both direct and functional biomarkers. The direct measurement of serum total vitamin B12 (using microbiological assay or automated competitive protein binding assays) has been the standard clinical test for many years, with B12 deficiency generally identified at B12 concentrations <148 pmol/L, albeit this can vary between laboratories [44]. The sensitivity of total B12 assays has caused some concern, however, with false normal results reported in patients with pernicious anemia [41]. About 80% of total vitamin B12 is metabolically inert, therefore measurement of holotranscobalamin (holoTC), or "active B12," is theoretically attractive because it represents only the metabolically active fraction (20%) of total B12 that is available for cellular processes. Although widely considered to be a robust biomarker of B12 status, serum HoloTC is not generally available in clinical settings.

The metabolites of B12-dependent reactions can be measured in blood to provide functional indicators of vitamin B12 status. With vitamin B12 depletion, the activity of the B-12 dependent enzyme methionine synthase is impaired, in turn leading to elevated homocysteine. Plasma homocysteine is however influenced by other vitamins (particularly folate) and non-nutrient factors (including renal function); therefore, it is not specific to vitamin B12 thus limiting its use as a biomarker of B12 status. Also, with B12 depletion, the activity of the second B-12 dependent enzyme in humans—methylmalonyl CoA mutase—is reduced, leading to an accumulation of the by-product methylmalonic acid (MMA). Measurement of MMA, unlike homocysteine, provides a specific and sensitive biomarker of B12 status, but limitations include the fact that it is greatly influenced by renal dysfunction and genetic variation, along with high running costs [44].

Given the limitations of each of the direct and functional B12 biomarkers, there is general agreement that two or more biomarkers should be used to more accurately diagnose B12 deficiency so that early intervention can be implemented, and any adverse health consequences prevented [45].

Consequences of Deficient B12 Status

Vitamin B12 deficiency in humans results in impaired activities of the two vitamin B12 dependent enzymes. The extent of functional deficiency and related adverse health outcomes that may arise will depend on the extent of B12 depletion.

Severe Deficiency: Anemia and Neuropathy

Severe vitamin B12 deficiency causes anemia which is reversible with treatment, and irreversible neurological disease leading to death if untreated.

Hematologically, a deficiency of B12 will be manifested as megaloblastic anemia, characterized by megaloblasts in the bone marrow and macrocytes in peripheral blood, and reflecting an underlying biochemical defect of impaired DNA synthesis. The explanation as to why the clinical sign of megaloblastic anemia is identical for a deficiency of either folate or vitamin B12 is because DNA synthesis will be impaired in either case. In B12 deficiency, folate recycling becomes impaired because of a decrease in the activity of the B12-dependent enzyme methionine synthase, therefore 5-methyltetrahydrofolate cannot be converted to tetrahydrofolate. Thus, folate cofactors becomes "trapped" in a form that cannot be used for DNA synthesis and, as a result, DNA synthesis becomes impaired—just like in folate deficiency. The mechanism to explain the occurrence of an identical anemia with folate or B12 deficiency is referred to as the "methyl trap hypothesis."

In addition to megaloblastic anemia, B12 deficiency affects the nervous system resulting in demyelination of peripheral and central neurons and neurological complications, including neuropathy and subacute combined degeneration of the spinal cord [40]. The progression of neurological complications is generally gradual and not reversible with treatment. The neurological manifestations of B12 deficiency can precede the appearance of hematological changes and may even occur in the absence of hematological complications [44].

Other Manifestations of Insufficient B12 Status

Emerging evidence indicates that low, though not necessarily deficient, vitamin B12 status is associated with increased risk of various diseases of aging including CVD (as discussed above), neuropsychiatric dysfunction, and osteoporosis.

Neuropsychiatric dysfunction: The reported neuropsychiatric effects of folate deficiency are remarkably similar to those described for vitamin B12 deficiency [31]. Both vitamins are required for the activity of methionine synthase, thus providing methyl groups for numerous central nervous system (CNS) reactions, and may therefore have overlapping roles in the prevention of disorders of CNS development and mood disorders, and in older people, cognitive dysfunction, and dementia (i.e., Alzheimer's disease and vascular dementia). Vitamin B12 deficiency, like folate deficiency, leads to decreased synthesis of S-adenosylmethionine thereby adversely affecting methylation reactions essential for the metabolism of components of the myelin sheath of nerve cells as well as for synthesis of neurotransmitters [44]. Randomized trials show that intervention with vitamin B12 in combination with folic acid and vitamin B6 can help to prevent cognitive decline in aging, and slow the rate of brain atrophy in older patients with mild cognitive impairment [3, 29, 30]. As observed in folate deficiency, low B12 status is also associated with an increased risk of depression [31], and both vitamins may have roles in the long-term management of depression [46].

Osteoporosis: Low vitamin B12 status is linked with poor bone health, with evidence from large cohort studies showing lower than average BMD in middle-aged adults with low plasma B12 concentrations <148 pmol/L [47, 48]. One meta-analysis reported a modest association of lower B12 concentrations with a higher fracture risk [49]. As with folate, mechanisms to explain the relationship of B12 with bone health may be via homocysteine, higher concentrations of which are linked with increased bone resorption and interference with collagen cross-linking. Vitamin B12 may also have a direct effect on bone, with evidence that osteoblast activity is dependent on B12 and bone metabolism may be adversely affected by B12 deficiency [50].

Other B-Vitamins Implicated in Anemia

Apart from folate and B12, the B-vitamins most commonly implicated in anemia, riboflavin is another, often overlooked, B-vitamin that when deficient can lead to anemia. Riboflavin, in its cofactor forms flavin mononucleotide (FMN) and flavin dinucleotide (FAD), is essential for numerous oxidation-reduction reactions and plays a fundamental role in the metabolism of energy and in supporting cellular antioxidant potential. Also, riboflavin-dependent metabolism involves interaction with many other nutrients that are implicated in anemia, including iron, folate, and vitamin B6.

Interaction of Riboflavin with Iron

Riboflavin deficiency can alter iron metabolism though various mechanisms, such as impairing iron absorption, increasing intestinal loss of iron, and/or reducing the utilization of iron for the synthesis of hemoglobin. Riboflavin deficiency can thus contribute to iron deficiency anemia; for example, riboflavin supplementation of young women was shown to enhance circulating hemoglobin concentrations and improve the response of iron deficiency anemia to iron therapy [51]. Additionally, a randomized trial conducted in pregnant women with anemia in China showed that the inclusion of riboflavin (along with retinol) decreased the prevalence of anemia compared to supplementation with iron and folic acid only [52].

Interaction of Riboflavin with Folate

Riboflavin deficiency could contribute to megaloblastic anemia through its interaction with folate. Specifically, riboflavin acts as a cofactor for the key folate metabolizing enzyme methylenetetrahydrofolate reductase (MTHFR). The importance of riboflavin in folate metabolism is perhaps most evident in individuals homozygous for the C677T polymorphism in *MTHFR*, resulting in a thermolabile enzyme with reduced activity, thus impairing folate recycling. The homozygous variant *MTHFR* 677TT ("TT") genotype affects about 10% of people globally, but this figure is much higher in some countries, including Mexico where a reported 32% of the population are affected by the TT genotype [53].

Although the health concerns in relation to this polymorphism have predominantly focussed on homocysteine as the well described phenotype, arguably of greater relevance to public health is the more recent emergence of a blood pressure phenotype, and a modulating role of riboflavin (as the MTHFR cofactor), in determining the risk of hypertension in affected individuals [53]. Three randomized trials to date in hypertensive patients showed that intervention with low-dose riboflavin (1.6 mg/day) results in lowering systolic blood pressure (by 6–14 mmHg), specifically in those with the variant TT genotype in *MTHFR* [53]. Moreover, very recent evidence from a large cohort of over 6000 Irish adults showed that the variant TT genotype in *MTHFR* was associated with higher blood pressure and an increased risk of hypertension from 18 years, whilst better biomarker status of riboflavin reduced this genetic risk [54]. The impact of this gene-nutrient effect may be particularly relevant in preventing adverse pregnancy outcomes, including gestational hypertension and preeclampsia, linked with this common folate polymorphism [17], but this remains to be demonstrated.

Riboflavin deficiency is a significant problem in low-middle income countries. Across the developed world also, deficient riboflavin status may be widespread, but this is largely undocumented as biomarker status is rarely measured in population-based studies [3]. The UK is in fact one of the very few countries worldwide to include a riboflavin biomarker as part of its rolling national nutrition survey. Riboflavin deficiency in pregnancy may be a particular concern across countries globally and, given its importance in both iron and folate metabolism, further research is needed investigating riboflavin-related anemia in pregnancy and the potential role of riboflavin in hypertensive disorders of pregnancy.

Interaction of Riboflavin with Vitamin B6

The conversion of vitamin B6 to the metabolically active form in tissues, pyridoxal 5′-phosphate (PLP), is dependent on riboflavin in the cofactor form FMN. Riboflavin is thus an important determinant of vitamin B6 status throughout the lifecycle, with recent evidence indicating that riboflavin may be the limiting nutrient for maintaining PLP in older people [55]. PLP, in turn, functions as a coenzyme of 5-aminolevulinic acid synthase, which is involved in the synthesis of heme, the iron-containing component of hemoglobin. Vitamin B6 deficiency may thus impair hemoglobin synthesis and lead to microcytic anemia.

Public Health Measures to Address B-Vitamin Insufficiency and Related Policy

Reduction of anemia is one of the World Health Assembly Global Nutrition Targets for 2025 [1]. There are particular concerns regarding tackling anemia in women of reproductive age and pregnant women, and a recent WHO report (2020) has reiterated the critical importance of addressing anemia in these target groups and particularly in low-middle income countries.

Addressing Folate Insufficiency

Advice for individuals: For the prevention of NTD, women globally are recommended to take 400 μg/day folic acid as a supplement from preconception until the end of the first trimester of pregnancy. Some women are considered to be at higher risk (e.g., those with a previous pregnancy affected by NTD; those taking certain anticonvulsant drugs) and thus are recommended to take higher folic acid doses (4–5 mg/day).

Folic acid supplements provide a highly effective means to optimize folate status in individual women who take their supplements as recommended. However, supplementation is not an effective public health strategy for populations because in practice very few women correctly follow the recommendations, as discussed below.

Folic acid-fortified foods, like folic acid supplements, are highly effective as a means of optimizing folate status in women who are regular consumers of fortified foods. In countries with voluntary fortification in place, folic acid-fortified foods such as breakfast cereals are found to have very significant impacts on dietary intakes and folate biomarkers [56].

Public health challenges: Implementation of current folic acid policy to prevent NTD is problematic. For over 25 years, policy in many countries has been based on recommending women to take a supplement containing folic acid (0.4 mg/day) from before conceiving until the 12th week of pregnancy. As a sole public health measure (as is the case in European countries), however, supplementation has had little or no impact in preventing NTD, despite active health promotion campaigns over many years. The lack of success of this measure is primarily because women typically start taking folic acid after the period of neural tube closure (i.e., the 3rd to 4th week of pregnancy) [3]. This has resulted in unacceptably high rates of NTD in Europeans countries, estimated to be 1.6 times higher than in regions of the world with mandatory folic acid fortification policies in place [57].

Food Fortification

Food fortification is the process of adding essential micronutrients to foods. Food fortification can be conducted on a mandatory (i.e., regulated) or a voluntary (i.e., at the discretion of individual food manufacturers) basis. When folic acid fortification is undertaken via mandatory fortification of staple foods, it has resulted in a population-wide increase in folate status and decreased prevalence of anemia [2]. Over 85 countries worldwide to date (including North America, most of South America and Australia) have implemented mandatory folic acid fortification. In such countries, folate status is found to be optimal and this is reflected in, not only a much lower prevalence of anemia, but also a lower risk of NTD, with evidence that rates of NTD have declined by between 27 and 50% in the US, Canada and Chile in response to mandatory folic acid fortification [57].

Although the UK and Ireland have led the way in Europe in terms of considering folic acid fortification on a mandatory basis, for more than a decade both governments have delayed decisions to introduce mandatory fortification due to concerns relating to possible health risks. However, two extensive government-commissioned reports from Ireland and UK recently provided the basis for reforming folic acid policy [58, 59], with the balance of scientific evidence in both reports indicating that there are no health risks associated with the low levels of folic acid being proposed. Of note, rates of NTD in Ireland are among the highest in the world and there is particular concern that NTD trends have been increasing in recent years [58]. Although voluntary folic acid fortification is permitted in Ireland and appears to be beneficial in terms of reducing NTD to some extent, the benefit will only be achieved by consumers who choose to eat fortified food products. Mandatory folic acid fortification, in contrast, would reach all women, including those who have not planned their pregnancy, will not be taking FA supplements in early pregnancy and therefore are not protecting against NTDs in their babies. Moreover, an expert international panel tasked with reviewing all aspects of folate biology, recently concluded that the proven benefits of folic acid fortification would outweigh any potential risks [2].

Summary and Recommendations

Severe deficiency of either folate or vitamin B12 leads to megaloblastic anemia. Insufficiency of either of these vitamins, even if not severe enough to cause anemia, can be a major cause of ill health globally, especially for women of reproductive age (folate) and older adults (B12). Much less well recognized is that riboflavin deficiency can also contribute to anemia through adversely affecting the metabolism of iron and folate.

Folate is essential in one-carbon metabolism and is thus required for critical biological processes. A large body of evidence links folate insufficiency with adverse health outcomes from early to late life, however, the driver of public health policy worldwide relates to NTD where folic acid supplementation of mothers before and in early pregnancy has a proven preventative effect. Despite this, preventable NTDs are not being prevented in many countries. Implementation of a policy of mandatory folic acid fortification of staple foods would be highly effective in preventing NTD in regions without such policy in place.

Metabolically, vitamin B12 interacts closely with folate, and deficiency manifests in an identical anemia, along with irreversible neuropathy. In addition to these clinical signs of deficiency, B12 insufficiency is associated with increased risk of diseases of aging including CVD, neuropsychiatric dysfunction, and osteoporosis.

Riboflavin has several essential roles, including in folate metabolism. Deficiency is widespread but goes undetected in almost all countries. The recent emergence of a novel interaction between a common folate polymorphism and riboflavin status with impacts for blood pressure is potentially important in preventing hypertension in sub-populations globally, and may offer new insights into mechanisms linking impaired folate with disease outcomes throughout life.

In summary, folate, vitamin B12, and riboflavin are important throughout the lifecycle. More rigorous assessment and prevention of insufficient status of these nutrients should be prioritized and based on measurement of biomarkers rather than relying on dietary data only. In older populations, routine monitoring of vitamin B12 status will identify those with deficiency and enable early intervention. Fortified foods provide a bioavailable source of folate and other B-vitamins and offer a practical and highly effective means of improving status.

References

1. WHO Global Nutrition Targets 2025. Anaemia policy brief. Geneva: World Health Organization; 2014 (WHO/NMH/NHD/14.4). https://www.who.int/nutrition/publications/globaltargets2025_policybrief_anaemia/en/.
2. Bailey LB, Stover PJ, McNulty H, et al. Biomarkers of nutrition for development—folate review. J Nutr. 2015;145:1636S–80S.
3. McNulty H, Ward M, Hoey L, Hughes CF, Pentieva K. Addressing optimal folate and related B vitamin status through the lifecycle: health impacts and challenges. Proc Nutr Soc. 2019;78(3):449–62.
4. Institute of Medicine. Dietary Reference Intakes for Thiamin, Riboflavin, Niacin, Vitamin B6, Folate, Vitamin B12, Pantothenic Acid, Biotin, and Choline. Washington (DC): National Academies Press (US); 1998.
5. European Food Safety Authority (EFSA) Panel on Dietetic Products, Nutrition and Allergies (NDA). Scientific opinion on dietary reference values for folate. EFSA J. 2014;12(11):3893.
6. Gibson RS. Assessment of folate and vitamin B12 status. In: Principles of nutritional assessment. 2nd ed. New York, NY: Oxford University Press; 2005. p. 595–640.
7. Refsum H, Smith AD, Ueland PM, et al. Facts and recommendations about total homocysteine determinations: an expert opinion. Clin Chem. 2004;50:3–32.
8. Rogers LM, Cordero AM, Pfeiffer CM, et al. Global folate status in women of reproductive age: a systematic review with emphasis on methodological issues. Ann N Y Acad Sci. 2018;1431:35–57.
9. McNulty B, McNulty H, Marshall B, et al. Impact of continuing folic acid after the first trimester of pregnancy: findings of a randomized trial of folic acid supplementation in the second and third trimesters. Am J Clin Nutr. 2013;98:92–8.
10. Blot I, Papiernik E, Kaltwasser JP, et al. Influence of routine administration of folic acid and iron during pregnancy. Gynecol Obstet Investig. 1981;12:294–304.
11. MRC Vitamin Study Research Group. Prevention of neural tube defects: results of the Medical Council Vitamin Study. Lancet. 1991;338:131–7.
12. Czeizel AE, Dudas I. Prevention of the first occurrence of neural-tube defects by periconceptional vitamin supplementation. N Engl J Med. 1992;327:1832–5.
13. Vollset E, Botto LD. Neural tube defects, other congenital malformations and single nucleotide polymorphisms in the 5,10-methylenetetrahydrofolate reductase (MTHFR) gene. In: Ueland P, Rozen R, editors. MTHFR polymorphisms and disease. Georgetown, TX: Landes Bioscience; 2004. p. 127–45.
14. Rothenberg SP, da Costa MP, Sequeira JM, et al. Autoantibodies against folate receptors in women with a pregnancy complicated by a neural-tube defect. N Engl J Med. 2004;350:134–42.
15. Molloy AM, Kirke PN, Troendle JF, Burke H, Brody LC, Scott JM, Mills JL. Maternal vitamin B12 status and risk of neural tube defects in a population with high neural tube defects and no folic acid supplementation. Pediatrics. 2009;123:917–23.
16. Van Beynum IM, Kapusta L, Bakker MK, et al. Protective effect of periconceptional folic acid supplements on the risk of congenital heart defects: a registry-based case-control study in the northern Netherlands. Eur Heart J. 2010;31:464–71.
17. Psara E, Pentieva K, Ward M, McNulty H. Critical review of nutrition, blood pressure and risk of hypertension through the lifecycle: do B vitamins play a role? Biochimie. 2020;173:76–90.
18. De Ocampo MPG, Araneta MRG, Macera CA, Alcaraz JE, Moore TRCC. Folic acid supplement use and the risk of gestational hypertension and preeclampsia. Women Birth. 2018;31:e77–83.
19. Wen SW, White RR, Rybak N, Gaudet LM, et al. Effect of high dose folic acid supplementation in pregnancy on pre-eclampsia (FACT): double blind, phase III, randomised controlled, international, multicentre trial. BMJ. 2018;362:k3478.
20. Caffrey A, McNulty H, Irwin RE, et al. Maternal folate nutrition and offspring health: evidence and current controversies. Proc Nutr Soc. 2019;78:208–20.
21. James P, Sajjadi S, Tomar AS, et al. Candidate genes linking maternal nutrient exposure to offspring health via DNA methylation: a review of existing evidence in humans with specific focus on one-carbon metabolism. Int J Epidemiol. 2018;47(6):1910–37.
22. McNulty H, Strain JJ, Pentieva K, Ward M. One-carbon metabolism and CVD outcomes in older adults. Proc Nutr Soc. 2012;71:213–21.
23. Wang X, Qin X, Demirtas H, et al. Efficacy of folic acid supplementation in stroke prevention: a meta-analysis. Lancet. 2007;369:1876–82.
24. Yang Q, Botto LD, Erickson JD, et al. Improvement in stroke mortality in Canada and the United States, 1990 to 2002. Circulation. 2006;113:1335–43.
25. Lonn E, Yusuf S, Arnold MJ, et al. Homocysteine lowering with folic acid and B vitamins in vascular disease. N Engl J Med. 2006;354:1567–77.
26. Saposnik G, Ray JG, Sheridan P, et al. the HOPE 2 Investigators. Homcysteine-lowering therapy and stroke risk, severity, and disability: additional findings from the HOPE 2 trial. Stroke. 2009;40:1365–72.
27. Rosenblatt DS. Inherited disorders of folate transport and metabolism. In: Scriver CR, Beaudet AL, Sly WS, et al., editors. The metabolic basis of inherited disease. New York: Mc Graw; 1995. p. 3111–28.
28. Porter K, Hoey L, Hughes CF, et al. Causes, consequences and public health implications of low B-vitamin status in ageing. Nutrients. 2016;8:1–29.
29. Smith AD, Smith SM, de Jager CA, et al. Homocysteine-lowering by B-vitamins slows the

rate of accelerated brain atrophy in mild cognitive impairment: a randomized controlled trial. PLoS One. 2010;5:e12244.

30. Douaud G, Refsum H, de Jager CA, et al. Preventing Alzheimer's disease-related gray matter atrophy by B-vitamin treatment. Proc Natl Acad Sci. 2013;110:9523–8.
31. Reynolds E. Vitamin B12, folic acid, and the nervous system. Lancet Neurol. 2006;5:949–60.
32. Gilbody S, Lightfoot T, Sheldon T. Is low folate a risk factor for depression? A meta-analysis and exploration of heterogeneity. J Epidemiol Comm Hlth. 2007;61:631–7.
33. Moore K, Hughes CF, Hoey L, et al. B-vitamins in relation to depression in older adults over 60 years of age: the TUDA Cohort study. JAMDA. 2019;20(2):551–7.
34. Gjesdal CG, Vollset SE, Ueland PM, et al. Plasma homocysteine, folate, and vitamin B 12 and the risk of hip fracture: the Hordaland Homocysteine Study. J Bone Miner Res. 2007;22:747–56.
35. van Meurs JB, Dhonukshe-Rutten RA, Pluijm SM, et al. Homocysteine levels and the risk of osteoporotic fracture. N Engl J Med. 2004;350:2033–41.
36. Kim Y-I. Folate and carcinogenesis: evidence, mechanisms, and implications. J Nutr Biochem. 1999;10:66–88.
37. Blount BC, Mack MM, Wehr CM, et al. Folate deficiency causes uracil misincorporation into human DNA and chromosome breakage: implications for cancer and neuronal damage. Proc Natl Acad Sci U S A. 1997;94:3290–5.
38. Cole BF, Baron JA, Sandler RS, et al. Folic acid for the prevention of colorectal adenomas: a randomized clinical trial. JAMA. 2007;297:2351–9.
39. Allen LH, Miller JW, de Groot L, Rosenberg IH, Smith AD, Refsum H, Raiten DJ. Biomarkers of nutrition for development (BOND): vitamin B-12 review. J Nutr. 2018;148:1995S–2027S.
40. Stabler SP. Vitamin B12 deficiency. New Engl J Med. 2013;368:2041–2.
41. Carmel R. Diagnosis and management of clinical and subclinical cobalamin deficiencies: why controversies persist in the age of sensitive metabolic testing. Biochimie. 2013;95:1047–55.
42. Lam JR, Schneider JL, Zhao W, Corley DA. Proton pump inhibitor and histamine 2 receptor antagonist use and vitamin B12 deficiency. JAMA. 2013;310:2435–42.
43. Porter KM, Ward M, Hughes CF. Hyperglycemia and metformin use are associated with B vitamin deficiency and cognitive dysfunction in older adults. J Clin Endocrinol Metab. 2019;104:4837–47.
44. Green R, Allen LH, Bjorke-Monsen AL, et al. Vitamin B12 deficiency. Nat Rev Dis Primers. 2017;3:17040.
45. Hughes CF, McNulty. Assessing biomarker status of vitamin B12 in the laboratory: no simple solution. Ann Clin Biochem. 2018;55:188–9.
46. Almeida OP, Ford AH, Flicker L. Systematic review and meta-analysis of randomized placebo-controlled trials of folate and vitamin B12 for depression. Int Psychogeriatr. 2015;27:727–37.
47. Tucker KL, Hannan MT, Qiao N, et al. Low plasma vitamin B12 is associated with lower BMD: the Framingham Osteoporosis study. J Bone Miner Res. 2005;20:152–8.
48. Morris M, Jacques P. Selhub J Relation between homocysteine and B-vitamin status indicators and bone mineral density in older Americans. Bone. 2005;37:234–42.
49. van Wijngaarden JP, Doets EL, Szczecinska A, et al. Vitamin B12, folate, homocysteine, and bone health in adults and elderly people: a systematic review with meta-analyses. J Nutr Metab. 2013;2013:486186.
50. Carmel R, Lau K, Baylink D, et al. Cobalamin and osteoblast-specific proteins. N Engl J Med. 1988;319:70–5.
51. Powers HJ, Hill MH, Mushtaq S, et al. Correcting a marginal riboflavin deficiency improves hematologic status in young women in the United Kingdom (RIBOFEM). Am J Clin Nutr. 2011;93:1274–84.
52. Ma AG, Schouten EG, Zhang FZ, et al. Retinol and riboflavin supplementation decreases the prevalence of anemia in Chinese pregnant women taking iron and folic Acid supplements. J Nutr. 2008;138:1946–50.
53. McNulty H, Strain JJ, Hughes CF, Pentieva K, Ward M. Evidence of a role for one-carbon metabolism in blood pressure: can B vitamin intervention address the genetic risk of hypertension owing to a common folate polymorphism. Curr Dev Nutr. 2020;4(1):nzz102.
54. Ward M, Hughes C, Strain JJ, al. Impact of the common MTHFR 677C→T polymorphism on blood pressure in adulthood and role of riboflavin in modifying the genetic risk of hypertension: evidence from the JINGO project. BMC Med. 2020;18:318.
55. Jungert A, McNulty H, Hoey L, et al. Riboflavin is an important determinant of vitamin B6 status in healthy adults. J Nutr. 2020;150:2699–706.
56. Hopkins SM, Gibney MJ, Nugent AP, et al. Impact of voluntary fortification and supplement use on dietary intakes and biomarker status of folate and vitamin B12 in Irish adults. Am J Clin Nutr. 2015;101:1163–72.
57. Khoshnood B, Loane M, Dolk H, et al. Long term trends in prevalence of neural tube defects in Europe: population based study. BMJ (Online). 2015;351:1–5.
58. Food Safety Authority of Ireland FSAI. Update report on folic acid and the prevention of birth defects in Ireland. 2016. https://www.fsai.ie/news_centre/press_releases/folic_acid_report_04052016.html.
59. Scientific Advisory Committee on Nutrition (SACN) Folate and Disease Prevention Report (2006) and Folic acid updated SACN recommendations (2017). Available at https://www.gov.uk/government/publications/sacn-folate-and-disease-prevention-report https://www.gov.uk/government/publications/folic-acid-updated-sacn-recommendations.

14 The Role of Zinc in the Etiology of Anemia

David W. Killilea and Jonathan H. Siekmann

Keywords

Zinc · Anemia · Hemoglobin · Iron homeostasis · Micronutrients

Coexistence of Anemia and Zinc Deficiency

Zinc is an essential mineral that is required in nearly every stage of cellular and systemic metabolism [1]. Zinc has structural, regulatory, and catalytic roles in hundreds of transcription factors and enzymes involved in cell division, tissue growth, and immune function. Because less is known about zinc storage in the body compared to other essential minerals, a regular threshold of adequate dietary zinc intake is thought to be necessary to support and maintain normal metabolism and immune system function. Failure to maintain a regular threshold of adequate dietary zinc intake can lead to zinc deficiency, which manifests in complex ways that are not easy to measure, yet have clear effects on many aspects of metabolism [1]. Zinc deficiency ultimately reduces the ability of the individual to thrive.

There are uncertainties around who and how many people are deficient in zinc [2–4]. To date, country-level plasma/serum zinc data for any population group exist for only 26 countries [2]. Much of the world population is also at risk for anemia, with the latest estimates from the World Health Organization (WHO) suggesting that anemia affects around 800 million children and women [5]. Although there are presently no direct country-level comparisons of anemia and zinc deficiency available, the latest available data reveal considerable overlap at country level, with countries in sub-Saharan African, South and Southeast Asia, and Latin America generally showing the highest prevalence of both anemia and inadequate zinc intake. Wessells and Brown estimate inadequate zinc intake in 17.3% of the global population [6]. The latest estimates of anemia from WHO range from 29.0% in non-pregnant women of reproductive age to 42.6% in preschool-age children [5].

Measurement of serum or plasma zinc concentration is considered the best biomarker for assessing population-level zinc deficiency [1], and for confirming suspected zinc deficiency based on estimates of inadequate zinc intake [7]. The International Zinc Nutrition Consultative Group (IZiNCG) considers zinc deficiency as serum or plasma zinc concentration <65 μg/dL

D. W. Killilea
UCSF Benioff Children's Hospital Oakland, Oakland, CA, USA
e-mail: David.Killilea@ucsf.edu

J. H. Siekmann (✉)
Department of Biological Sciences, City College of San Francisco, San Francisco, CA, USA
e-mail: jsiekmann@ccsf.edu

C. D. Karakochuk et al. (eds.), *Nutritional Anemia*, Nutrition and Health,
https://doi.org/10.1007/978-3-031-14521-6_14

(<10 μmol/L), and this cut-point is used by most countries [2]. The WHO Micronutrient Database contains the most recent country-level data on low serum or plasma zinc concentrations [3]. Additionally, a recent paper by Gupta and colleagues presents plasma zinc concentrations for women of reproductive age and/or children in 25 countries [8]. For children, the prevalence of zinc deficiency was >20% in all but 7 of the 24 countries with data [8]. For the 18 countries that collected data on women of reproductive age, all but one (Fiji) had a prevalence of zinc deficiency >20% [8]. The International Zinc Nutrition Consultative Group (IZiNCG) website features a map with data for preschool-age children in 24 of these countries, and planned updates to the map will include data from other countries, including Nepal and India [2]. As measurement of serum or plasma zinc concentration increasingly becomes a component of national nutrition surveys, additional country-level data on plasma or serum zinc concentrations will permit further study of the relationship between zinc and anemia.

Despite the lack of available country-level data, several studies confirm the coexistence of anemia and zinc deficiency in a number of countries. For example, a systematic review of iron and zinc status and intakes in children and adolescents aged 0–19 years in Ethiopia, Kenya, Nigeria, and South Africa revealed a prevalence of anemia ranging from 25 to 53% and zinc deficiency ranging from 32 to 63%, as assessed by serum zinc concentration <65 μg/dL [9]. Another study that mapped micronutrient deficiencies in five Southeast Asian countries (Cambodia, Indonesia, Lao PDR, Thailand, and Vietnam) found high levels of anemia in all five countries, despite low levels of iron deficiency in Cambodia, and high levels of zinc deficiency, as assessed by serum zinc concentration, in the four countries where it was measured [10]. In summary, there is documented coexistence of zinc deficiency and anemia, suggesting a potential role for zinc in the etiology of anemia.

Associations Between Zinc Deficiency and Anemia

Analysis of data from a number of studies has revealed associations between plasma or serum zinc concentrations and hemoglobin, with zinc being one of the most statistically significant predictors of anemia in some cases. These associations between zinc deficiency and anemia have been found in school-age children in Cambodia [11] and New Zealand [12], and in pregnant women in Ethiopia [13]. A recent analysis of data from preschool-age children (PSC) and women of reproductive age (WRA) in 13 countries found that zinc concentrations were independently and positively associated with hemoglobin concentrations in 7 out of 13 countries for PSC and 5 out of 12 countries for WRA [14]. In roughly half the countries studied, there was an association between zinc and hemoglobin concentrations, even when controlling for iron status. Additionally, zinc deficiency was significantly associated with a higher prevalence of anemia in 5 out of 13 countries (for PSC) and 4 out of 12 countries (for WRA). Furthermore, in women of reproductive age, the association between zinc and hemoglobin concentrations was stronger when the overall anemia prevalence in the country was lower [14]. By way of explanation, the authors posited that the contribution of zinc deficiency to overall anemia prevalence might become more important if other causes of anemia, especially iron deficiency, are less prevalent.

Other studies have found positive associations between anemia and zinc deficiency in children in Turkey [15], in pregnant women in China [16] and Ethiopia [17], and in adults in Turkey [18]. When comparing a group of children with iron deficiency anemia to a group of controls, Ece and colleagues found that mean serum zinc concentration was significantly lower in children with iron deficiency anemia [15]. In a study of a large population of pregnant women in China, marginal zinc deficiency (defined as serum zinc concentration <70 μg/dL) was found in 51% of anemic and 45% non-anemic women in their third trimester [16]. Additionally, serum zinc concentration increased in this population as hemoglobin increased [16]. Gebremedhin and colleagues also found hemoglobin and serum zinc levels to be positively correlated in pregnant women in southern Ethiopia, and the association persisted after adjustments for potential nutritional and non-nutritional confounders [17]. In Turkey, a case-control study comparing adult patients with iron deficiency anemia to gender-matched healthy controls also found lower serum zinc levels in the anemic patients [18].

Three additional studies support associations between zinc status and anemia. A recent study in Guatemala found a strong association between zinc deficiency and anemia in infants/toddlers aged 6–24 months: The odds of anemia were >3 times greater for infants and toddlers with zinc deficiency (OR = 3.40; 95% CI [1.54, 7.47]) [19]. Another recent study in schoolchildren in Turkey that examined the relationship between zinc status, ferritin and hemoglobin, together with other estimates of anemia, found that zinc deficiency was the strongest predictor of observed anemia [20]. Using regression analysis, zinc was a stronger predictor of anemia than ferritin in the school children studied. In another study in pregnant women, Shamim and colleagues [21] found that zinc status had a positive association with hemoglobin concentration. The increase in hemoglobin was greatest when comparing the lowest to the upper quartiles of zinc status. The authors posited that there might be a level above which the role of zinc in hematopoiesis is minimized.

How Could Zinc Deficiency Contribute to Anemia?

Although it is unclear how zinc deficiency could induce anemia, there are several interesting connections between zinc metabolism and the synthesis or regulation of hemoglobin, as shown in Fig. 14.1. The following examples illustrate potential connections between zinc and hemoglobin production, but should not be considered an exhaustive list of all possibilities. In fact, only a few of these associations have been assessed in vivo, and it is possible that at least some of these essential zinc-dependent metabolic functions are likely to be conserved even during a shortage of zinc from the diet [22]. Therefore, the following sections serve primarily as suggestions for further research.

Direct Mechanisms

Heme Synthesis

Heme synthesis is a complex eight-step process that takes place predominantly within bone marrow and liver cells [23]. Synthesis begins in the mitochondria, continues in the cytoplasm, then returns to the mitochondria for the incorporation of iron into the protoporphyrin ring. The mature heme is then transported back to the cytoplasm to be complexed with the globin protein subunits before assembly into the target heme-proteins, including hemoglobin. The second enzyme in the synthetic pathway is known as aminolevulinate dehydratase (ALAD) or porphobilinogen synthase (EC 4.2.1.24) and catalyzes the condensation of two 5-aminolevulinate molecules to create porphobilinogen [23]. ALAD from archaea, yeast, and metazoa (including humans) all contain essential zinc cofactors at the active site of function [24]. Because the active form of ALAD in humans is an octomer, eight zinc ions are required for each single holoenzyme and thus could be sensitive to a drop in zinc concentration. However, it has not yet been shown if decreases in zinc status can result in loss of ALAD activity.

Superoxide Dismutase

Zinc is an integral cofactor in Cu-Zn superoxide dismutase (EC 1.15.1.1), also known as superoxide dismutase 1 (SOD1) [25]. SOD1 is one of three SOD isoforms in human physiology with a major role in detoxifying superoxide radicals in the cytoplasmic and mitochondrial intermembrane space compartments of most cell types. Because heme synthesis is coordinated with both

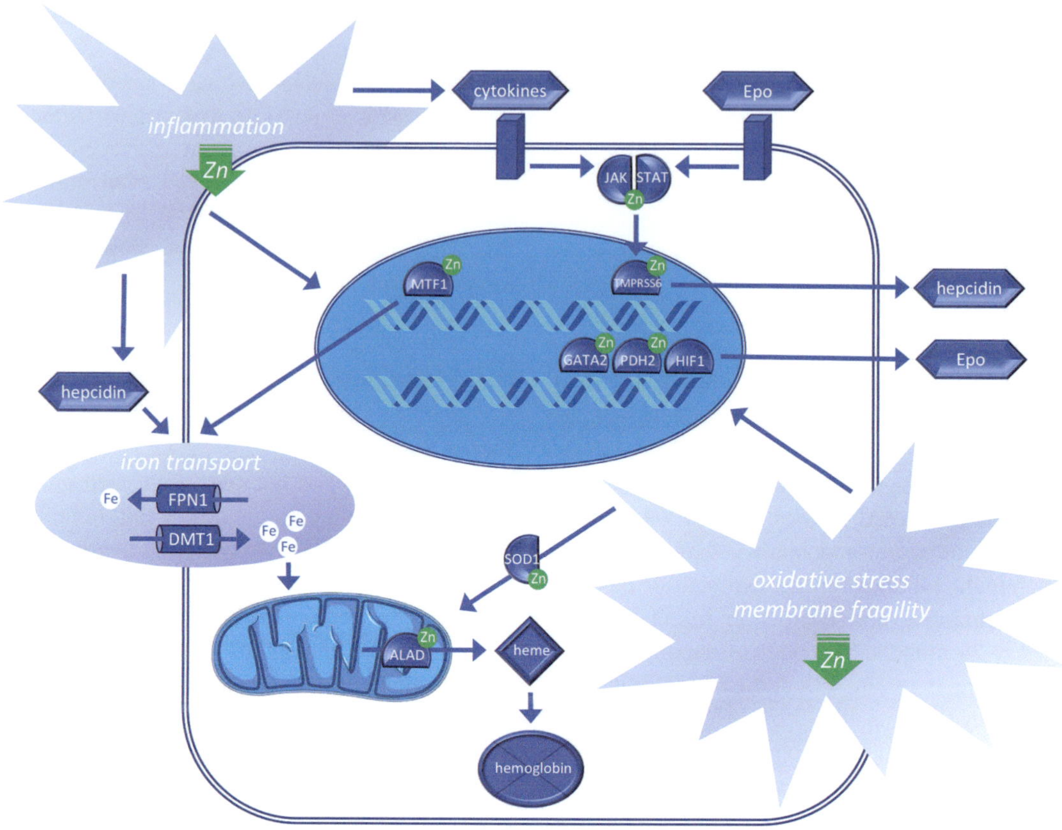

Fig. 14.1 Zinc has numerous roles in the regulation of hemoglobin synthesis. This illustration highlights some of the pathways in which zinc (green circles and arrows) is required within the cellular pathways that control hemoglobin production. Directly, zinc (green circles) is required for proper function of many proteins (blue semi-circles) including transcription factors, signaling kinases, oxidant defense proteins, and the heme biosynthetic enzyme, ALAD. Key regulatory proteins like hepcidin and erythropoietin (Epo) also require zinc for both their own upstream regulatory mechanisms and downstream signalling cascades. Indirectly, zinc availability (green arrows) influences many metabolic states that alter cellular function, including inflammation, iron transport, oxidative stress, and membrane fragility. Abbreviations and details for specific pathways are defined in the text. Note that this illustration is not intended to represent a specific cell type or show all steps involved in hemoglobin synthesis; the figure is simply meant to depict some of the ways in which zinc availability might influence anemia

mitochondrial and cytoplasmic enzymes, maintaining proper redox balance within each cellular compartment is essential [25]. Decreases in SOD1 activity within erythrocytes have been shown to disrupt hemoglobin synthesis and ultimately cause anemia [26]. However, it has not yet been shown if decreases in zinc availability can result in loss of SOD1 activity.

Erythropoietin

Erythropoietin (Epo) is an essential cytokine for maintaining adequate levels of hematopoiesis, predominantly in response to changes in oxygen availability [32]. Two key transcription factors that regulate Epo production are GATA-binding factor 2 (GATA-2) and hypoxia-inducible factor 1 (HIF-1) [33]. GATA-2 has two zinc-finger structural motifs essential for function, and HIF-1 is regulated by several zinc-finger proteins, including PDH2 and PDHZFHX32. Thus, it is plausible that changes in zinc availability could affect the activity of these transcription factors and their downstream targets. However, it has not yet been shown if decreases in zinc availability can result in loss of GATA-2 or HIF-1 associated protein activities. In addition, Epo receptors communicate through the Janus kinases (JAK) and signal transducer and activator of transcription proteins (STAT) intracellular protein kinase cascade, collectively called the JAK-STAT pathway. The JAK-STAT cascade requires zinc as a cofactor for signal transduction.

Hepcidin

The hepatic peptide hormone hepcidin is the central regulator of systemic iron homeostasis. It regulates iron absorption and controls iron release from cells that recycle or store iron [27]. Hepcidin exerts its effect by binding to the major iron export protein, ferroportin (FPN1), resulting in decreased iron absorption and trapping iron within macrophages and liver cells [28]. Knez and colleagues have proposed that zinc availability can modulate hepcidin levels through the upstream protein TMPRSS6, which requires zinc cofactors to function [29]. Low concentrations of zinc could depress the activity of TMPRSS6 so that a key regulatory protein, hemojuvelin, is not activated, resulting in increased hepcidin synthesis and consequently reduced iron uptake. In addition, zinc deficiency has been shown to enhance the acute phase response through the JAK-STAT pathway, which directly regulates hepcidin expression [30]. These are possible ways in which zinc could regulate iron availability and subsequently hemoglobin concentration, but neither mechanism has yet been shown to result in anemia due to dietary zinc deficiency.

Indirect Mechanisms

Iron Absorption

Divalent metal transporter 1 (DMT1) and FPN1 are essential metal transporters in human physiology that play a major role in absorption of iron into the body and tissues, shuttling ionic iron through cellular and organelle membranes. Reduced levels of DMT1 and FPN1 can result in reduced iron status or trapped iron in sequestered stores. The concentration of zinc within the cell has been shown to influence the expression of DMT1 and FPN1, at least partially through metal transcription factor-1 (MTF1), which is sensitive to cellular zinc concentration [31]. Several studies have shown that animal models or human cells placed in zinc-deficient conditions have reduced concentrations of both zinc and iron [31]. However, it has not yet been shown if decreases in zinc availability can cause anemia through this mechanism.

Oxidative Stress and Membrane Fragility

Along with SOD1, zinc ions are important in a number of protein systems involved in reduction of oxidative stress and repair of oxidative damage to cellular macromolecules [34]. Additionally, zinc has been shown to have a structural role in the boundary between the membrane and cytoplasmic compartments, including the membranes of erythrocytes [35]. Some of the membrane-associated zinc might actually be bound to the cytoskeletal proteins like actin and vimentin that support the erythrocyte membrane [36]. Loss of this zinc might result in reduced erythrocyte pliability and increased likelihood of rupture [37]. However, it has not yet been shown if decreases in zinc availability can specifically cause changes in oxidative stress and membrane fragility that results in anemia.

Inflammation

Immune function is arguably the best-studied role of zinc within the body. When zinc availability decreases, immune tone becomes compromised, allowing inflammation to become more easily established [38]. Inflammation is a well-known trigger for alterations in iron homeostasis, with body iron stores shifted into storage as ferritin to make it inaccessible to potentially pathogenic bacteria [39]. If the inflammation is severe or persists in a chronic state, this mechanism is known to cause anemia [40]. However, the pathways leading from reduced zinc availability to inflammation to anemia are complex and not so easily demonstrated. This topic is covered extensively in other literature [41], as well as in Chap. 5 of this book, *The Effect of Inflammation on the Biomarkers of Nutritional Anemia*.

Zinc Supplementation

Animals and Cell Culture

To test whether zinc availability could be a contributing factor to anemia, a few studies have examined the effects of zinc supplementation on hemoglobin production. Chen and colleagues found that exogenous zinc stimulated hematopoiesis in several different species of fish [42]. The same group later found that supplemental zinc also stimulated hematopoiesis in phenylhydrazine-treated anemic rats [43]. When bone marrow from these rats was cultured ex vivo in serum-free media, supplementation with exogenous zinc and transferrin was sufficient to induce a 1.6-fold proliferation of new red blood cells after 1 day [43]. Thus, zinc appears to stimulate hematopoiesis in different animal and cell models.

Humans

A number of systematic reviews and meta-analyses examined the results of zinc supplementation trials in humans. In a 2009 review, Brown and colleagues examined the effect of zinc supplementation on hemoglobin concentration in children from 11 zinc supplementation trials with doses ranging from 1 to 70 mg per dose (median 10 mg, with one dose unknown) in which the supplements differed only by the presence or absence of zinc [44]. They found no overall effect of zinc supplementation on change in hemoglobin concentrations. Additionally, zinc supplementation was not associated with changes in iron status, including serum or plasma ferritin concentrations.

Other literature showed that receiving 10–20 mg doses of zinc for extended durations had no significant effect on hemoglobin concentration in children [45]. Mayo-Wilson and colleagues examined preventive zinc supplementation for children and found no evidence of an effect of zinc supplementation on hemoglobin (27 trials) or on prevalence of anemia (13 trials) [46]. The daily doses, where reported, were 0–5 mg (5 studies), 5–10 mg (19 studies), 10–15 mg (30 studies), 15–20 mg (8 studies), and 20 mg or more (12 studies) [46]. Furthermore, Petry and colleagues found that iron and zinc given together to older infants and young children, resulted in smaller increases in serum ferritin compared with giving iron alone [47]. Only studies where the daily iron dose for children did not exceed 15 mg and the daily zinc dose did not exceed 10 mg were included in this analysis [47]. The effect of zinc intake on hemoglobin concentrations or anemia was not assessed in this review, but the ferritin findings did not support the idea that zinc supplementation would increase hemoglobin or reduce anemia. Finally, a 2018 review of systematic reviews of effective approaches for addressing micronutrient deficiencies in children aged 0–5 years found that neither zinc supplementation nor zinc fortification had a significant effect on hemoglobin, serum ferritin, or the risk of anemia [48]. Zinc supplementation alone resulted in a lower mean hemoglobin and higher risk of anemia compared with combined iron and zinc supplementation [48].

Since those four reviews were published, more recent findings from studies in Lao PDR [49] and Tanzania [50] support the idea that zinc supplementation does not increase hemoglobin concentrations or reduce anemia prevalence in humans. In the Lao PDR study, neither therapeutic zinc treatment nor preventive zinc supplements showed significant increases in hemoglobin or reductions in anemia over 32–40 weeks, compared with a control or a micronutrient powder containing iron and zinc [49]. Only the micronutrient powder containing both iron and zinc was found to marginally improve iron status and reduce anemia, and this was observed only in children who were anemic at baseline. In the Tanzania study, participating pregnant women who received zinc actually had a significant reduction in their mean hemoglobin concentration compared with those who received no zinc [50].

Conclusion

In principle, zinc could play a mechanistic role in the regulation of hemoglobin concentrations in vivo. However, there are at present not enough data to demonstrate a clear causal role of zinc in the etiology of anemia in humans. The studies showing an association between zinc availability and hemoglobin concentrations in experimental animal and cell models are intriguing and warrant further investigation.

Disclaimers Neither of the authors declare a conflict of interest with regard to this manuscript. The findings and conclusions in this report are those of the authors and do not necessarily represent the official position of UCSF or City College of San Francisco.

References

1. King JC, Brown KH, Gibson RS, Krebs NF, Lowe NM, Siekmann JH, et al. Biomarkers of Nutrition for Development (BOND)-Zinc Review. J Nutr. 2015;146(4):858S–85S.
2. International Zinc Nutrition Consultative Group (IZiNCG). International Zinc Nutrition Consultative Group (IZiNCG) website. https://www.izincg.org/riskzincdeficiency.
3. World Health Organization (WHO). Micronutrient Database. https://www.who.int/vmnis/database/en/.
4. Development Initiatives Poverty Research Ltd. 2020 global nutrition report: action on equity to end malnutrition. Bristol, UK: Development Initiatives; 2020. https://globalnutritionreport.org/reports/global-nutrition-report-2018/three-issues-critical-need-attention/.
5. World Health Organization (WHO). The global prevalence of anaemia in 2011. Geneva: World Health Organization (WHO); 2015. https://apps.who.int/iris/bitstream/handle/10665/177094/9789241564960_eng.pdf;jsessionid=78BE360BA88056636E540876AD4D2D37?sequence=1.
6. Wessells KR, Brown KH. Estimating the global prevalence of zinc deficiency: results based on zinc availability in national food supplies and the prevalence of stunting. PLoS One. 2012;7(11):e50568.
7. Hess SY. National risk of zinc deficiency as estimated by national surveys. Food Nutr Bull. 2017;38(1):3–17.
8. Gupta S, Brazier AKM, Lowe NM. Zinc deficiency in low- and middle-income countries: prevalence and approaches for mitigation. J Hum Nutr Diet. 2020;33(5):624–43.
9. Harika R, Faber M, Samuel F, Mulugeta A, Kimiywe J, Eilander A. Are low intakes and deficiencies in iron, vitamin A, zinc, and iodine of public health concern in Ethiopian, Kenyan, Nigerian, and South African children and adolescents? Food Nutr Bull. 2017;38(3):405–27.
10. Roos N, Ponce MC, Doak CM, Dijkhuizen M, Polman K, Chamnan C, et al. Micronutrient status of populations and preventive nutrition interventions in South East Asia. Matern Child Health J. 2019;23(S1):29–45.
11. Wieringa F, Dahl M, Chamnan C, Poirot E, Kuong K, Sophonneary P, et al. The high prevalence of anemia in Cambodian children and women cannot be satisfactorily explained by nutritional deficiencies or hemoglobin disorders. Nutrients. 2016;8(6):348.
12. Houghton LA, Parnell WR, Thomson CD, Green TJ, Gibson RS. Serum zinc is a major predictor of anemia and mediates the effect of selenium on hemoglobin in school-aged children in a nationally representative survey in New Zealand. J Nutr. 2016;146(9):1670–6.
13. Gibson RS, Abebe Y, Stabler S, Allen RH, Westcott JE, Stoecker BJ, et al. Zinc, gravida, infection, and iron, but not vitamin B-12 or folate status, predict hemoglobin during pregnancy in Southern Ethiopia. J Nutr. 2008;138(3):581–6.
14. Greffeuille V, Fortin S, Gibson R, Rohner F, Williams A, Young MF, et al. Associations between zinc and hemoglobin concentrations in preschool children and women of reproductive age: an analysis of representative survey data from the Biomarkers Reflecting Inflammation and Nutritional Determinants of Anemia (BRINDA) project. Pending.
15. Ece A, Uyanik BS, Işcan A, Ertan P, Yiğitoğlu MR. Increased serum copper and decreased serum zinc levels in children with iron deficiency anemia. Biol Trace Elem Res. 1997;59(1–3):31–9.
16. Ma A-G, Chen X-C, Xu R-X, Zheng M-C, Wang Y, Li J-S. Comparison of serum levels of iron, zinc and copper in anaemic and non-anaemic pregnant women in China. Asia Pac J Clin Nutr. 2004;13(4):348–52.
17. Gebremedhin S, Enquselassie F, Umeta M. Prevalence of prenatal zinc deficiency and its association with socio-demographic, dietary and health care related factors in rural Sidama, Southern Ethiopia: a cross-sectional study. BMC Public Health. 2011;11:898.
18. Kelkitli E, Ozturk N, Aslan NA, Kilic-Baygutalp N, Bayraktutan Z, Kurt N, et al. Serum zinc levels in patients with iron deficiency anemia and its association with symptoms of iron deficiency anemia. Ann Hematol. 2016;95(5):751–6.
19. Palacios AM, Hurley KM, De-Ponce S, Alfonso V, Tilton N, Lambden KB, et al. Zinc deficiency associated with anaemia among young children in rural Guatemala. Matern Child Nutr. 2020;16(1):e12885.
20. Atasoy HI, Bugdayci G. Zinc deficiency and its predictive capacity for anemia: unique model in school children. Pediatr Int. 2018;60(8):703–9.
21. Shamim AA, Kabir A, Merrill RD, Ali H, Rashid M, Schulze K, et al. Plasma zinc, vitamin B(12) and α-tocopherol are positively and plasma γ-tocopherol is negatively associated with Hb concentration in early pregnancy in north-west Bangladesh. Public Health Nutr. 2013;16(8):1354–61.

22. Ames BN. Low micronutrient intake may accelerate the degenerative diseases of aging through allocation of scarce micronutrients by triage. Proc Natl Acad Sci U S A. 2006;103(47):17589–94.
23. Ferreira GC. Heme synthesis. In: Encyclopedia of biological chemistry. 2nd edn. 2013.
24. Information on EC 4.2.1.24—porphobilinogen synthase. BRENDA—the comprehensive enzyme information system. https://www.brenda-enzymes.org/enzyme.php?ecno=4.2.1.24.
25. Information on EC 1.15.1.1—superoxide dismutase. BRENDA—the comprehensive enzyme information system. https://www.brenda-enzymes.org/enzyme.php?ecno=1.15.1.1&UniProtAcc=Q9YE27&OrganismID=171.
26. Iuchi Y, Okada F, Onuma K, Onoda T, Asao H, Kobayashi M, et al. Elevated oxidative stress in erythrocytes due to a SOD1 deficiency causes anaemia and triggers autoantibody production. Biochem J. 2007;402(2):219–27.
27. Sangkhae V, Nemeth E. Regulation of the Iron Homeostatic Hormone Hepcidin123. Adv Nutr. 2017;8(1):126–36.
28. Ginzburg YZ. Hepcidin-Ferroportin axis in health and disease. In Vitamins and hormones. Elsevier; 2019. p. 17–45. https://linkinghub.elsevier.com/retrieve/pii/S0083672919300020.
29. Knez M, Graham RD, Welch RM, Stangoulis JCR. New perspectives on the regulation of iron absorption via cellular zinc concentrations in humans. Crit Rev Food Sci Nutr. 2017;57(10):2128–43.
30. Liu M-J, Bao S, Napolitano JR, Burris DL, Yu L, Tridandapani S, et al. Zinc regulates the acute phase response and serum amyloid A production in response to sepsis through JAK-STAT3 signaling. PLoS One. 2014;9(4):e94934.
31. Kondaiah P, Yaduvanshi PS, Sharp PA, Pullakhandam R. Iron and zinc homeostasis and interactions: does enteric zinc excretion cross-talk with intestinal iron absorption? Nutrients. 2019;11(8)
32. Zhang Y, Wang L, Dey S, Alnaeeli M, Suresh S, Rogers H, et al. Erythropoietin action in stress response, tissue maintenance and metabolism. Int J Mol Sci. 2014;15(6):10296–333.
33. Haase VH. Regulation of erythropoiesis by hypoxia-inducible factors. Blood Rev. 2013;27(1):41–53.
34. Lee SR. Critical role of zinc as either an antioxidant or a prooxidant in cellular systems. Oxid Med Cell Longev. 2018. https://www.ncbi.nlm.nih.gov/pmc/articles/PMC5884210/.
35. Maret W. Zinc biochemistry: from a single zinc enzyme to a key element of life12. Adv Nutr. 2013;4(1):82–91.
36. Liem RKH. Cytoskeletal integrators: the spectrin superfamily. Cold Spring Harb Perspect Biol. 2016;8(10):a018259.
37. Paterson PG, Card RT. The effect of zinc deficiency on erythrocyte deformability in the rat. J Nutr Biochem. 1993;4(4):250–5.
38. Maywald M, Wessels I, Rink L. Zinc signals and immunity. Int J Mol Sci. 2017;18(10). https://www.ncbi.nlm.nih.gov/pmc/articles/PMC5666901/.
39. Weiss G, Goodnough LT. Anemia of chronic disease. N Engl J Med. 2005;352(10):1011–23.
40. Kassebaum NJ. The global burden of anemia. Hematol Clin. 2016;30(2):247–308.
41. World Health Organization (WHO). Nutritional anaemias: tools for effective prevention and control. 2017. 96p. https://www.who.int/publications/i/item/9789241513067.
42. Chen Y-H, Shiu J-R, Ho C-L, Jeng S-S. Zinc as a signal to stimulate red blood cell formation in fish. Int J Mol Sci. 2017;18(1).
43. Chen Y-H, Feng H-L, Jeng S-S. Zinc supplementation stimulates red blood cell formation in rats. Int J Mol Sci. 2018;19(9).
44. Brown KH, Peerson JM, Baker SK, Hess SY. Preventive zinc supplementation among infants, preschoolers, and older prepubertal children. Food Nutr Bull. 2009;30(1 Suppl):S12–40.
45. Dekker LH, Villamor E. Zinc supplementation in children is not associated with decreases in hemoglobin concentrations. J Nutr. 2010;140(5):1035–40.
46. Mayo-Wilson E, Imdad A, Junior J, Dean S, Bhutta ZA. Preventive zinc supplementation for children, and the effect of additional iron: a systematic review and meta-analysis. BMJ Open. 2014;4(6):e004647.
47. Petry N, Olofin I, Boy E, Donahue Angel M, Rohner F. The effect of low dose iron and zinc intake on child micronutrient status and development during the first 1000 days of life: a systematic review and meta-analysis. Nutrients. 2016;8(12).
48. Campos Ponce M, Polman K, Roos N, Wieringa FT, Berger J, Doak CM. What approaches are most effective at addressing micronutrient deficiency in children 0–5 years? A review of systematic reviews. Matern Child Health J. 2019;23(Suppl 1):4–17.
49. Barffour MA, Hinnouho G-M, Kounnavong S, Wessells KR, Ratsavong K, Bounheuang B, et al. Effects of daily zinc, daily multiple micronutrient powder, or therapeutic zinc supplementation for diarrhea prevention on physical growth, anemia, and micronutrient status in rural Laotian children: a randomized controlled trial. J Pediatr. 2019;207:80–89.e2.
50. Noor RA, Abioye AI, Darling AM, Hertzmark E, Aboud S, Premji Z, et al. Prenatal zinc and vitamin a reduce the benefit of iron on maternal hematologic and micronutrient status at delivery in Tanzania. J Nutr. 2020;150(2):240–8.

15 The Role of Vitamin D in Anemia

Merryn J. Netting, Karen P. Best, and Tim J. Green

Keywords

Vitamin D · Anemia · 25hydroxyvitamin D · Iron · Inflammation · Hepcidin · Observational studies · Randomized control trials

Introduction

Vitamin D deficiency and anemia are common conditions worldwide [1, 2]. Vitamin D deficiency and anemia often coexist in populations, suggesting that vitamin D deficiency may play a role in the etiology of anemia [3]. The leading theory is that vitamin D is an essential regulator of hepcidin, a key hormone involved in systemic iron metabolism [4]. Here we explore the emerging role of vitamin D in anemia, starting with a brief overview of vitamin D, an examination of the mechanistic evidence linking vitamin D to anemia, followed by a review of the human observational studies and randomized control trials of vitamin D and anemia and related biomarkers.

M. J. Netting · K. P. Best · T. J. Green (✉)
SAHMRI Women and Kids, SAHMRI, Adelaide, SA, Australia

School of Medicine, The University of Adelaide, Adelaide, SA, Australia
e-mail: tim.green@sahmri.com

Vitamin D

Vitamin D can be obtained exogenously from a few foods, such as oily fish, eggs, and mushrooms where it is found naturally, and fortified foods such as milk and vitamin supplements [5]. However, most people are dependent on endogenous synthesis for vitamin D, when ultraviolet (UV) light from the sun converts 7-dehydrocholesterol in the skin into vitamin D [6]. Anything that limits the amount of UV light reaching and penetrating the skin will affect vitamin D status, including season, latitude, time of day, the amount of melanin in the skin, and amount of skin exposed to the sun (e.g., covering up for religious or cultural regions). Regardless of the source, vitamin D is hydroxylated in the liver, forming 25-hydroxyvitamin D (25OHD), the primary circulating form of vitamin D and the best biomarker of status [7, 8]. However, there is considerable disagreement about the appropriate cut-off (20–100 nmol/L), which explains, in part, the vastly different prevalence estimates for vitamin D deficiency.

The best described role of vitamin D is maintaining serum calcium concentrations within a narrow range. When serum calcium levels drop, parathyroid hormone (PTH) is released, which activates 25OHD-1α-hydroxylase in the kidney, converting 25OHD to 1,25-dihydroxyvitamin D (1,25OH$_2$D) [8]. This active form of vitamin D increases intestinal calcium absorption, calcium

C. D. Karakochuk et al. (eds.), *Nutritional Anemia*, Nutrition and Health,
https://doi.org/10.1007/978-3-031-14521-6_15

release from bone, and calcium reabsorption in the kidney, thereby increasing serum calcium concentration and shutting off the process. $1{,}25OH_2D$ binds to a vitamin D receptor on the plasma membrane of cells in the intestine, bone, and kidney, forming a complex that binds to the vitamin D responsive element (VDRE) in the promoter region of target genes to exert genomic effects [8]. The vitamin D receptor is expressed in many other tissues and cells, including hematopoietic and immune cells, indicating that vitamin D has roles beyond calcium homeostasis. Some of these cells also express the enzyme 25OHD-1α-hydroxylase, suggesting an autocrine or paracrine role for vitamin D [7].

Vitamin D and Anemia Mechanisms

Vitamin D may influence hemoglobin through an effect on erythropoiesis. Vitamin D, as $1{,}25OH_2D$, has been shown to increase erythropoiesis by promoting the proliferation of erythroid precursors and augmenting the impact of erythropoietin [9, 10]. In kidney disease, an elevated PTH concentration leads to decreased erythropoiesis and reduced hemoglobin concentration. Thus, vitamin D may promote erythropoiesis by suppressing PTH production [11]. However, the leading theory is that vitamin D protects against anemia by reducing inflammation. It is proposed that vitamin D is an essential regulator of hepcidin, a key hormone involved in systemic iron metabolism [12] (Fig. 15.1). Chronic inflammation caused by infection, autoimmune disease, cancer, obesity, or even lifestyle factors such as smoking and alcohol use can decrease hemoglobin synthesis due to a lack of available iron [13]. Vitamin D may counter the effect of inflammation by reducing levels of proinflammatory cytokines and hepcidin, the primary regulator of systemic iron homeostasis. Cytokines, released in response to inflammation, particularly interleukin 6, suppress erythropoiesis, diminish the effect of erythropoietin, and reduce erythrocyte survival time. Interleukin 6 also induces the transcription of the hepcidin gene through Janus kinase (JAK)2/signal transducer and activator of transcription (STAT)3 pathway, increasing hepatic hepcidin synthesis [14]. Hepcidin binds to a receptor on

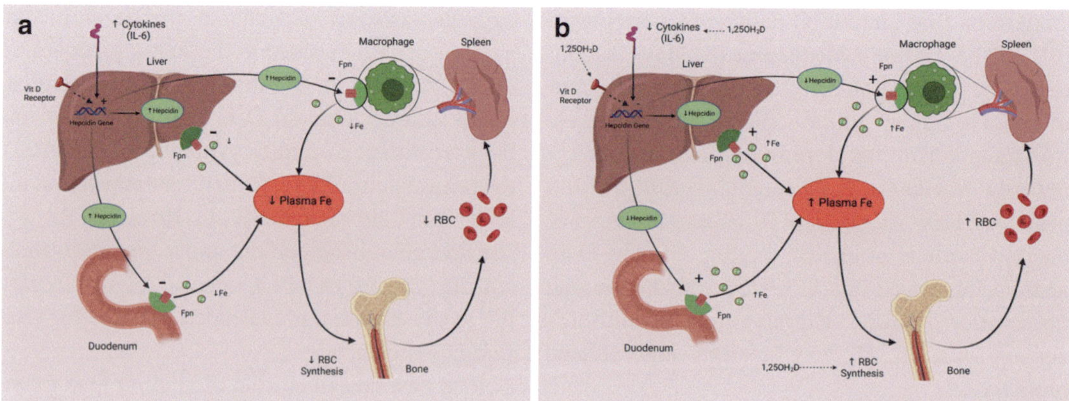

Fig. 15.1 Potential mechanisms by which vitamin D modifies anemia of inflammation. Panel (**a**): In inflammation, cytokines released, especially interleukin 6 (IL-6), bind to the promoter region of the gene encoding for hepcidin, causing an increase in hepatic hepcidin production. Hepcidin binds to ferroportin, found on the plasma membrane of macrophages, enterocytes, and hepatocytes, blocking iron release into serum. Consequently, the amount of iron available for erythropoiesis in the bone marrow reduces red blood cell count and anemia. Panel (**b**): Vitamin D, as 1,25 dihydroxyvitamin D ($1{,}25OH_2D$), may promote erythropoiesis by reducing cytokine production or stimulating red blood cell synthesis in the bone marrow. The prevailing theory is that $1{,}25OH_2D$ binds to a vitamin D receptor on the plasma membrane, forming a complex that binds to the promoter region on the hepatic hepcidin gene, inhibiting hepcidin synthesis. A decrease in hepcidin allows iron export from ferroportin, increasing serum iron, making iron available for erythropoiesis

ferroportin, the sole cellular transmembrane iron exporter, blocking the export of iron from the cell. Hepcidin binds to ferroportin on the plasma membranes of enterocytes, macrophages, and hepatocytes and reduces the amount of iron released into circulation, limiting the amount of iron available for erythropoiesis [13]. Vitamin D, specifically 1,25OH$_2$D, binds to a VDRE located in the promotor region of the hepcidin gene and downregulates hepcidin transcription, reducing hepcidin, allowing ferroportin to export iron, making it available for erythropoiesis [15].

Iron and Inflammation Indices

Iron-deficiency anemia occurs in stages starting with depleted iron stores, characterized by high serum soluble transferrin receptor (sTfR) and low ferritin and hepcidin [16, 17]. Once stores are depleted, erythropoiesis becomes impaired; serum transferrin increases, and serum iron and transferrin saturation drops [16]. As iron deficiency progresses, hemoglobin synthesis is reduced, leading to anemia. In contrast, anemia of inflammation is characterized by high serum ferritin and hepcidin, low serum iron and transferrin saturation, and a normal sTfR. The anemia of iron deficiency is microcytic and hypochromic, whereas the anemia of inflammation is normocytic and normochromic [13]. Studies of vitamin D and iron biomarkers are difficult to interpret, particularly when iron deficiency and inflammation coexist. For example, serum ferritin is typically low in individuals with iron deficiency and elevated in the presence of inflammation.

Observational Studies

Observational Studies in Children and Adolescents

Anemia rates were higher in children/adolescents with lower 25OHD in population-representative surveys conducted in the USA, South Korea, and Tehran [18–20] (Table 15.1). In the US National Health and Nutrition Examination Survey (NHANES) 2001–2006, children and adolescents (1–21 years) with a 25OHD <75 nmol/L were at a twofold greater risk of anemia than those with a higher 25OHD [18, 19]. Anemia prevalence was seven times higher in "Blacks" than "Whites" (14% vs. 2%); yet, in "Blacks," only a 25OHD less than 30 nmol/L was associated with lower hemoglobin. In "Whites," this threshold was 50 nmol/L [18]. Similar racial variation in 25OHD cut-offs has been observed for other health outcomes between "Blacks" and "Whites" [21]. In the Korean NHANES 2010–2012, adolescents (10–20 years) with a 25OHD <37.5 nmol/L versus ≥50 nmol/L had a 1.8- and 2.3-fold greater risk of anemia and iron deficiency anemia (ferritin <12 μg/L and transferrin saturation <16% with anemia), respectively [19]. Yet when data were stratified by sex, these associations remained significant for females only, possibly because anemia rates were higher in females than males (6.8% versus 1.4%) [19]. In pregnant American adolescents, anemia was eightfold higher at delivery in those with a 25OHD <50 nmol/L compared with ≥50 nmol/L [22].

In both NHANES studies, 25OHD was inversely associated with hemoglobin concentrations [18, 19, 23]. The magnitude of the association was small in both studies; in the US study, for example, there was only a 2 g/L difference between the top three quartiles of 25OHD compared with the lowest quartile (<50 nmol/L) [18]. Moreover, the relationship between hemoglobin and 25OHD was not continuous; above a 25OHD of 50 nmol/L, further increases in hemoglobin were not observed. In contrast, 25OHD was inversely associated with hemoglobin concentration in a population-based survey of German adolescents (11–17 years), with the authors suggesting an inhibitory effect of vitamin D on erythropoiesis [24]. In a study of pregnant adolescents in the USA, hemoglobin at delivery was 9 g/L higher in women with a ≥50 compared to <50 nmol/L [22]. Plasma volume increases in late pregnancy; therefore, this large difference in hemoglobin may reflect differences in hemodilution [25].

Table 15.1 Observational studies of vitamin D status and anemia, hemoglobin, biomarkers of iron and inflammation in children and adolescents

Study/ country	Survey/sample/age	Comparison/adjustment	Results
Atkinson, US [18]	NHANES (2001–2006). $N = 10,410/1–21$ years	25OHD and anemia risk by logistic regression adjusted for age, sex, race, obesity, CRP, serum B_{12}, and folate	25OHD <75 nmol/L associated with increased risk of anemia, OR 1.9 (95% CI, 1.2–3.1), $p = 0.006$, and <25 nmol/L, OR 1.5 (95% CI 1.1–1.9), $p = 0.004$
Doudin, Germany [24]	Nationally representative sample. $N = 5066/11–17$ years	Correlations between 25OHD and Hb, sTfR, or ferritin. Multinomial regression with adjustment for age, sex, BMI, socioeconomic status, and self-rated total quality of life	25OHD was inversely associated with Hb ($r = -0.04$, $p = 0.003$), and sTfR ($r = -0.1$, $p < 0.001$) but was not associated with ferritin ($r = 0.02$, $p = 0.172$). Multinomial regression indicated similar findings
Lee, Korea [19]	NHANES (2010–2012). $N = 2526/10–20$ years	25OHD and anemia (WHO cut-offs), iron deficiency (ferritin <12 μg/L and transferrin saturation <16%), and IDA (ID + anemia). Adjusted for age, BMI, and low household income	Vit D deficiency associated with increased risk for anemia, OR 1.8 (95% CI, 1.1–2.9), $p = 0.013$, ID OR 1.94 (95% CI, 1.3–3.0), $p = 0.002$ and IDA OR 2.3 (95% CI, 1.2–4.2), $p = 0.01$
Moran-Lev, US [26]	Hospitalized Patients. $N = 90/1–16$ years	Children were divided into three groups: acute infection with anemia ($n = 32$), acute infection without anemia ($n = 30$), and controls ($n = 28$; no infection). Blood was obtained within 72 h of admission, and biomarkers were measured	Hepcidin, ferritin, IL-6 were significantly higher, and 25OHD, serum iron and transferrin were significantly lower in those with infection and anemia
Nikooyeh, Iran [20]	A random sample of 60 schools in Tehran grades 4 and 5. $N = 937/9–12$ years	The difference in 25OHD in anemic and nonanemic children (Hb <115 g/L). Vit D def (25OHD <25 nmol/L) and risk of anemia after adjustment for sex, age, BMI, and PTH	Mean ± SD 25OHD lower in anemic vs. nonanemic (19.6 ± 13.3 vs. 24.0 ± 23.1 nmol/L; $p = 0.003$). Vit D deficient children were more likely to be anemic; OR 3.5 (95% CI, 1.2–9.8)
Thomas, US [22]	A prospective longitudinal study of pregnant adolescents. $N = 158/<19$ years	Maternal 25OHD, hemoglobin adjusted for maternal race and age at enrolment	Anemia was 8.0 times greater in adolescents with delivery 25OHD concentrations, <50 nmol/L than in those with 25OHD concentrations ≥50 nmol/L ($p < 0.001$)

Abbreviations: *25OHD* 25hydroxyvitamin D; *BMI* body mass index; *CI* confidence interval; *CRP* C-reactive protein; *Hb* hemoglobin; *IDA* iron deficiency anemia; *IL-6* interleukin 6; *OR* odds ratio; *PTH* parathyroid hormone; *sTfR* soluble transferrin receptor; *NHANES* National Health and Nutrition Examination Survey; *Vit D* Vitamin D; *WHO* World Health Organization

Only two studies have included measures of iron and inflammation biomarkers with mixed results. Thomas found no association between 25OHD and ferritin, sTfR, or hepcidin in pregnant adolescents [22]. Moran-Lev et al. divided hospitalized children into three groups: acute infection with anemia (n = 32), acute infection without anemia (n = 30), and controls (n = 28; no infection) [26]. Serum 25OHD was lower, and interleukin 6 (IL-6), hepcidin, and ferritin concentrations were higher in the anemic children with infectious disease, consistent with vitamin D's purported role as immunomodulator anemia chronic disease.

Observational Studies in Adults

Findings in adults were similar to children and adolescents. In the US NHANES (2001–2006), individuals (≥17 years) with a 25OHD concentration <50 nmol/L were 1.6 times more likely to be anemic [27] (Table 15.2). In a large group of predominately adult patients (>17 years), members of an integrated health plan in the USA, 25OHD <75 nmol/L was associated with a nearly 2-times increase in anemia; however, 65% of patients had chronic kidney disease [28]. Sim et al. reported a significant modifying effect of race on the relationship between anemia and 25OHD. There was no relationship in White Americans, but African-Americans with a 25OHD <50 versus ≥50 nmol/L had a 6.4 times higher risk of anemia. Black Americans with a 25OHD <50 nmol/L were at 8.4 times greater risk if they had anemia with inflammation [29]. There was an inverse association between hemoglobin and 25OHD concentration up to 50 nmol/L. In the Korean NHANES (2010–2011), hemoglobin concentration began to decrease in adults (>20 years) as 25OHD fell below 66 nmol/L [30]. When the association was analyzed by sex and menstrual status, the corresponding 25OHD concentrations were 69, 30, and 34 nmol/L for males, premenopausal wmen, and postmenopausal women, respectively.

Table 15.2 Observational studies of vitamin D status and anemia, hemoglobin, biomarkers of iron and inflammation in adults

Study/country	Survey/sample/age	Comparison/adjustment	Results
De la Cruz, Mexico [32]	A convenience sample of older adults. *N* = 783/>60 years	Tertile of the log of hepcidin by 25OHD <25 nmol/L; adjusted for sex, age, inflammation, ferritin, sTfR, BMI, renal disease, anemia, frailty, and smoking	Hepcidin tertile was not associated with vitamin D deficiency; OR 0.74 (95% CI, 0.42–1.28)
Han, Korea [23]	NHANES (2010–2011). *N* = 11,206/>20 years	A generalized additive model was used to examine Hb and 25OHD, adjusted OR for anemia by quartile of 25OHD. Examined overall and by sex and menstrual status	Hb decreased linearly when 25OHD <69, 30, and 34 nmol/L for males, pre- and postmenopausal females, respectively. Anemia risk associated with 25OHD in females only
Malczewska, Poland [31]	Female professional athletes. *N* = 219/14–34 years	Logistic regression 25OHD <75 nmol/L and ID (ferritin <16 μg/L) or IDA (ferritin <16 μg/L, sTfR >8.3 mg/L, TIBC >390 μg/dL, and Hb <120 g/L) adjusted for length of time spent outdoors, and age	Having a 25OHD <75 nmol/L was associated with an increased risk of ID, OR 2.7 (95% CI, 1.3–5.6), $p = 0.007$ and IDA, OR 4.2 (95% CI, 1.8–11.7), $p < 0.01$
Monlezun, US [27]	NHANES (2001–2006). *N* = 5456/≥17 years	Regression analysis, adjusted for age, sex, race, BMI, presence of kidney disease, CRP, ferritin, vitamin B12, folic acid, and iron levels	Adults with 25OHD <50 nmol/L were more likely to be anemic; OR 1.6 (95% CI, 1.1–2.5), $p = 0.03$
Sim, US [28]	Patients from an integrated health plan with hemoglobin and 25OHD measurement; *N* = 554/>17 years	Hb was stratified by 25OHD using logistic regression, adjusted for age, gender, erythrocyte-stimulating agent, and chronic kidney disease	25OHD <75 vs. ≥75 nmol/L was associated with increased risk of anemia) OR 1.9 (95% CI, 1.3–2.7)
Smith, US [29]	A convenience sample of healthy adults working at a university. *N* = 638/>17 years	Multivariate logistic regression to determine the association between anemia and 25OHD (<50 vs. ≥50 nmol/) stratified by race. Further analysis by anemia of inflammation (CRP >3 mg/L or IL-6 >1.76 pg/mL)	No association in whites. Anemia by 25OHD in African-Americans, OR 6.4 (95% CI, 1.9–22.0). Anemia including infection by 25OHD OR 8.3 (95% CI, 2.0–36.2)

Abbreviations: *25OHD* 25hydroxyvitamin D; *BMI* body mass index; *CI* confidence interval; *CRP* C-reactive protein; *Hb* hemoglobin; *ID* iron deficiency; *IDA* iron deficiency anemia; *IL-6* interleukin 6; *OR* odds ratio; *sTfR* soluble transferrin receptor; *Vit D* Vitamin D

Women, but not men, in the lowest quartile of 25OHD were at greater risk of anemia.

The association between 25OHD and iron deficiency, iron deficiency anemia, and biomarkers of iron has not been well studied. In professional female athletes, a 25OHD <75 nmol/L was not associated with anemia but was associated with a 2.7- and a 4.2-fold higher risk of iron deficiency and iron-deficiency anemia, respectively [31]. In a large study (n = 783) of 783 older Mexican adults (>60 years), there was no association between 25OHD and hepcidin. Although anemia was high (36%), less than 10% of participants had a 25OHD <50 nmol/L [32].

Overall, evidence from the observational studies in children, adolescents, and adults suggests that 25OHD is associated with anemia. The magnitude of difference in hemoglobin between the high and low 25OHD is small, with a threshold effect for 25OHD ~50 nmol/L. This association is influenced by the prevalence of vitamin D deficiency and anemia. Other factors are possibly involved, including the criteria to define anemia, the cut-off used for 25OHD, and the method used to measure 25OHD and hemoglobin. The complex relationship between iron and inflammation biomarkers in iron deficiency anemia and anemia of chronic disease complicates the interpretation of studies. There is a suggestion that higher 25OHD is associated with lower hepcidin in a population with an increased burden of inflammation, but this is not consistent. Ferritin is not related to 25OHD, but is a biomarker of iron status and inflammation.

Randomized Control Trials

Ultimately, randomized control trials (RCTs) are required as it is impossible to rule out residual confounding and infer causation from observational studies (Table 15.3).

Anemia

Nine studies were found in which participants were randomized to vitamin D supplementation or placebo with anemia, hemoglobin, or related biomarkers as outcomes [30, 33–40]. Three studies were in healthy participants [29, 36, 37], including one study in pregnant women [30]; one trial in iron-deficient women [33] and another study in anemic patients [40]; three studies were in populations with chronic disease [34, 35, 41], and one study was in mechanically ventilated critically ill patients [39]. The number of participants in the trials ranged from 28 to 250 [37, 38] and were between 1 week [38] and 3 years in duration [42]. Vitamin D was given as oral vitamin D_3 and in daily doses from 10 to 250 μg up to a single bolus dose of 15,000 μg given intramuscularly [40]. Most studies report a higher 25OHD at follow-up between those receiving vitamin D than placebo.

In the RCTs that included hemoglobin as an outcome, two trials reported that hemoglobin was higher in those randomized to vitamin D supplementation than placebo [33, 39], four trials did not [34, 35, 40]. In one study, women (n = 50) with marginal iron deficiency were asked to consume an iron-fortified breakfast cereal containing 9 mg of elemental iron for 8 weeks and randomized to receive 38 μg/day vitamin D_3 or placebo. The women who received vitamin D had a 7 g/L higher hemoglobin. In contrast, adding a single bolus intramuscular vitamin D to parenteral iron in Indian patients with iron deficiency anemia did not result in higher hemoglobin at 12-weeks follow-up. Likewise, participants (n = 251) with low 25OHD from North Africa, South and South-East Asia, and living in Norway in the winter were randomized to one of three groups: 10 or 25 μg vitamin D or placebo. Neither group receiving vitamin D had a higher mean hemoglobin after 16 weeks compared to placebo. Ernst et al.

Table 15.3 Randomized control trials of vitamin D supplementation and anemia, hemoglobin (Hb) biomarkers of iron and inflammation in adults

Study/ country	Participants	Intervention	Outcomes
Ahmad, UK [33]	Premenopausal women with marginal iron deficiency (ferritin <20 μg/L), $N = 50/19–49$ years	Iron-fortified breakfast cereal (15 mg/100 g) with and without 38 μg vitamin D_3/day for 8 weeks	Significant mean ± SD increase in Hb from baseline in D_3 group vs. placebo 4 ± 7 vs. −3 ± 12, $p = 0.037$. No effect on ferritin and hepcidin
Braithwaite, UK [30]	Pregnant women. $N = 195/30 \pm 5$ years	25 μg/day vitamin D_3 vs. placebo from ~14 weeks gestation until delivery	At 34 weeks gestation, no differences in hepcidin, ferritin, CRP, and α1-acid glycoprotein
Ernst, Austria [35]	Patients with heart failure. $N = 200/{>}18$ years	70 μg/day vitamin D_3 vs. placebo for 8 weeks	No effect on Hb
Ernst, Germany [34]	Patients with heart failure. $N = 172/{>}18–79$ years	100 μg/day vitamin D_3 vs. placebo for 3 years	No effect on Hb
Kasprowicz, Poland [36]	Male ultra-marathon runners. $N = 20/41 \pm 5$ years	250 μg vitamin D_3 vs. placebo daily for 2 weeks before a 100 km ultra-marathon. Blood was collected at baseline, pre-, post, and 12 h post-run	There were no differences among hepcidin, IL-6, sTFR, TIBC, or ferritin groups
Madar, Norway [37]	Healthy adults of South Asian, Middle Eastern, and African descent living in Norway. $N = 251/18–50$ years	10 μg D_3, or 25 μg vitamin D_3 vs. placebo daily for 16 weeks during winter	No difference in mean Hb −2 (95% CI, −12, 9) g/L; ferritin 1.9 (95% CI, −3.2, 7.0) μg/L; between those receiving vitamin D_3 versus placebo
Smith, US [38]	Healthy adults. $N = 28/18–65$ years	6250 μg D_3 as single bolus vs. placebo	Mean (95%CI) hepcidin was lower in the vitamin D_3 group than placebo at 1 week, 73% (95% CI, 4–92%), $p = 0.04$. No difference in ferritin or cytokines between groups
Smith, US [39]	Critically ill, ventilated adults. $N = 30/{>}18$ years	1250 or 2500 μg vitamin D_3 vs. placebo daily for 5 days. Blood was collected at baseline and weekly for 4 weeks	At 3 weeks mean Hb was higher in 2500 μg/day versus placebo 113 (9, 14) vs. 82 g/L [7, 9], ($p = 0.03$)]. Hepcidin was lower in the 2500 μg D_3 group ($p = 0.007$). No effect of 1250 μg
Sooragonda, India [40]	Adults with iron deficiency anemia (ferritin <15 μg/L and anemia) $N = 30/41 \pm 11$ years	Intravenous iron with bolus Vitamin D_3 (15,000 μg) or placebo administered intramuscularly. Follow-up after 12-weeks	No difference between mean ± SD Hb between groups (118 ± 15 vs. 121 ± 15 g/L, $p = 0.6$). No difference in ferritin or 25OHD between groups

Abbreviations: *25OHD* 25hydroxyvitamin D; *BMI* body mass index; *CI* confidence interval; *CRP* C-reactive protein; *Hb* hemoglobin; *ID* iron deficiency; *IDA* iron deficiency anemia; *IL-6* interleukin 6; *OR* odds ratio; *sTfR* soluble transferrin receptor; *TIBC* total iron binding capacity; *Vit D* Vitamin D

showed no effect of vitamin D on hemoglobin in two studies of patients with cardiovascular disease [34, 35]. One of these two studies included 172 participants with heart failure who received 100 μg/day vitamin D_3 or placebo for 3 years [34].

Iron Status and Inflammation Indices

Vitamin D lowered hepcidin in 2 of 5 studies reporting changes in hepcidin as an outcome. Plasma hepcidin was lower in healthy adults ($n = 28$) randomized to a single bolus of vitamin

D_3 (6250 μg/day) than placebo after 1 week [38]. In a small study, 30 critically ill ventilated subjects were randomized to 1250 μg/day, 2500 μg/day, or placebo for 1 week. After 4-weeks, patients receiving 2500 μg/day vitamin D_3 but not 1250 μg/day had lower hepcidin and higher hemoglobin than those receiving the placebo [39]. However, only four patients remained in the study after 4 weeks. Anemia is common in elite athletes, potentially due to exercise-induced inflammation, and vitamin D might improve hemoglobin by decreasing inflammation and lowering hepcidin. However, in a study of male marathon runners ($n = 20$) training for an ultramarathon, 250 μg/day vitamin D_3 for 2 weeks prerace did not reduce inflammatory cytokines or hepcidin concentrations compared to placebo post-race [36]. Braithwaite et al. [30] randomized pregnant women to 25 μg/day vitamin D_3 or placebo at ~14 weeks gestation. In late pregnancy, there was no difference between the two groups in hepcidin, ferritin, and inflammatory markers.

Overall, RCTs conducted to date do not support a role for vitamin D in improving hemoglobin. Most studies were small and underpowered and had heterogeneity in participant characteristics, vitamin D dose, duration of supplementation, and follow-up. Several RCTs were conducted against a low background rate of anemia and vitamin D deficiency. Given that observational studies suggest a 25OHD concentration above which no further increases are not associated with higher hemoglobin, an improvement in hemoglobin with vitamin D supplementation should not be expected. If vitamin D improves anemia by decreasing hepcidin, then an improvement in anemia would only be expected in those with anemia of inflammation. Careful consideration should be given to the design of future studies. Populations with a high background of inflammation and anemia and low 25OHD that are sufficiently powered are most likely to show an effect of vitamin D.

Conclusions

Vitamin D deficiency and anemia frequently coexist in populations. There is mechanistic evidence to support a role for vitamin D supplementation in anemia reduction, most likely through vitamin D's anti-inflammatory role as a regulator of the hepcidin-ferroportin axis. Most observational studies in children and adults show an association between 25OHD and hemoglobin. Still, the effect size is small and is modified by sex, ethnicity, and background rates of inflammation and anemia. RCT evidence does not support giving vitamin D to reduce anemia, but current trial evidence is insufficient.

Blanket iron supplementation is often recommended for women of reproductive age and children under five in low-resource countries where the background prevalence of anemia is high [43]. However, iron deficiency and inflammation often coexist [44]. Iron supplementation will not reduce anemia unless inflammation is reduced. Vitamin D supplementation may help reduce inflammation, thereby making more iron available for erythropoiesis, but more robust RCT evidence is required.

References

1. Amrein K, Scherkl M, Hoffmann M, Neuwersch-Sommeregger S, Köstenberger M, Tmava Berisha A, Martucci G, Pilz S, Malle O. Vitamin D deficiency 2.0: an update on the current status worldwide. Eur J Clin Nutr. 2020;74(11):1498–513.
2. McLean E, Cogswell M, Egli I, Wojdyla D, Benoist B. Worldwide prevalence of anaemia, WHO Vitamin and Mineral Nutrition Information System, 1993–2005. Public Health Nutr. 2008;12:444–54.
3. Azizi-Soleiman F, Vafa M, Abiri B, Safavi M. Effects of iron on vitamin D metabolism: a systematic review. Int J Prev Med. 2016;7:126.
4. Bacchetta J, Zaritsky JJ, Sea JL, Chun RF, Lisse TS, Zavala K, Nayak A, Wesseling-Perry K, Westerman M, Hollis BW, Salusky IB, Hewison M. Suppression of iron-regulatory hepcidin by vitamin D. J Am Soc Nephrol. 2014;25(3):564–72.

5. Vatanparast H, Calvo MS, Green TJ, Whiting SJ. Despite mandatory fortification of staple foods, vitamin D intakes of Canadian children and adults are inadequate. J Steroid Biochem Mol Biol. 2010;121(1–2):301–3.
6. Rockell JE, Skeaff CM, Williams SM, Green TJ. Association between quantitative measures of skin color and plasma 25-hydroxyvitamin D. Osteoporos Int. 2008;19(11):1639–42.
7. Holick MF, Vitamin D. Deficiency. N Engl J Med. 2007;357(3):266–81.
8. Dusso AS, Brown AJ, Slatopolsky E. Vitamin D. Am J Physiol Renal Physiol. 2005;289(1):F8–28.
9. Aucella F, Scalzulli RP, Gatta G, Vigilante M, Carella AM, Stallone C. Calcitriol increases burst-forming unit-erythroid proliferation in chronic renal failure. Nephron Clin Pract. 2003;95(4):c121–c7.
10. Alon DB, Chaimovitz C, Dvilansky A, Lugassy G, Douvdevani A, Shany S, Nathan I. Novel role of 1,25(OH)2D3 in induction of erythroid progenitor cell proliferation. Exp Hematol. 2002;30(5):403–9.
11. Tanaka M, Komaba H, Fukagawa M. Emerging association between parathyroid hormone and anemia in hemodialysis patients. Ther Apher Dial. 2018;22(3):242–5.
12. Madu AJ, Ughasoro MD. Anaemia of chronic disease: an in-depth review. Med Princ Pract. 2017;26(1):1–9.
13. Ganz T. Anemia of inflammation. N Engl J Med. 2019;381(12):1148–57.
14. Nemeth E, Rivera S, Gabayan V, Keller C, Taudorf S, Pedersen BK, Ganz T. IL-6 mediates hypoferremia of inflammation by inducing the synthesis of the iron regulatory hormone hepcidin. J Clin Invest. 2004;113(9):1271–6.
15. Zughaier SM, Alvarez JA, Sloan JH, Konrad RJ, Tangpricha V. The role of vitamin D in regulating the iron-hepcidin-ferroportin axis in monocytes. J Clin Transl Endocrinol. 2014;1(1):19–25.
16. DeLoughery TG. Microcytic anemia. N Engl J Med. 2014;371(14):1324–31.
17. Camaschella C, Nai A, Silvestri L. Iron metabolism and iron disorders revisited in the hepcidin era. Haematologica. 2020;105(2):260–72.
18. Atkinson MA, Melamed ML, Kumar J, Roy CN, Miller ER 3rd, Furth SL, Fadrowski JJ. Vitamin D, race, and risk for anemia in children. J Pediatr. 2014;164(1):153–8 e1.
19. Lee JA, Hwang JS, Hwang IT, Kim DH, Seo JH, Lim JS. Low vitamin D levels are associated with both iron deficiency and anemia in children and adolescents. Pediatr Hematol Oncol. 2015;32(2):99–108.
20. Nikooyeh B, Neyestani TR. Poor vitamin D status increases the risk of anemia in school children: National Food and Nutrition Surveillance. Nutrition. 2018;47:69–74.
21. Aloia JF, Chen DG, Chen H. The 25(OH)D/PTH threshold in black women. J Clin Endocrinol Metab. 2010;95(11):5069–73.
22. Thomas CE, Guillet R, Queenan RA, Cooper EM, Kent TR, Pressman EK, Vermeylen FM, Roberson MS, O'Brien KO. Vitamin D status is inversely associated with anemia and serum erythropoietin during pregnancy. Am J Clin Nutr. 2015;102(5):1088–95.
23. Han SS, Kim M, Kim H, Lee SM, Oh YJ, Lee JP, Kim S, Joo KW, Lim CS, Kim YS, Kim DK. Non-linear relationship between serum 25-hydroxyvitamin D and hemoglobin in Korean females: the Korean National Health and Nutrition Examination Survey 2010-2011. PLoS One. 2013;8(8):e72605.
24. Doudin A, Becker A, Rothenberger A, Meyer T. Relationship between serum 25-hydroxyvitamin D and red blood cell indices in German adolescents. Eur J Pediatr. 2018;177(4):583–91.
25. Takaoka N, Nishida K, Sairenchi T, Umesawa M, Noguchi R, Someya K, Kobashi G. Changes in vitamin D status considering hemodilution factors in Japanese pregnant women according to trimester: a longitudinal survey. PLoS One. 2020;15(10):e0239954.
26. Moran-Lev H, Weisman Y, Cohen S, Deutsch V, Cipok M, Bondar E, Lubetzky R, Mandel D. The interrelationship between hepcidin, vitamin D, and anemia in children with acute infectious disease. Pediatr Res. 2018;84(1):62–5.
27. Monlezun DJ, Camargo CA Jr, Mullen JT, Quraishi SA. Vitamin D status and the risk of anemia in community-dwelling adults: results from the National Health and Nutrition Examination Survey 2001-2006. Medicine (Baltimore). 2015;94(50):e1799.
28. Sim JJ, Lac PT, Liu IL, Meguerditchian SO, Kumar VA, Kujubu DA, Rasgon SA. Vitamin D deficiency and anemia: a cross-sectional study. Ann Hematol. 2010;89(5):447–52.
29. Smith EM, Alvarez JA, Martin GS, Zughaier SM, Ziegler TR, Tangpricha V. Vitamin D deficiency is associated with anaemia among African Americans in a US cohort. Br J Nutr. 2015;113(11):1732–40.
30. Braithwaite VS, Crozier SR, D'Angelo S, Prentice A, Cooper C, Harvey NC, Jones KS, Group MT. The effect of vitamin D supplementation on hepcidin, iron status, and inflammation in pregnant women in the United Kingdom. Nutrients. 2019;11(1).
31. Malczewska-Lenczowska J, Sitkowski D, Surala O, Orysiak J, Szczepanska B, Witek K. The association between iron and vitamin D status in female elite athletes. Nutrients. 2018;10(2).
32. De la Cruz-Góngora V, Salinas-Rodríguez A, Flores-Aldana M, Villalpando S. Etiology of anemia in older mexican adults: the role of hepcidin, vitamin A and vitamin D. Nutrients. 2021;13(11):3814.
33. Ahmad Fuzi SF, Mushtaq S. Vitamin D3 supplementation for 8 weeks leads to improved haematological status following the consumption of an iron-fortified breakfast cereal: a double-blind randomised controlled trial in iron-deficient women. Br J Nutr. 2019;121(10):1146–57.
34. Ernst JB, Prokop S, Fuchs U, Dreier J, Kuhn J, Knabbe C, Berthold HK, Pilz S, Gouni-Berthold I, Gummert JF, Börgermann J, Zittermann A. Randomized supplementation of 4000 IU vitamin D(3) daily vs placebo on the prevalence of anemia in advanced heart failure: the EVITA trial. Nutr J. 2017;16(1):49.

35. Ernst JB, Tomaschitz A, Grübler MR, Gaksch M, Kienreich K, Verheyen N, März W, Pilz S, Zittermann A. Vitamin D supplementation and hemoglobin levels in hypertensive patients: a randomized controlled trial. Int J Endocrinol. 2016;2016:6836402.
36. Kasprowicz K, Ratkowski W, Wolyniec W, Kaczmarczyk M, Witek K, Zmijewski P, Renke M, Jastrzebski Z, Rosemann T, Nikolaidis PT, Knechtle B. The effect of vitamin D3 supplementation on hepcidin, iron, and IL-6 responses after a 100 km ultra-marathon. Int J Environ Res Public Health. 2020;17(8).
37. Madar AA, Stene LC, Meyer HE, Brekke M, Lagerlov P, Knutsen KV. Effect of vitamin D3 supplementation on iron status: a randomized, double-blind, placebo-controlled trial among ethnic minorities living in Norway. Nutr J. 2016;15(1):74.
38. Smith EM, Alvarez JA, Kearns MD, Hao L, Sloan JH, Konrad RJ, Ziegler TR, Zughaier SM, Tangpricha V. High-dose vitamin D3 reduces circulating hepcidin concentrations: a pilot, randomized, double-blind, placebo-controlled trial in healthy adults. Clin Nutr. 2017;36(4):980–5.
39. Smith EM, Jones JL, Han JE, Alvarez JA, Sloan JH, Konrad RJ, Zughaier SM, Martin GS, Ziegler TR, Tangpricha V. High-dose vitamin D3 administration is associated with increases in hemoglobin concentrations in mechanically ventilated critically Ill adults: a pilot double-blind, randomized, placebo-controlled trial. JPEN J Parenter Enteral Nutr. 2018;42(1):87–94.
40. Sooragonda B, Bhadada SK, Shah VN, Malhotra P, Ahluwalia J, Sachdeva N. Effect of vitamin D replacement on hemoglobin concentration in subjects with concurrent iron-deficiency anemia and vitamin D deficiency: a randomized, single-blinded, placebo-controlled trial. Acta Haematol. 2015;133(1):31–5.
41. Panwar B, McCann D, Olbina G, Westerman M, Gutierrez OM. Effect of calcitriol on serum hepcidin in individuals with chronic kidney disease: a randomized controlled trial. BMC Nephrol. 2018;19(1):35.
42. Eloqayli H, Al-Yousef A, Jaradat R. Vitamin D and ferritin correlation with chronic neck pain using standard statistics and a novel artificial neural network prediction model. Br J Neurosurg. 2018;32(2):172–6.
43. Samson KLI, Loh SP, Lee SS, Sulistyoningrum DC, Khor GL, Shariff ZBM, Ismai IZ, Yelland LN, Leemaqz S, Makrides M, Hutcheon JA, Roche ML, Karakochuk CD, Green TJ. Weekly iron–folic acid supplements containing 2.8 mg folic acid are associated with a lower risk of neural tube defects than the current practice of 0.4 mg: a randomised controlled trial in Malaysia. BMJ Glob Health. 2020;5(12):e003897.
44. Harvey-Leeson S, Karakochuk CD, Hawes M, Tugirimana PL, Bahizire E, Akilimali PZ, Michaux KD, Lynd LD, Whitfield KC, Moursi M, Boy E, Foley J, McLean J, Houghton LA, Gibson RS, Green TJ. Anemia and micronutrient status of women of childbearing age and children 6–59 months in the Democratic Republic of the Congo. Nutrients. 2016;8(2):98.

Oxidative Stress and Vitamin E in Anemia

16

Maret G. Traber and Afaf Kamal-Eldin

Abbreviations

AVED	Ataxia with isolated vitamin E deficiency
Hb	Hemoglobin
HIV/AIDS	Human immunodeficiency virus/acquired immunodeficiency syndrome
met-Hb	Met-hemoglobin
NAD(P)H	Reducing equivalents
O_2	Oxygen
PEM	Protein energy malnutrition
R	Carbon centered radical
RBC	Red blood cell/erythrocyte
ROO	Peroxyl radical
ROOH	Lipid hydroperoxides
ROS	Reactive oxygen species
α-TO·	α-Tocopheroxyl radical
α-TOH	α-tocopherol
α-TTP	α-tocopherol transfer protein

M. G. Traber (✉)
Linus Pauling Institute and College of Health and Human Sciences, Oregon State University, Corvallis, OR, USA
e-mail: maret.traber@oregonstate.edu

A. Kamal-Eldin
Department of Food Science, United Arab Emirates University, AlAin, UAE

Introduction

Anemia is characterized by a low number of healthy circulating erythrocytes/red blood cells (RBCs) due to inadequate production or excessive destruction. Anemia can result from nutritional deficiencies (e.g., iron deficiency, vitamin B12 deficiency, and vitamin E deficiency), inherited disorders (hemolytic anemia), and/or from infections or exposure to certain toxins and medications (aplastic anemia). Hemolytic anemia, prevalent in inherited diseases such as sickle cell anemia, thalassemia, glucose-6-phosphate dehydrogenase (EC 1.1.1.49) deficiency, and superoxide dismutase-2 (EC 1.15.1.1) deficiency, occur due to destruction of premature or defective RBCs. **Aplastic anemia** occurs when the bone marrow capacity to produce RBCs is compromised due to viral infections and/or exposure to toxic chemicals, radiation, or medications (such as antibiotics, antiseizure drugs, and some cancer treatments). Anemia can lead to a variety of health problems, since the oxygen required by the body is carried by RBCs and because oxidative stress can be generated by the iron released from damaged RBCs. Oxidative distress, caused by overproduction of reactive oxygen species (ROS) and impaired antioxidant potential, is associated with anemia. Several enzymatic and nonenzymatic components, including vitamin E, are protective against oxidative stress.

C. D. Karakochuk et al. (eds.), *Nutritional Anemia*, Nutrition and Health,
https://doi.org/10.1007/978-3-031-14521-6_16

Oxidative Distress and Anemia

Oxidative Distress Definition, Free Radicals, and Reactive Oxygen Species

The term oxidative distress denotes *a disturbance in the prooxidant-antioxidant balance in favor of the former*. ROS include several free radical and nonradical molecular species generated during normal oxygen metabolism leading to damage in "oxidative distress" [1]. Examples of ROS include triplet oxygen (·↑O=O↑·), singlet oxygen (·↑O=O↓·), hydrogen peroxide (H_2O_2), and superoxide anion (O_2·–) and hydroxyl (HO·) radicals (Fig. 16.1). Transition metal ions, such as iron and/or copper, can act as catalysts, generating radicals from lipid hydroperoxides, for example, via the Fenton reaction. Free radicals and ROS react and cause damage and dysfunction of lipids, proteins, and DNA nucleotides. Lipid peroxidation is especially dangerous as it creates more radicals, causes a chain reaction, damages numerous polyunsaturated fatty acids, and generates toxic aldehydes.

Oxidative Distress and Destruction of Erythrocytes

RBCs are particularly prone to oxidative damage, and related complications, because of their high concentrations of polyunsaturated fatty acids, iron, and oxygen. ROS cause the oxidation of RBCs membrane lipids leading to their deformation and destruction, but α-tocopherol is the vitamin E enriched in these membranes. During the binding of oxygen to hemoglobin (Hb) iron to form oxy-hemoglobin, an electron is transferred from iron to the bound oxygen and a ferric-superoxide anion complex is formed [2]. If this electron is not returned to iron during deoxygenation, the oxygen will transform to a superoxide anion radical (O_2·–) and Hb will adopt a met-hemoglobin status (met-Hb):

$$\text{Hb}\left(\text{Fe}^{2+}\right)\text{O}_2 \rightarrow \text{met-Hb}\left(\text{Fe}^{3+}\right)+\text{O}_2\cdot-$$

This reaction affects 0.5–3% of Hb daily and is followed by dismutation of the O_2·– to H_2O_2, which may react with met-Hb to form a hypervalent ferryl-Hb radical that is able to initiate lipid oxidation:

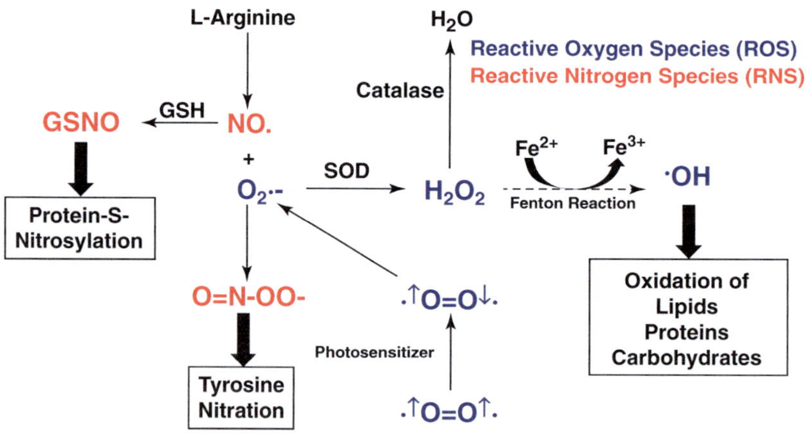

Fig. 16.1 Reactive oxygen species (ROS) and reactive nitrogen species (RNO) and their oxidative damage to lipids, proteins, and carbohydrates. ROS can be formed from singlet oxygen (·↑O=O↓·) and RNS from the oxidation of L-arginine. The antioxidant enzymes, superoxide dismutase (SOD) and catalase, neutralize the superoxide anion radical (O_2·–) and hydrogen peroxide (H_2O_2), respectively. In the presence of iron and other transition metal ions, hydrogen peroxide is split into very reactive hydroxyl radicals (HO·) that react instantaneously with lipids, proteins, and carbohydrates

$$\text{met-Hb}\left(\text{Fe}^{3+}\right) + \text{H}_2\text{O}_2 \rightarrow \text{Hb.}-\left(\text{Fe}^{4+}\right) = \text{O} + \text{H}_2\text{O}$$

met-Hb is also produced by the attack of Hb by other oxidants including H_2O_2, NO·, and ·OH. Several antioxidant systems exist in the RBC to protect them against oxidation [3]:

- Antioxidant molecules, namely, glutathione, ascorbic acid (vitamin C), and α-tocopherol (vitamin E).
- Sources of the redox equivalents NADH and NADPH, that is, the pentose phosphate cycle and glucose-6-phosphate dehydrogenase.
- Antioxidant enzymes including superoxide dismutase, catalase (EC 1.11.1.6), glutathione peroxidase (EC 1.11.1.9), and peroxiredoxins (EC 1.11. 1.15).

If the antioxidant machinery fails to combat the ROS generation, production of met-Hb and its participation in further oxidation reactions will lead to oxidative distress. The disruption of membrane phospholipids enhances the exposure of phosphatidylserine on the outer cell surface [4], enabling its engulfment by macrophages having phosphatidyl serine-specific receptors, which will lead to RBC destruction. During these processes, met-Hb undergoes slow denaturation generating hemichromes that form tight associations with the cytoplasmic domain of the major erythrocyte membrane protein. This process results in oxidation and clusterization and finally the triggering of phagocytosis-mediated erythrocyte removal [2]. Importantly, increased RBC's α-tocopherol concentrations decrease phosphatidyl serine externalization and their procoagulability [5].

Vitamin E Antioxidant Activity

Vitamin E Definitions

Vitamin E is the collective name for plant-synthesized molecules having a chromanol head and a phytyl tail (tocopherols) or an isoprenoid tail (tocotrienols), all scavenging peroxyl radicals and exhibiting the antioxidant activity of α-tocopherol [6]. Eight molecules (α-, β-, γ-, and δ-tocopherols and α-, β-, γ-, and δ-tocotrienols) vary in the number of methyl groups on the chromanol ring (Fig. 16.2). Unlike most other vitamins, chemically synthesized α-tocopherol is not identical to the natural form synthesized by plants, that is, *RRR*-α-tocopherol (on labels: d-α-tocopherol), is only one of the eight stereoisomers present in synthetic *all-rac*-α-tocopherol. The Food and Nutrition Board [7] defined vitamin E for human requirements as only 2*R*-α-tocopherol; thus, only half of the stereoisomers in *all-rac*-α-tocopherol meet the vitamin E requirement. With regard to human nutrition, natural α-tocopherol (*RRR* or *d* form) is provided by

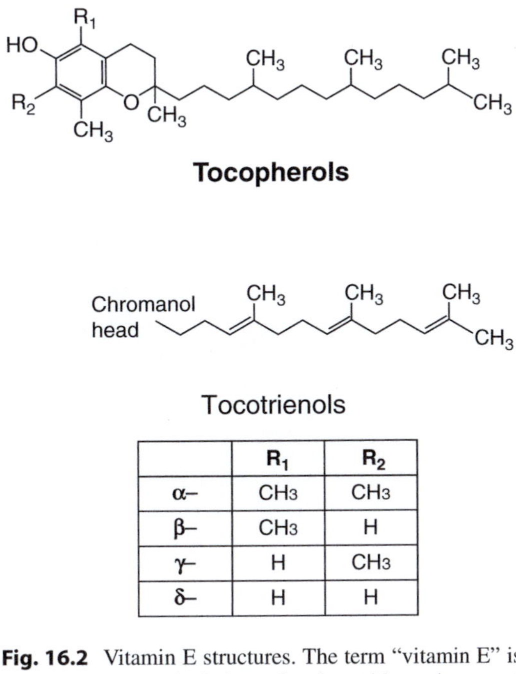

	R_1	R_2
α–	CH_3	CH_3
β–	CH_3	H
γ–	H	CH_3
δ–	H	H

Fig. 16.2 Vitamin E structures. The term "vitamin E" is usually meant to include molecules with a chromanol head and a phytyl tail (tocopherols) or an isoprenoid tail (tocotrienols). Eight molecules form the family (α-, β-, γ-, and δ-tocopherols and α-, β-, γ-, and δ-tocotrienols) based on the number of methyl groups on the chromanol ring, as indicated

foods or supplements, while *all-rac*-α-tocopherol (or *d,l*-α-tocopherol) is obtained by food fortification or supplementation.

Antioxidant Functions

Vitamin E, particularly α-tocopherol, functions in vivo as a lipid-soluble peroxyl radical scavenger and chain-breaking antioxidant [8]. α-Tocopherol (TOH) reacts with peroxyl radicals (ROO·) 1000-times faster than polyunsaturated fatty acids (RH) and, thus, protects these acids from auto-oxidation. The phenolic group of the chromanol ring reacts with the ROO· to form corresponding hydroperoxides and the vitamin E radical (TO·):

$$\text{In the presence of vitamin E: } ROO\cdot + TOH \rightarrow ROOH + TO\cdot$$

$$\text{In the absence of vitamin E: } ROO\cdot + RH \rightarrow ROOH + R\cdot$$

$$R\cdot + O_2 \rightarrow ROO\cdot$$

TO· Is recycled back to tocopherol with ascorbate (vitamin C), thiols especially glutathione, or other reductants serving as hydrogen donors (AH) [9].

$$TO\cdot + AH \rightarrow TOH + A\cdot$$

The regeneration of tocopherol from the tocopheroxyl radical in the RBC membrane (Fig. 16.3) is especially relevant to the discussion of oxidative distress, causing RBC destruction and ultimately anemia. A number of antioxidant enzymes, including superoxide dismutase, glutathione peroxidase, and catalase, are also involved in the protection of RBCs against oxidative stress and the sparing of vitamin E [10].

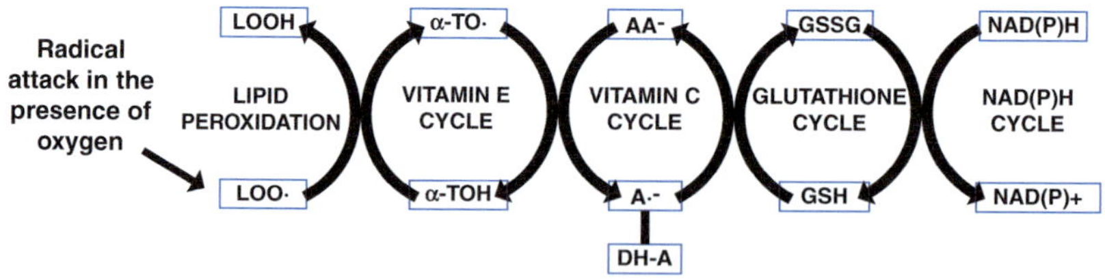

Fig. 16.3 Vitamin E, antioxidant network, and membrane lipid oxidation. As part of the antioxidant network, α-tocopherol (α-TOH) forms a tocopheroxyl radical (α-TO·) when it intercepts a peroxyl radical (LOO·) in a cell membrane. In the absence of vitamin E, these LOO· can abstract a hydrogen from polyunsaturated fatty acids (LH) and generate both a hydroperoxide (LOOH) and another carbon centered radical (L·), which in the presence of oxygen (O_2) will form an LOO· and thus a lipid peroxidation chain reaction occurs. If α-TOH is present, it intercepts the radical 1000 times faster than the radical reacts with polyunsaturated fatty acids, and both an ROOH and an α-TO· are formed. This α-TO· radical can be detoxified and α-TOH regenerated by intracellular antioxidants including vitamin C, glutathione, and reducing equivalents (NAD(P)H) derived from oxidative metabolism

Vitamin E Deficiency Symptoms in Humans

Low serum or plasma vitamin E concentrations are indicative of vitamin E deficiency. The Food and Nutrition Board of the US Institute of Medicine [7] defined the lower limit of plasma α-tocopherol at 12 μmol/L for normal, healthy, adult humans. However, measurements of plasma α-tocopherol levels alone may be insufficient for patients with cholestatic liver disease. These patients have elevated serum lipids and α-tocopherol concentrations in the apparently "normal" range, but these may not be sufficient to protect tissues due to abnormal lipoprotein metabolism [11]. Calculation of effective plasma vitamin E concentrations needs to take into account these high lipid (sum of plasma total cholesterol and triglyceride) levels. Patients with cholestatic liver disease, characterized by extraordinarily high lipid levels, also had neurologic symptoms related to vitamin E deficiency while plasma α-tocopherol concentrations were in the normal range [11]. There is a controversy with respect to the adequacy of α-tocopherol/lipids; if circulating lipid levels are low, there is insufficient lipoprotein carrier for vitamin E. In this case, the absolute plasma α-tocopherol concentrations may be a more reliable biomarker of vitamin E status than their lipid ratio. Certainly, it is worthwhile to present both forms of the data.

Tocopherol levels in RBCs are generally lower than those observed in plasma. For example, plasma α- and γ-tocopherol concentrations in healthy Japanese university students (n = 12) were 19.6 and 0.12 μmol/L compared with 2.2 and 0.02 μmol/L in packed RBC, respectively [12]. Kinetic studies have shown that newly absorbed α-tocopherol is enriched in the RBC with a maximum occurring in less than 24 h after dosing compared to about 12 h in plasma [13].

A major vitamin E deficiency symptom in humans was described as a peripheral neuropathy characterized by the degeneration of the large caliber axons in the sensory neurons of persons with fat malabsorption syndromes [14]. This neurodegeneration is apparently the cause of the ataxia with vitamin E deficiency (AVED), [15] which results from α-tocopherol transfer protein (α-TTP) genetic defects [16]. In α-tocopherol deficiency, anemia occurs as a result of free radical damage to erythrocyte membranes [17]. Similarly, peripheral neuropathy is likely due to α-tocopherol depletion and subsequent free radical damage to the nerves [18].

Underconsumption of fruits and vegetables, evaluated in 702 school children (4–10 years) in the western Brazilian Amazon, was found in 5% of the children, along with 9% vitamin E deficiency and incidences of 6.3% anemia and 33% multiple nutritional deficiencies. Anemia is not the only consequence of vitamin E deficiency. Chronic underconsumption of vitamin E will lead to overt vitamin E deficiency symptoms if the α-tocopherol levels in target tissues (e.g., peripheral nerves) are depleted [18]. Thus, children historically have been the susceptible population in which vitamin E deficiency has been observed, for example, one quarter of the newborns in the tropical region of northeastern Brazil are vitamin E deficient [19]. In Algeria, both small for gestational age and large birth weight newborns have increased oxidative stress and low vitamin C and E concentrations compared with average weight newborns [20]. There is an increasing appreciation of oxidative distress in the newborn [21] but no clear approaches to improve their antioxidant status. As shown in basic science studies using a zebrafish embryo model, vitamin E and α-TTP are critical for brain development [22, 23]. Moreover, inadequate vitamin E availability during this critical developmental window results in long-term cognitive deficits [24]. It is unclear if the same is true for human embryos and if low vitamin E status causes increased anemia. Importantly, a micronutrient-enriched spread (with 143% the vitamin E DRI), not one lacking micronutrients, was shown to reverse anemia and stunting in Saharawi refugee children (n = 374) aged 3–5 years [25]. These findings emphasize that a combination of micronutrients, not just vitamin A and iron, may be necessary to reduce anemia.

Vitamin E Deficiency Syndromes

In addition to genetic defects in α-TTP [15], vitamin E deficiency can occur secondary to fat malabsorption, because intestinal vitamin E absorption requires biliary and pancreatic secretions. Failure of micellar solubilization and malabsorption of dietary lipids leads to vitamin E deficiency in children with chronic cholestatic hepatobiliary disorders, including disease of the liver and anomalies of intrahepatic and extrahepatic bile ducts [14]. Children with cystic fibrosis can also become vitamin E deficient, because the impaired secretion of pancreatic digestive enzymes causes steatorrhea and vitamin E malabsorption, even when pancreatic enzyme supplements are administered orally [14]. It should be emphasized that any disorder that causes chronic fat malabsorption can lead to vitamin E deficiency. Thus, generally poor intake of nutrients in combination with chronic diarrhea in children could lead to vitamin E deficiency, if the fat malabsorption is sufficiently severe and the child has low α-tocopherol body stores.

Vitamin E Deficiency Caused by Defects in Lipoprotein Synthesis

Vitamin E deficiency is also caused by genetic defects in lipoprotein synthesis that result in fat malabsorption. Studies of patients with hypobetalipoproteinemia or abetalipoproteinemia (low to nondetectable circulating chylomicrons, very low-density lipoprotein, or low-density lipoprotein) have demonstrated that lipoproteins containing apolipoprotein B are necessary for effective absorption and plasma transport of lipids, especially vitamin E [26]. Clinical features include retarded growth, acanthocytosis, retinitis pigmentosa, and a chronic progressive neurological disorder with ataxia. The acanthocytosis is a spicule shape to the erythrocytes, likely due to abnormal cholesterol distribution in the membrane. Nonetheless, it is important to note that this disorder, which is associated with poor vitamin E status, is also associated with abnormalities in erythrocyte function. Clinically, persons with hypobetalipoproteinemia or abetalipoproteinemia can become vitamin E deficient and develop a characteristic neurologic syndrome, a progressive peripheral neuropathy, if they are not given large vitamin E supplements (approximately 10 g/day) [26]. Despite low plasma concentrations, adipose tissue α-tocopherol concentrations reach normal levels in patients given large (10 g/day) vitamin E doses [27].

Vitamin E Malnourishment

Vitamin E status in humans is compromised during anemia as a result of the oxidative distress caused by RBC hemolysis. Antioxidant molecules and enzymes, mentioned above, critically maintain the redox balance in the erythrocytes that contain high hemoglobin-bound iron concentrations. Anemia, especially during release of free iron in hemolytic anemia, increases the oxidative stress and iron toxicity [28].

Protein Energy Malnutrition (PEM)

Vitamin E deficiency symptoms were reported in children with severely limited food intake, which limits the vitamin E available for absorption, as well as the amino acids required to synthesize the hepatic α-TTP necessary for regulation of plasma α-tocopherol (Table 16.1). PEM patients, having low plasma α-tocopherol concentrations and low α-tocopherol/lipid ratios, had neurologic abnormalities characteristic of vitamin E deficiency [29]. Remarkably, 92% of the children with neurologic abnormalities had plasma α-tocopherol concentrations of 8 μmol/L or less, a value observed in many children with PEM [30]. In a follow-up study with 6 weeks of vitamin E supplementation, the subjects' circulating α-tocopherol levels were normalized and their neurologic abnormalities were improved [31].

The degree to which vitamin E deficiency is associated with kwashiorkor and/or marasmus is not clear, because evaluation of vitamin E status in malnourished children is difficult. Although plasma triglycerides are sometimes increased and

Table 16.1 Plasma α-tocopherol in children with protein energy malnutrition (PEM, e.g., kwashiorkor or marasmus)

Country (median, mean, or range, error)	Age, *n*	Status	α-tocopherol (μmol/L)	α-tocopherol/lipids (units)	Ref.
India	3–8 years, *n* = 50	Control	9.5 ± 2.1	0.72 ± 0.12 mg/g	[29]
(mean ± SD)	3–8 years, *n* = 100	PEM	6.0 ± 2.6	0.47 ± 0.14 mg/g	[29]
Nigeria	22 months, *n* = 18	Control	7.4	0.70 mg/g	[85]
(median)	24 months, *n* = 12	Kwashiorkor	3.8	0.48 mg/g	[85]
	14 months, *n* = 8	Severe marasmus	6.9	0.70 mg/g	[85]
	17 months, *n* = 15	Marasmus	5.3	0.66 mg/g	[85]
Nigeria (mean ± SD)	24 months, 1–4 years, *n* = 10	Control	17.4 ± 4.0	1.8 ± 0.4 mg/g	[86]
	15 months, 1–4 years, *n* = 26	Marasmus	8.8 ± 0.5	1.0 ± 0.2 mg/g	[86]
	28 months, 1–4 years, *n* = 11	Marasmic-kwashiorkor	7.9 ± 1.0	0.8 ± 0.2 mg/g	[86]
	36 months, 1–4 years, *n* = 10	Kwashiorkor	10.7 ± 3.4	1.2 ± 0.4 mg/g	[86]
Kenya	3.4 ± 1.3 years, *n* = 39	Control	11.6 ± 4.2	1.6 ± 0.3 mmol/mol	[87]
(mean ± SD)	3.1 ± 1.5 years, *n* = 30	Kwashiorkor	4.6 ± 4.2	1.1 ± 0.7 mmol/mol	[87]
	2.5 ± 1.1 years, *n* = 16	Marasmus	9.3 ± 4.2	1.4 ± 0.8 mmol/mol	[87]
Sudan	21 months, *n* = 14	Marasmus	9.4 (5.0–17.7)	1.0 (0.5–1.7) mg/g	[88]
(median, range)	24 months, *n* = 11	Marasmic-kwashiorkor	8.5 (1.6–9.9)	0.86 (0.2–1.3) mg/g	[88]
	24 months, *n* = 5	Kwashiorkor	9.1 (4.9–26.5)	0.87 (0.4–3.0) mg/g	[88]
Egypt (mean ± SE)	13 ± 2 months, *n* = 22	Control	16.5 ± 0.8	–	[89]
	13 ± 2 months, *n* = 26	Kwashiorkor	11.6 ± 0.7	–	[89]
	12 ± 1 months, *n* = 20	Marasmus	11.5 ± 1	–	[89]

sometimes not, children with kwashiorkor uniformly appear to have low plasma cholesterol concentrations [32]. Moreover, elevated circulating triglycerides and fatty liver of PEM appear to be a result of dysregulation of lipid metabolism [32]. Protein depletion in PEM can be so severe that there is insufficient protein for synthesis of lipolytic enzymes to digest fat, which complicates evaluation of vitamin E nutrition. The transport and delivery of vitamin E is critically dependent on the hepatic secretion of lipoproteins and their uptake by peripheral tissues. Indeed, if α-tocopherol is trapped in triglyceride-rich lipoproteins that cannot be effectively catabolized, then the α-tocopherol is not available to the target tissues and oxidative distress can ensue. Indeed, lipid peroxidation can lead to further damage and a damaging chain reaction can occur in membranes, such as RBCs.

Iron Deficiency Anemia

Inadequate nutrition is also associated with iron deficiency anemia. This disorder is associated with decreased production of hemoglobin (Hb) and other iron-containing proteins such as myoglobin, catalase, peroxidase, and cytochromes. The RBC membranes, with their high polyunsaturated fatty acid concentrations, are also more susceptible to oxidative damage during iron deficiency anemia [33]. Studies in Nigeria have shown that RBCs from school children with iron deficiency anemia have increased lipid peroxidation and decreased antioxidant enzyme capacity [34].

Iron supplementation to iron-deficient individuals was found to increase the oxidative stress [i.e., increased malondialdehyde (MDA) levels and compromised antioxidant enzyme activities] [35]. Indeed, high levels of free iron may enhance radical production via the Fenton and Haber-Weiss reactions. Importantly, treatment of iron-deficient patients with a combination of iron and vitamins A, C, and E proved effective in normalizing the oxidative distress [35].

Oxidative Distress in Anemia Caused by Inherited and Transmitted Diseases

Thalassemia and Sickle Cell Anemia

Thalassemia and sickle cell diseases are inherited blood Hb disorders that cause anemia with wide variability according to the heterogeneity of the disease [36]. The mild to severe anemia associated with the different types of thalassemia results from oxidative distress that damages erythrocyte membranes resulting in decreased deformability and hemolysis, as well as to increased recognition and removal by immune cells [37]. These erythrocytes contain a lower ratio of unsaturated-to-saturated fatty acids, a 50% decrease in titratable-thiol groups, as well as decreased plasma concentrations of vitamins A, C, E and carotenoids. Compared with healthy controls, α-thalassemic patients had lower ($P < 0.001$) plasma vitamin C (13.2 ± 1.2 vs. 6.7 ± 1.4 μg/mL), vitamin E (7.8 ± 0.5 vs. 6.6 ± 0.2 μg/mL), and vitamin A concentrations (76 ± 5 vs 56 ± 4 μg/dL) [37]. The mechanisms responsible for increased oxidative distress in thalassemia and sickle cell anemia have been partially explored [38]. Patients with thalassemia had significantly decreased NADPH/NADP ratios, catalase activities, and glutathione concentrations similar to the case of severe glucose-6-phosphate dehydrogenase-deficiency anemia [39]. RBC vitamin E in α-thalassemic patients was lower than in controls (56 vs. 67 μg/dL, respectively). Increased protein oxidation in both Eβ- and β-thalassemic patients leads to protein degradation as reflected by increased tyrosine release [40]. Thalassemia is also characterized by decreased catalase, glutathione peroxidase, and glutathione reductase and elevated superoxide dismutase activities that were all normalized by vitamin E treatment [40].

Patients with sickle cell anemia are more prone to oxidative stress, because (i) Hb S oxidizes at a higher rate than Hb A and Hb F, (ii) the activity of xanthine oxidase activity in their aortic endothelium is increased, and (iii) they have higher number of leucocytes that produce higher fluxes of superoxide than healthy individuals [41]. Increased production of ROS leads to inflammation, endothelial dysfunction, and erythrocyte adhesion to blood vessel walls. Thus, sickle cell disease is a chronic inflammatory disease characterized by elevated levels of tumor necrosis factor-α and interleukin-6. Sickle cell RBCs are unstable and produce large amounts of ROS as a result of Hb deoxygenation and subsequent RBC rupture. Compared with healthy controls, individuals with sickle cell disease may have higher levels of homocysteine, which also contributes to oxidative stress. As a result, low levels of antioxidant vitamins C and E and carotenoids have been reported in sickle cell disease. Notably, patients with sickle cell anemia [42] and β-thalassemia [43] have lower serum lipids than healthy controls. Nonetheless, low plasma vitamin E levels are highlighted here, because vitamin E supplements appear to counteract the sickling process [44]. However, in a more recent study, plasma vitamins E and C increased with supplementation, but anemia did not decrease [45]. Vitamin E supplementation raises plasma α-tocopherol concentrations, but the extent of the increase is largely dependent upon the starting vitamin E status (Table 16.2). In one study, supplementation of sickle cell anemic children with vitamin E was shown to reduce sickled erythrocytes, to increase their resistance to lysis, and to enhance Hb concentration [46]. If the subject is severely nutritionally compromised, then vitamin

Table 16.2 Plasma α-tocopherol concentrations in children and adults with thalassemia and sickle cell disease

Country (mean, range, error)	Age, n	Status	α-tocopherol (μmol/L)	Ref.
India	$n = 6$	Normal	4.0 ± 0.4	[40]
(mean ± SE)	$n = 9$	Eβ-thalassemia	2.7 ± 0.4	[40]
		4 week vitamin E supplementation	5.1 ± 0.4	[40]
	$n = 8$	β-thalassemia	2.9 ± 1.5	[40]
		4 week vitamin E supplementation	2.9 ± 1.4	[40]
Egypt	9 ± 4 years, 2–18 years, $n = 63$	Control	14.0 ± 3.8	[90]
(mean ± SD)	9 ± 5 years, 2–18 years, $n = 64$	Thalassemia	11.9 ± 3.3	[90]
Saudi Arabia (mean ± SD)	30 ± 13 years, $n = 25$	Severe sickle cell anemia	4.7 ± 1.7	[91]
	29 ± 8 years, $n = 25$	Control	10.0 ± 2.3	[91]
Nigeria (mean ± SE)	23 ± 1 years, $n = 10$	Sickle cell anemia	4.0 ± 0.2	[92]
Netherlands (mean ± SD)	9 ± 5 years, $n = 13$	Sickle cell disease, baseline	13.9 ± 4.8	[93]
		8 month supplementation 1 (460 mg α-tocopherol + others),	23.1 ± 8.5	[93]
		Followed by 7 month supplementation 2 (400 mg mixed α-tocopherol + others)	25.7 ± 7.4	[93]

E supplementation may have to be accompanied by a strong dietary program to achieve the optimal outcome [47].

Thalassemia and sickle cell disease are treated in some cases by blood transfusion, which leads to iron overload and to oxidative distress *inter alia* in RBC [48]. A study from Thailand showed that 20 children with β-thalassemia major who received packed red cells blood transfusions without iron chelation therapy had low vitamin C and vitamin E levels and high oxidative stress [49]. They recommended supplementation of β-thalassemia patients with both nutrients [49].

Glucose-6-Phosphate Dehydrogenase Deficiency

Glucose-6-phosphate dehydrogenase, the enzyme that catalyzes the rate-limiting step in the hexose monophosphate pathway, is an important enzyme for RBC functionality. Glucose-6-phosphate dehydrogenase deficiency is an inherited defect, with a great variability, that affects about 400 million people worldwide, mainly in tropical areas [50]. Glucose-6-phosphate dehydrogenase is associated with oxidative stress because of its involvement in the production of NAD(P)H, which is important for maintaining adequate redox levels of glutathione and other sulfhydryl groups (Fig. 16.4). Glucose-6-phosphate dehydrogenase deficiency leads to Hb oxidation to methemoglobin, Heinz body formation, membrane damage, and anemia due to increased removal of damaged erythrocytes from the circulation. Vitamin E administration restored the inactivation of glucose-6-phosphate dehydrogenase activity due to nicotine administration in various rat tissues in vivo and in vitro [51]. In glucose-6-phosphate dehydrogenase–deficient subjects with a history of hemolysis, a 16-week course of oral vitamin E therapy (800 IU/day) increased plasma vitamin E concentrations, improved blood Hb levels, and decreased reticulocytosis and hemolysis [52].

Superoxide Dismutase-2 Deficiency

Genetic superoxide dismutase-2 deficiency causes a persistent hematopoietic anemia similar to morphologic sideroblastic anemia and is pri-

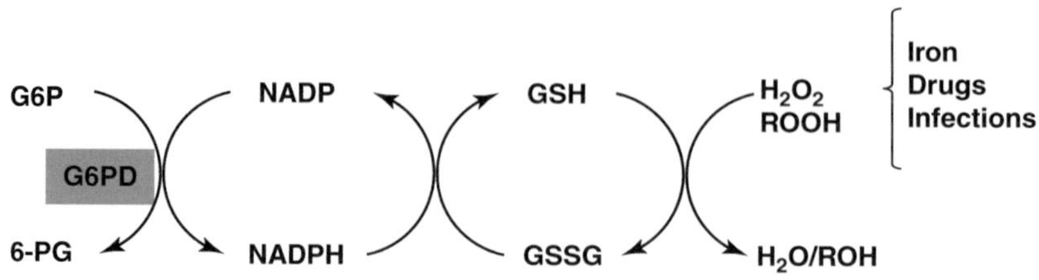

Fig. 16.4 Role of glucose-6-phosphate dehydrogenase in oxidative stress. Glucose-6-phosphate dehydrogenase (G6PD) regenerates NAD(P)H using glutathione (GSH) and therefore is important in the deactivation of reactive oxygen species such as hydrogen peroxide (H_2O_2) and other hydroperoxides (ROOH)

marily manifested in reticulocytes and in immature erythrocytes. Superoxide dismutase-2 deficiency leads to severe mitochondrial dysfunction characterized by impaired activity of the oxidation-sensitive iron-sulfur cluster enzyme complexes I and II and the tricarboxylic acid cycle enzyme, aconitase [53]. Superoxide dismutase-2–deficient erythrocytes contain high levels of a number of chaperone-like proteins involved *inter alia* in redox regulation and adenosine triphosphate (ATP) synthesis. Superoxide dismutase/catalase antioxidant therapy led to extended erythrocyte lifespan [54]. Vitamin E supplementation was found to counteract superoxide dismutase deficiency and improve the Hb levels [55].

Malaria

Malaria is a common disease in the tropics, annually accounting for 500 million episodes and about 2.7 million deaths [56]. In 50 children with severe and 50 with mild malaria along with 50 age- and sex-matched control subjects, the concentrations of glutathione, α-tocopherol, retinol, and carotenoid were lower in the patients than in the controls ($P < 0.001$) [57]. Malaria alone was reported to exert greater influence on plasma antioxidants than does malnutrition [58]. Although plasma α-tocopherol concentrations may not change, erythrocyte concentrations are markedly depleted during malarial episodes [59]. Similarly, plasma ascorbic acid levels were lower in children infected with malaria compared with healthy children [60].

According to Sherman et al. [61], the human malaria parasite, *P. falciparum*, causes the erythrocyte to age. The malaria-infected cell is osmotically fragile and more permeable to a wide variety of molecules. There are declines in sialic acid, reduced glutathione, α-tocopherol, and ATP levels. Interestingly, α-tocopherol may have a critical role in regulating cell responses by regulating the externalization of phosphatidyl serine, a key step in the initiation of apoptosis [5]. Although ascorbic acid or α-tocopherol do not inhibit *P. falciparum* growth in vitro [62], they can reduce malaria-associated endothelial damage by neutrophil secretory products [63]. Paradoxically, malaria resistance in mice is increased with vitamin E deficiency [64], while the opposite appears to occur in people. In humans, antioxidant status decreases with increased disease severity and the decrease in plasma α-tocopherol declines with recovery from disease [65, 66]. A potential explanation for the decline in plasma α-tocopherol observed in many studies during malarial episodes arises from studies by Guha et al. [67] who found that malarial infection induces hepatic apoptosis through augmentation of oxidative stress. Importantly, the hepatic dysfunction will further cause diminution of the secretion of α-tocopherol from the liver [68], causing further limitations in plasma and tissue antioxidant defenses with increasing severity of the disease [69, 70].

Interestingly, antimalarial drugs function by forming complexes with free heme; these complexes disturb the redox equilibrium and can kill the parasite [71]. Moreover, chloroquine treatment does not only increase the oxidative stress but also diminishes the antioxidant enzymes [72]. The parasite reacts by producing extra glutathione to counter the oxidative stress [71]. Drugs that reduce cellular glutathione levels enhanced the antimalarial action of chloroquine in mice [73]. Hence, a level of oxidative stress may be important during treatment although it contributes negatively to the general health, possibly inducing anemia as a result of RBC destruction. The infected individual, suffering from enhanced oxidative stress during the incubation period and the malaria episode as well as during treatment, may benefit from a posttreatment vitamin E supplementation.

HIV and AIDS

Human immunodeficiency virus/acquired immunodeficiency syndrome (HIV/AIDS) is associated with numerous hematologic disorders, especially anemia [74]. A Cochrane review of clinical trials suggested that currently, there are no useful therapeutic strategies to decrease anemia in HIV/AIDS patients [75].

Reactive oxygen species (ROS) are believed to play a critical role in the activation of NF-κB transcription factor and the stimulation of HIV infections [76, 77]. HIV-positive patients in Toronto experienced increased oxidative distress and reduced plasma antioxidants compared with healthy subjects, suggesting chronic oxidative stress caused by infection [77]. The role of malnutrition in immune function has been suggested to be important in viral infections by affecting the patient's health and influencing virus virulence [78]. Immune function was found to improve with vitamin E supplementation in elderly institutionalized humans [79, 80].

Concluding Remarks

Although anemia was an early classic symptom of vitamin E deficiency in children [81], it is clear that neurologic abnormalities, especially ataxia, are now considered the first unequivocal symptom of vitamin E deficiency in humans [7]. It is likely that if neurologic testing were carried out in more children, then more children would be found with obvious vitamin E deficiency symptoms. The complication in evaluating vitamin E status during malnutrition is the difficulty in evaluating α-tocopherol intakes because of the variability in oil vitamin E contents, as well as the limitation in accurate food vitamin E measurements. The problem of low vitamin E status may not be solely due to a limitation in α-tocopherol intakes, for example, severe PEM is associated not only with poor vitamin E status but also with essential fatty acid deficiency [82].

The formulation of a nutritional supplement containing the unoxidizable vitamin E form, α-tocopheryl acetate, may be critical, because vitamin E is not well absorbed in the absence of dietary fat [83]. Remarkably, Faber et al. [84] reported on anemia in infants aged 6–12 mo ($n = 361$), who were randomly assigned to receive maize-meal porridge for 6 months that was either unfortified (control group) or fortified with β-carotene, iron, zinc, ascorbic acid, copper, selenium, riboflavin, vitamin B_6, vitamin B_{12}, and vitamin E. The proportion of infants with anemia decreased from 45% to 17% in the fortified-porridge group, whereas it remained >40% in the control group. These findings suggest that the combination of nutrients as a supplement to food may be the best strategy for ameliorating anemia in at risk children.

Taken together, many of the various types of anemia reported herein seem to be accompanied by low vitamin E status that may be also associated with neurologic symptoms characteristic of α-tocopherol deficiency. While the α-tocopherol deficiency in malnutrition may be caused by inadequate food intakes, other anemias related to genetic malfunctions or viral infections may result in a α-tocopherol deficiency caused either by impaired vitamin E absorption, or increased oxidative distress. In the latter cases, α-tocopherol deficiency may occur in the absence of deficiencies of other nutrients. In any case, the severity of the neurologic abnormalities that result from α-tocopherol deficiency, as well as the immunologic dysregulation reported to occur with inadequate α-tocopherol intakes, emphasizes the critical need not only for vitamin E supplementation but also adequate dietary support with respect to all nutrients.

References

1. Sies H, Jones DP. Reactive oxygen species (ROS) as pleiotropic physiological signalling agents. Nat Rev Mol Cell Biol. 2020;21(7):363–83. https://doi.org/10.1038/s41580-020-0230-3.
2. Iuchi Y. In: Silverberg DS, editor. Anemia caused by oxidative stress. IntechOpen: Anemia; 2012.
3. Kuhn V, Diederich L, Keller TCS, Kramer CM, Luckstadt W, Panknin C, et al. Red blood cell function and dysfunction: redox regulation, nitric oxide metabolism, anemia. Antioxid Redox Signal. 2017;26(13):718–42. https://doi.org/10.1089/ars.2016.6954.
4. Hannemann A, Rees DC, Brewin JN, Noe A, Low B, Gibson JS. Oxidative stress and phosphatidylserine exposure in red cells from patients with sickle cell anaemia. Br J Haematol. 2018;182(4):567–78. https://doi.org/10.1111/bjh.15441.
5. Klein A, Deckert V, Schneider M, Dutrillaux F, Hammann A, Athias A, et al. Alpha-tocopherol modulates phosphatidylserine externalization in erythrocytes: relevance in phospholipid transfer protein-deficient mice. Arterioscler Thromb Vasc Biol. 2006;26(9):2160–7. https://doi.org/10.1161/01.ATV.0000235699.98024.11.
6. DellaPenna D. A decade of progress in understanding vitamin E synthesis in plants. J Plant Physiol. 2005;162(7):729–37. https://doi.org/10.1016/j.jplph.2005.04.004.
7. Food and Nutrition Board, Institute of Medicine. Dietary reference intakes for vitamin C, vitamin E, selenium, and carotenoids. Washington, DC: National Academy Press; 2000. https://www.ncbi.nlm.nih.gov/pubmed/25077263. https://doi.org/10.17226/9810.
8. Niki E. Role of vitamin E as a lipid-soluble peroxyl radical scavenger: in vitro and in vivo evidence. Free Radic Biol Med. 2014;66:3–12. https://doi.org/10.1016/j.freeradbiomed.2013.03.022.
9. Buettner GR. The pecking order of free radicals and antioxidants: lipid peroxidation, alpha-tocopherol, and ascorbate. Arch Biochem Biophys. 1993;300(2):535–43. https://doi.org/10.1006/abbi.1993.1074.
10. Attri S, Sharma N, Jahagirdar S, Thapa BR, Prasad R. Erythrocyte metabolism and antioxidant status of patients with Wilson disease with hemolytic anemia. Pediatr Res. 2006;59(4 Pt 1):593–7. https://doi.org/10.1203/01.pdr.0000203098.77573.39.
11. Sokol RJ, Heubi JE, Iannaccone ST, Bove KE, Balistreri WF. Vitamin E deficiency with normal serum vitamin E concentrations in children with chronic cholestasis. N Engl J Med. 1984;310(19):1209–12. https://doi.org/10.1056/NEJM198405103101901.
12. Saito M, Nakatsugawa K, Oh-Hashi A, Nishimuta M, Kodama N. Comparison of vitamin E levels in human plasma, red blood cells, and platelets following varying intakes of vitamin E. J Clin Biochem Nutr. 1992;12(1):59–68. https://doi.org/10.3164/jcbn.12.59.
13. Traber MG, Leonard SW, Ebenuwa I, Violet PC, Wang Y, Niyyati M, et al. Vitamin E absorption and kinetics in healthy women, as modulated by food and by fat, studied using 2 deuterium-labeled alpha-tocopherols in a 3-phase crossover design. Am J Clin Nutr. 2019;110(5):1148–67. https://doi.org/10.1093/ajcn/nqz172.
14. Sokol RJ. Vitamin E deficiency and neurological disorders. In: Packer L, Fuchs J, editors. Vitamin E in health and disease. New York, NY: Marcel Dekker, Inc.; 1993. p. 815–49.
15. Di Donato I, Bianchi S, Federico A. Ataxia with vitamin E deficiency: update of molecular diagnosis. Neurol Sci. 2010;31(4):511–5. https://doi.org/10.1007/s10072-010-0261-1.
16. Ouahchi K, Arita M, Kayden H, Hentati F, Ben Hamida M, Sokol R, et al. Ataxia with isolated vitamin E deficiency is caused by mutations in the alpha-tocopherol transfer protein. Nat Genet. 1995;9(2):141–5.
17. Kayden HJ, Silber R, Kossmann CE. The role of vitamin E deficiency in the abnormal autohemolysis of acanthocytosis. Trans Assoc Am Phys. 1965;78:334–42.
18. Traber MG, Sokol RJ, Ringel SP, Neville HE, Thellman CA, Kayden HJ. Lack of tocopherol in peripheral nerves of vitamin E-deficient patients with peripheral neuropathy. N Engl J Med. 1987;317(5):262–5. https://doi.org/10.1056/NEJM198707303170502.
19. Barros MF, Leger CL, Lira PI, Lima MC, Carbonneau MA, Descomps B, et al. Cord blood essential fatty acid and alpha-tocopherol in full-term newborns in a Northeast Brazil area. Int J Vitam Nutr Res. 2002;72(3):155–60. https://doi.org/10.1024/0300-9831.72.3.155.
20. Saker M, Soulimane Mokhtari N, Merzouk SA, Merzouk H, Belarbi B, Narce M. Oxidant and antioxidant status in mothers and their newborns according to birthweight. Eur J Obstet Gynecol Reprod Biol. 2008;141(2):95–9. https://doi.org/10.1016/j.ejogrb.2008.07.013.
21. Perez M, Robbins ME, Revhaug C, Saugstad OD. Oxygen radical disease in the newborn, revisited: oxidative stress and disease in the newborn period. Free Radic Biol Med. 2019;142:61–72. https://doi.org/10.1016/j.freeradbiomed.2019.03.035.
22. Head B, La Du J, Tanguay RL, Kioussi C, Traber MG. Vitamin E is necessary for zebrafish nervous system development. Sci Rep. 2020;10(1):15028. https://doi.org/10.1038/s41598-020-71760-x.
23. Miller GW, Ulatowski L, Labut EM, Lebold KM, Manor D, Atkinson J, et al. The alpha-tocopherol transfer protein is essential for vertebrate embryogenesis. PLoS One. 2012;7(10):e47402. https://doi.org/10.1371/journal.pone.0047402.

24. McDougall M, Choi J, Truong L, Tanguay R, Traber MG. Vitamin E deficiency during embryogenesis in zebrafish causes lasting metabolic and cognitive impairments despite refeeding adequate diets. Free Radic Biol Med. 2017;110:250–60. https://doi.org/10.1016/j.freeradbiomed.2017.06.012.
25. Lopriore C, Guidoum Y, Briend A, Branca F. Spread fortified with vitamins and minerals induces catch-up growth and eradicates severe anemia in stunted refugee children aged 3-6 y. Am J Clin Nutr. 2004;80(4):973–81. https://doi.org/10.1093/ajcn/80.4.973.
26. Rader DJ, Brewer HB. Abetalipoproteinemia - new insights into lipoprotein assembly and vitamin-E metabolism from a rare genetic disease. JAMA. 1993;270(7):865–9.
27. Traber MG, Rader D, Acuff R, Brewer HB, Kayden HJ. Discrimination between RRR- and all rac-a-tocopherols labeled with deuterium by patients with abetalipoproteinemia. Atherosclerosis. 1994;108:27–37.
28. Coates TD. Physiology and pathophysiology of iron in hemoglobin-associated diseases. Free Radic Biol Med. 2014;72:23–40. https://doi.org/10.1016/j.freeradbiomed.2014.03.039.
29. Kalra V, Grover J, Ahuja GK, Rathi S, Khurana DS. Vitamin E deficiency and associated neurological deficits in children with protein-energy malnutrition. J Trop Pediatr. 1998;44(5):291–5. https://doi.org/10.1093/tropej/44.5.291.
30. Traber MG. Vitamin E inadequacy in humans: causes and consequences. Adv Nutr. 2014;5(5):503–14. https://doi.org/10.3945/an.114.006254.
31. Kalra V, Grover JK, Ahuja GK, Rathi S, Gulati S, Kalra N. Vitamin E administration and reversal of neurological deficits in protein-energy malnutrition. J Trop Pediatr. 2001;47(1):39–45. https://doi.org/10.1093/tropej/47.1.39.
32. Dhansay MA, Benade AJ, Donald PR. Plasma lecithin-cholesterol acyltransferase activity and plasma lipoprotein composition and concentrations in kwashiorkor. Am J Clin Nutr. 1991;53(2):512–9. https://doi.org/10.1093/ajcn/53.2.512.
33. Kumerova A, Lece A, Skesters A, Silova A, Petuhovs V. Anaemia and antioxidant defence of the red blood cells. Mater Med Pol. 1998;30(1–2):12–5.
34. Sharif Usman S, Dahiru M, Abdullahi B, Abdullahi SB, Maigari UM, Ibrahim UA. Status of malondialdehyde, catalase and superoxide dismutase levels/activities in schoolchildren with iron deficiency and iron-deficiency anemia of Kashere and its environs in Gombe State, Nigeria. Heliyon. 2019;5(8):e02214. https://doi.org/10.1016/j.heliyon.2019.e02214.
35. Gadjeva V, Kuchukova D, Georgieva R. Vitamin combinations reduce oxidative stress and improve antioxidant status in patients with iron deficiency anemia. Comp Clin Path. 2005;14:99–104.
36. Schrier SL. Pathophysiology of thalassemia. Curr Opin Hematol. 2002;9(2):123–6. https://doi.org/10.1097/00062752-200203000-00007.
37. Cheng ML, Ho HY, Tseng HC, Lee CH, Shih LY, Chiu DT. Antioxidant deficit and enhanced susceptibility to oxidative damage in individuals with different forms of alpha-thalassaemia. Br J Haematol. 2005;128(1):119–27. https://doi.org/10.1111/j.1365-2141.2004.05257.x.
38. Queiroz RF, Lima ES. Oxidative stress in sickle cell disease. Rev Bras Hematol Hemoter. 2013;35(1):16–7. https://doi.org/10.5581/1516-8484.20130008.
39. Scott MD. H2O2 injury in beta thalassemic erythrocytes: protective role of catalase and the prooxidant effects of GSH. Free Radic Biol Med. 2006;40(7):1264–72. https://doi.org/10.1016/j.freeradbiomed.2005.11.017.
40. Das N, Das Chowdhury T, Chattopadhyay A, Datta AG. Attenuation of oxidative stress-induced changes in thalassemic erythrocytes by vitamin E. Pol J Pharmacol. 2004;56(1):85–96.
41. Silva DGH, Belini Junior E, de Almeida EA, Bonini-Domingos CR. Oxidative stress in sickle cell disease: an overview of erythrocyte redox metabolism and current antioxidant therapeutic strategies. Free Radic Biol Med. 2013;65:1101–9. https://doi.org/10.1016/j.freeradbiomed.2013.08.181.
42. Rahimi Z, Merat A, Haghshenass M, Madani H, Rezaei M, Nagel RL. Plasma lipids in Iranians with sickle cell disease: hypocholesterolemia in sickle cell anemia and increase of HDL-cholesterol in sickle cell trait. Clin Chim Acta. 2006;365(1–2):217–20. https://doi.org/10.1016/j.cca.2005.08.022.
43. Zannos-Mariolea L, Papagregoriou-Theodoridou M, Costantzas N, Matsaniotis N. Relationship between tocopherols and serum lipid levels in children with beta-thalassemia major. Am J Clin Nutr. 1978;31(2):259–63.
44. Natta CL, Machlin LJ, Brin M. A decrease in irreversibly sickled erythrocytes in sicle cell anemia patients given vitamin E. Am J Clin Nutr. 1980;33(5):968–71. https://doi.org/10.1093/ajcn/33.5.968.
45. Arruda MM, Mecabo G, Rodrigues CA, Matsuda SS, Rabelo IB, Figueiredo MS. Antioxidant vitamins C and E supplementation increases markers of haemolysis in sickle cell anaemia patients: a randomized, double-blind, placebo-controlled trial. Br J Haematol. 2013;160(5):688–700. https://doi.org/10.1111/bjh.12185.
46. Jilani T, Iqbal MP. Does vitamin E have a role in treatment and prevention of anemia? Pak J Pharm Sci. 2011;24(2):237–42.
47. Rachmilewitz EA, Shifter A, Kahane I. Vitamin E deficiency in beta-thalassemia major: changes in hematological and biochemical parameters after a therapeutic trial with alpha-tocopherol. Am J Clin Nutr. 1979;32(9):1850–8. https://doi.org/10.1093/ajcn/32.9.1850.
48. Sadrzadeh SM, Graf E, Panter SS, Hallaway PE, Eaton JW. Hemoglobin. A biologic Fenton reagent. J Biol Chem. 1984;259(23):14354–6.
49. Dissayabutra T, Tosukhowong P, Seksan P. The benefits of vitamin C and vitamin E in children with beta-thalassemia with high oxidative stress. J Med Assoc Thail. 2005;88(Suppl 4):S317–21.

50. Beutler E. Glucose-6-phosphate dehydrogenase deficiency. N Engl J Med. 1991;324(3):169–74.
51. Gumustekin K, Ciftci M, Coban A, Altikat S, Aktas O, Gul M, et al. Effects of nicotine and vitamin E on glucose 6-phosphate dehydrogenase activity in some rat tissues in vivo and in vitro. J Enzyme Inhib Med Chem. 2005;20(5):497–502.
52. Eldamhougy S, Elhelw Z, Yamamah G, Hussein L, Fayyad I, Fawzy D. The vitamin E status among glucose-6 phosphate dehydrogenase deficient patients and effectiveness of oral vitamin E. Int J Vitam Nutr Res. 1988;58(2):184–8.
53. Melov S, Coskun P, Patel M, Tuinstra R, Cottrell B, Jun AS, et al. Mitochondrial disease in superoxide dismutase 2 mutant mice. Proc Natl Acad Sci U S A. 1999;96(3):846–51. https://doi.org/10.1073/pnas.96.3.846.
54. Friedman JS, Lopez MF, Fleming MD, Rivera A, Martin FM, Welsh ML, et al. SOD2-deficiency anemia: protein oxidation and altered protein expression reveal targets of damage, stress response, and antioxidant responsiveness. Blood. 2004;104(8):2565–73. https://doi.org/10.1182/blood-2003-11-3858.
55. Rusu A, Rusu F, Zalutchi D, Muresan A, Gherman Caprioara M, Kacso I. The influence of vitamin E supplementation on erythropoietin responsiveness in chronic hemodialysis patients with low levels of erythrocyte superoxide dismutase. Int Urol Nephrol. 2013;45(2):495–501. https://doi.org/10.1007/s11255-012-0175-3.
56. Snow RW, Guerra CA, Noor AM, Myint HY, Hay SI. The global distribution of clinical episodes of plasmodium falciparum malaria. Nature. 2005;434(7030):214–7. https://doi.org/10.1038/nature03342.
57. Das BS, Thurnham DI, Das DB. Plasma alpha-tocopherol, retinol, and carotenoids in children with falciparum malaria. Am J Clin Nutr. 1996;64(1):94–100. https://doi.org/10.1093/ajcn/64.1.94.
58. Adelekan DA, Adeodu OO, Thurnham DI. Comparative effects of malaria and malnutrition on plasma concentrations of antioxidant micronutrients in children. Ann Trop Paediatr. 1997;17(3):223–7. https://doi.org/10.1080/02724936.1997.11747890.
59. Griffiths MJ, Ndungu F, Baird KL, Muller DP, Marsh K, Newton CR. Oxidative stress and erythrocyte damage in Kenyan children with severe Plasmodium falciparum malaria. Br J Haematol. 2001;113(2):486–91. https://doi.org/10.1046/j.1365-2141.2001.02758.x.
60. Hassan GI, Gregory U, Maryam H. Serum ascorbic acid concentration in patients with acute falciparum malaria infection: possible significance. Braz J Infect Dis. 2004;8(5):378–81. https://doi.org/10.1590/s1413-86702004000500007.
61. Sherman IW, Eda S, Winograd E. Erythrocyte aging and malaria. Cell Mol Biol (Noisy-le-Grand). 2004;50(2):159–69.
62. Geary TG, Boland MT, Jensen JB. Antioxidants do not prevent the in vitro induction of plasmodium falciparum crisis forms by human malaria-immune, TB or rabbit TNF serum. Am J Trop Med Hyg. 1986;35(4):704–7.
63. Hemmer CJ, Lehr HA, Westphal K, Unverricht M, Kratzius M, Reisinger EC. Plasmodium falciparum malaria: reduction of endothelial cell apoptosis in vitro. Infect Immun. 2005;73(3):1764–70. https://doi.org/10.1128/IAI.73.3.1764-1770.2005.
64. Levander OA, Ager AL Jr, Morris VC, May RG. Menhaden-fish oil in a vitamin E-deficient diet: protection against chloroquine-resistant malaria in mice. Am J Clin Nutr. 1989;50(6):1237–9. https://doi.org/10.1093/ajcn/50.6.1237.
65. Metzger A, Mukasa G, Shankar AH, Ndeezi G, Melikian G, Semba RD. Antioxidant status and acute malaria in children in Kampala, Uganda. Am J Trop Med Hyg. 2001;65(2):115–9. https://doi.org/10.4269/ajtmh.2001.65.115.
66. Nussenblatt V, Mukasa G, Metzger A, Ndeezi G, Eisinger W, Semba RD. Relationship between carotenoids and anaemia during acute uncomplicated Plasmodium falciparum malaria in children. J Health Popul Nutr. 2002;20(3):205–14.
67. Guha M, Kumar S, Choubey V, Maity P, Bandyopadhyay U. Apoptosis in liver during malaria: role of oxidative stress and implication of mitochondrial pathway. FASEB J. 2006;20(8):1224–6. https://doi.org/10.1096/fj.05-5338fje.
68. Herbas MS, Okazaki M, Terao E, Xuan X, Arai H, Suzuki H. Alpha-tocopherol transfer protein inhibition is effective in the prevention of cerebral malaria in mice. Am J Clin Nutr. 2010;91(1):200–7. https://doi.org/10.3945/ajcn.2009.28260.
69. Simoes AP, van den Berg JJ, Roelofsen B, Op den Kamp JA. Lipid peroxidation in Plasmodium falciparum-parasitized human erythrocytes. Arch Biochem Biophys. 1992;298(2):651–7. https://doi.org/10.1016/0003-9861(92)90462-6.
70. Mohan K, Ganguly NK, Dubey ML, Mahajan RC. Oxidative damage of erythrocytes infected with Plasmodium falciparum. An in vitro study. Ann Hematol. 1992;65(3):131–4. https://doi.org/10.1007/BF01695812.
71. Becker K, Tilley L, Vennerstrom JL, Roberts D, Rogerson S, Ginsburg H. Oxidative stress in malaria parasite-infected erythrocytes: host-parasite interactions. Int J Parasitol. 2004;34(2):163–89. https://doi.org/10.1016/j.ijpara.2003.09.011.
72. Magwere T, Naik YS, Hasler JA. Effects of chloroquine treatment on antioxidant enzymes in rat liver and kidney. Free Radic Biol Med. 1997;22(1–2):321–7. https://doi.org/10.1016/s0891-5849(96)00285-7.
73. Deharo E, Barkan D, Krugliak M, Golenser J, Ginsburg H. Potentiation of the antimalarial action of chloroquine in rodent malaria by drugs known to reduce cellular glutathione levels. Biochem Pharmacol. 2003;66(5):809–17. https://doi.org/10.1016/s0006-2952(03)00396-4.
74. Adias TC, Uko E, Erhabor O. Anaemia in human immunodeficiency virus infection: a review. Niger J

Med. 2006;15(3):203–6. https://doi.org/10.4314/njm.v15i3.37203.
75. Marti-Carvajal AJ, Sola I, Pena-Marti GE, Comunian-Carrasco G. Treatment for anemia in people with AIDS. Cochrane Database Syst Rev. 2011;(10):CD004776. https://doi.org/10.1002/14651858.CD004776.pub3.
76. Schreck R, Rieber P, Baeuerle PA. Reactive oxygen intermediates as apparently widely used messengers in the activation of the NF-kappa B transcription factor and HIV-1. EMBO J. 1991;10(8):2247–58.
77. Allard JP, Aghdassi E, Chau J, Salit I, Walmsley S. Oxidative stress and plasma antioxidant micronutrients in humans with HIV infection. Am J Clin Nutr. 1998;67(1):143–7. https://doi.org/10.1093/ajcn/67.1.143.
78. Beck MA, Handy J, Levander OA. Host nutritional status: the neglected virulence factor. Trends Microbiol. 2004;12(9):417–23. https://doi.org/10.1016/j.tim.2004.07.007.
79. Meydani SN, Meydani M, Blumberg JB, Leka LS, Siber G, Loszewski R, et al. Vitamin E supplementation and in vivo immune response in healthy elderly subjects. A randomized controlled trial. JAMA. 1997;277(17):1380–6. https://doi.org/10.1001/jama.1997.03540410058031.
80. Meydani SN, Leka LS, Fine BC, Dallal GE, Keusch GT, Singh MF, et al. Vitamin E and respiratory tract infections in elderly nursing home residents: a randomized controlled trial. JAMA. 2004;292(7):828–36. https://doi.org/10.1001/jama.292.7.828.
81. Farrell PM, Bieri JG, Fratantoni JF, Wood RE, di Sant'Agnese PA. The occurrence and effects of human vitamin E deficiency. A study in patients with cystic fibrosis. J Clin Invest. 1977;60(1):233–41. https://doi.org/10.1172/JCI108760.
82. Squali Houssaini FZ, Foulon T, Payen N, Iraqi MR, Arnaud J, Groslambert P. Plasma fatty acid status in Moroccan children: increased lipid peroxidation and impaired polyunsaturated fatty acid metabolism in protein-calorie malnutrition. Biomed Pharmacother. 2001;55(3):155–62. https://doi.org/10.1016/s0753-3322(01)00041-5.
83. Bruno RS, Leonard SW, Park S-I, Zhao Y, Traber MG. Human vitamin E requirements assessed with the use of apples fortified with deuterium-labeled α-tocopheryl acetate. Am J Clin Nutr. 2006;83(2):299–304.
84. Faber M, Kvalsvig JD, Lombard CJ, Benade AJ. Effect of a fortified maize-meal porridge on anemia, micronutrient status, and motor development of infants. Am J Clin Nutr. 2005;82(5):1032–9. https://doi.org/10.1093/ajcn/82.5.1032.
85. Becker K, Botticher D, Leichsenring M. Antioxidant vitamins in malnourished Nigerian children. Int J Vitam Nutr Res. 1994;64(4):306–10.
86. Laditan AA, Ette SI. Plasma alpha-tocopherol (vitamin E) levels and tocopherol-lipid ratio among children with protein-energy malnutrition (PEM). Ann Trop Paediatr. 1982;2(2):85–8.
87. Sauerwein RW, Mulder JA, Mulder L, Lowe B, Peshu N, Demacker PN, et al. Inflammatory mediators in children with protein-energy malnutrition. Am J Clin Nutr. 1997;65(5):1534–9. https://doi.org/10.1093/ajcn/65.5.1534.
88. Ahmed HM, Laryea MD, el-Karib AO, el-Amin EO, Biggemann B, Leichsenring M, et al. Vitamin E status in Sudanese children with protein-energy malnutrition. Z Ernahrungswiss. 1990;29(1):47–53. https://doi.org/10.1007/BF02019534.
89. Ashour MN, Salem SI, El-Gadban HM, Elwan NM, Basu TK. Antioxidant status in children with protein-energy malnutrition (PEM) living in Cairo, Egypt. Eur J Clin Nutr. 1999;53(8):669–73. https://doi.org/10.1038/sj.ejcn.1600830.
90. Nasr MR, Ali S, Shaker M, Elgabry E. Antioxidant micronutrients in children with thalassaemia in Egypt. East Mediterr Health J. 2002;8(4–5):490–5.
91. Hasanato RM. Zinc and antioxidant vitamin deficiency in patients with severe sickle cell anemia. Ann Saudi Med. 2006;26(1):17–21. https://doi.org/10.5144/0256-4947.2006.17.
92. Gbenebitse S, Jaja SI, Kehinde MO. Effect of changes in plasma vitamin E level of vascular responses and lipid peroxidation in sickle cell anaemia subjects. Niger Postgrad Med J. 2005;12(2):81–4.
93. Muskiet FA, Muskiet FD, Meiborg G, Schermer JG. Supplementation of patients with homozygous sickle cell disease with zinc, alpha-tocopherol, vitamin C, soybean oil, and fish oil. Am J Clin Nutr. 1991;54(4):736–44. https://doi.org/10.1093/ajcn/54.4.736.

Part V

Physiological Consequences and Significance of Iron Deficiency and Anemia

17 Iron Deficiency and Anemia Associated with Infectious and Inflammatory Diseases

Alexander Hoffmann, Lara Valente de Souza, and Günter Weiss

Keywords

Iron · Anemia · Anemia of inflammation · Infection · Bacteria · Intracellular microbes · Extracellular bacteria · Erythropoietin · Transfusion · Iron supplementation

Introduction

An intact iron metabolism is an integral part of a healthy living organism as balanced iron ensures many biological processes, while iron disturbances are accompanied with several diseases. Adequate iron homeostasis is required for erythropoiesis, various enzymatic functions, cell viability, and proliferation. The largest part of total body iron (3–4 g) is stored in hemoglobin as part of erythroid cells. Only 1–2 mg is daily absorbed in the duodenum from the diet to compensate for iron loss due to epidermal desquamation. The bone marrow requires 25 mg of iron every day for production of erythrocytes, which originates from iron recycling of senescent red blood cells (RBCs) by splenic and circulating macrophages [1].

The master iron regulator is the hepatic hormone hepcidin. It can bind to the only known cellular iron exporter ferroportin (FPN1), which leads to its internalization and lysosomal degradation. As FPN1 is densely present in duodenal enterocytes and in macrophages, the hepcidin-FPN1 interaction regulates iron absorption and iron efflux. Under steady-state conditions, hepcidin expression is regulated in response to circulating iron levels by bone morphogenetic proteins (BMPs), specifically BMP6 and BMP2, produced by hepatic iron-sensing sinusoidal endothelial cells [2]. Erythroid requirement for iron or hypoxia can suppress hepcidin expression by mechanisms involving inhibition of BMP6 signaling pathway via the hormone erythroferrone (ERFE), platelet-derived growth factors (PDGF-BB) or hypoxia-inducible factor 1 (HIF-1) [3, 4].

The two major hepcidin signaling routs are the iron-dependent BMP-SMA and mothers against decapentaplegic (SMAD) pathway and the inflammatory interleukin-6 – janus kinase/ signal transducer and activator of transcription – 3 (IL-6 - JAK/STAT3) pathway [2]. Inflammatory cytokines, such as interleukin (IL)-6 or IL-1β,

Alexander Hoffmann and Lara Valente de Souza contributed equally with all other contributors.

A. Hoffmann · L. Valente de Souza · G. Weiss (✉)
Department of Internal Medicine II, Infectious Diseases, Immunology, Rheumatology, Medical University of Innsbruck, Innsbruck, Austria

Christian Doppler Laboratory for Iron Metabolism and Anemia Research, Medical University of Innsbruck, Innsbruck, Austria
e-mail: alexander.hoffmann@i-med.ac.at; lara.valente@i-med.ac.at; guenter.weiss@i-med.ac.at

C. D. Karakochuk et al. (eds.), *Nutritional Anemia*, Nutrition and Health, https://doi.org/10.1007/978-3-031-14521-6_17

activate JAK1/2 to phosphorylate STAT3, which subsequently binds to the promoter region of hepcidin and induces subsequent hepcidin expression [2]. By stimulating hepcidin expression, inflammatory signals cause iron retention in macrophages and reduce dietary iron absorption [5]. In addition, cytokines and bacterial products affect macrophage iron retention and FPN1 expression by hepcidin-independent transcriptional and posttranscriptional pathways [6–8].

Alterations of Iron Homeostasis in Inflammation and Infection

Regulating Iron Metabolism During Infection

Most of the human-pathogenic microbes, like bacteria, certain viruses, parasites, and fungi, need a sufficient supply of iron for their metabolism, multiplication, and pathogenicity. Hence, beside an active immune response by the host, further resistance mechanisms exist to prevent pathogens from accessing necessary nutrients, thereby limiting microbial growth and virulence, a process called "nutritional immunity" [9]. To limit the availability of free reactive toxic iron in the plasma, iron-binding proteins (IBPs) like transferrin and lactoferrin have a low saturation to immediately buffer and bind iron entering the system. In the case of an infection, this mechanism withdraws iron from pathogens [9–11]. Likewise, host's haptoglobin and hemopexin are acute phase proteins and scavenge extracellular hemoglobin and labile heme in the plasma [9, 11].

To maintain their fitness and pathogenicity, invading pathogens are strongly dependent on iron acquisition. A direct bacterial iron acquisition mechanism is the uptake of host IBPs. *Staphylococcus aureus* has a specific hemoglobin receptor (IsdB), *Escherichia coli* has a heme receptor that binds and promotes heme degradation, [12] and Neisseriaceae, Pasteurellaceae, and Moraxellaceae express transferrin receptors [13]. In addition, bacteria can acquire either ferrous or ferric iron via specific transporters [10, 14]. Moreover, Gram-negative bacteria or fungi can secrete peptides called hemophores to acquire heme, or siderophores to obtain molecular iron from their environment. Notably, both can be taken up by ferric-chelate-specific transporters. In a further mechanism, the ferric iron of these structures is reduced to ferrous iron, being picked up by membranous ferrous transporters [14].

The host's general reaction to bacterial infections is to reduce serum iron in order to keep it away from invading pathogens. It is an effective reaction against extracellular pathogens, but increased intracellular iron could enhance the growth of intracellular bacteria like *Salmonella, Chlamydia, Legionella,* and *Mycobacterium* [14, 15]. Of interest, iron overload was associated with a worse outcome in infections (e.g., malaria and tuberculosis) [14, 15], and iron supplementation in endemic areas with a high burden of infection showed an increase in morbidity and mortality [16, 17]. On the contrary, iron deficiency and anemia have a negative effect on proliferation and differentiation of T cells and immune cell proliferation, which may result in an adverse clinical course of infections [18], whereas mild anemia could even be protective against clinical malaria [19]. Further, intracellular iron concentrations can modulate macrophage polarization, specifically their response to interferon gamma (IFN-γ), a central cytokine for coordinating host responses to infection [15].

Differences in Infections with Intra- and Extracellular Pathogens

Modifications of Iron Metabolism Against Extracellular Pathogens

The induction of hypoferremia by upregulating cellular iron import and downregulating its export is the main strategy to reduce iron accessibility to extracellular pathogens (Fig. 17.1). Hepcidin is capable of reducing iron export and is either produced by hepatocytes for systemical use [20] or, in small quantities, autocrine by macrophages [21]. Beside the posttranscriptionally regulation of FPN1 by hepcidin, IFN-γ can repress FPN1 tran-

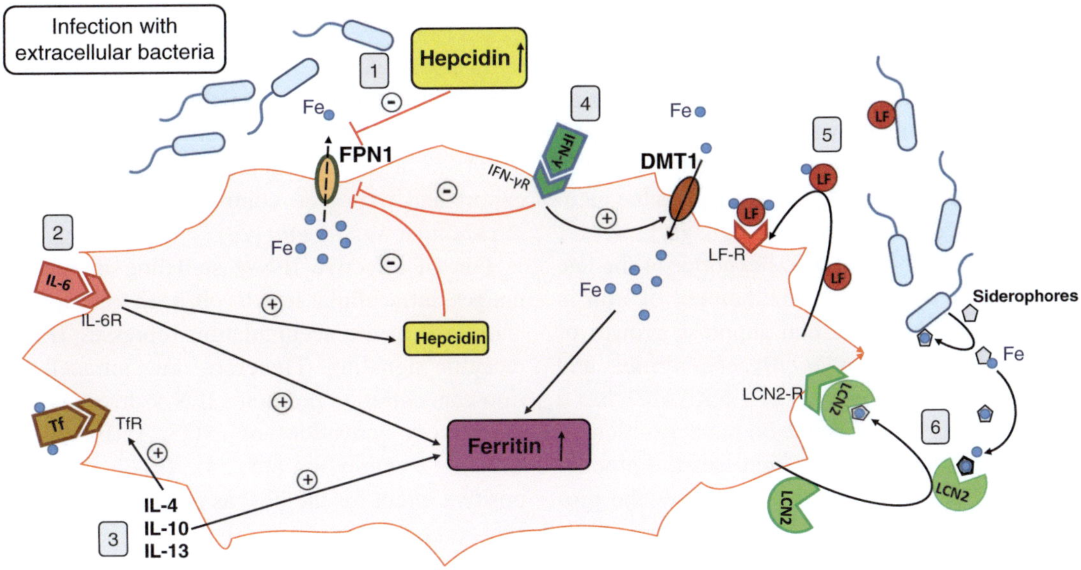

Fig. 17.1 Modifications of iron metabolism against extracellular pathogens. (1) High levels of hepatic hepcidin inhibit cellular iron export by ferroportin (FPN1) degradation. (2) The proinflammatory cytokine interleukin (IL)-6 binds to its receptor and stimulates autocrine hepcidin and ferritin production. (3) The anti-inflammatory cytokines IL-4, IL-10, IL-13 upregulate transferrin receptor (TfR) and ferritin expression and therefore support the cellular iron uptake and storage to reduce extracellular iron concentration. (4) Interferon gamma (IFN-γ) signaling increases the expression of the divalent metal transporter 1 (DMT1) and represses FPN1 expression. (5) Lactoferrin (LF) has a dual role as it can scavenge iron and has a direct antimicrobial effect. (6) Lipocalin-2 (LCN2) is a secreted protein that binds bacterial siderophores and is taken up by the LCN2 receptor (LCN2-R) of the host cell. Siderophores are peptides secreted and taken up by bacteria to scavenge extrabacterial iron

scription in macrophages [6]. The iron regulatory protein–iron responsive element (IRP – IRE) system is able to posttranslationally regulate iron uptake, storage, and export [2]. With high intracellular iron levels, the binding of IRPs to IREs is inhibited, resulting in supported iron export and suppressed iron import. Nitric oxide (NO), which is produced in excess during infection by the enzyme inducible NO synthase (iNOS), can circumvent this mechanism and increase the binding affinities of IRPs to IREs on the mRNA of genes like transferrin receptor (TfR), ferritin, and FPN1, thereby promoting iron accumulation in the macrophages [22, 23]. Further, IFN-γ is capable of inducing expression of divalent metal transporter (DMT1), which acts as an iron importer [6]. Likewise, other cytokines like IL-4, IL-10, and IL-13 are able to upregulate TfR and ferritin and promote cellular iron retention [24].

A further resistance mechanism against extracellular bacteria is the secretion of lactoferrin by macrophages, monocytes, or neutrophil granulocytes. Lactoferrin is a member of the transferrin family and binds iron with an even higher affinity than transferrin. Hence, it reduces the accessibility of extracellular iron to pathogens, beside its direct antimicrobial effect [25].

Lipocalin (LCN2 or NGAL), a carrier protein, is produced by macrophages, monocytes, and neutrophil granulocytes, and can bind catechol type siderophores secreted by bacteria. Due to siderophore sequestration by LCN2, iron availability for bacteria decreases. The LCN2-siderophore complex is delivered to the LCN2 receptor and taken up by the host cell. Of note, LCN2 contributes to systemic iron regulation and controls host immune responses [26].

Modifications of Iron Metabolism Against Intracellular Pathogens

Infections with intracellular pathogens lead to an opposite mechanism, with induction of cellular iron export and decreased iron import (Fig. 17.2). An important protein for this strategy is the natural resistance–associated macrophage protein 1 (NRAMP1), a divalent metal exporter of the late phagosome. By reducing the amount of iron in the late phagosome, it can suppress growth of bacteria like *Salmonella*, *Mycobacterium,* and parasites like *Leishmania* [27]. NRAMP1 has a direct impact on the local immune reaction of infected macrophage as it increases the production of TNF-α and NO and suppresses the production of IL-10 by promotion of cellular iron egress [28].

In addition, NO formation by macrophages stimulates nuclear factor erythroid 2-related factor 2 (Nrf2) expression, which induces the transcription of FPN1, resulting in cellular iron export and improved control of infection with intracellular *Salmonella* [29].

For an effective IFN-γ signaling in macrophages, intracellular iron levels need to be low or "normal," as its accumulation represses IFN-γ receptor signaling. Therefore, low intracellular iron concentration promotes IFN-γ-driven proinflammatory activations of iNOS, TNF-α, IL-6, and IL-12 expression [15, 24]. This is a double positive effect for the host as reduced intracellu-

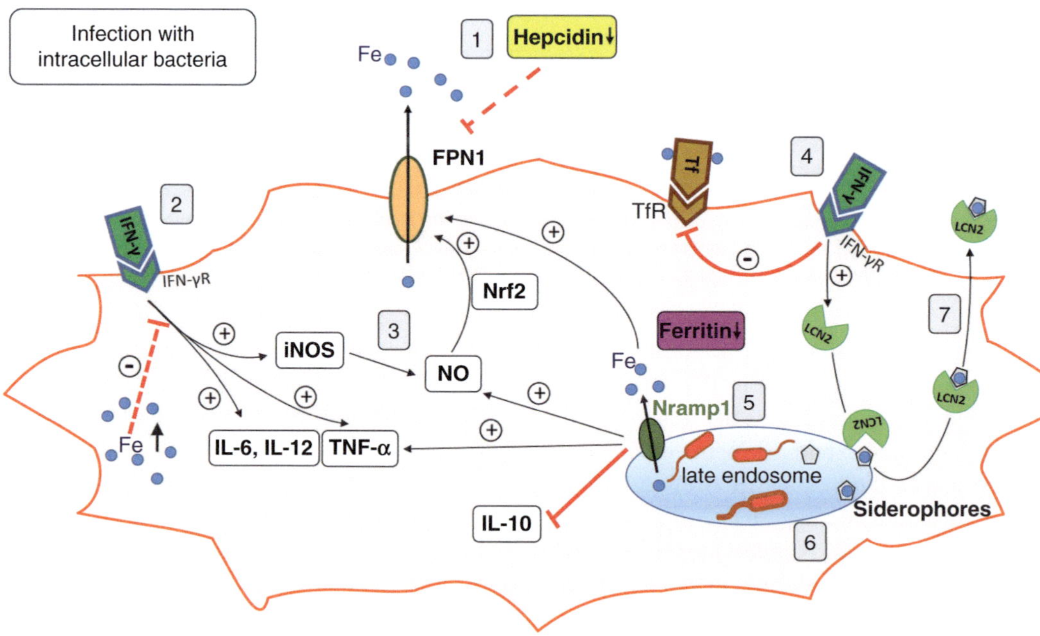

Fig. 17.2 Modifications of the iron metabolism against intracellular pathogens. (1) Hepatic hepcidin levels remain relatively low; therefore, cellular iron export via ferroportin (FPN1) is not affected. (2) Interferon gamma (IFN-γ) signaling increases the expression of proinflammatory cytokines like tumor necrosis factor alpha (TNF-α), interleukin (IL)-6, IL-12, and the inducible nitric oxide-synthase (iNOS). (3) The iNOS product nitric oxide (NO) activates the transcription factor nuclear factor erythroid 2-related factor 2 (Nrf2), which further enhances FPN1 expression. (4) Furthermore, IFN-γ signaling inhibits the transferrin receptor (TfR) expression but activates the production of lipocalin-2 (LCN2). (5) The late endosome, where bacteria like *Salmonella* are localized, expresses the iron transporter natural resistance–associated macrophage protein 1 (Nramp1), which exports iron from the compartment and therefore reduces iron availability for the pathogen. Nramp1 functionality indirectly increases NO, TNF-α and suppresses the production of the anti-inflammatory cytokine IL-10 via modulating cellular iron levels. (6) Bacteria in the late endosome can secrete siderophores to scavenge extrabacterial iron and these siderophores are neutralized when bound by LCN2. (7) The host cell can also secrete LCN2 and therefore participate in iron export

lar iron content on the one hand starves the pathogen and, on the other hand, drives pro inflammatory events. Further IFN-γ stimulates the production of LCN2, which was primarily identified as a secreted antimicrobial protein that binds siderophores from pathogens, but it may also affect cellular iron homeostasis upon binding mammalian siderophores [11]. In addition, IFN-γ limits iron access to intracellular microbes by reducing TfR expression [30].

While the host developed mechanisms to starve and fight pathogens, microbes build various strategies to counteract them. *Salmonella* preferentially targets macrophages that phagocytose erythrocytes, as they carry more iron [31]. This may be linked to the fact that iron-loaded macrophages present a niche for the bacteria to have access to the nutrient iron, whereas bacteria may also benefit from immune-deactivating effects of iron [15]. The latter is in line with the observation that phagocytosis of RBCs can impair the ability of phagocytes to kill intracellular pathogens, as shown in infection-associated hemophagocytic syndromes [32].

Infectious organisms may find a way to evade immune surveillance, but they cannot escape their basic iron requirement for growth. If the host can scavenge iron from particular niches, the resulting inhibition of pathogen growth may allow time for immunity to develop and control infections before rapid microbial replication overwhelms the host. In addition, several other mechanisms contribute to alterations of iron homeostasis and immune controls of infection with various pathogens, which have been recently nicely reviewed [14, 15].

Anemia of Inflammation with or without Combined Iron Deficiency

Definition, Etiology, and Epidemiology

Anemia is a highly prevalent condition that affects around 30% of the world's population. Among them, pregnant women, children, and the elderly are at higher risk [33]. It is an important determinant of morbidity and has been associated with worsened outcomes in several diseases, such as cancer, renal failure, and heart failure (not including myocardial infarction) [34]. Among its different causes, iron-deficiency anemia (IDA) is the most common, accounting for more than half of all anemias. Its prevalence decreased between 1990 and 2010, mainly due to lower numbers in North America and Western Europe. This suggests that IDA is a major issue in third world countries, correlating with malnutrition and poor health [35]. The second most frequent is anemia of inflammation (AI) with a prevalence of 40%, being the main cause of anemia in hospitalized patients [36].

IDA results from low levels of total body iron, leading to iron-restricted erythropoiesis. It can be a consequence of inadequate iron intake, impaired absorption, increased iron demand, or excess iron loss (primarily due to urogenital or gastrointestinal bleeding) [37].

Iron deficiency (ID) results in insufficient iron supply for erythropoiesis and thus anemia. However, ID also causes impaired metabolic activity, reduced mitochondrial respiration, and decrease in cell proliferation [37]. Therefore, ID can occur without anemia, having prognostic implications in cardiovascular diseases and being independently associated with all-cause mortality [1, 38].

AI develops along with inflammatory stimuli, and it is common in immune-mediated diseases, malignancies, inflammatory diseases, and infections (Fig. 17.3). In these cases, pro-inflammatory cytokines like IL-6 and IL-1β activate the JAK/STAT3 hepcidin signaling pathway. Due to increased hepcidin and lower FPN1 expression, iron is retained in macrophages and is less absorbed from the diet by duodenal enterocytes. In addition, IL-1, IL-6, IL-10, and TNF-α promote iron acquisition into macrophages and its storage within ferritin, while IFN-γ and lipopolysaccharide (LPS) block the transcription of FPN1 and further reduce iron efflux [36]. The major source of iron in inflamed macrophages, however, is the increased phagocytosis of damaged RBCs due to immune activation. Consequently, hypoferremia and hyperferretinemia develop and

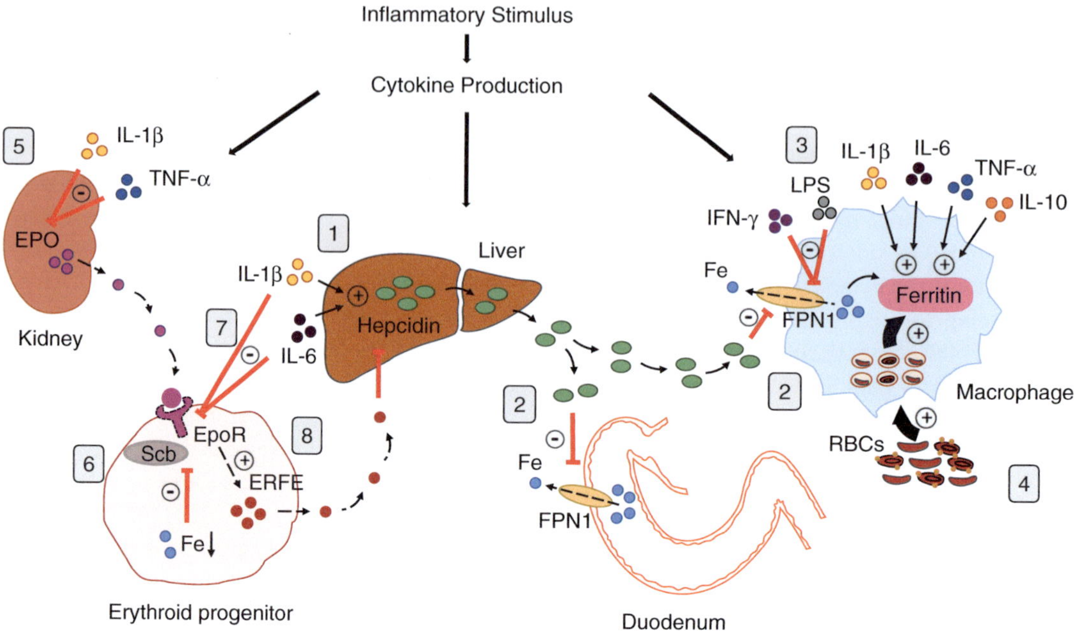

Fig. 17.3 Mechanisms of anemia of inflammation (AI). During infection or inflammation, many cytokines such as interleukin (IL)-6, IL-1β, IL-10, tumor necrosis factor alpha (TNF-α), interferon gamma (IFN-γ) are produced in order to orchestrate the immune response, which can have a great impact on iron homeostasis. (1) IL-6 and IL-1β stimulate hepcidin production in the liver. (2) Hepcidin promotes iron accumulation in macrophages and less iron absorption in the duodenum by degrading ferroportin (FPN1), thus causing hypoferremia. (3) Further, IL-6, IL-1β, IL-10, and TNF-α promote iron acquisition into macrophages, while IFN-γ and lipopolysaccharide (LPS) diminish iron export by FPN1. (4) A major source for increased iron acquisition by macrophages is the phagocytic ingestion of senescent and immune radical damaged erythrocytes. These mechanisms lead to increased intracellular iron levels, reflected by hyperferritinemia, and low circulating iron, termed as hypoferremia. (5) IL-1β and TNF-α further inhibit the formation of erythropoietin (EPO) in the kidney. (6) Moreover, the interaction between erythropoietin receptor (EpoR) and Scribble is compromised by erythroid iron deficiency. (7) IL-1β and IL-6 negatively affect signaling via EpoR, thereby contributing to EPO hyporesponsiveness. (8) Production of erythroferrone (ERFE) in response to EPO is diminished, thus leading to higher hepcidin levels and iron retention. Finally, cytokines exert various negative effects on proliferation and differentiation of erythroid progenitors

the iron restriction for erythroid progenitors impairs the production of RBCs. Moreover, the biological activity of erythropoietin (EPO), a hormone produced by the kidney that induces the differentiation of erythroid progenitors, is reduced in the setting of inflammation [36]. Inflammatory cytokines such as IL-1 and tumor necrosis factor alpha (TNF-α) inhibit EPO formation, while IL-1, IL-6, or IFN-γ cause EPO-receptor (EpoR) hyporesponsiveness [1]. Moreover, Scribble is a receptor control element important for maintaining surface presentation of EpoR on erythroid progenitors. Upon iron deficiency, Scribble is less available for EpoR binding, leading to reduced activation of the EPO signaling pathway [39]. The reduced EPO activity also blunts ERFE formation, thereby increasing hepcidin expression and further limiting iron access for erythroid cells [36, 40].

Due to the nonaccessibility of body iron, AI characterizes with functional ID. Often, absolute and functional IDs (AI/IDA) coexist, such as in patients with malignancies or autoimmune diseases associated with gastrointestinal or urogenital bleeding [36]. Table 17.1 summarizes pathophysiology and consequences of ID, IDA, AI, and AI/IDA.

Despite the documented high prevalence and association of AI with disease progression, the involvement of anemia in the underlying disease

Table 17.1 Main pathophysiological mechanisms and consequences in ID, IDA, AI, AI/IDA

	Pathophysiology
ID (absolute ID)	• Insufficient iron availability relative to the body's need due to increased iron losses (bleeding), increased iron needs (growth, pregnancy), or reduced iron absorption (e.g., dietary, genetic, achlorhydria, celiac disease) • Impaired metabolic and cellular functions despite efficient erythropoiesis
IDA (absolute ID)	• Same mechanism as in ID • More severe ID leading to insufficient iron for erythropoiesis and development of microcytic and hypochromic anemia
AI (functional ID)	• Inflammatory cytokines induce hepcidin expression, synergistically causing iron retention in the RES and reduced dietary iron absorption with limited iron availability for erythropoiesis • Diminished biological activity of EPO • Reduced erythrocyte half-life via enhanced erythrophagocytosis • Cytokine-mediated antiproliferative effects on erythroid progenitors
AI/IDA (functional and absolute ID)	• Same mechanism as in AI • Additional iron absolute ID due to chronic urogenital or gastrointestinal bleeding (e.g., menstruation, gastrointestinal lesions in inflammatory bowel disease, carcinoma, duodenal ulcers; helminth infestations), iatrogenic blood losses (e.g., dialysis), or inefficient iron absorption

ID iron deficiency, *IDA* iron deficiency anemia, *AI* anemia of inflammation, *EPO* erythropoietin, *RES* reticuloendothelial system

is yet not fully understood, leading to the question if AI is a marker or a causative factor of disease severity and progression. As nutritional immunity causes iron retention in order to restrict its access to pathogens, it is a major component of AI during acute and chronic infections [14, 15, 36]. AI's prevalence increases in individuals affected with other comorbidities, being higher among hospitalized patients (40–45%), patients in intensive care unit (ICU) (up to 100%), subjects suffering from tuberculosis (62%), and also individuals hospitalized for severe COVID-19 infection [41]. Mild ID and IDA may be protective against malaria's development and associated death, while a more severe anemia in the course of infection correlates with a worse prognosis [1]. All these factors bring about the complex interaction between iron, infection, and immunity and the open questions on the best management of anemia when associated with infectious and inflammatory diseases.

Diagnosis

Due to the high prevalence of anemia and ID and its association with morbidity, a correct diagnosis of the specific type of anemia is mandatory. In particular, differentiation between AI and AI/IDA is of importance due to divergent subsequent diagnostic steps and therapeutic strategies. On the one hand, iron misbalances in AI can act as a host defense strategy, in which iron supplementation may be harmful to the progression of the underlying disease, specifically in the case of infections and possibly also in association with cancer. On the other hand, individuals with coexisting absolute ID (AI/IDA) may benefit from repletion of iron stores, as they need iron for their intracellular basic metabolic pathways. Several laboratory markers are available to help with the diagnosis (Table 17.2) although there is no single marker that can differentiate these two features in an easy and precise form [36, 37].

Absolute ID is characterized by low ferritin levels, low serum iron, and often reduced transferrin saturation (TfS). In addition to these, IDA presents with low hemoglobin, microcytic and hypochromic RBCs, and often increased transferrin levels. In contrast, AI shows low serum iron and TfS, but high ferritin and low transferrin levels, whereas mean corpuscular volume (MCV) and mean corpuscular hemoglobin (MCH) are mostly normal. AI/IDA also presents with low TfS and low serum iron, while serum ferritin can be normal, MCV and MCH can be normal or slightly reduced. A number of other markers and indices have been proposed and introduced into clinical practice to help with the differential diagnosis, such as reticulocyte hemoglobin content (CHr), sTfR ferritin index, or hepcidin levels.

Table 17.2 Available parameters for establishing differential diagnosis among ID, IDA, AI, and AI/IDA

Parameters	Normal values	ID	IDA	AI	AI/IDA
Hb (g/dl)	Men: >13 Women: >12	Normal	Low	Low	Low
MCV (fl)	80–95	Normal to low	Low	Normal	Low to normal
MCH (pg)	27–34	Normal to low	Low	Normal	Low to normal
Serum iron (μmol/L)	10–30	Low	Low	Low	Low
Ferritin (μg/L)	Men: 40–300 Women: 20–200	Low	Low	Normal to high	Low to normal
Transferrin (mg/dl)	220–400	Normal to high	High	Low	Low to normal
TfS (%)	>16 to <45	Normal to low	Low	Low	Low
sTfR (mg/L)	2–5	Normal to high	High	Normal	Normal to high
Hepcidin	Variable[a]	Low	Low	High	Low to normal
CHr (pg)	31.2 ± 1.6	Low	Low	Low to normal	Low
sTfR-F index[b]	Variable	NA	High	Low	High

IDA iron deficiency anemia, *AI* anemia of inflammation, *Hb* hemoglobin, *MCV* mean corpuscular volume, *MCH* mean corpuscular hemoglobin, *TfS* transferrin saturation, *sTfR* soluble transferrin receptor, *CHr* reticulocyte hemoglobin content, *sTfR-F index* soluble transferrin receptor – ferritin index

[a] Hepcidin and sTfR-F index values vary according to the method used

[b] sTfR-F index: sTfR/log ferritin

However, none of these can be independently used for that purpose [36, 37].

Current and Emerging Treatment Strategies

Anemia as well as ID result in a number of symptoms including fatigue, reduced physical activity, impaired cardio-pulmonary performance, or impaired cognitive function.

The initial approach is the identification of the underlying cause of anemia and its correction, if possible. Only in severe and life-threatening cases of anemia with hemoglobin levels below 8 g/dl, immediate correction by blood transfusions may be justified. This includes patients with acutely developing anemia, hemodynamic instability, and/or with comorbidities, such as coronary heart disease or advanced pulmonary dysfunction. However, transfusions have been associated with increased mortality and risk for postsurgical infections in several studies [1, 42]. A restrictive rather than liberal use of RBC transfusion was correlated with lower mortality in patients at ICU and after surgery or trauma [42].

In subjects with ID and IDA, and no pathologies impairing iron absorption, replenishment of iron stores is performed by iron supplementation. In AI, curing the underlying disease would mostly lead to resolution of anemia over time, with normal iron redistribution once inflammatory stimuli diminish. However, when cure of the disease associated with AI cannot be achieved, treatment of AI or AI/IDA is warranted [36, 43].

Generally, repletion of iron stores is obtained with oral or intravenous (i.v.) iron supplementation. This decision is based on many elements, like type and severity of anemia, the underlying disease, the degree of inflammation, the costs and availability of the drugs, as well as the convenience to the patient. Oral iron is cheap and easy to administrate, although it may cause undesired gastrointestinal side effects. As mentioned above, hepcidin inversely controls intestinal iron absorption. The latter increases with iron deficiency but lowers upon inflammation [5]. While oral iron supplementation is effective to treat absolute ID and IDA, its efficiency in AI decreases with more advanced inflammation. However, in AI with mild inflammation, due to lower hepcidin levels, and in AI/IDA, where the ID-mediated hepcidin inhibition overcomes the inflammation-driven hepcidin stimulation, this treatment may be successful in ameliorating anemia [1, 36, 43].

Indications of i.v. iron include undesired side effects and ineffective treatment with oral compounds, besides severe anemia needing urgent iron repletion. Parenteral iron bypasses the hepcidin blockage in the duodenum. However, macrophages phagocytose iron-carbohydrate complexes, which accumulate in the reticuloendothelial system (RES), being once more susceptible to the hepcidin-FPN1 interaction. Therefore, the efficiency of IV iron is likewise higher in AI/IDA and AI with mild inflammation. It is not completely comprehended how the iron accumulation in the RES may influence the underlying disease or if it can have an impact on the risk to infections. Limitations of i.v. iron preparations are a higher price, the need for i.v. administration and potential side effects, such as hypophosphatemia or an infrequent risk for anaphylaxis [1, 43].

Once iron supplements are no longer efficient, adding erythropoiesis-stimulating agents (ESAs) becomes an alternative to improve hematopoiesis. The efficiency of ESAs is built upon iron stores, and thus, both treatments are often combined. However, its administration can downregulate proinflammatory immune pathways and may be associated with increased thromboembolic events, specifically with higher dosages [1, 36]. Of interest, there is a lack of evidence concerning the use of iron supplementation and ESAs upon chronic and acute infections, as most data originate from studies in autoimmune diseases, such inflammatory bowel disease (IBD), chronic kidney disease (CKD), or congestive heart failure [1].

Since hepcidin is the major controller of iron homeostasis and responsible for iron efflux, new therapies to AI intend to target this hormone mainly aiming redistribution of iron trapped in the RES. Therapeutics include antibodies directed against hepcidin or drugs and antibodies either against components of the BMP-SMAD pathway (mostly BMP6) or adjunct molecules, such as hemojuvelin. Furthermore, antibodies that stabilize FPN1 are an interesting approach to neutralize hepcidin activity. Such therapies may be combined with ESAs in order to achieve a better therapeutic efficacy with reduced side effects, as hepcidin-modifying strategies increase iron availability and thus may decrease the needed ESAs dosages [36, 43, 44].

Notably, preservation of HIF-1 promotes EPO production and impacts on iron homeostasis [4]. The novel therapy with HIF-prolyl hydroxylase inhibitors (HIF-PHIs), which stabilizes HIF thus ameliorating anemia, is currently in phase 3 clinical trials [36, 43].

There are still many aspects to consider concerning anemia treatment during inflammation and infection. On the one hand, several studies showed association between iron supplementation and increased risk of infections (tuberculosis, malaria, brucellosis), infection-related hospitalization and mortality, diarrhea, change in microbiota and fecal metabolites [16, 45–48]. On the other hand, high iron levels in the gut may reduce virulence to specific bacteria, such as *Citrobacter* [49]. Further, the location of iron in the cell and its traffic during infection and inflammation can play an essential role for the risk of infections or their exacerbation with extra- and intracellular bacteria [11, 50]. In addition, we lack information from in vivo studies on the thresholds of iron availability for immune function and antimicrobial host responses. Further, the influence of anemia and/or ID on the course of underlying disease is insufficiently known. This gives rise to the complexity of iron supplementation and redistribution in the setting of inflammation and infection, including cause of the disease and character of the pathogen, highlighting the importance of precise diagnosis and an individual approach [36].

Outlook and Perspectives

Anemia and ID are frequently associated with inflammatory diseases and infections, leading to higher morbidity and mortality. The human body holds several mechanisms in order to avoid and control infections, a major one termed nutritional immunity, by which the host retains iron and limits its availability for pathogens. Meanwhile, microbes developed numerous mechanisms that evade the host's iron restriction to assure their growth and proliferation. While we have acquired important knowhow over the last years regarding the mechanisms of these interactions, there is still a large lack of knowledge related to diagnosis of different forms of anemia in these settings and their optimal therapy. More specifically, differentiating AI from AI/IDA gains importance due to its different treatment approaches, while reliable biomarkers to precise iron homeostasis in the setting on anemia and inflammation are missing. In addition, there is much knowledge to acquire concerning information on the optimal start and end points of therapy and on the influence of treatment toward the underlying inflammatory disease or infection. Taking into account the prevalence of these iron disturbances and its detrimental consequences to patients´ quality of life, further scientific investigations are urgently needed and of major importance for human health.

References

1. Valente de Souza L, Hoffmann A, Weiss G. Impact of bacterial infections on erythropoiesis. Expert Rev Anti-Infect Ther. 2020;1-15 https://doi.org/10.1080/14787210.2021.1841636.
2. Muckenthaler MU, Rivella S, Hentze MW, Galy B. A red carpet for iron metabolism. Cell. 2017;168(3):344–61. https://doi.org/10.1016/j.cell.2016.12.034.
3. Sonnweber T, Nachbaur D, Schroll A, Nairz M, Seifert M, Demetz E, et al. Hypoxia induced downregulation of hepcidin is mediated by platelet derived growth factor BB. Gut. 2014;63(12):1951–9. https://doi.org/10.1136/gutjnl-2013-305317.
4. Peyssonnaux C, Zinkernagel AS, Schuepbach RA, Rankin E, Vaulont S, Haase VH, et al. Regulation of iron homeostasis by the hypoxia-inducible transcription factors (HIFs). J Clin Invest. 2007;117(7):1926–32. https://doi.org/10.1172/jci31370.
5. Theurl I, Aigner E, Theurl M, Nairz M, Seifert M, Schroll A, et al. Regulation of iron homeostasis in anemia of chronic disease and iron deficiency anemia: diagnostic and therapeutic implications. Blood. 2009;113(21):5277–86. https://doi.org/10.1182/blood-2008-12-195651.
6. Ludwiczek S, Aigner E, Theurl I, Weiss G. Cytokine-mediated regulation of iron transport in human monocytic cells. Blood. 2003;101(10):4148–54. https://doi.org/10.1182/blood-2002-08-2459.
7. Guida C, Altamura S, Klein FA, Galy B, Boutros M, Ulmer AJ, et al. A novel inflammatory pathway mediating rapid hepcidin-independent hypoferremia. Blood. 2015;125(14):2265–75. https://doi.org/10.1182/blood-2014-08-595256.
8. Tilg H, Ulmer H, Kaser A, Weiss G. Role of IL-10 for induction of anemia during inflammation. J Immunol. 2002;169(4):2204–9. https://doi.org/10.4049/jimmunol.169.4.2204.
9. Weinberg ED. Iron availability and infection. Biochim Biophys Acta. 2009;1790(7):600–5. https://doi.org/10.1016/j.bbagen.2008.07.002.
10. Cassat JE, Skaar EP. Iron in infection and immunity. Cell Host Microbe. 2013;13(5):509–19. https://doi.org/10.1016/j.chom.2013.04.010.
11. Soares MP, Weiss G. The iron age of host-microbe interactions. EMBO Rep. 2015;16(11):1482–500. https://doi.org/10.15252/embr.201540558.
12. Turlin E, Débarbouillé M, Augustyniak K, Gilles AM, Wandersman C. Staphylococcus aureus FepA and FepB proteins drive heme iron utilization in Escherichia coli. PLoS One. 2013;8(2):e56529. https://doi.org/10.1371/journal.pone.0056529.
13. Pogoutse AK, Moraes TF. Iron acquisition through the bacterial transferrin receptor. Crit Rev Biochem Mol Biol. 2017;52(3):314–26. https://doi.org/10.1080/10409238.2017.1293606.
14. Gerner RR, Nuccio SP, Raffatellu M. Iron at the host-microbe interface. Mol Asp Med. 2020;75:100895. https://doi.org/10.1016/j.mam.2020.100895.
15. Nairz M, Weiss G. Iron in infection and immunity. Mol Asp Med. 2020;75:100864. https://doi.org/10.1016/j.mam.2020.100864.
16. Sazawal S, Black RE, Ramsan M, Chwaya HM, Stoltzfus RJ, Dutta A, et al. Effects of routine prophylactic supplementation with iron and folic acid on admission to hospital and mortality in preschool children in a high malaria transmission setting: community-based, randomised, placebo-controlled trial. Lancet. 2006;367(9505):133–43. https://doi.org/10.1016/s0140-6736(06)67962-2.
17. Soofi S, Cousens S, Iqbal SP, Akhund T, Khan J, Ahmed I, et al. Effect of provision of daily zinc and iron with several micronutrients on growth and morbidity among young children in Pakistan: a cluster-randomised trial. Lancet. 2013;382(9886):29–40. https://doi.org/10.1016/s0140-6736(13)60437-7.
18. Brekelmans P, van Soest P, Leenen PJ, van Ewijk W. Inhibition of proliferation and differentiation during early T cell development by anti-transferrin receptor antibody. Eur J Immunol. 1994;24(11):2896–902. https://doi.org/10.1002/eji.1830241147.
19. Nyakeriga AM, Troye-Blomberg M, Dorfman JR, Alexander ND, Bäck R, Kortok M, et al. Iron deficiency and malaria among children living on the coast of Kenya. J Infect Dis. 2004;190(3):439–47. https://doi.org/10.1086/422331.
20. Nemeth E, Tuttle MS, Powelson J, Vaughn MB, Donovan A, Ward DM, et al. Hepcidin regulates cellular iron efflux by binding to ferroportin and inducing its internalization. Science. 2004;306(5704):2090–3. https://doi.org/10.1126/science.1104742.
21. Theurl I, Theurl M, Seifert M, Mair S, Nairz M, Rumpold H, et al. Autocrine formation of hepcidin induces iron retention in human monocytes.

Blood. 2008;111(4):2392–9. https://doi.org/10.1182/blood-2007-05-090019.
22. Weiss G, Goossen B, Doppler W, Fuchs D, Pantopoulos K, Werner-Felmayer G, et al. Translational regulation via iron-responsive elements by the nitric oxide/NO-synthase pathway. EMBO J. 1993;12(9):3651–7.
23. Drapier JC, Hirling H, Wietzerbin J, Kaldy P, Kuhn LC. Biosynthesis of nitric oxide activates iron regulatory factor in macrophages. EMBO J. 1993;12(9):3643–9.
24. Weiss G, Schett G. Anaemia in inflammatory rheumatic diseases. Nat Rev Rheumatol. 2013;9(4):205–15. https://doi.org/10.1038/nrrheum.2012.183.
25. Giansanti F, Panella G, Leboffe L, Antonini G. Lactoferrin from Milk: nutraceutical and pharmacological properties. Pharmaceuticals. 2016;9(4) https://doi.org/10.3390/ph9040061.
26. Nairz M, Schroll A, Haschka D, Dichtl S, Sonnweber T, Theurl I, et al. Lipocalin-2 ensures host defense against salmonella typhimurium by controlling macrophage iron homeostasis and immune response. Eur J Immunol. 2015;45(11):3073–86. https://doi.org/10.1002/eji.201545569.
27. Forbes JR, Gros P. Divalent-metal transport by NRAMP proteins at the interface of host-pathogen interactions. Trends Microbiol. 2001;9(8):397–403. https://doi.org/10.1016/s0966-842x(01)02098-4.
28. Fritsche G, Nairz M, Werner ER, Barton HC, Weiss G. Nramp1-functionality increases iNOS expression via repression of IL-10 formation. Eur J Immunol. 2008;38(11):3060–7. https://doi.org/10.1002/eji.200838449.
29. Nairz M, Schleicher U, Schroll A, Sonnweber T, Theurl I, Ludwiczek S, et al. Nitric oxide-mediated regulation of ferroportin-1 controls macrophage iron homeostasis and immune function in salmonella infection. J Exp Med. 2013;210(5):855–73. https://doi.org/10.1084/jem.20121946.
30. Byrd TF, Horwitz MA. Regulation of transferrin receptor expression and ferritin content in human mononuclear phagocytes. Coordinate upregulation by iron transferrin and downregulation by interferon gamma. J Clin Invest. 1993;91(3):969–76. https://doi.org/10.1172/jci116318.
31. Nix RN, Altschuler SE, Henson PM, Detweiler CS. Hemophagocytic macrophages harbor salmonella enterica during persistent infection. PLoS Pathog. 2007;3(12):e193. https://doi.org/10.1371/journal.ppat.0030193.
32. Silva-Herzog E, Detweiler CS. Intracellular microbes and haemophagocytosis. Cell Microbiol. 2008;10(11):2151–8. https://doi.org/10.1111/j.1462-5822.2008.01192.x.
33. Kassebaum NJ, Collaborators GBDA. The global burden of anemia. Hematol Oncol Clin North Am. 2016;30(2):247–308. https://doi.org/10.1016/j.hoc.2015.11.002.
34. Martinsson A, Andersson C, Andell P, Koul S, Engstrom G, Smith JG. Anemia in the general population: prevalence, clinical correlates and prognostic impact. Eur J Epidemiol. 2014;29(7):489–98. https://doi.org/10.1007/s10654-014-9929-9.
35. Schumann K, Solomons NW. Perspective: what makes it so difficult to mitigate worldwide anemia prevalence? Adv Nutr. 2017;8(3):401–8. https://doi.org/10.3945/an.116.013847.
36. Weiss G, Ganz T, Goodnough LT. Anemia of inflammation. Blood. 2019;133(1):40–50. https://doi.org/10.1182/blood-2018-06-856500.
37. Camaschella C. Iron-deficiency anemia. N Engl J Med. 2015;372(19):1832–43. https://doi.org/10.1056/NEJMra1401038.
38. Cappellini MD, Comin-Colet J, de Francisco A, Dignass A, Doehner W, Lam CS, et al. Iron deficiency across chronic inflammatory conditions: international expert opinion on definition, diagnosis, and management. Am J Hematol. 2017;92(10):1068–78. https://doi.org/10.1002/ajh.24820.
39. Khalil S, Delehanty L, Grado S, Holy M, White Z 3rd, Freeman K, et al. Iron modulation of erythropoiesis is associated with scribble-mediated control of the erythropoietin receptor. J Exp Med. 2018;215(2):661–79. https://doi.org/10.1084/jem.20170396.
40. Arezes J, Foy N, McHugh K, Sawant A, Quinkert D, Terraube V, et al. Erythroferrone inhibits the induction of hepcidin by BMP6. Blood. 2018;132(14):1473–7. https://doi.org/10.1182/blood-2018-06-857995.
41. Bellmann-Weiler R, Lanser L, Barket R, Rangger L, Schapfl A, Schaber M, et al. Prevalence and predictive value of anemia and dysregulated iron homeostasis in patients with COVID-19 infection. J Clin Med. 2020;9(8) https://doi.org/10.3390/jcm9082429.
42. Villanueva C, Colomo A, Bosch A, Concepcion M, Hernandez-Gea V, Aracil C, et al. Transfusion strategies for acute upper gastrointestinal bleeding. N Engl J Med. 2013;368(1):11–21. https://doi.org/10.1056/NEJMoa1211801.
43. Petzer V, Theurl I, Weiss G. Established and emerging concepts to treat imbalances of iron homeostasis in inflammatory diseases. Pharmaceuticals. 2018;11(4) https://doi.org/10.3390/ph11040135.
44. Sheetz M, Barrington P, Callies S, Berg PH, McColm J, Marbury T, et al. Targeting the hepcidin-ferroportin pathway in anaemia of chronic kidney disease. Br J Clin Pharmacol. 2019;85(5):935–48. https://doi.org/10.1111/bcp.13877.
45. Zimmermann MB, Chassard C, Rohner F, N'Goran EK, Nindjin C, Dostal A, et al. The effects of iron fortification on the gut microbiota in African children: a randomized controlled trial in cote d'Ivoire. Am J Clin Nutr. 2010;92(6):1406–15. https://doi.org/10.3945/ajcn.110.004564.
46. Das NK, Schwartz AJ, Barthel G, Inohara N, Liu Q, Sankar A, et al. Microbial metabolite signaling is required for systemic iron homeostasis. Cell Metab. 2020;31(1):115–30 e6. https://doi.org/10.1016/j.cmet.2019.10.005.
47. Murray MJ, Murray AB, Murray MB, Murray CJ. The adverse effect of iron repletion on the course

of certain infections. Br Med J. 1978;2(6145):1113–5. https://doi.org/10.1136/bmj.2.6145.1113.

48. Isanaka S, Mugusi F, Urassa W, Willett WC, Bosch RJ, Villamor E, et al. Iron deficiency and anemia predict mortality in patients with tuberculosis. J Nutr. 2012;142(2):350–7. https://doi.org/10.3945/jn.111.144287.
49. Sanchez KK, Chen GY, Schieber AMP, Redford SE, Shokhirev MN, Leblanc M, et al. Cooperative metabolic adaptations in the host can favor asymptomatic infection and select for attenuated virulence in an enteric pathogen. Cell. 2018;175(1):146–58 e15. https://doi.org/10.1016/j.cell.2018.07.016.
50. Nairz M, Haschka D, Demetz E, Weiss G. Iron at the interface of immunity and infection. Front Pharmacol. 2014;5:152. https://doi.org/10.3389/fphar.2014.00152.

Iron Deficiency, Anemia, and the Immune System

18

Anna-Maria Mitterstiller, Laura von Raffay, and Manfred Nairz

Keywords

Iron · Iron deficiency · Iron deficiency anemia Anemia · Anemia of inflammation · Immune system · Hepcidin · Viral infection · Allergy

Introduction

Iron Is Essential But Potentially Toxic

The balance of iron is essential to all forms of life, as iron-containing proteins play a role in oxygen transport, electron transfer, DNA synthesis, enzymatic processes, and cellular metabolism. In its free state, iron participates in redox reactions. Excess free iron can lead to an uncontrolled production of free radicals, which may damage cellular membranes, proteins, or DNA. Therefore, iron homeostatic mechanisms have evolved to avoid potential toxicity and to tightly control the iron content at a cellular level. Similar mechanisms also keep the uptake of iron from the environment, its recycling by macrophages, and its storage in macrophages or hepatocytes in systemic balance. Various factors of genetic, physiological, or environmental nature may disrupt these highly organized and regulated pathways, and lead to the development of either iron overload or iron deficiency (ID) conditions [1].

Iron Deficiency Can Cause Anemia

Anemia is characterized by a decreased total amount of red blood cells (RBCs) in terms of volume or number, or a reduced hemoglobin (Hb) content and thus entails a reduced ability of the blood to carry oxygen. The consequences of anemia are as diverse as its underlying causes, and they depend, besides gender and age, on individual factors and on the severity of anemia. Subtle signs and symptoms of anemia include reduced oxygen and energy metabolism, which often cause tiredness, fatigue and loss of energy, difficulty concentrating, and decreased work capacity [2]. Severe anemia, however, impairs the function of vital organs such as the brain and the heart and may become life-threatening, especially when the decline in Hb levels comes fast and remains uncorrected.

Absolute and Functional Iron Deficiency Differs from Each Other

Two major forms of ID exist, absolute and functional ID. Absolute ID, defined as depleted body

A.-M. Mitterstiller (✉) · L. von Raffay · M. Nairz (✉)
Department of Internal Medicine II, Infectious Diseases, Immunology, Rheumatology, Pneumology, Medical University of Innsbruck, Innsbruck, Austria
e-mail: anna.mitterstiller@i-med.ac.at

C. D. Karakochuk et al. (eds.), *Nutritional Anemia*, Nutrition and Health,
https://doi.org/10.1007/978-3-031-14521-6_18

iron stores, results from low intake or impaired assimilation of iron, high iron demand, or chronic blood—and thus iron—loss. The second most prevalent form, functional ID, occurs in several chronic diseases, including chronic kidney disease, chronic heart failure, cancer, autoimmune disease, and other inflammatory diseases. These chronic conditions are associated with inflammation-driven retention of iron in innate immune cells, which inevitably leads to iron-limited erythropoiesis. When persisting, prolonged immune activation thus causes anemia of inflammation (AI), which is globally the second most frequent anemia and the most frequent anemia in hospitalized and chronically ill patients. Furthermore, absolute ID often coexists with other chronic disorders, which have an inflammatory component. Therefore, the interactions of these causes and conditions, especially inflammation-driven ones, make the differential diagnosis of ID challenging [3].

Basic Principles of Iron Deficiency and Iron Deficiency Anemia

ID occurs when body iron levels are low or insufficient to maintain normal physiologic functions. Unrecognized or untreated ID may finally lead to ineffective erythropoiesis and smoothly transit into anemia. Strict division between absolute and functional ID is difficult as various combinations exist.

Absolute ID usually develops when release of recycled iron from senescent erythrocytes and the absorption of dietary iron in the gut cannot reimburse for growing iron needs (e.g., during growth, frequent blood donations, bleedings, or infections). This leads to decreased or exhausted body iron stores, and finally results in IDA [4], which develops slowly [2, 5].

In contrast, functional ID occurs when body iron stores in the form of iron-laden ferritin (Ft) present in the macrophages of the liver, spleen, and bone marrow are normal or increased. In this scenario, iron is barely mobilized from stores as the immune system is activated, triggered by danger signals derived from damaged tissues or from pathogens. Moreover, the trafficking of iron from enterocytes and macrophages to the circulation is terminated, which leads to its accumulation within macrophages, for example, as a result of chronic inflammation and infections. When these functional disturbances persist, they subsequently lead to AI. Furthermore, states of increased erythropoiesis, such as during therapy with erythropoiesis-stimulating agents (ESAs) or after major blood loss followed by an endogenous erythropoietin (EPO) response, might create divergent states between iron demand and its supply [6].

Causes and Consequences of Iron Deficiency and Iron Deficiency Anemia

The causes of IDA vary based on gender, age, and socioeconomic status. ID may result from low nutritional iron intake, insufficient absorption, or blood loss (Table 18.1). Genetic variants or defects, with or without inflammation, might be another cause (Table 18.2). In western societies, healthy individuals may be susceptible to ID due to special eating habits (e.g., vegan diet), dietary restrictions, or frequent blood donations. Most of all, chronic bleeding, often in combination with reduced iron absorption, is another common cause of ID in high-income countries [2, 7].

In low- and middle-income countries (LMICs), ID and IDA typically result from malnutrition or diets poor in bioavailable iron and are often associated with infections with parasites (e.g., hookworm infestation or schistosomiasis), causing hemorrhages [8].

While ID is most prevalent, and sometimes severe, in young children and women of reproductive age, it is also a concern for elderly people. It is assumed that 50% of pregnant women and 40% of preschool children in LMICs are iron deficient [9]. Infants and young children have increased iron needs during rapid growth periods. In these groups, IDA is related to poorer cognition, along with delayed motor and cognitive development, and all of these conditions are

Table 18.1 Common causes of absolute and functional iron deficiency (ID) are shown [2, 6, 7, 19]

Common causes of ID	
Absolute ID/ IDA	**Depletion of iron stores**
High iron demand	• Pregnancy (second and third trimester) due to mutual expansion of erythroid mass • Fast-growing infants/children
Low nutritional iron intake	• Malnutrition (due to poverty; developing countries) • Vegetarian and vegan diet • Eating disorder
Insufficient iron absorption In the gut	• Environmental enteric dysfunction • Antinutritional factors (phytate, tannins, caffeine) • Surgery (duodenal/gastric bypass, gastrectomy, bariatric surgery) • Medical conditions/instances (*helicobacter pylori*, atrophic gastritis, autoimmune gastritis) • Parasitic infection • Proton pump inhibitors and H2 blockers
Protracted and chronic blood loss	• Menstruation • Genito-urinary bleeding • Frequent donation of blood • Elite athletes • Gastrointestinal bleeding (e.g., hookworms, esophagitis, intestinal cancer, drugs like anticoagulants and antiplatelet compounds, peptic ulcers) • Intravascular hemolysis (paroxysmal nocturnal hemoglobinuria (PNH), autoimmune hemolytic anemia, damaged heart valves) • Systemic blood loss due to defects of hemostasis
Functional ID/ AI	**Sequestration of iron in stores, iron supply is inadequate**
Inflammation	• High levels of hepcidin due to, e.g., autoimmune diseases, chronic infections, cancer, chronic kidney disease (CKD), chronic heart failure (CHF), chronic pulmonary disease (CPD), inflammatory bowel disease (IBD) • Parasitic infection
Chronic diseases	• Chronic kidney disease (CKD), chronic heart failure (CHF), chronic pulmonary disease (CPD)

Table 18.2 Additional causes of iron deficiency (ID) are shown [2, 6, 19]

Other causes of ID	
Genetic reasons leading to impaired signaling pathways	• Impaired genes involved in uptake, mobilization, and utilization, like DMT1 (SLC11A2), ceruloplasmin (CP), transferrin (TF) • IRIDA (iron-refractory iron deficiency anemia) leading to high hepcidin levels
ESA (erythropoiesis-stimulating agents) therapy	• Massive erythropoiesis leading to impaired iron demand
Obesity	• Reduced iron absorption • Immune-driven dysregulation of iron metabolism due to hepcidin and adipocytokines
Postoperative state	• Intraoperative blood loss • Immune-driven dysregulation of iron metabolism after surgery
Aging	• Low intake and reduced absorption • Gastrointestinal blood loss (drugs and unintended drug interactions, ulcers, cancer)

highly prevalent in LMICs [10]. Efforts to avoid such developmental defects in children aim to supplementing iron. Importantly, the unbiased treatment with iron supplements in tropical regions resulted in a significant increase in morbidity and mortality from infectious diseases [11, 12]. These unexpected yet detrimental effects of iron substitution supplementation programs might be due to the relevance of the metal to the lifecycle of parasites or the proliferation of bacteria [13]. Conversely, infants and pregnant women with mild ID were shown to be partly protected from malaria, which might be linked to starving circulating pathogens from the nutrient iron, an reduced susceptibility to infection or an effect of iron on immune response and remains an important clinical question [14, 15].

Intriguingly, anemia also affects the development of the immune system as shown in a study with young children living in Tanzania and Mozambique. The immune system dynamically changes during the first years of life, when maternal-derived immune mediators such as antibodies are lost and the thymus takes over its key role in the development of T lymphocytes and thus in the immune response. Anemia in infants is related to altered composition of the immune system, as affected children showed lower recent thymic emigrant CD4$^+$ T cells, IgG$^+$ memory B cells, as well as lower production of antibodies and plasmablasts compared to nonanemic children. This is directly linked to the bioavailability of iron and to comorbidities and nutritional status, causing anemia [16]. Furthermore, data suggest a negative effect on the development of the adaptive immune cells in children suffering from anemia [17].

In western societies, the number of patients with absolute ID is increasing as a result of enhanced life expectancy and as a consequence of comorbidities and, possibly, medications. The causes of anemia in the elderly are manifold. Specifically, age-related disorders such as coronary artery disease, congestive heart failure (CHF), type 2 diabetes mellitus, chronic kidney disease (CKD), and chronic obstructive pulmonary disease (COPD) are linked to absolute ID, which is associated with increased risk of hospitalization and morbidity [18]. Furthermore, cognitive decline and increased risk of dementia in elderly have associations with ID and IDA [19].

Taken together, the causes of IDA can vary depending on gender, age, and socioeconomic circumstances, because IDA can result from low nutritional iron intake, insufficient absorption, blood loss, inflammation/infections, or rare genetic defects.

Pathophysiology of Iron Deficiency and Iron Deficiency Anemia

Iron metabolism (Fig. 18.1) is tightly regulated, to avoid both iron excess and ID and as a consequence IDA. Hepcidin acts as the liver-derived master regulator to control the entry of iron into the circulation. This is achieved by modulating

Fig. 18.1 Maintenance of systemic iron homeostasis and mechanism of iron deficiency anemia (IDA). (**a**) Cells involved in systemic iron regulation are shown. Dietary iron absorption starts at the brush-border membrane of duodenal enterocytes. Ferric iron (Fe^{3+}) is reduced to ferrous (Fe^{2+}) iron by duodenal cytochrome B (DcytB) and is transported across the membrane via divalent metal transporter 1 (Dmt1). Ferroportin (Fpn) at the basolateral membrane cooperates with hephaestin (Hp) that oxidizes Fe^{2+} to Fe^{3+}. Ferric iron circulates in the blood bound to transferrin (Tf). Tf-bound iron supplies all cells with iron by binding to the transferrin receptor1 (TfR1) and subsequent endocytosis. Fe^{2+} in the cytosol is collectively referred to as the "labile iron pool" (LIP). Hepatocytes and macrophages store high amounts of iron in ferritin. When required, iron is exported from the LIP via Fpn back to circulation (after reoxidation of Fe^{2+} to Fe^{3+} by ceruloplasmin (CP)). Iron of old erythrocytes is recycled from macrophages via heme oxygenase 1 (HO-1). Upon iron loading, bone morphogenetic protein 6 (BMP6) secreted by endothelial cells stimulates hepcidin expression in the hepatocytes. BMP6 binds to the BMP receptor (BMPR)/hemojuvelin (HJV) complex, phosphorylates SMAD proteins, and *trans*-activates the promoter of the *Hamp* (for hepcidin gene). The HFE protein/transferrin receptor 2 (TfR2) complex is involved in iron sensing. Hepcidin produced by hepatocytes decreases cellular iron export by binding to Fpn and inducing its endocytosis, resulting in decreased intestinal iron absorption and iron release from macrophages. TfR1 is highly expressed on erythroblasts. Iron from erythrocytes is recycled by macrophage via HO-1 and Fpn. Under iron sufficient conditions, T_H1 cells expansion is promoted as is the secretion of cytokines like IFN-γ and TNF [26]. (**b**) Mechanisms of adaptation to iron deficiency are displayed. In mild iron deficiency, TfR2 is lost from the erythroblast surface, thereby increasing EPO sensitivity. In addition, iron deficiency and hypoxia increase Epo, which enhances erythropoiesis. This in turn suppresses the generation of hepcidin through erythroferrone (ERFE) produced by erythroblasts. ERFE antagonizes BMP signaling in hepatocytes, thus lowering circulating hepcidin levels and enabling iron to be transferred from the gut to the blood [1]. Anemia per se stimulates the proliferation of erythroid progenitors and ERFE [49]. Several cofactors expressed on the hepatocyte cell membrane such as HFE, hemojuvelin (HJV), or TfR2 impact on hepcidin expression via the BMP-SMAD pathway [25]. Low liver iron content increases transmembrane protease serine 6 (TMPRSS6), which cleaves iron-sensing complexes to reduce the expression of hepcidin. HJV exists, beside its membrane-bound form, also in a circulating soluble form (sHJV), which acts as an antagonist of BMP signaling and was shown to be increased in vivo during iron deficiency [50]. Histone deacetylase 3 (HDAC3) participates in hepcidin suppression by erasing activation markers at the *Hamp* locus [51]. Iron is released by Fpn into the circulation. If iron stores are exhausted, iron availability remains low, which consequently prevents the uptake of iron by all cells and organs (e.g., heart, skeletal muscle) [52]. Under limited iron supply, T_H2 cells will expand and secrete IL-4 and IL-13 [26]

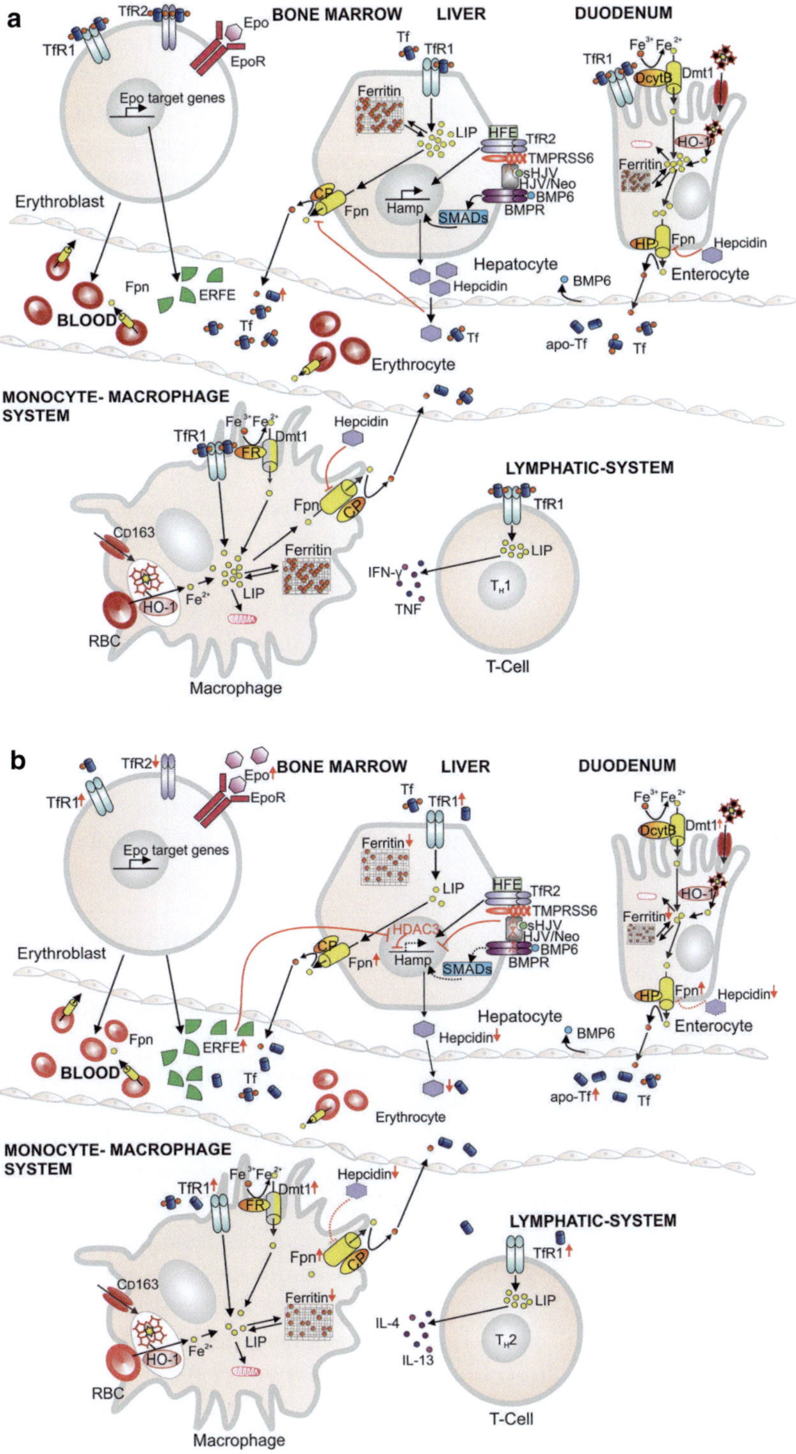
a
BONE MARROW
LIVER
DUODENUM
TfR1
TfR2
Epo
EpoR
Epo target genes
Erythroblast
Tf
Ferritin
LIP
HFE
TfR2
TMPRSS6
sHJV
HJV/Neo
BMP6
BMPR
Hamp
SMADs
CP
Fpn
Hepatocyte
Hepcidin
Fe3+ Fe2+
DcytB
Dmt1
HO-1
HP
Enterocyte
BLOOD
ERFE
apo-Tf
Erythrocyte
MONOCYTE- MACROPHAGE SYSTEM
FR
CD163
Fe2+
RBC
Macrophage
LYMPHATIC-SYSTEM
IFN-γ
TNF
TH1
T-Cell
b
HDAC3
IL-4
IL-13
TH2

the expression of ferroportin (Fpn) on phagocytes that recycle iron from aged red blood cells (RBCs) and on duodenal enterocytes that absorb dietary iron from the intestinal lumen. Iron circulates bound to transferrin (Tf) to different cells; yet, most iron is used by the bone marrow to synthesize Hb in RBC precursors, which possess high levels of transferrin receptor 1 (TfR1). Cell types, such as hepatocytes and macrophages of the mononuclear phagocyte system (MPS), are considered to be major iron storage sites. To meet physiological requirements, iron is released from the stores to maintain plasma iron levels and supply the erythron. During ID (Fig. 18.1), or increased erythropoietic needs (as in childhood, pregnancy, or in hypoxic conditions, e.g., at high altitude), adaptive mechanisms aim to optimize the usage of iron for erythropoiesis and to maximize its absorption [1].

Functional Iron Deficiency Due to Inflammatory Processes

Inflammatory signals evoked by pathogens, autoimmune tissue damage, or cancer-induced alterations in systemic iron fluxes, especially in the MPS, are regulated by systemic iron levels and culminate in increased requirements and sequestration of iron in innate immune cells. The functional ID that results is thus characterized by the presence of adequate or increased iron stores but insufficient iron mobilization, two of the hallmarks of the AI. The underlying pathophysiology of AI is more complex, though, and comprises at least three main pathways: (a) iron retention in the MPS, (b) suppression of erythropoiesis combined with a reduction of the activity of the hormone EPO, and (c) diminished erythrocyte survival [6].

Specifically, interleukin 6 (IL-6) and IL-1β, as well as lipopolysaccharide (LPS), present in the cell wall of Gram-negative bacteria, induce Ft and hepcidin to counterregulate Fpn-mediated iron export from the MPS. Therefore, in the systemic circulation, increased Ft and hepcidin levels can be found as both markers of AI and mediators of macrophage iron retention. However, inflammatory cytokines such as IL-1 and tumor necrosis factor (TNF) not only alter iron distribution, but also directly impair the renal production of EPO and thus erythropoiesis. In physiologic conditions, EPO stimulates cell proliferation and differentiation of erythroid progenitors. However, in AI, erythroid EPOR expression and EPOR-mediated signaling are inhibited by different cytokines [1, 6].

Moreover, erythrocytes have been shown to have a shortened survival during inflammation in general, and in certain infections, specifically. Inflammation-born radicals damage lipids in the RBC membrane, thus enhancing erythrophagocytosis [6]. A range of pathogens directly target RBC as well. On the one hand, malaria and babesiosis are characterized by infection of RBC and the presence of intracellular microbes [20]. On the other hand, Gram-positive bacteria such as *Staphylococci* and *Streptococci* produce hemolysins that damage or destroy RBC [21].

In summary, the combination of many immune-mediated regulatory effects leads to iron retention in monocytes and macrophages, shown by low Fpn expression and increased Ft levels in the cells and in the systemic circulation.

Iron and the Immune System

Iron and the Innate Immune System

Iron is an essential nutrient for both humans and pathogens. Therefore, iron deprivation serves as an innate immune mechanism against invading microbes. On the other hand, pathogens have evolved refined strategies to obtain iron and other micronutrients from the host [22, 23]. Not only do macrophages play a key role in iron homeostasis, they also form an indispensable part of the innate immune control against pathogens and both functions appear to be linked. Macrophages can be exposed to different microenvironmental conditions such as the inflammatory cytokine milieu, damaged RBCs, living pathogens, and iron gradients. As a result, macrophages can embrace different functions and phenotypes, many more than the dichotomous model of proinflammatory (M1-like) and anti-inflammatory (M2-like) populations would suggest. Monocytes and macrophages fulfill a spectrum of functions including RBC and iron recycling. Nevertheless, M1-like and M2-like macrophages not only differ in their molecular signature, these phagocytic cells were also shown to observe distinct patterns of iron gene expression [3].

Classically activated M1-like cells secrete proinflammatory cytokines and favor iron sequestration via Fpn repression and Ft heavy chain induction. Possibly, this phenotype aims at limiting the availability of the essential metal for circulating pathogens [3]. At the same time, however, macrophage iron retention may directly be involved in the pathogenesis of chronic inflammatory and autoimmune diseases [24]. Moreover, the cytokine milieu can directly modulate iron metabolism in immune cells including macrophages. This is facilitated in a coordinated fashion to reduce the size of the intracellular labile iron pool (LIP) via reduction of TfR1 on the cell surface and increased synthesis of Ft for iron storage. Then again, small amounts of hepcidin are also produced by immune cells and can exert autocrine or paracrine functions, which are mediated by fine-tuning of the intracellular LIP, too [25].

In contrast, M2-like macrophages exert anti-inflammatory functions in tissues. Moreover, these cells have a lower iron content but are highly specialized for iron recycling from senescent erythrocytes [17]. Thereby, they represent the key cellular system responsible for supplying iron essential for erythropoiesis and may themselves be unable to store iron. In vitro, M2-polarized macrophages show high Fpn and lower Ft levels, thereby allowing iron recirculation and support of iron expensive tissue-healing processes [3]. Many other functions of macrophages, however, critically depend on the production of specific effector molecules such as antimicrobial peptides and toxic radicals.

Iron handling by macrophages is bidirectionally linked to the production of reactive nitrogen intermediates, above all NO. NO has high affinity for iron and was shown to control intracellular iron trafficking by regulating critical genes of iron metabolism via the cytoplasmatic iron sensors—the iron regulatory proteins (IRPs). The formation of NO by macrophages is negatively regulated by iron and is very important for immune control of infections and cancer. Interestingly, the iron exporter of the phagolysosome, known as natural resistance associated macrophage protein-1 (Nramp1), lowers the intracellular labile iron pool of macrophages, thus promoting NO production [13].

During ID, the bactericidal activity of macrophages is reduced, although phagocytosis is unaffected. Furthermore, neutrophils show lower killing activity under low iron conditions due to reduced activity of the iron containing enzyme, myeloperoxidase [3]. In summary, monocytes and macrophages have key functions in systemic iron homeostasis. Additionally, the intracellular iron content in these phagocytic cells has direct effects on their immune functions and thus needs to be tightly regulated by IRPs, NO, hepcidin, Nramp1, and other pathways for adequate host response to infections and other insults [13].

Iron and the Adaptive Immune System

T cells, together with antibody-producing B cells, are the two major lymphocyte populations and the main components of the adaptive immune system. Lymphocytes express a range of iron proteins, because their development and proliferation requires iron, whose uptake is mainly mediated via TfR1. As a consequence, reduced transferrin iron saturation may lower cell-mediated immune responses [3, 26].

More recently, it was shown that lymphocytes express hepcidin and that its production increases after activation. Hepcidin controls lymphocyte iron homeostasis in an autocrine and paracrine loop. Low hepcidin expression impairs normal lymphocyte proliferation [25]. TfR1 associates with HFE, which is a nonclassical MHC-I molecule and yet another candidate through which iron homeostasis affects T cell functions. The classical *HFE* mutation, *C282Y*, results in quantitative and functional alterations of T cell subsets and the iron storage disorder hereditary hemochromatosis [26]. Poly(rC)-binding protein 1 (Pcbp1), which may function as iron-stabilizing cytoplasmatic chaperone, is linked to T cell function as well. Concretely, intracellular iron stabilizes Pcbp1 protein and, in turn, prolonse translation of IL-2 and of granulocyte macrophage colony–stimulating factor (GM-CSF) [27]. Vice versa, iron depletion diminishes the production of these two cytokines associated with T_H1 and T_H17 type responses and counteracts autoimmunity in a model of multiple sclerosis [28]. Similarly, the absence of TfR1 on $CD4^+$ T cells protects from autoimmunity due to reduced production of IL-2, GM-CSF, and IFN-γ [3].

In line with these observations in mice, mutations in *TFRC gene*, encoding TfR1, in human subjects result in an inherited immune deficiency syndrome characterized by impaired function of T and B lymphocytes [1].

B lymphocyte function is largely dependent on signals from T lymphocytes and is influenced by iron, too. At the same time, resting B cells express lower levels of TfR1 than T cells and their proliferation and differentiation to plasma cells is less affected by iron. On the other side, iron seems to inhibit cytidine deaminase, an important enzyme involved in immunoglobulin class switching . ID may therefore facilitate IgE class switching in the presence of T_H2-associated cytokines like IL-4 and IL-13. B-cells have also been shown to be stimulated by TGF-β to secrete IgA. Furthermore, the iron-binding protein lactoferrin, known to participate in host defense against microbial pathogens, is also able to initiate class-switching to IgA and IgG2b [29]. Human subjects with ID show preserved antibody production in response to immunization with various antigens. In contrast, IDA may result in significantly weakened antibody responses to vaccination [22, 30, 31].

Taken together, evidence is accumulating that the iron content of the microenvironment surrounding T cells and iron uptake via Tfr1 shape T cell immunity. Low serum iron could furthermore limit the ability of lymphocytes to acquire iron to support clonal expansions and the development of adaptive responses.

The Effect of the Hosts Iron Status on Vaccination Success

Every year, more than five million children in LMICs die before the age of five. Most fatalities are due to preventable causes including infections, as children do not have access to medication or immunization [32]. Vaccination programs against diseases, like diphtheria, pertussis, polio, and measles, significantly contribute to reducing childhood morbidity and mortality [30]. Immune responses to vaccines and natural antigen challenges may differ between lower- and higher-income countries. In low-income countries, a strong link of inadequate nutritional status, including ID, to poor vaccination response exists [10]. In African infants, IDA at the time of vaccination was associated with reduced response to diphtheria, pneumococcal, and pertussis vaccines. In contrast, infants who received iron at the time of measles vaccination had higher concentrations of anti-measles IgG and IgG avidity [31]. In high-income countries, antibody production to influenza vaccine was independent of inflammation and iron status in dialysis patients but was associated with previous vaccination and age [33]. Still, treatment with iron during vaccination might be seen critical, as iron promotes the growth of pathogens like *Mycobacterium tuberculosis* and was shown to contribute to an increased risk of tuberculosis (TB) or a worsened TB outcome [22].

In summary, a better understanding of the interconnections of iron homeostasis and immune response to vaccination may help to increase the efficacy of programs, especially in LMICs, and should be taken into account in future vaccine studies.

Iron in Viral Infections

Iron is involved in many fundamental biological processes including DNA and RNA synthesis or ATP generation. As viruses exploit these metabolic pathways in infected cells, the iron content of host cells critically determines the course of viral infection (Fig. 18.2). This has been demonstrated

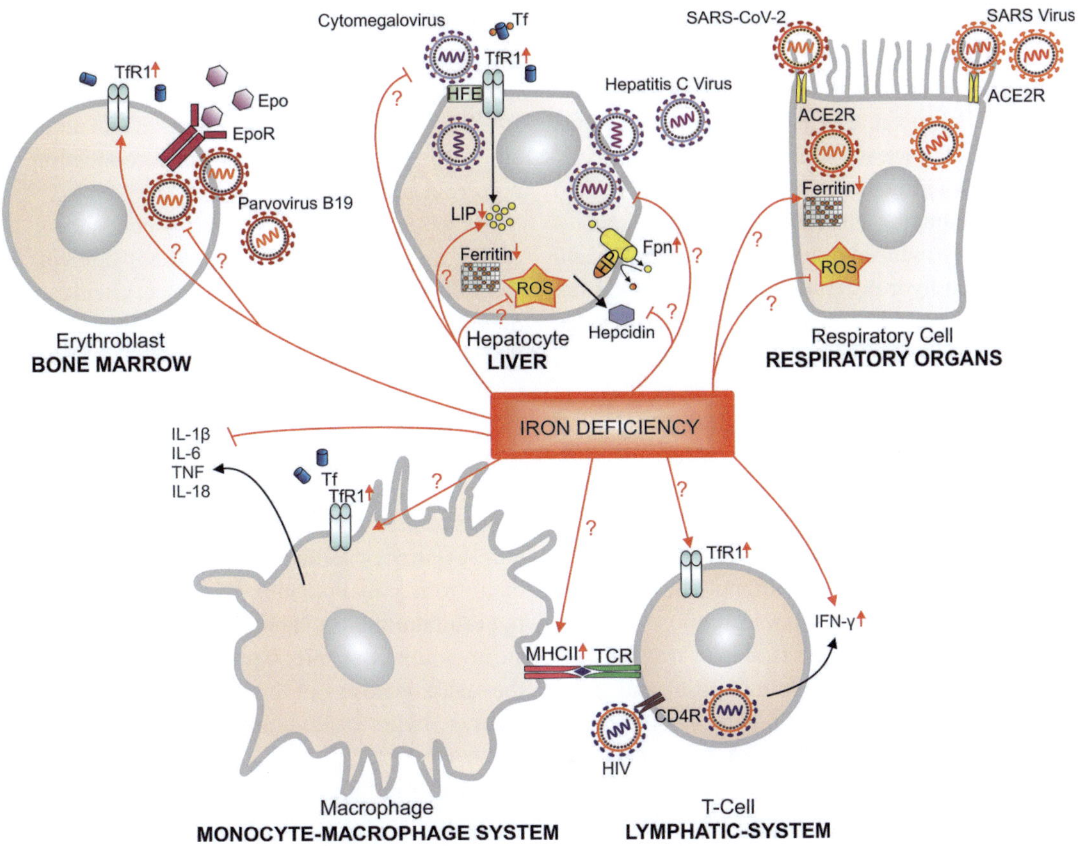

Fig. 18.2 Putative effects of iron deficiency (ID) on the course of viral infections. Parvovirus B19 mainly infects cells of the erythroid lineage and thus depends on EPO for survival and replication [53]. Hepatitis C virus (HCV) alters iron metabolism by reducing the level of hepcidin, leading to iron accumulation in hepatocytes and is related to production of reactive oxygen species (ROS) and liver damage [54]. Cytomegalovirus (CMV) facilitates iron accumulation in the tissue via degradation of HFE, a competitor of the transferrin Receptor 1 (TfR1) [55]. Severe acute respiratory syndrome coronavirus 2 (SARS-CoV-2) causes hyperinflammation with cytokine storm and systemic iron dysregulation. Reported intracellular ferritin excess, due to iron overload, leads to generation of ROS and finally to ferroptosis and is linked to tissue damage and organ failure [35]. SARS Virus and SARS-CoV2 are likely to use host metabolic pathways and enzymes, which depend on iron [37]. Iron is required for Human deficiency Virus (HIV) replication [34]. The virus is known to infect T cells via interaction with CD4 receptor [34]. Putative effects of ID during virus infection (shown in red) might limit the iron availability for the invading virus and reduce the deleterious effects of excess intracellular iron via ROS production and inflammation. Reduction of intracellular iron by chelation is known to have an inhibitory effect on the production of TNF and other cytokines involved in hyperinflammation [35]. Additionally, IFN-γ modulates the iron pool and immune functions by promoting the synthesis of nitric oxide and might thereby contribute to an antiviral effect of this cytokine. Therefore, mild iron deficiency may reduce viral replication [13]

for human immune deficiency virus (HIV) infection and viral hepatitis, but is also suggested for coronavirus disease-2019 (COVID-19) [34, 35].

In HIV-1 infection, iron is involved in several key steps of viral reproduction [34]. For example, the ATPase involved in assembly of the HIV capsid binds iron. Strikingly, also the ATP hydrolases necessary to unwind the severe acute respiratory syndrome coronavirus (SARS-CoV) and Middle East respiratory syndrome coronavirus (MERS-CoV) [36] genome during viral replication bind iron [37].

Importantly, interactions between iron homeostasis and the course of viral infection not only exist at the cellular level, but also at the systemic levels with clinical implications. For instance, iron accumulation and alterations in the mitochondrial electron transport system have been observed in patients with chronic hepatitis C virus (HCV) infection. The liver injury is related to the production of reactive oxygen species (ROS), ROS-induced mitochondrial damage, and iron-derived hydroxyl radical production via the Fenton reaction [38]. Many studies explored the connection between iron and HCV life cycle with controversial results. Some studies show that iron promotes HCV replication, while others found that iron suppresses HCV replication [38–40]. Some reports also indicate that anemia is associated with poor outcome of HIV infection [34].

Conversely, data from patients with hepatitis B virus (HBV) and HCV infection link conditions of iron overload to a poor prognosis [41]. In accordance with this, increased liver iron is commonly observed in HCV infection and may become a driver of disease progression, because increased iron accumulation in hepatocytes is associated with alterations in iron metabolism and reduced levels of hepcidin [38]. This is in line with the increased mortality from HIV-1 infection reported in another study. Changes in iron metabolism toward iron overload are also achieved by cytomegalovirus (CMV) where the viral protein US2 leads to degradation of HFE protein after binding to it. Similarly, during HIV infection, Nef protein important for the progression to AIDS downregulates HFE, a competitor of TfR1 to bind Tf, thereby increasing iron accumulation [34]. Besides, TfR1 was identified as the cellular receptor for some of the New World hemorrhagic fever arenaviruses [42].

Regarding parvovirus B19 (B19V), known to mainly infect erythroid progenitor cells, little is known in context of iron metabolism. B19V can cause a variety of mild to severe hematological disorders, including aplastic crisis in patients with hemolytic anemia or persistent anemia in immunosuppressed patients. Interestingly, EPO/EPOR signaling, regulated by hypoxia, is not only essential for differentiation and development of erythroid progenitors and the production of mature RBCs, but is also crucial for B19V DNA replication. While the underlying mechanisms have not systematically been explored, it is tempting to speculate that the EPO response to B19V-induced anemia stimulates TfR1 expression, iron uptake, and thus virus replication in erythroid cells [43].

Recently, SARS-CoV-2 has been shown to cause a severe respiratory illness known as COVID-19, which leads to a worldwide pandemic starting in 2020. In susceptible cohorts, SARS-CoV-2 can rapidly cause high mortality rates due to hypoxemia and multiorgan failure [35]. In a closely related disorder, SARS, increased levels of proinflammatory cytokines including IL-1β, IL-6, and IFN-γ have been shown to be coupled to pulmonary inflammation and respiratory failure. In accordance with this, data from patients with COVID-19 show that hyperinflammation, and the resulting cytokine storm with massive IL-6 production, are linked to the pathogenesis of multiorgan failure [44]. Further, hyperferritinemia is a second hallmark of severe COVID-19 and reported to increase patients' mortality risk [35]. Vice versa, low serum iron was, in the face of comparable Ft levels, associated with low lymphocyte numbers and severe hypoxemia in critically ill COVID-19 patients, and again it remains unidentified if ID is a risk factor for impaired immunity against SARS-CoV-2 or a surrogate indicating poor clinical course in COVID-19 patients [45]. However, hyperinflammation, in association with altered iron homeostasis, has been suggested to play a key role in the pathogenesis of inflammatory diseases including viral infections [34, 38].

IL-6 is well known as key mediator of inflammation-driven iron management, thereby inducing hepcidin, which regulates iron transport. Inflammation therefore leads to functional ID as reflected by hyperferritinemia and low serum iron levels. Especially severe COVID-19 causes prolonged alterations of iron homeostasis, also at systemic levels with persisting lung pathologies and impaired physical performance, as was shown in an observational study. In addition, hyperferritinemia and increased expression of hepcidin and inflammation markers, such as IL-6 and C-reactive protein, were still found

2 months after COVID-19 onset in a pertinent proportion of these patients [46]. Mechanistic suggestions link hyperferritinemia and alterations in hepcidin regulation to iron toxicity, which may lead to end-organ damage in COVID-19 [35]. This is supported by data demonstrating that inflammation induces ferroptosis, an iron-dependent cellular pathway that finally leads to cell death that involves iron-dependent accumulation of lipid peroxides [47].

As treatment for severe disease is still suboptimal, uncovering the role of iron homeostasis and ferroptosis in multiple organ involvement could open avenues to new treatment strategies.

A plethora of enzymatic processes require iron and viruses exploit such cellular pathways for their entry into host cells or replication therein, implying that iron metabolism affects viral diseases. While much progress has been made to characterize the interconnections between iron homeostasis and viral infections at a molecular level, we are only just beginning to understand what these interconnections mean for clinical outcome or how we can manipulate iron levels to treat infections with known or emerging viruses. For example, treatment with iron chelators like deferiprone inhibited virus proliferation and induced apoptosis in HIV infection [34, 38]. Thus, depriving iron supply might also be a promising therapeutic option in COVID-19 [35].

Iron and Allergy as Immune-Mediated Disease

Allergies are immune-mediated diseases caused by a hypersensitivity of the immune system towards exogenous, usually harmless antigens derived from animal dander, house dust mites, insect venom, and pollen as well as from food components. In particular, in western societies, the prevalence of allergy seems to increase, with approximately 20% of adults in Germany being currently affected by at least one allergy [29].

Several studies associate ID and IDA with the development of allergic diseases and the onset of allergy. As such, poor iron status of mother and child can increase the risk of developing allergic diseases, for instance, wheezing and asthma [29]. Immune activation under low iron status may result in the expansion of T_H2 cells due to their larger intracellular iron pool, the induction of class-switching in B cells, and a reduction in the anti-inflammatory role of M2-like macrophages [26]. Moreover, both the use of iron fortification and supplementation and the incidence of allergies are increasing, implying that the interconnections between iron metabolism and T_H2 immunity are incompletely understood. Furthermore, diverse allergens have lipocalin-like protein folds, and were shown to bind iron via siderophores [29].

Furthermore, atopic diseases like food allergies might lead to avoidance of suspected food and thus might lead to malnutrition. Together with chronic inflammation and use of systemic immunosuppressant medications, these factors are associated with IDA [29].

In conclusion, despite the increasing prevalence of allergies in high-income countries, little is known about how iron homeostasis and the different types of hypersensitivity reactions are interconnected.

Summary and Outlook

ID is a frequent clinical condition and, if long-lasting and severe, has a plethora of systemic consequences, which are not limited to the erythropoietic system, extending to the immune system as well. Therefore, a complex network exists that links iron homeostasis and the function of the immune system. The interconnections are reciprocal and relevant for both cellular pathways and clinical outcomes. In the last decades, we have characterized the key players of iron homeostasis and the main effects that immune activation has on systemic iron metabolism. Recently, we have also begun to investigate the interconnections between cellular iron and energy metabolism and how this affects the function of immune cell populations, for instance, during infections [48].

While new pathogens, which dysregulate iron homeostasis, such as SARS-CoV-2, are entering the field, we still lack a fundamental understanding of how altered iron metabolism affects the pathophysiologic processes of inflammatory diseases. In order to better fight off invading pathogens and malignant cells, we need to learn how to pharmacologically fine-tune host iron metabolism so that the clinical course of infectious and neoplastic diseases can be improved in affected individuals. The pathophysiology and pharmacology of AI are excellent examples, since we have an increasing armamentarium of iron-targeting therapies at hand, but we know little about their potential effects on the disorders, which underlie the AI.

References

1. Muckenthaler MU, Rivella S, Hentze MW, Galy B. A red carpet for iron metabolism. Cell. 2017;168(3):344–61. https://doi.org/10.1016/j.cell.2016.12.034.
2. Lopez A, Cacoub P, Macdougall IC, Peyrin-Biroulet L. Iron deficiency anaemia. Lancet. 2016;387(10021):907–16. https://doi.org/10.1016/S0140-6736(15)60865-0.
3. Cronin SJF, Woolf CJ, Weiss G, Penninger JM. The role of iron regulation in immunometabolism and immune-related disease. Front Mol Biosci. 2019;6:116. https://doi.org/10.3389/fmolb.2019.00116.
4. Nairz M, Theurl I, Wolf D, Weiss G. Iron deficiency or anemia of inflammation? Differential diagnosis and mechanisms of anemia of inflammation. Wien Med Wochenschr. 2016;166(13–14):411–23. https://doi.org/10.1007/s10354-016-0505-7.
5. Auerbach M, Adamson JW. How we diagnose and treat iron deficiency anemia. Am J Hematol. 2016;91(1):31–8. https://doi.org/10.1002/ajh.24201.
6. Weiss G, Ganz T, Goodnough LT. Anemia of inflammation. Blood. 2019;133(1):40–50. https://doi.org/10.1182/blood-2018-06-856500.
7. Camaschella C. Iron deficiency. Blood. 2019;133(1):30–9. https://doi.org/10.1182/blood-2018-05-815944.
8. Shaw JG, Friedman JF. Iron deficiency anemia: focus on infectious diseases in lesser developed countries. Anemia. 2011;2011:260380. https://doi.org/10.1155/2011/260380.
9. Kassebaum NJ, Jasrasaria R, Naghavi M, Wulf SK, Johns N, Lozano R, et al. A systematic analysis of global anemia burden from 1990 to 2010. Blood. 2014;123(5):615–24. https://doi.org/10.1182/blood-2013-06-508325.
10. Armitage AE, Moretti D. The importance of iron status for young children in low- and middle-income countries: a narrative review. Pharmaceuticals (Basel). 2019;12(2) https://doi.org/10.3390/ph12020059.
11. Sazawal S, Black RE, Ramsan M, Chwaya HM, Stoltzfus RJ, Dutta A, et al. Effects of routine prophylactic supplementation with iron and folic acid on admission to hospital and mortality in preschool children in a high malaria transmission setting: community-based, randomised, placebo-controlled trial. Lancet. 2006;367(9505):133–43. https://doi.org/10.1016/S0140-6736(06)67962-2.
12. Soofi S, Cousens S, Iqbal SP, Akhund T, Khan J, Ahmed I, et al. Effect of provision of daily zinc and iron with several micronutrients on growth and morbidity among young children in Pakistan: a cluster-randomised trial. Lancet. 2013;382(9886):29–40. https://doi.org/10.1016/S0140-6736(13)60437-7.
13. Nairz M, Ferring-Appel D, Casarrubea D, Sonnweber T, Viatte L, Schroll A, et al. Iron regulatory proteins mediate host resistance to salmonella infection. Cell Host Microbe. 2015;18(2):254–61. https://doi.org/10.1016/j.chom.2015.06.017.
14. Gwamaka M, Kurtis JD, Sorensen BE, Holte S, Morrison R, Mutabingwa TK, et al. Iron deficiency protects against severe Plasmodium falciparum malaria and death in young children. Clin Infect Dis. 2012;54(8):1137–44. https://doi.org/10.1093/cid/cis010.
15. Kabyemela ER, Fried M, Kurtis JD, Mutabingwa TK, Duffy PE. Decreased susceptibility to plasmodium falciparum infection in pregnant women with iron deficiency. J Infect Dis. 2008;198(2):163–6. https://doi.org/10.1086/589512.
16. Hill DL, Carr EJ, Rutishauser T, Moncunill G, Campo JJ, Innocentin S, et al. Immune system development varies according to age, location, and anemia in African children. Sci Transl Med. 2020;12(529) https://doi.org/10.1126/scitranslmed.aaw9522.
17. Petzer V, Theurl I, Weiss G. Established and emerging concepts to treat imbalances of iron homeostasis in inflammatory diseases. Pharmaceuticals (Basel). 2018;11(4) https://doi.org/10.3390/ph11040135.
18. Culleton BF, Manns BJ, Zhang J, Tonelli M, Klarenbach S, Hemmelgarn BR. Impact of anemia on hospitalization and mortality in older adults. Blood. 2006;107(10):3841–6. https://doi.org/10.1182/blood-2005-10-4308.
19. Andro M, Le Squere P, Estivin S, Gentric A. Anaemia and cognitive performances in the elderly: a systematic review. Eur J Neurol. 2013;20(9):1234–40. https://doi.org/10.1111/ene.12175.
20. Homer MJ, Aguilar-Delfin I, Telford SR 3rd, Krause PJ, Persing DH. Babesiosis. Clin Microbiol Rev. 2000;13(3):451–69. https://doi.org/10.1128/cmr.13.3.451-469.2000.
21. Sheldon JR, Heinrichs DE. Recent developments in understanding the iron acquisition strategies of gram positive pathogens. FEMS Microbiol Rev. 2015;39(4):592–630. https://doi.org/10.1093/femsre/fuv009.

22. Cassat JE, Skaar EP. Iron in infection and immunity. Cell Host Microbe. 2013;13(5):509–19. https://doi.org/10.1016/j.chom.2013.04.010.
23. Schaible UE, Kaufmann SH. Iron and microbial infection. Nat Rev Microbiol. 2004;2(12):946–53. https://doi.org/10.1038/nrmicro1046.
24. Recalcati S, Locati M, Gammella E, Invernizzi P, Cairo G. Iron levels in polarized macrophages: regulation of immunity and autoimmunity. Autoimmun Rev. 2012;11(12):883–9. https://doi.org/10.1016/j.autrev.2012.03.003.
25. Drakesmith H, Prentice AM. Hepcidin and the iron-infection axis. Science. 2012;338(6108):768–72. https://doi.org/10.1126/science.1224577.
26. Weiss G. Iron and immunity: a double-edged sword. Eur J Clin Investig. 2002;32(Suppl 1):70–8. https://doi.org/10.1046/j.1365-2362.2002.0320s1070.x.
27. Arezes J, Foy N, McHugh K, Sawant A, Quinkert D, Terraube V, et al. Erythroferrone inhibits the induction of hepcidin by BMP6. Blood. 2018;132(14):1473–7. https://doi.org/10.1182/blood-2018-06-857995.
28. Weigel KJ, Lynch SG, LeVine SM. Iron chelation and multiple sclerosis. ASN Neuro. 2014;6(1):e00136. https://doi.org/10.1042/AN20130037.
29. Roth-Walter F, Pacios LF, Bianchini R, Jensen-Jarolim E. Linking iron-deficiency with allergy: role of molecular allergens and the microbiome. Metallomics. 2017;9(12):1676–92. https://doi.org/10.1039/c7mt00241f.
30. Savy M, Edmond K, Fine PE, Hall A, Hennig BJ, Moore SE, et al. Landscape analysis of interactions between nutrition and vaccine responses in children. J Nutr. 2009;139(11):2154S–218S. https://doi.org/10.3945/jn.109.105312.
31. Zimmermann M, Stoffel N, Uyoga M, Karanja S. Effects of anaemia and iron supplementation on vaccine response: a birth cohort study and a randomized trial follow-up study in Kenyan infants. Curr Dev Nutr. 2020;4(Supplement_2):1115. https://doi.org/10.1093/cdn/nzaa054_187.
32. WHO. Fact sheet - Children: improving survival and well-being. https://www.who.int/news-room/fact-sheets/detail/children-reducing-mortality2020.
33. Eiselt J, Kielberger L, Rajdl D, Racek J, Pazdiora P, Malanova L. Previous vaccination and age are more important predictors of immune response to influenza vaccine than inflammation and iron status in dialysis patients. Kidney Blood Press Res. 2016;41(2):139–47. https://doi.org/10.1159/000443416.
34. Drakesmith H, Prentice A. Viral infection and iron metabolism. Nat Rev Microbiol. 2008;6(7):541–52. https://doi.org/10.1038/nrmicro1930.
35. Edeas M, Saleh J, Peyssonnaux C. Iron: innocent bystander or vicious culprit in COVID-19 pathogenesis? Int J Infect Dis. 2020; https://doi.org/10.1016/j.ijid.2020.05.110.
36. Desai MR, Holtz TH, Helfand R, Terlouw DJ, Wannemuehler KA, Kariuki SK, et al. Relationship of measles vaccination with anaemia and malaria in western Kenya. Tropical Med Int Health. 2005;10(11):1099–107. https://doi.org/10.1111/j.1365-3156.2005.01494.x.
37. Liu W, Zhang S, Nekhai S, Liu S. Depriving iron supply to the virus represents a promising adjuvant therapeutic against viral survival. Curr Clin Microbiol Rep. 2020:1–7. https://doi.org/10.1007/s40588-020-00140-w.
38. Schmidt SM. The role of iron in viral infections. Front Biosci (Landmark Ed). 2020;25:893–911.
39. Foka P, Dimitriadis A, Karamichali E, Kyratzopoulou E, Giannimaras D, Koskinas J, et al. Alterations in the iron homeostasis network: a driving force for macrophage-mediated hepatitis C virus persistency. Virulence. 2016;7(6):679–90. https://doi.org/10.1080/21505594.2016.1175700.
40. Fillebeen C, Pantopoulos K. Iron inhibits replication of infectious hepatitis C virus in permissive Huh7.5.1 cells. J Hepatol. 2010;53(6):995–9. https://doi.org/10.1016/j.jhep.2010.04.044.
41. Fujita N, Sugimoto R, Urawa N, Araki J, Mifuji R, Yamamoto M, et al. Hepatic iron accumulation is associated with disease progression and resistance to interferon/ribavirin combination therapy in chronic hepatitis C. J Gastroenterol Hepatol. 2007;22(11):1886–93. https://doi.org/10.1111/j.1440-1746.2006.04759.x.
42. Radoshitzky SR, Abraham J, Spiropoulou CF, Kuhn JH, Nguyen D, Li W, et al. Transferrin receptor 1 is a cellular receptor for New World haemorrhagic fever arenaviruses. Nature. 2007;446(7131):92–6. https://doi.org/10.1038/nature05539.
43. Luo Y, Qiu J. Human parvovirus B19: a mechanistic overview of infection and DNA replication. Future Virol. 2015;10(2):155–67. https://doi.org/10.2217/fvl.14.103.
44. Huang C, Wang Y, Li X, Ren L, Zhao J, Hu Y, et al. Clinical features of patients infected with 2019 novel coronavirus in Wuhan, China. Lancet. 2020;395(10223):497–506. https://doi.org/10.1016/S0140-6736(20)30183-5.
45. Shah A, Frost JN, Aaron L, Donovan K, Drakesmith H, Collaborators. Systemic hypoferremia and severity of hypoxemic respiratory failure in COVID-19. Crit Care. 2020;24(1):320. https://doi.org/10.1186/s13054-020-03051-w.
46. Sonnweber T, Boehm A, Sahanic S, Pizzini A, Aichner M, Sonnweber B, et al. Persisting alterations of iron homeostasis in COVID-19 are associated with non-resolving lung pathologies and poor patients' performance: a prospective observational cohort study. Respir Res. 2020;21(1):276. https://doi.org/10.1186/s12931-020-01546-2.
47. Yang M, Lai CL. SARS-CoV-2 infection: can ferroptosis be a potential treatment target for multiple organ involvement? Cell Death Discov. 2020;6(1):130. https://doi.org/10.1038/s41420-020-00369-w.
48. Telser J, Volani C, Hilbe R, Seifert M, Brigo N, Paglia G, et al. Metabolic reprogramming of salmonella infected macrophages and its modulation by iron availability and the mTOR pathway. Microb

Cell. 2019;6(12):531–43. https://doi.org/10.15698/mic2019.12.700.
49. Kautz L, Jung G, Valore EV, Rivella S, Nemeth E, Ganz T. Identification of erythroferrone as an erythroid regulator of iron metabolism. Nat Genet. 2014;46(7):678–84. https://doi.org/10.1038/ng.2996.
50. Zhang AS, Anderson SA, Meyers KR, Hernandez C, Eisenstein RS, Enns CA. Evidence that inhibition of hemojuvelin shedding in response to iron is mediated through neogenin. J Biol Chem. 2007;282(17):12547–56. https://doi.org/10.1074/jbc.M608788200.
51. Pasricha SR, Lim PJ, Duarte TL, Casu C, Oosterhuis D, Mleczko-Sanecka K, et al. Hepcidin is regulated by promoter-associated histone acetylation and HDAC3. Nat Commun. 2017;8(1):403. https://doi.org/10.1038/s41467-017-00500-z.
52. Weiss G, Goodnough LT. Anemia of chronic disease. N Engl J Med. 2005;352(10):1011–23. https://doi.org/10.1056/NEJMra041809.
53. Chen AY, Guan W, Lou S, Liu Z, Kleiboeker S, Qiu J. Role of erythropoietin receptor signaling in parvovirus B19 replication in human erythroid progenitor cells. J Virol. 2010;84(23):12385–96. https://doi.org/10.1128/JVI.01229-10.
54. Nishina S, Hino K, Korenaga M, Vecchi C, Pietrangelo A, Mizukami Y, et al. Hepatitis C virus-induced reactive oxygen species raise hepatic iron level in mice by reducing hepcidin transcription. Gastroenterology. 2008;134(1):226–38. https://doi.org/10.1053/j.gastro.2007.10.011.
55. Vahdati-Ben Arieh S, Laham N, Schechter C, Yewdell JW, Coligan JE, Ehrlich R. A single viral protein HCMV US2 affects antigen presentation and intracellular iron homeostasis by degradation of classical HLA class I and HFE molecules. Blood. 2003;101(7):2858–64. https://doi.org/10.1182/blood-2002-07-2158.

19 Genetic Hemoglobin Disorders and Their Association with Hemoglobin Concentration and Biomarkers of Nutritional Anemia

Crystal D. Karakochuk, Aviva I. Rappaport, and Brock A. Williams

Hemoglobin and its Structure, Function and Synthesis

Hemoglobin is a protein molecule in red blood cells (RBCs) that primarily functions to carry oxygen from the lungs to the tissues, and consequently, to carry carbon dioxide from the tissues back to the lungs [1].

Hemoglobin has a quaternary protein structure containing four globin proteins (also referred to as globin chains) and four iron-containing heme molecules [2]. Normal adult hemoglobin (called hemoglobin A, depicted as $\alpha_2\beta_2$) is composed of two α-globin proteins, two β-globin proteins and four heme molecules (Fig. 19.1). Across the lifespan, other forms of hemoglobin can also exist. For example, in fetuses and infants, the hemoglobin molecule contains two α-globin proteins and two γ-proteins (called fetal hemoglobin or hemoglobin F, depicted as $\alpha_2{}^{G}\gamma_2$) [2]. As the infant grows, the γ-globin proteins are gradually replaced by β-globin proteins, forming the adult hemoglobin structure. There are also other less common species of hemoglobin that exist in humans, either during early intrauterine life (e.g. Gower 1, Portland 1) or adulthood (hemoglobin A_2).

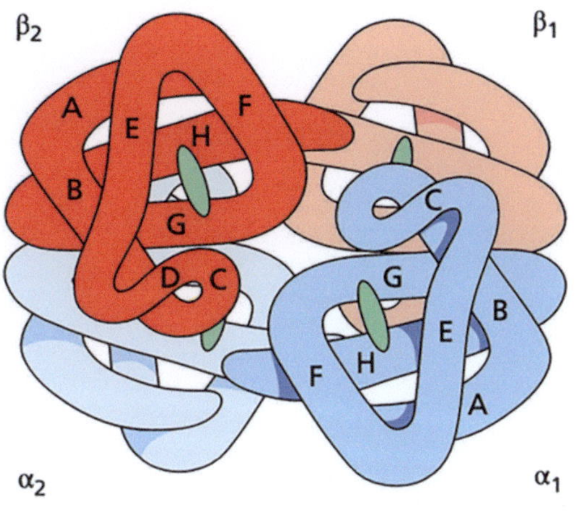

Fig. 19.1 Quaternary structure of a normal adult hemoglobin A molecule (Bains B) [2]. Permission obtained from Rightslink

Supplementary Information The online version contains supplementary material available at https://doi.org/10.1007/978-3-031-14521-6_19.

C. D. Karakochuk (✉)
Human Nutrition, The University of British Columbia, Vancouver, BC, Canada
e-mail: crystal.karakochuk@ubc.ca

B. A. Williams
Food Nutrition and Health, The University of British Columbia, Vancouver, BC, Canada

BC Children's Hospital Research Institute, Vancouver, BC, Canada

A. I. Rappaport
School of Human Nutrition, McGill University, Sainte-Anne-de-Bellevue, QC, Canada

C. D. Karakochuk et al. (eds.), *Nutritional Anemia*, Nutrition and Health,
https://doi.org/10.1007/978-3-031-14521-6_19

Genetic Hemoglobin Disorders

The α-globin and β-globin proteins of hemoglobin are encoded by four α-genes and two β-genes, respectively. Deletions and/or point mutations in these α- and/or β-genes can result in a decreased production of hemoglobin or structurally variant forms of hemoglobin, that are collectively referred to as genetic hemoglobin disorders or hemoglobinopathies. Genetic hemoglobin disorders are generally categorized as either structural hemoglobin variants or thalassemia (Table 19.1) [3].

Genetic hemoglobin disorders can result from one or multiple combinations of point mutations, insertions, or deletions that occur in single, compound, and/or coinherited forms, thus, characterizing the abnormalities of globin gene synthesis can be complicated. The consequences of point mutations (alterations of a single nucleotide) varies widely and can result in no effect on the amino acid sequence, or can have varying impact on the characteristics of the hemoglobin molecule, depending on the site of the mutation [2].

Table 19.1 Two major types of genetic hemoglobin disorders

	Structural hemoglobin variants	Thalassemias
Pathophysiology	A point mutation in one or more genes encoding the α-globin or β-globin protein	A deletion or duplication in one or more genes encoding the α-globin or β-globin protein
Consequence(s)	Structurally altered hemoglobin molecule; potential and varying effect on stability, oxygen affinity, solubility or other critical characteristic of the hemoglobin molecule	Impaired or reduced rate of synthesis of one or more of the globin protein molecules
Examples	Hb S (sickle cell), Hb E, Hb C, Hb Constant Spring, Hb Paksé	α-or β-thalassemia

Genetic hemoglobin disorders can result in diverse clinical outcomes depending on the inheritance pattern and severity of the disorder. Genetic hemoglobin disorders are autosomal-recessive conditions, which means they are passed down from parent(s) to their offspring. Individuals who inherit an affected chromosome from only one parent are termed heterozygous, also referred to as carriers or traits (e.g., sickle cell trait or α-thalassemia minor), whereas individuals who inherit affected chromosomes from both parents are termed homozygous (e.g., sickle cell disease or β-thalassemia major). Homozygous disorders result in a more severe phenotype (e.g., more severe anemia and associated complications). The clinical outcomes of these disorders can range from relatively asymptomatic (e.g., α-thalassemia minor) to extremely severe (e.g., Bart's Hydrops Fetalis) [4]. Some individuals with severe homozygous disorders (e.g., β-thalassemia major) require life-long blood transfusions to prevent further morbidity and/or mortality [5].

Laboratory Methodologies for Diagnosis

The diagnosis of genetic hemoglobin disorders can be complex and often require more than one technique for detection and/or diagnosis. A genetic DNA test is often required for definitive diagnosis. High-performance liquid chromatography (HPLC) is an automated and high-throughput technique that can identify many variant hemoglobin types from normal hemoglobin. However, this method requires an established laboratory, expensive equipment and reagents, and skilled technicians. Hemoglobin electrophoresis and isoelectric focusing are other common methods to detect structural hemoglobin variants. Some small automated benchtop equipment provide a high-throughput option for hemoglobin electrophoresis, including specialized programs to differentiate between hemoglobin molecules. For example, use of the Sebia MINICAP analyzer and a specialized Hemoglobin E program can detect both normal hemoglobin and hemoglobin variants (e.g., E, H, Constant Spring), and has an additional advantage of being able to differentiate between Hb A_2 and E, both of which are common in some areas of Southeast Asia. Polymerase chain reaction (PCR) assays can also be used to detect α-or β-thalassemia in samples of extracted DNA; however, these techniques can be complex and require skilled technicians and established laboratories. Relatively easy-to-use kits have also been developed (StripAssay Kit, Vienna-Lab Diagnostics) that can detect multiple different gene deletions and point mutations on test strips that generate test results by enzymatic color reaction that are visible to the naked eye for diagnosis of α-or β-thalassemia. Lastly, some simplified solubility tests exist for the detection of Hb sickle cell and are available in commercially available, relatively easy-to-use kits. Ultimately, the detection and diagnosis of genetic hemoglobin disorders remains a challenge in many low-resource countries due to limited access to specialized laboratory methods, skilled technicians, and the high-cost of many of these techniques.

Global Distribution of Genetic Hemoglobin Disorders

Genetic hemoglobin disorders are one of the most common monogenic disorders in the world. The high gene frequencies for these disorders are attributable to the theory of natural selection. Many types of these genetic mutations conferred protection against severe malaria, this "natural selection" is the predominant reason for the high prevalence observed in historically malaria-endemic areas of the world [6]. Although these genetic disorders have historically been most frequent in tropical regions, increased global migration has translated to an increasing disease burden worldwide.

Certain genetic hemoglobin disorders are more common in different regions of the world. For example, sickle cell disease is one of the most common disorders, with an estimated 300,000 affected infants born each year globally [7]. Table 19.2 summarizes the global distribution of some of the more common genetic hemoglobin disorders worldwide. The prevalence of Hb S (sickle cell) and many of the other hemoglobin disorders are highest in sub-Saharan Africa, although accurate global and national estimates of all the hemoglobin disorders are difficult to obtain due to inherent limitations in diagnostic testing and reporting in low- and middle-income countries.

Table 19.2 Pathophysiology and global distribution of some common genetic hemoglobin disorders[a]

Type	Pathophysiology	Global distribution	References
Hb S (sickle cell)	Point mutation in a β-gene encoding the β-globin protein of hemoglobin, causing reduced solubility and a sickle-shaped hemoglobin molecule	Three well-known β-globin haplotypes are thought to have arisen in Africa: Senegal, Central African Republic and southern Africa (Bantu or CAR type), and Benin, Central, West and North Africa (Benin type). Migration from sub-Saharan Africa has led to high prevalence of Hb S in certain parts of Africa (Nigeria and DR Congo), India, the Middle East, the Mediterranean, the Caribbean, Europe, and the Americas. Hb S an also be coinherited with the Hb C (Hb SC), commonly found in north-west African regions	Bain et al. [2] Piel et al. [8] Wastnedge et al. [9]
Hb E	Point mutation in a β-gene encoding the β-globin protein of hemoglobin, causing a reduced rate of synthesis of β-globin and an unstable hemoglobin molecule	Most common in South-East Asia; highest prevalence found in Thailand, Cambodia, and Laos but also detected in South Asia (India, Sri Lanka, Pakistan, Bangladesh) and other parts of South-East Asia (the Philippines, Indonesia) and Europe (Turkey)	Bain et al. [2] Rees et al. [10]
α-Thalassemia	Typically due to a deletion or duplication of one or more genes, gene fusion, or loss of a gene that cause a reduced rate of synthesis of α-globin	α-Thalassemia deletions are highly prevalent worldwide. Most common are the -$\alpha^{3.7}$ and -$\alpha^{4.2}$, affecting populations in Africa, the Middle East, parts of Europe (Cypress, Greece, Italy), the Caribbean (Jamaica), South Asia (Pakistan, Nepal, India), South East Asia (Thailand, Cambodia, Laos) in varying prevalence rates Certain types of other α-thalassemia mutations are specific to certain ethnic groups (e.g., --^{SEA}, --^{FIL}, and --^{THAI} are common in South-East Asia and southern China, and --^{MED} is more common in the Mediterranean and Middle East)	Bain et al. [2] Piel et al. [11]
β-Thalassemia	Typically due to point mutations, or a deletion or duplication of one or more genes that cause a reduced rate of synthesis of β-globin	β-Thalassemia deletions are rarer than α-thalassemia, and can be found in India, the Mediterranean, Middle East (Saudi Arabia), South-East Asia, Africa, and parts of Europe (Greece, Cypress, Italy)	Bain et al. [2] Kattamis et al. [12]

[a] Genetic hemoglobin disorders can be coinherited; thus, individuals with these genetic disorders can carry more than one, resulting in different phenotypes and biological/clinical implications

Genetic Hemoglobin Disorders and their Association with Hemoglobin Concentration

It is well established that individuals with some genetic hemoglobin disorders have lower hemoglobin concentrations, regardless of iron status. The impact of a hemoglobin disorder on hemoglobin concentration typically correlates with the severity of the disorder (heterozygous vs. homozygous) and the physiological consequence of the disorder on the synthesis, structure, and/or function of hemoglobin. Genetic hemoglobin disorders can cause a reduced rate of synthesis of the hemoglobin molecule (leading to lower concentrations) or cause a dysfunctional hemoglobin structure that has a shorter lifespan. For example, in one study in Cambodia, hemoglobin concentrations were significantly lower among Cambodian women with the homozygous Hb EE disorder (n = 31, 109 ± 7.3 g/L) as compared to women with the normal (wildtype) hemoglobin genotype ($n = 195$, 130 ± 8.9 g/L; $p < 0.05$) [13]. This is an important consideration from a nutrition and public health perspective, as in individuals with genetic hemoglobin disorders, anemia may persist regardless of iron status, and iron or other nutritional interventions may not be effective to reduce, treat, or prevent anemia in these individuals.

Genetic Hemoglobin Disorders and their Association with Biomarkers of Nutritional Anemia

Certain genetic hemoglobin disorders can cause higher red blood cell turnover, due to chronic hemolysis and increased erythropoiesis seen in hereditary hemolytic conditions. Requirements of nutrients involved in erythropoiesis, including iron, soluble transferrin receptor (sTfR), zinc, folate, vitamins B_6 and B_{12}, and riboflavin are therefore thought to be increased in individuals with genetic hemoglobin disorders, especially if dietary intake is marginal. Conversely, deficiencies of these micronutrients can contribute to significant alterations in erythropoiesis. Deficiencies of folate, vitamins B_6 and B_{12}, and riboflavin can affect nucleic acid synthesis decreasing hemoglobin concentrations and cellular proliferation, and causing megaloblastic anemia [14]. This highlights the complex interplay among micronutrient deficiencies, hemoglobin disorders, and anemia, all of which may coexist in the same individual.

We systematically reviewed the literature for studies that measured ferritin, sTfR, zinc, folate, vitamin B_{12}, vitamin B_6, and riboflavin concentrations in individuals with genetic hemoglobin disorders as compared to controls. Full details of the search strategies and flow charts of inclusion are found in Online Supplementary File 1. Included studies are summarized below in Tables 19.3, 19.4, 19.5, 19.6, 19.7, 19.8, and 19.9: the arrows and symbols in these tables indicate whether or not the study populations in each of the listed studies demonstrated significantly higher or lower mean or median concentrations of each nutritional biomarker (or no significant difference) as compared to control subjects. Full citations for each listed reference in Tables 19.3, 19.4, 19.5, 19.6, 19.7, 19.8, and 19.9 are found in Online Supplementary File 2.

Table 19.3 Ferritin concentrations in study populations with genetic hemoglobin disorders compared to controls[a]

Genetic hemoglobin disorder	Study population	Fasted?	Ferritin concentrations	References[b]
Hb SS (sickle cell disease)	Pediatric, USA[c] Pediatric, Nigeria Adult, India[d]		↑ ↑ ↑	Lulla et al. (2010) Akodu et al. (2013) Mohanty et al. (2017)
Hb AS (sickle cell trait)	Pregnant women, The Gambia Pediatric, Cameroon Pediatric, Kenya		↑ ↑ –	Menendez et al. (1995) Engle-Stone et al. (2017) Byrd et al. (2018)
Mixed SCD genotypes	Adult, USA Pediatric, UK Pregnant women, Nigeria Adult, Nigeria Adult, Nigeria Adult, UK Adult, Nigeria Pediatric, Benin	Yes	↑ ↑ – ↑ ↑ ↑ ↑ ↑	Peterson et al. (1975) Hussain et al. (1978) Oluboyede et al. (1980) Oluboyede et al. (1983) Abudu et al. (1990) Ezeh (2005) Sani et al. (2015) Gomez et al. (2016)

(continued)

Table 19.3 (continued)

Genetic hemoglobin disorder	Study population	Fasted?	Ferritin concentrations	References[b]
Hb AE (heterozygous)	Pregnant women, Thailand		↑	Sanchaisuriya et al. (2007)
	Pediatric, Cambodia		–	George et al. (2012)
	Pediatric, Thailand		–	Nanta et al. (2021)
Hb EE (homozygous)	Pediatric, Thailand		↑	Thurlow et al. (2005)
	Pregnant women, Thailand		↑	Sanchaisuriya et al. (2007)
	Pediatric, Cambodia		–	George et al. (2012)
	Adult, Cambodia	Yes	↑	Karakochuk et al. (2015)
	Adult, Thailand		↑	Jamnok et al. (2020)
α-thalassemia trait	Pregnant women, Yemen/UAE/Oman		–	White et al. (1986)
	Adult, Spain	Yes	↑	Vaya et al. (2011)
	Pediatric, Kenya		–	Byrd et al. (2018)
	Pediatric, Cambodia		–	George et al. (2012)
	Adult, Thailand		↑	Jamnok et al. (2020)
Homozygous α-thalassemia	Pediatric, Vanuatu		–	Rees et al. (1998)
Hb E trait/α-thalassemia trait	Pregnant women, Thailand		↑	Sanchaisuriya et al. (2007)
	Pediatric, Cambodia		–	George et al. (2012)
Heterozygous β-thalassemia (minor)	Adult, UK		↑	Hussein et al. (1976)
	Pediatric, Greece		↑	Lagos et al. (1980)
	Pregnant women, Yemen/UAE/Oman		↑	White et al. (1986)
	Adult, India		–	Madan et al. (1996)
	Adult, Iran		–	Hashemi et al. (2007)
	Adult, Thailand	Yes	↑	Zimmermann et al. (2008)
	Pediatric, Turkey		↑	Canatan et al. (2012)
	Adult, Georgia	Yes	↑	Asadov et al. (2016)
Homozygous β-thalassemia (major)	Pediatric, Italy,	Yes	–	Galanello et al. (1980)
	Pediatric, India[d]		↑	Saraya et al. (1985)
	Adult, Melanesia		–	Bowden et al. (1987)
	Adult, India[d]		↑	Mehta et al. (1987)
	Pediatric & Adult, Germany[d]		↑	Cario et al. (2000)
	Pediatric, Egypt		↑	Ragab et al. (2002)
	Pediatric, Tunisia[d]	Yes	↑	Kassab-Chekir et al. (2003)
	Pediatric, India		↑	Naithani et al. (2006)
	Pediatric, Egypt[d]		↑	Shehata et al. (2010)
	Pediatric, Turkey		↑	Canatan et al. (2012)
	Pediatric, India[d]		↑	Bhagat et al. (2013)
	Pediatric, Iran	Yes	↑	Shahramian et al. (2013)
	Adult, Brazil		↑	Guimaraes et al. (2015)
	Pediatric, Iran		↑	Jahromi et al. (2015)
	Pediatric, India		↑	Behera et al. (2014)
	Pediatric, Egypt[d]		↑	Hagag et al. (2016)
	Pediatric, Egypt	Yes	↑	Kaddah et al. (2017)
	Adult, Gaza[d]		↑	Ayyash et al. (2018)
	Pediatric, Egypt		↑	Ismail et al. (2019)
	Pediatric, Indonesia		↑	Susanah et al. (2021)
β-thalassemia/HbE	Adult, Thailand	Yes	↑	Zimmermann et al. (2008)
	Pediatric, India		↑	Chakraborty et al. (2010)

[a]↑ symbol indicates that concentrations in those with the disorder were significantly higher as compared to control subjects; – symbol indicates no significant difference in concentration between case and control subjects

[b]Full citations for each listed reference are found in Online Supplementary File 2

[c]In comparison to Hb AS (heterozygous) genotype

[d]Study participants receiving red blood cell transfusions

Table 19.4 Soluble transferrin receptor (sTfR) concentrations in study populations with genetic hemoglobin disorders compared to controls[a]

Genetic hemoglobin disorder	Study population	Fasted?	sTfR concentrations	References[b]
Hb SS (sickle cell disease)	Pediatric, Jamaica		↑	Singhal et al. (1993)
	Adult, USA		↑	Croizat et al. (1999)
	Adult, Brazil		↑	Grotto et al. (1999)
	Pediatric, USA[c]		↑	Lulla et al. (2010)
	Adult, Nigeria[d]		–	Sani et al. (2015)
	Pediatric, Benin[d]		↑	Gomez et al. (2016)
	Pediatric, DR Congo[c]		↑	Barker et al. (2017)
Hb AE (heterozygous)	Pediatric, Cambodia		↑	George et al. (2012)
	Adult, Cambodia	Yes	↑	Karakochuk et al. (2015b)
	Pregnant women, Thailand		↑	Uaprasert et al. (2019)
Hb EE (homozygous)	Pediatric, Thailand		↑	Thurlow et al. (2005)
	Pediatric, Cambodia		↑	George et al. (2012)
	Adult, Cambodia	Yes	↑	Karakochuk et al. (2015a)
	Adult, Cambodia	Yes	↑	Karakochuk et al. (2015b)
HB CS	Adult, Cambodia	Yes	↑	Karakochuk et al. (2015a)
	Adult, Cambodia	Yes	↑	Karakochuk et al. (2015b)
α-Thalassemia trait	Pediatric, Vanuatu		↑	Rees et al. (1998)
	Pregnant women, Thailand		–	Uaprasert et al. (2009)
	Pediatric, Cambodia		↑	George et al. (2012)
	Adult, Cambodia	Yes	–	Karakochuk et al. (2015a)
Homozygous α-thalassemia	Pediatric, Vanuatu		↑	Rees et al. (1998)
	Adult, Cambodia	Yes	–	Karakochuk et al. (2015a)
Hb E trait/α-thalassemia trait	Pregnant women, Thailand		–	Uaprasert et al. (2009)
	Pediatric, Cambodia		↑	George et al. (2012)
	Adult, Cambodia		–	Karakochuk et al. (2015a)
Heterozygous β-thalassemia (minor)	Pediatric, Turkey		↑	Polat et al. (2002)
	Pediatric, Egypt		↑	Ragab et al. (2002)
	Adult, Greece		↑	Skarmoutsou et al. (2003)
	Pediatric, Turkey		↑	Demir et al. (2004)
	Adult, Malaysia		–	Jayaranee et al. (2006)
	Adult, USA[c,d]		↑	Origa et al. (2007)
	Adult, Italy		↑	Camberlein et al. (2008)
	Pediatric, Italy		↑	Danise et al. (2008)
	Pediatric, Greece		–	Chouliaras et al. (2009)
	Pediatric, Egypt		↑	Montaser et al. (2011)
	Adult, Iran		–	Jalali et al. (2012)
	Adult, Italy		↑	Ricchi et al. (2012)
Homozygous β-thalassemia (major)	Pediatric, Italy		↑	Musto et al. (1993)
	Adult, Italy[d]		↑	Dore et al. (1996)
	Adult, Italy		↑	Bianco et al. (2000)
	Pediatric, Thailand		↑	Bhokaisawan et al. (2002)
	Adult, Thailand[d]	Yes	↑	Dedoussis et al. (2002)
	Pediatric, Egypt		↑	Ragab et al. (2002)
	Adult, Italy		↑	Camberlein et al. (2008)
	Pediatric, Egypt[d]		↑	Shehata et al. (2010)
	Pediatric, Egypt		↑	Montaser et al. (2011)
	Adult, Italy		↑	Ricchi et al. (2012)
β-thalassemia/HbE	Pediatric, Thailand		↑	Bhokaisawan et al. (2002)
HbH (Hb Bart)	Pediatric, Greece		↑	Papassotiriou et al. (1998)

[a]↑ symbol indicates that concentrations in those with the disorder were significantly higher as compared to control subjects; – symbol indicates no significant difference in concentration between case and control subjects
[b]Full citations for each listed reference are found in Online Supplementary File 2
[c]In comparison to heterozygous genotype
[d]Study participants receiving red blood cell transfusions

Table 19.5 Plasma or serum zinc concentrations in study populations with genetic hemoglobin disorders compared to controls[a]

Genetic hemoglobin disorder	Study population	Fasted?	Serum/plasma zinc concentrations	References[b]
Hb SS (homozygous sickle cell)	Adult, USA		↓	Karayalcin et al. (1974)
	Adult, USA		↓	Prasad et al. (1975)
	Adult, USA		↓	Prasad et al. (1976)
	Adult, USA		↓	Niell et al. (1979)
	Pediatric, Netherlands		↓	Muskiet et al. (1984)
	Pediatric, USA		↓	Prasad et al. (1984)
	Pediatric, USA		–	Daeschner et al. (1985)
	Adult, Turkey		–	Donma et al. (1986)
	Pediatric, USA	Yes	–	Abshire et al. (1988)
	Pediatric, USA		↓	Phebus et al. (1988)
	Pediatric, Jordan		↓	Bashir et al. (1995)
	Adult, Turkey	Yes	↓	Arcasoy et al. (2001)
	Pediatric, Brazil		↓	Oliveira et al. (2001)
	Adults, Saudi Arabia	Yes	–	Hasanato et al. (2006)
	Pediatric, USA		–	Kuvibidilia et al. (2006)
	Adult, USA		↓	Bao et al. (2008)
	Pediatric, Nigeria		↓	Temiye et al. (2011)
	Pediatric, Nigeria		↓	Onukwuli et al. (2017)
	Pediatric, Democratic Republic of the Congo		↓	Sungu et al. (2018)
	Pediatric, Iraq		↓	Yousif et al. (2018)
	Pediatric, Nigeria		↓	Emokpae et al. (2019)
	Pediatric, Nigeria		↓	Kudirat et al. (2019)
Hb SC (heterozygous sickle cell)	Adult, USA		↓	Karayalcin et al. (1974)
	Pediatric, Brazil		↓	Oliveira et al. (2001)
Heterozygous β-thalassemia (minor)	Adults, Turkey	Yes	↓	Arcasoy et al. (2001)
Homozygous β-thalassemia (major)	Pediatric, USA		↓	Prasad et al. (1965)
	Pediatric, Turkey		↓[c]	Arcasoy et al. (1987)
	Pediatric, Jordan		↓	Bashir et al. (1995)
	Pediatric & adult, Turkey	Yes	↓	Arcasoy et al. (2001)
	Pediatric, Tunisia	Yes	↓[c]	Kassab-Chekir et al. (2003)
	Pediatric, Iran	Yes	↓[c]	Mashhadi et al. (2014)
	Pediatric, Pakistan		–[c]	El Missiry et al. (2014)
	Pediatric, India	Yes	↓[c]	Nidumuru et al. (2017)
	Pediatric, Sri Lanka		↓[c]	Karunaratna et al. (2018)
	Pediatric, Egypt	Yes	↓[c]	Sherief et al. (2014)

[a]↑ symbol indicates that mean/median concentrations in those with the disorder were significantly higher as compared to control subjects; "–"symbol indicates no significant difference in concentration between case and control subjects; ↓ symbol indicates that concentrations in those with the disorder were significantly lower as compared to control subjects

[b]Full citations for each listed reference are found in Online Supplementary File 2

[c]Study participants receiving red blood cell transfusions

Table 19.6 Folate concentrations in study populations with genetic hemoglobin disorders compared to controls[a]

Genetic hemoglobin disorder	Study population	Fasted?	Serum/plasma folate concentrations	References[b]
Hb SS (homozygous sickle cell)	Pediatric & adult, USA Pediatric, USA Adult, USA Pediatric, Nigeria[c] Pediatric, USA Pediatric, Curaçao Pediatric, USA Pediatric, Curaçao[d] Pediatric, USA Pediatric, Ghana[c] Adult, Saudi Arabia	Unknown Unknown Unknown Unknown Unknown Yes Unknown Yes Yes Unknown No	↓ ↓ ↓ ↑ – – – ↓ – ↑ –	Pearson et al. (1964) Liu (1974) Liu (1975) Osifo et al. (1984) Gray et al. (1992) van der Dijs et al. (1998) Rodriguez-Cortes et al. (1999) van der Dijs et al. (2002) Segal et al. (2004) Adjei et al. (2020) Kamal et al. (2021)
Hb SC (heterozygous sickle cell)	Pediatric, Curaçao	Yes	–	van der Dijs et al. (1998)
Hb AS (sickle cell trait)	Pediatric, USA Adult, USA	Unknown Unknown	↓ –	Liu (1974) Liu (1975)
Mixed SCD genotypes	Adult, USA[c] Adult, USA[c,e]	No Unknown	↑ ↑	Lowenthal et al. (2000) Ajayi et al. (2013)
Hb EE (homozygous)	Pediatric, Thailand	No	–	Thurlow et al. (2005)
Hb AE (heterozygous)	Pediatric, Thailand	No	–	Thurlow et al. (2005)
Homozygous β-thalassemia (major)	Pediatric & adult, India Pediatric & adult, Iran[f] Pediatric & adult, Turkey[c,f] Pediatric, Egypt[c,f] Adult, Brazil	Unknown Unknown Yes Yes Yes	↓ – ↑ ↑ ↓	Kumar et al. (1985) Mojtahedzadeh et al. (2006) Ozdem et al. (2008) Sherief et al. (2014) Paniz et al. (2020)
Heterozygous β-Thalassemia (minor)	Adult, Italy Pediatric & adult, India Pediatric & adult, Brazil Adult, Italy	Yes Unknown Yes Unknown	↓ ↓ – –	Castaldi et al. (1983) Saraya et al. (1984) Silva et al. (1989) Gallerani et al. (1990)
β-thalassemia/HbE	Pediatric & adult, Thailand	Unknown	↓	Vatanavicharn et al. (1979)
HbH (Hb Bart)	Pediatric & adult, Thailand	Unknown	↓	Vatanavicharn et al. (1979)
Genetic hemoglobin disorder	**Study population**	**Fasted?**	**RBC folate concentrations**	**References[b]**
Hb SS (homozygous sickle cell)	Pediatric, USA Adult, USA Pediatric, Nigeria[c] Pediatric, USA Pediatric, USA Pediatric, Curaçao[d] Pediatric, USA Pediatric, USA	Unknown Unknown Unknown Unknown Unknown Yes Yes Yes	– ↑ ↑ – – – ↑ –	Liu (1974) Liu (1975) Osifo et al. (1984) Gray et al. (1992) Rodriguez-Cortes et al. (1999) van der Dijs et al. (2002) Balasa et al. (2002) Segal et al. (2004)
Hb AS (sickle cell trait)	Pediatric, USA Adult, USA	Unknown Unknown	– –	Liu (1974) Liu (1975)
Hb EE (homozygous)	Pediatric, Thailand	No	–	Thurlow et al. (2005)
Hb AE (heterozygous)	Pediatric, Thailand	No	–	Thurlow et al. (2005)
Homozygous β-thalassemia (major)	Pediatric & adult, India	Unknown	↑	Kumar et al. (1985)

(continued)

Table 19.6 (continued)

Genetic hemoglobin disorder	Study population	Fasted?	RBC folate concentrations	References[b]
Heterozygous β-thalassemia (minor)	Adult, Italy	Yes	↓	Castaldi et al. (1983)
	Pediatric & adult, India	Unknown	↓	Saraya et al. (1984)
	Pediatric & adult, Israel	Unknown	–	Froom et al. (1985)
β-thalassemia/HbE	Pediatric & adult, Thailand	Unknown	↓	Vatanavicharn et al. (1979)
HbH (Hb Bart)	Pediatric & adult, Thailand	Unknown	–	Vatanavicharn et al. (1979)

[a]↑ symbol indicates that mean/median concentrations in those with the disorder were significantly higher as compared to control subjects; – symbol indicates no significant difference in concentration between case and control subjects; ↓ symbol indicates that concentrations in those with the disorder were significantly lower as compared to control subjects. RBC, red blood cells; SCD, sickle cell disease

[b]Full citations for each listed reference are found in Online Supplementary File 2

[c]Majority (>50%) of participants supplemented with routine folic acid (1–5 mg/d)

[d]In comparison to individuals with Hb SC genotype

[e]Significant number of participants treated with hydroxyurea (hydroxycarbamide)

[f]Study participants receiving red blood cell transfusions

Table 19.7 Plasma or serum vitamin B12 concentrations in study populations with genetic hemoglobin disorders compared to controls[a]

Genetic hemoglobin disorder	Study population	Fasted?	Vitamin B12 concentrations	References[b]
Hb SS (homozygous sickle cell)	Pediatric, Nigeria	Unknown	↓	Osifo et al. (1983)
	Pediatric, Nigeria	Unknown	↓	Osifo et al. (1984)
	Adult, Nigeria	Unknown	↓	Osifo et al., (1989)
	Pediatric, Curaçao[c]	Yes	–	van der Dijs et al. (1998)
	Pediatric, Curaçao[c]	Yes	–	van der Dijs et al. (2002)
	Pediatric, USA	Yes	–	Segal et al. (2004)
	Adult, Saudi Arabia	No	↓	Kamal et al. (2021)
Hb SC (heterozygous sickle cell)	Pediatric, Curaçao	Yes	↓	van der Dijs et al. (1998)
Mixed SCD genotypes	Pediatric & adult, Saudi Arabia	Unknown	↓	Al-Momen (1995)
	Adult, USA	No	–	Lowenthal et al. (2000)
	Adult, USA	No	–	Kamineni et al. (2006)
	Adult, USA[d]	Unknown	↓	Ajayi et al. (2013)
Hb EE (homozygous)	Pediatric, Thailand	No	–	Thurlow et al. (2005)
Hb AE (heterozygous)	Pediatric, Thailand	No	–	Thurlow et al. (2005)
Homozygous β-thalassemia (major)	Pediatric, India	Unknown	↑	Kumar et al. (1985)
	Pediatric & adult, Turkey[e]	Yes	–	Ozdem et al. (2008)
	Pediatric, Egypt[e]	Yes	↓	Sherief et al. (2014)
	Adult, Brazil	Yes	–	Paniz et al. (2020)
Heterozygous β-Thalassemia (minor)	Pediatric & adult, India	Unknown	↓	Saraya et al. (1984)
	Pediatric & adult, Brazil	Yes	–	Silva et al. (1989)
	Adult, Italy	Unknown	–	Gallerani et al. (1990)

[a]↑ symbol indicates that mean/median concentrations in those with the disorder were significantly higher as compared to control subjects; – symbol indicates no significant difference in concentration between case and control subjects; ↓ symbol indicates that concentrations in those with the disorder were significantly lower as compared to control subjects

[b]Full citations for each listed reference are found in Online Supplementary File 2

[c]In comparison to individuals with Hb SC genotype

[d]Participants treated with hydroxyurea (hydroxycarbamide)

[e]Study participants receiving red blood cell transfusions

Table 19.8 Plasma or whole blood vitamin B6 concentrations in study populations with genetic hemoglobin disorders compared to controls[a]

Genetic hemoglobin disorder	Study population	Fasted?	Vitamin B6 concentrations	References[b]
Hb SS (homozygous sickle cell)	Pediatric & adult, USA Pediatric, Curaçao[c] Pediatric, Curaçao[c] Pediatric, USA Pediatric, USA	Yes (cases) Yes Yes Yes Yes	↓ ↓ – ↓ ↓	Natta et al. (1984) van der Dijs et al. (1998) van der Dijs et al. (2002) Balasa et al. (2002) Segal et al., (2004)
Hb SC (heterozygous sickle cell)	Pediatric, Curaçao	Yes	–	van der Dijs et al. (1998)
Mixed SCD genotypes	Pediatric, USA	Unknown	–	Flores et al. (1988)

[a]↓ symbol indicates that mean/median concentrations in those with the disorder were significantly lower as compared to control subjects; – symbol indicates no significant difference in concentration between case and control subjects
[b]Full citations for each listed reference are found in Online Supplementary File 2
[c]In comparison to individuals with Hb SC genotype

Table 19.9 Riboflavin coefficients in study populations with genetic hemoglobin disorders compared to controls[a]

Genetic hemoglobin disorder	Study population	Fasted?	Riboflavin (EGRac) coefficients	References[b]
Hb SS (homozygous sickle cell)	Pediatric, Nigeria Pediatric, Nigeria	Unknown Unknown	– ↑	Adelekan et al. (1987) Adelekan et al. (1989)
Hb EE (homozygous)	Adult, Cambodia	Yes	↑	Williams et al. (2020)
Hb AE (heterozygous)	Adult, Cambodia	Yes	–	Williams et al. (2020)
α-thalassemia trait	Adult, Cambodia	Yes	–	Williams et al. (2020)
Hb E trait/α-thalassemia trait	Adult, Cambodia	Yes	–	Williams et al. (2020)
Heterozygous β-thalassemia (minor)	Adult, Italy	Unknown	↑	Anderson et al. (1989)

[a]↑ symbol indicates that values in those with the disorder were significantly higher as compared to control subjects; – symbol indicates no significant difference in values between case and control subjects. *EGRac* erythrocyte glutathione reductase activation coefficient
[b]Full citations for each listed reference are found in Online Supplementary File 2

Ferritin Concentrations

We found 27 studies in children and adolescents and 22 studies in adults, and 1 study in children and adults, which compared mean or median ferritin concentrations in study populations with genetic hemoglobin disorders compared to study controls (Table 19.3). Twenty-two of the 27 studies in children and adolescents and 18 of the 22 studies in adults demonstrated that study populations with genetic hemoglobin disorders had higher mean or median ferritin concentrations as compared to study controls; the remaining studies showed no difference between the two groups and no studies showed that ferritin concentrations were lower among those with genetic hemoglobin disorders compared to study controls.

Ferritin concentrations may be elevated in individuals with certain genetic hemoglobin disorders for several reasons. Some severe forms of hemoglobin disorders are associated with altered iron metabolism, induced by chronic erythropoietic stimuli, where hepcidin concentrations, the main regulator of iron metabolism, are lowered [15]. This can result in iron overload and/or high ferritin concentrations. Inflammation may also be a factor that is contributing to higher ferritin concentrations in those with certain genetic hemoglobin disorders where inflammation may coexist. In these cases, the inflammatory response stimulates the production of hepcidin, which binds to and degrades ferroportin, a transport protein on the wall of the macrophage, sequestering iron in the macrophage and preventing it from being accessible for red blood cell synthesis [16]. This results in "functional iron deficiency" and is thought to be a protective mechanism to prevent pathogenic organisms from using iron in circulation, and can also potentially contribute to increased ferritin concentrations (iron stores) [17]. For example, in sickle cell disease, the inflammatory process can often be initiated in individuals as a consequence of the associated comorbidities of the disease (e.g., vaso-occlusion, acute chest syndrome, pulmonary hypertension, leg ulcers) [18]. It is well established that ferritin concentration increases in the presence of inflammation [19]. Thus, in some cases, individuals with certain genetic hemoglobin disorders may have increased ferritin concentrations as a result of inflammation that is associated with comorbidities of the genetic disorder itself. Ultimately, it is important to note that in individuals with some genetic hemoglobin disorders, ferritin concentrations may not accurately represent an individual's iron status and that iron deficiency may be underestimated in populations with a high prevalence of hemoglobin disorders and/or inflammation. In some cases, provision of iron to individuals with genetic hemoglobin disorders may in fact be harmful, as iron absorption may be inopportunely increased, and excess iron can cause oxidative stress and cell damage [20]. Population-level iron interventions should always be cautiously assessed with both safety and potential impact in consideration [21, 22].

Soluble Transferrin Receptor Concentrations

We found 17 studies in children and adolescents and 15 studies in adults which compared mean or median sTfR concentrations in study populations with genetic hemoglobin disorders compared to study controls (Table 19.4). Sixteen of the 17 studies in children and adolescents and 12 of the 15 studies in adults demonstrated that study populations with genetic hemoglobin disorders had higher mean or median sTfR concentrations as compared to study controls; the remaining studies showed no difference between the two groups (no studies showed that sTfR concentrations were lower among those with genetic hemoglobin disorders compared to study controls).

STfR is an indicator of iron status that reflects the demand for iron or increased erythropoietic activity [23]. STfR is also thought to be influenced by the presence of inflammation, but to a lesser degree than ferritin [19]. STfR can be elevated in individuals with hemolytic conditions, which may be associated with some genetic hemoglobin disorders or inherited conditions (e.g., sickle cell disease or glucose-6-phosphate dehydrogenase deficiency) [8, 24, 25]. Similarly to ferritin, it is important to note that in individuals with some genetic hemoglobin disorders, sTfR concentrations may not accurately represent an individual's iron status and that population-level iron deficiency may be overestimated when sTfR is used to assess iron status in populations with a high prevalence of hemoglobin disorders and/or inflammation.

Zinc Concentrations

We found 23 studies in children and adolescents and 8 studies in adults, which compared either plasma or serum zinc concentrations in study populations with genetic hemoglobin disorders compared to study controls (Table 19.4). Nineteen of the 23 studies in children and adolescents and 6 of the 8 studies in adults demonstrated that study populations with genetic hemoglobin disorders had lower mean or median serum or plasma zinc concentrations as compared to study controls; the remaining studies showed no difference between the two groups (no studies showed that zinc concentrations were higher among those with genetic hemoglobin disorders compared to study controls).

Zinc is a negative acute phase protein; thus, it is decreased in the presence of inflammation [26]. Thus, in some cases, individuals with certain genetic hemoglobin disorders may have decreased zinc concentrations as a result of inflammation that is associated with comorbidities of the genetic disorder itself. Similarly to the markers of iron status, it is important to note that in individuals with some genetic hemoglobin disorders, zinc concentrations may not accurately represent an individual's zinc status and that population-level zinc deficiency may be underestimated when serum or plasma zinc is used to assess zinc status in populations with a high prevalence of hemoglobin disorders and/or inflammation.

Folate Concentrations

Of the B vitamins involved in the folate and methionine cycles (folate, riboflavin, vitamin B_6 and vitamin B_{12}), folate is the most widely studied micronutrient in relation to hemoglobinopathies. Evidence of folate deficiency in individuals with sickle cell disease emerged in case studies as early as the 1950s [27–29] and many studies since have illustrated the association between sickle cell disease and decreased folate concentrations (Table 19.6). Studies in the 1960s and 1970s illustrated that increased rates of folate deficiency were seen in populations with sickle cell disease not supplemented with folic acid (synthetic folate), either through diet or pharmaceutical supplements [30–32].

We found a total of 25 studies (11 in in children and adolescents, 6 in adults, and 8 in both children and adults), which compared either serum/plasma or RBC folate concentrations in study populations with genetic hemoglobin disorders compared to study controls (Table 19.6). Since the earlier studies in the 1960s and onward, many changes in food systems and clinical care for individuals with hemoglobinopathies have occurred. It is now widely common clinical practice to recommend that individuals with sickle cell disease and other hemolytic anemias receive daily folic acid supplementation of 1–5 mg/d. Additionally, the introduction of national programs of folic acid fortification of refined grains in many countries around the world has also contributed to increased dietary intake of folate.

There is now emerging evidence of high folate concentrations and detectable levels of unmetabolized folic acid (folic acid that circulates in plasma when enzymatic capacity is limited or when the liver is fully saturated with folate), in individuals with hemoglobinopathies receiving high-dose folic acid supplementation [33–35], especially in populations that have national programs of refined-grain folic acid fortification [14, 36]. Thus, suggesting that some folic acid-supplemented individuals with hemoglobin disorders may receive excess amounts of folic acid, although the health consequences of this are not fully elucidated [37, 38].

Beyond the association of lower folate concentrations in individuals with sickle cell disease, this association has also been demonstrated among individuals with β-thalassemia, β-thalassemia/Hb E, and Hb H genotypes (Table 19.6).

Vitamin B_{12} and B_6 and Riboflavin Concentrations

A similar association has also been shown among sickle cell disease, β-thalassemia, and decreased plasma concentrations of vitamins B_{12} (Table 19.7) and B_6 (commonly measured as concentrations of pyridoxal 5′-phosphate, the coenzyme form of B_6) (Table 19.8). Both of these B-vitamins, in addition to riboflavin, are needed in adequate amounts for folate cycle activity, one-carbon metabolism, and methylation reactions. Despite evidence of decreased concentrations of plasma vitamin B_{12} in individuals with SCD and β-thalassemia, there is limited evidence of a corresponding increase in the rates of vitamin B_{12} deficiency [39–41]. On the other hand, decreased concentrations of vitamin B_6 have been associated with poorer B_6 status in individuals with hemoglobinopathies [39, 42], likely due to increased oxidative stress and oxidative damage [43]. There is also a small but inconclusive body of evidence regarding the association between deficiencies of thiamin [39] and riboflavin (commonly determined by erythrocyte glutathione reductase activation coefficients, a functional measure of riboflavin status) (Table 19.9) and hemoglobinopathies in adults [44–46].

Continuing advancements in the medical care for individuals with hemoglobinopathies may further alter B-vitamin requirements. In sickle cell disease, for example, the prophylactic use of hydroxyurea (hydroxycarbamide), a medication, which significantly extends the average lifespan of red blood cells through the promotion of fetal hemoglobin (Hb F) [47], transfusion medicine, and emerging gene therapies, may decrease the need for B-vitamins, especially folate, due to reduced red blood cell production and turnover. As medical care advances, continued reassessment of routine B-vitamin supplementation practices will be warranted and the association between genetic hemoglobin disorders and biomarkers of nutritional anemia may change.

Newborn Genetic Screening Programs

Newborn genetic screening programs have been initiated in many regions of the world and can identify babies with treatable genetic disorders with use of a small blood sample collected at the time of birth. Early detection of these disorders allows for early intervention treatment that may prevent severe morbidity, mental handicap, growth faltering, and/or sudden infant death [48]. Newborns screened positive for severe sickle cell hemoglobinopathies are referred to health facilities for confirmation of diagnosis and long-term follow-up. For example, the province of British Columbia in Canada implemented a newborn screening program in 2000 that screens for 22 different disorders, including sickle cell, cystic fibrosis, and other certain endocrine and metabolic disorders [49]. A heel-prick blood sample is collected onto a blood spot card typically within 1–2 days of birth. Sickle cell hemoglobinopathies are detected using isoelectric focusing and results are recorded in a provincial database. Similar newborn screening programs have been established in many countries worldwide [50, 51]. These are critical public health programs that have the potential to reduce morbidity and mortality early in life in individuals with severe hemoglobinopathies.

Other Inherited Blood Disorders

In addition to genetic abnormalities in the hemoglobin molecule, other inherited blood disorders can also contribute to anemia and have serious hematological and clinical consequences for affected individuals. Some examples of these conditions include.

Glucose-6-phosphate dehydrogenase deficiency (G6PD): It is an X-linked, hereditary genetic defect due to one or more mutations in the G6PD gene, which encodes an enzyme responsible for a critical reaction in the pentose phosphate pathway. G6PD deficiency is the most common human enzyme defect worldwide [25]. Over 140 different mutations have been identified, which lead to a varying severity of clinical phenotypes [25]. G6PDA–, the most common type in sub-Saharan Africa, is characterized by the coinheritance of two variants (A376G and G202A). A common clinical manifestation of G6PD deficiency is acute hemolytic anemia, which is usually triggered by an external event (e.g., ingestion of fava beans, infection, or certain medications). Individuals with G6PD deficiency may have anemia regardless of iron status and their biomarkers of iron status may not accurately reflect their nutrition status. In a study in the DR Congo, Barker et al. found that two G6PD variant genotypes were associated with elevated sTfR concentrations in Congolese children, which limits the accuracy of sTfR as a biomarker of iron status in this population [52].

Fanconi anemia: It is the most frequent hereditary cause of bone marrow failure [53]. Bone marrow is the soft tissue in the center of bones that functions to produce blood cells and platelets. Fanconi anemia has been characterized by 15 different variant genes to date and leads to a decreased production of all types of blood cells. Fanconi anemia is the most common inherited form of aplastic anemia (a condition when the bone marrow does not synthesize adequate blood cells). Individuals with Fanconi anemia are also at an increased risk of acute myeloid leukemia as a result of this genetic disorder [53].

Thrombotic thrombocytopenic purpura (TTP): It is a rare blood disorder that increases the risk of blood clots forming in small blood vessels [54]. TPP causes an increased red blood cell turnover and leads to hemolytic anemia. TPP can be hereditary (caused by a variant in the ADAMTS13 gene) or acquired (triggered by certain conditions, events, or exposures such as medicines or infections) [54]. Common symptoms include blood clots, anemia, jaundice, low platelet count, or damaged red blood cells.

Hereditary spherocytosis: It is an inherited disorder associated with a variety of mutations that lead to defects in RBC membrane proteins [55]. A classic morphologic sign is the microspherocyte, which is caused by a loss of RBC membrane surface area. Individuals with hereditary spherocytosis have a varying range of clinical phenotypes, from asymptomatic conditions to severe hemolytic anemia.

Congenital pernicious anemia: It is a rare congenital disorder where infants are born lacking the ability to adequately synthesize the gastric intrinsic factor, which is critical for the absorption of vitamin B_{12} [56]. This disorder is characterized by vitamin B12 deficiency and megaloblastic anemia, and can result in severe or long-lasting pernicious anemia that can damage the heart, brain, and other organs in the body.

Conclusions

Individuals with genetic hemoglobin disorders may have anemia, regardless of iron status. Iron or other nutritional interventions may not be effective to reduce, treat, or prevent anemia in these individuals. Further, in individuals with some genetic hemoglobin disorders, biomarkers of nutritional anemia may not accurately represent an individual's nutritional status and nutritional deficiency prevalence may be falsely underestimated or overestimated in populations with genetic hemoglobin disorders.

References

1. Greer JP, Foerster J, Rodgers GM, Paraskevas F. Wintrobe's clinical hematology. 12th ed. Baltimore, MD: Lippincott Williams & Wilkins; 2009.
2. Bain BJ. Haemoglobinopathy diagnosis. 2nd ed. Oxford: Blackwell Publishing Ltd.; 2006.
3. Weatherall D, Akinyanju O, Fucharoen S, et al. Inherited disorders of hemoglobin. In: Jamison DT, Breman JG, Measham AR, et al., editors. Disease control priorities in developing countries [internet]. 2nd ed. New York: Oxford University Press; 2006. https://www.ncbi.nlm.nih.gov/books/NBK11727/.
4. King A, Higgs D. Potential new approaches to the management of the Hb Bart's hydrops fetalis syndrome: the most severe form of α-thalassemia. Hematol Am Soc Hematol Educ Progr. 2018;1:353–60.
5. Lal A, Wong T, Andrews J, Balasa V, Chung J, Forester C, Ikeda A, Keel S, Pagano M, Puthenveetil G, et al. Transfusion practices and complications in thalassemia. Transfusion. 2018;58:2826–35.
6. Allison A. Protection afforded by sickle-cell trait against subtertian malarial infection. Br Med J. 1954;1:290–4.
7. Piel FB, Patil AP, Howes RE, Nyangiri OA, Gething PW, Dewi M, Temperley WH, Williams TN, Weatherall DJ, Hay SI. Global epidemiology of sickle haemoglobin in neonates: a contemporary geostatistical model-based map and population estimates. Lancet. 2013;9861:142–51.
8. Piel F, Steinberg M, Rees D. Sickle cell disease. Lancet. 2017;390:311–23.
9. Wastnedge E, Waters D, Patel S, Morrison K, Goh MY, Adeloye D, Rudan I. The global burden of sickle cell disease in children under five years of age: a systematic review and meta-analysis. J Glob Health. 2018;8:1–9.
10. Rees D, Styles L, Vichinsky E, Clegg J, Weatherall D. The hemoglobin E syndromes. Ann N Y Acad Sci. 1998;850:334–43.
11. Piel F, Weatheral D. The α-thalassemias. N Engl J Med. 2014;371:1908–16.
12. Kattamis A, Forni G, Aydinok Y, Viprakasit V. Changing patterns in the epidemiology of β-thalassemia. Eur J Haematol. 2020;105:692–703.

13. Karakochuk CD, Whitfield KC, Barr SI, Lamers Y, Devlin AM, Vercauteren SM, Kroeun H, Talukder A, McLean J, Green TJ. Genetic hemoglobin disorders rather than iron deficiency are a major predictor of hemoglobin concentration in women of reproductive age in rural Prey Veng, Cambodia. J Nutr. 2015;145:134–42.
14. Williams BA, Mayer C, McCartney H, Devlin AM, Lamers Y, Vercauteren SM, Wu JK, Karakochuk CD. Detectable unmetabolized folic acid and elevated folate concentrations in folic acid-supplemented Canadian children with sickle cell disease. Front Nutr. 2021;8:642306.
15. Zimmermann MB, Fucharoen S, Winichagoon P, Sirankapracha P, Zeder C, Gowachirapant S, Judprasong K, Tanno T, Miller JL, Hurrell RF. Iron metabolism in heterozygotes for hemoglobin E (HbE), alpha-thalassemia 1, or beta-thalassemia and in compound heterozygotes for HbE/beta-thalassemia. Am J Clin Nutr. 2008;88:1026–31.
16. Nemeth E, Tuttle MS, Powelson J, Vaughn MB, Donovan A, Ward DM, Ganz T, Kaplan J. Hepcidin regulates cellular iron efflux by binding to ferroportin and inducing its internalization. Science. 2004;306:2090–3.
17. Baumann H, Gauldie J. The acute phase response. Immunol Today. 1994;15:74–80.
18. Conran N, Belcher J. Inflammation in sickle cell disease. Clin Hemorheol Microcirc. 2018;68:263–99.
19. Suchdev PS, Williams AM, Mei Z, Flores-Ayala R, Pasricha S-R, Rogers LM, Namaste SM. Assessment of iron status in settings of inflammation: challenges and potential approaches. Am J Clin Nutr. 2017;106:1626S–33S.
20. Schümann K, Ettle T, Szegner B, Elsenhans B, Solomons NW. On risks and benefits of iron supplementation recommendations for iron intake revisited. J Trace Elem Med Biol. 2007;21:147–68.
21. Baldi A, Larson L, Pasricha S. Balancing safety and potential for impact in universal iron interventions. Nestle Nutr Inst Work Ser. 2020;93:51–62.
22. Karakochuk CD. Iron supplementation in predominantly iron-replete populations: is there an emerging concern? Sight Life Mag. 2016:44–51.
23. Cook J, Dassenko S, Skikne B. Serum transferrin receptor as an index of iron absorption. Br J Haematol. 1990;75:603–9.
24. Mast AE, Blinder MA, Gronowski AM, Chumley C, Scott MG. Clinical utility of the soluble transferrin receptor and comparison with serum ferritin in several populations. Clin Chem. 1998;44:45–51.
25. Cappellini MD, Fiorelli G. Glucose-6-phosphate dehydrogenase deficiency. Lancet. 2008;371:64–74.
26. King JC, Brown KH, Gibson RS, Krebs NF, Lowe NM, Siekmann JH, Raiten DJ. Biomarkers of nutrition for development (BOND): zinc review. J Nutr. 2016;146:858S–85S.
27. Mabayoje JO. Sickle-cell anaemia; a major disease in West Africa. Br Med J. 1956;1:194–6.
28. Watson-Williams EJ. Folic acid deficiency in sickle-cell anaemia. East Afr Med J. 1962;39:213–21.
29. Lindenbaum J, Klipstein FA. Folic acid deficiency in sickle-cell anemia. N Engl J Med. 1963;269:875–82.
30. Tso S. Significance of subnormal red-cell folate in thalassaemia. J Clin Pathol. 1976;29:140–3.
31. Liu Y. Folic acid deficiency in sickle cell anaemia. Scand J Haematol. 1975;14:71–9.
32. Liu YK. Folate deficiency in children with sickle cell anemia: lack of relationship between folate deficiency and growth retardation in sickle cell anemia. Am J Dis Child. 1974;127:389–93.
33. Azzam M, Attalla S. Serum folate levels in patients with chronic hemolytic anemia on regular folic acid supplementation before and after dose modification. Indian Pediatr. 2019;56:845–8.
34. Tripathi G, Kalra M, Mahajan A. Folate supplementation in transfusion-dependent thalassemia: do we really need such high doses? Indian J Med Paediatr Oncol. 2016;37:305.
35. Al-Saqladi A-WM, Harper G, Delpisheh A, Fijnvandraat K, Bin-Gadeem HA, Brabin BJ. Frequency of the MTHFR C677T polymorphism in Yemeni children with sickle cell disease. Hemoglobin. 2010;34:67–77.
36. Paniz C, Lucena MR, Bertinato JF, dos Santos MNN, Gomes GW, Figueiredo MS, de Fátima Sonati M, Blaia-D Avila VLN, Green R, Guerra-Shinohara EM. Serum folate and cytokines in heterozygous β-thalassemia. Int J Lab Hematol. 2020;42:718–26.
37. Colapinto CK, O'Connor DL, Sampson M, Williams B, Tremblay MS. Systematic review of adverse health outcomes associated with high serum or red blood cell folate concentrations. J Public Health (Bangkok). 2016;38:e84–97.
38. Maruvada P, Stover PJ, Mason JB, Bailey RL, Davis CD, Field MS, Finnell RH, Garza C, Green R, Gueant J-L, et al. Knowledge gaps in understanding the metabolic and clinical effects of excess folates/folic acid: a summary, and perspectives, from an NIH workshop. Am J Clin Nutr. 2020;00:1–14.
39. Claster S, Wood JC, Noetzli L, Carson SM, Hofstra TC, Khanna R, Coates TD. Nutritional deficiencies in iron overloaded patients with hemoglobinopathies. Am J Hematol. 2009;84:344–8.
40. Martyres DJ, Vijenthira A, Barrowman N, Harris-Janz S, Chretien C, Klaassen RJ. Nutrient insufficiencies/deficiencies in children with sickle cell disease and its association with increased disease severity. Pediatr Blood Cancer. 2016;63:1060–4.
41. Kennedy TS, Fung EB, Kawchak DA, Zemel BS, Ohene-Frempong K, Stallings VA. Red blood cell folate and serum vitamin B12 status in children with sickle cell disease. J Pediatr Hematol Oncol. 2001;23:165–9.
42. Nelson MC, Zemel BS, Kawchak DA, Barden EM, Frongillo EAJ, Coburn SP, Ohene-Frempong K, Stallings VA. Vitamin B6 status of children

with sickle cell disease. J Pediatr Hematol Oncol. 2002;24

43. Telen MJ. Pyridoxamine: another vitamin for sickle cell disease? Haematologica. 2020;105:2348–50.
44. Varma R, Mankad V, Phelps D, Jenkins L, Suskind R. Depressed erythrocyte glutathione reductase activity in sickle cell disease. Am J Clin Nutr. 1983;38:884–7.
45. El-Hazmi M, Al-Swailem A, Warsy A. Case studies on haemoglobin S heterozygotes with severe clinical manifestations. J Trop Pediatr. 1990;36:223–9.
46. El-Hazmi M, Warsy A. Glutathione reductase in the south-western province of Saudi Arabia--genetic variation vs. acquired deficiency. Haematologia (Budap). 1989;22:37–42.
47. Steinberg MH, Chui DHK, Dover GJ, Sebastiani P, Alsultan A. Fetal hemoglobin in sickle cell anemia: a glass half full? Blood. 2014;123:481–5.
48. Dietzen D, Rinaldo P, Whitley R. National Academy of Clinical Biochemistry Laboratory Medicine Practice Guidelines: follow-up testing for metabolic disease identified by expanded newborn screening using tandem mass spectrometry. Clin Chem. 2009;55:1615–26.
49. Neonatal guideline 9: newborn screening. Vancouver, Canada; 2010.
50. Bain. Neonatal/newborn haemoglobinopathy screening in Europe and Africa. J Clin Pathol. 2009;62:53–6.
51. Padilla C, Therrell B. Newborn screening in the Asia Pacific region. J Inherit Metab Dis. 2007;30:490–506.
52. Barker KB, Henderson AM, Naguib K, Vercauteren SM, Devlin AM, Albert AY, Bahizire E, Tugirimana PL, Akilimali PZ, Boy E, et al. Serum soluble transferrin receptor concentrations are elevated among Congolese children with glucose-6-phosphate dehydrogenase variants, but not sickle cell variants or alpha-thalassemia. J Nutr. 2017;147:1785–94.
53. Soulier J. Fanconi anemia. Hematol Am Soc Hematol Educ Progr. 2011:492–7.
54. Hovinga J, George J. Hereditary thrombotic thrombocytopenic purpura. N Engl J Med. 2019;381:1653–62.
55. Hassoun H, Palek J. Hereditary spherocytosis: a review of the clinical and molecular aspects of the disease. Blood Rev. 1996;10:129–47.
56. Green R, Mitra A. Megaloblastic anemias: nutritional and other causes. Med Clin North Am. 2017;101:297–317.

Iron and the Human Gut Microbiota

20

Daniela Paganini, Mary A. Uyoga, and Michael B. Zimmermann

Keywords

Iron · Fortification · Supplementation · Infant Gut · Microbiota · Pathogens · Inflammation Prebiotic · Galacto-oligosaccharides

Introduction

Iron absorption from the diet, iron-fortified foods, or oral iron supplements is tightly regulated in humans, because there is no active pathway for iron excretion and excess body iron can be harmful [1, 2]. Circulating non-transferrin-bound iron can generate toxic free radicals, which can cause tissue damage [3] or be more available to infectious organisms than iron sequestered in transferrin [4]. Iron absorption from iron-fortified foods or oral iron supplements is generally low, with a fractional absorption typically <10% [5, 6]. In population groups with a high burden of infections, such as in rural African populations, iron absorption is likely to be even lower, as inflammation increases plasma hepcidin, which reduces iron absorption [7]. Thus, the majority of iron from oral iron supplements or fortificants passes unabsorbed into the colon where the iron is available to gut microbes and may potentially affect the gut microbiome. This chapter begins with a broad introduction on bacterial iron acquisition and metabolism. Thereafter, the main focus is on human studies examining the effects of oral iron on the gut microbiota. At the end, a short outlook is given on promising strategies to diminish the potentially harmful side effects of iron on the gut microbiota.

Iron Acquisition Is a Determinant of Bacterial Growth and Virulence

The ability of enteropathogens to acquire sufficient iron to support their growth and proliferation is an important virulence determinant [8, 9]. Gut bacteria have evolved a variety of mechanisms (including siderophores, Feo-uptake systems, and metal-transporting binding-protein-dependent ABC systems) to acquire iron even under conditions of limited iron availability [8–10]. Iron plays a crucial role in replication and virulence (e.g., adhesion, invasion, and induction of virulence factors) of many enteric Gram-negative bacteria (e.g., *Salmonella, Shigella,* or pathogenic *Escherichia coli*) [8, 9]. During iron-limiting conditions, such as during an inflammation when the host limits free extracellular iron, pathogenic bacteria can secrete

D. Paganini · M. A. Uyoga · M. B. Zimmermann (✉)
Laboratory of Human Nutrition, Institute of Food, Nutrition and Health, Zürich, Switzerland
e-mail: daniela.paganini@uzh.ch; mary.uyoga@hest.ethz.ch; michael.zimmermann@hest.ethz.ch

C. D. Karakochuk et al. (eds.), *Nutritional Anemia*, Nutrition and Health,
https://doi.org/10.1007/978-3-031-14521-6_20

iron-scavenging siderophores that bind iron with a much higher affinity than the host's iron-binding proteins [11, 12]. As an example of the substantial bacterial genomic investment in iron capture and metabolism, approximately 7% of the *Salmonella typhimurium* genome is directly or indirectly regulated by iron [13]. The iron-sensing transcriptional repressor *Fur* is central to iron homeostasis in most Gram-negative bacteria such as *Salmonella* [9]. During iron deficiency, lack of iron-bound *Fur* allows transcription of genes for iron uptake and storage [14]. *Fur*-mediated regulation of virulence genes contributes to the enhancement of *Salmonella* virulence in iron-rich conditions [15]. Another example of how the virulence of gut pathogens is enhanced by iron is the recent observation that cholera toxin enhances the growth of *Vibrio cholera* in the gut lumen by facilitating its iron acquisition [16]. Similar adaptations to iron deficiency occur in Gram-positive bacterial pathogens. The genome of *Clostridium difficile* encodes multiple ferric, ferrous, and siderophore-bound iron uptake systems that are *Fur*-regulated and highly responsive to changes in iron supply [17, 18]. The presence of these redundant iron-uptake systems highlights the importance of iron acquisition for clostridial growth. Low-iron conditions evoke a stress response in *C. difficile*, mediated through iron-binding sites for *Fur* [17]. This binding alters expression of iron transporters and increases iron uptake. *C. difficile* also modifies its cell wall in response to iron deficiency; this may protect it from other microbes or host immune responses [18].

Mammalian hosts have evolved several mechanisms to counter bacterial iron uptake in the gut. Recently, host production of calprotectin, a manganese/zinc-chelating protein and a marker of gut inflammation [19], was shown to limit bacterial iron acquisition via its capacity to bind iron [20]. The host can also produce the innate defense peptide lipocalin-2, which binds the ferric-siderophore complexes, thereby preventing its uptake by bacteria [21]. However, several pathogenic bacteria including *S. typhimurium*, pathogenic *E. coli*, *Klebsiella*, and *Shigella* can evade this host defense mechanism by the production of "stealth siderophores" (e.g., salmochelin and aerobactin), structurally modified siderophores that resist binding by host lipocalin-2 [8].

Notably, beneficial commensal gut bacteria, such as *Bifidobacteriaceae* and *Lactobacillaceae*, that provide an important barrier against colonization by enteropathogens, require very little or no iron [22, 23]. Several *Bifidobacterium* species, including *B. bifidum*, *B. longum*, *B. breve*, *B. pseudolongum,* and *B. pseudocatenulatum*, all species commonly found in the infant gut, grow well under iron-depleted conditions [23]. The ability of *Bifidobacterium* to grow in low iron conditions and efficiently sequester any available iron, thereby further limit iron available to gut pathogens, may provide a competitive advantage against enteropathogens [23, 24]. Lactobacilli do not produce siderophores to sequester iron and their growth is similar in media with and without iron [25]; they instead rely on manganese for growth [22]. Other commensal bacteria are also particularly well adapted to outcompete enteropathogens for iron in low-iron conditions. The nonpathogenic *E. coli Nissle* has multiple iron acquisition pathways and can secrete enterobactin, salmochelin, yersiniabactin, and aerobactin, allowing it to effectively acquire iron at the expense of *Salmonella* [26, 27]. Furthermore, *E. coli Nissle* specifically targets the uptake of siderophore-bound iron by pathogenic enterobacteria by secreting antibacterial molecules that damage enteropathogens by binding to their siderophore receptors [28].

Recent data on locally produced hepcidin in the intestinal mucosa further supports the importance of iron in determining microbial pathogenicity in the gut [29]. Systemically, hepcidin-mediated iron sequestration withholds iron from invading microorganisms and plays a key role in innate immune responses to infection [30]. Hepcidin production by mucosal dendritic cells sequesters iron into colonic myeloid cells, limiting increases in free iron released during gut inflammation and tissue damage. Failure to sequester iron locally resulted in dysbiosis, increased microbial translocation, and more severe gut inflammation [29].

The Gut Microbiota May Modulate Host Iron Absorption and Metabolism

When placed on a low-iron diet, compared to conventional mice, germ-free mice show milder iron deficiency-induced anemia, suggesting more efficient iron uptake in the absence of gut microbiota that may compete with the host for iron uptake [31]. Certain *Lactobacilli* sp. reduce host iron uptake through the production of small molecule metabolites, such as 1,3-diaminopropane (DAP), which inhibits HIF2 alpha and expression of iron uptake proteins in the enterocyte. Production of DAP by *Lactobacilli* was increased during dietary iron deficiency, suggesting the gut microbiota may modulate gut iron homeostasis and luminal iron availability [31]. In addition, the gut microbiota may affect the systemic inflammatory response, and thereby influence hepcidin synthesis, dietary iron absorption, and systemic hypoferremia [32].

The Effect of Increasing Iron Intake and the Human Gut Microbiota

Controlled Studies of Iron Fortification and Supplementation in Infants

The WHO recommends iron fortification with iron-containing micronutrient powders (MNPs) in infants aged 6–23 months [33]. Because iron absorption in African infants from these MNPs is only 4–8% [5], they are usually formulated to provide a high dose of iron (12.5 mg). The first studies investigating the effects of in-home fortification with iron-containing MNPs on the infant gut microbiota were two double-blind randomized controlled trials in 6-month-old infants in south coast Kenya (n = 115) [34]. Infants in the first trial consumed either an MNP containing 12.5 mg iron as ferrous fumarate or an MNP without iron daily for 4 months. Infants in the second trial consumed either a new low-iron dose MNP containing 2.5 mg iron as sodium iron ethylenediaminetetraacetate (NaFeEDTA) or an MNP without iron daily for 4 months. Overall, *Bifidobacteriaceae* was clearly the predominant bacterial family in these infants' gut microbiota. Interestingly, the authors reported an overall high prevalence of potential enteropathogens in the fecal samples (65% tested positive for enteropathogenic *E. coli* (EPEC), 49% for enterotoxigenic *E. coli* producing heat-labile toxin (ETEC LT), 7% for ETEC producing heat-stable toxin (ETEC ST), 10% for enterohemorrhagic *E. coli* producing shiga-like toxin 1 (EHEC stx1), 9% for EHEC producing shiga-like toxin 2 (EHEC stx2), 57% for *C. difficile*, 90% for members of the *Clostridium perfringens* group, and 22% for *Salmonella*) [34]. During the intervention, in the iron, compared to the no iron groups, there was a significant increase in enterobacteria, particularly *Escherichia/Shigella*, the enterobacteria/bifidobacteria ratio, and *Clostridium* spp. Moreover, there was a significant treatment effect on pathogenic *E. coli*, with higher abundances in the iron compared to the no iron groups at endpoint (Fig. 20.1). In addition, at endpoint of the study, fecal calprotectin was significantly higher in the iron compared to the no iron control group [34]

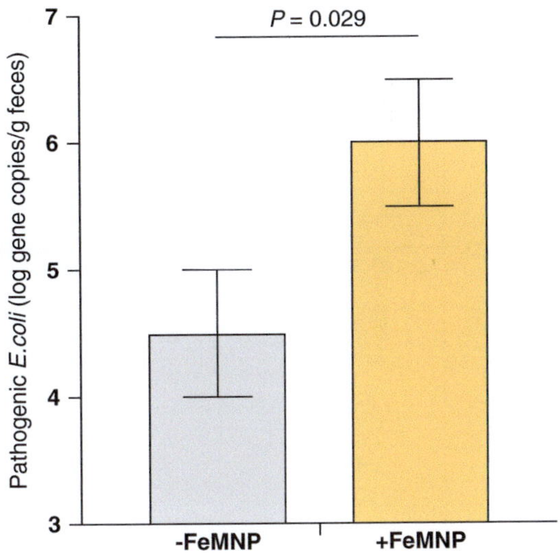

Fig. 20.1 Abundance of pathogenic *E. coli* at endpoint, by group in Kenyan infants (n = 115) receiving daily for 4 months a micronutrient powder containing either no iron (-FeMNP), or 2.5 mg or 12.5 mg iron (+FeMNP). Univariate general linear models with baseline values as covariates were used to estimate the intervention effect. Adapted from [34]

(Fig. 20.2). These controlled studies demonstrated for the first time that provision of iron-containing MNPs to African infants causes an adverse shift in the gut microbiota composition, increases abundances of enteropathogens and levels of gut inflammation.

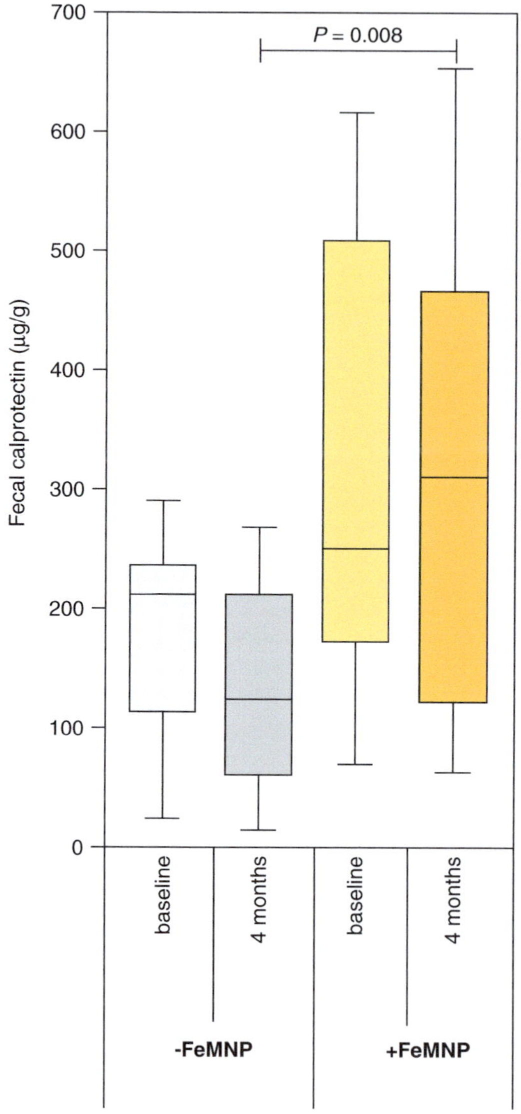

Fig. 20.2 Fecal calprotectin levels at baseline and 4 months, by group in Kenyan infants (n = 115) receiving daily for 4 months a micronutrient powder containing either no iron (-FeMNP); or containing 12.5 mg iron (+FeMNP). Differences were investigated using general linear models and baseline variables as covariates. Boxplots are shown with the 10–90th percentiles. Adapted from [34]

A subsequent 4-month, controlled, double-blind trial in the same study area investigating the effects of a new MNP containing 5 mg of iron on the infant gut microbiota reported similar results [35]. Infants aged 6.5–9.5 months (n = 155) were randomly assigned to receive daily (a) an MNP without iron (control group); (b) the identical MNP but with 5 mg iron (2.5 mg as NaFeEDTA and 2.5 mg as ferrous fumarate) (Fe group); or (c) the identical MNP as the Fe group but with 7.5 g galacto-oligosaccharides (GOS) (FeGOS group) [35]. The effects of coprovision of GOS (FeGOS group) are detailed later in this chapter. Similar to the studies described above [34], iron treatment (Fe group) had a major impact on the infant gut microbiota composition. After 4 months of intervention in the Fe group, compared to the control group, there were lower abundances of *Lactobacillus* and *Bifidobacterium* but higher abundances of *Clostridiales* and *Enterobacteriaceae* (Fig. 20.3a). Colonization rate of the infant gut with enteropathogens at baseline was high: EPEC was detected in 63%, ETEC LT in 26%, ETEC ST in 21%, EHEC stx2 in 18%, EHEC stx1 in 8%, *C. perfringens* in 65%, *C. difficile* in 35%, and *Salmonella* spp. in 4%. In the control group, there was a decrease in the sum of virulence and toxin genes (VTGs) of all these pathogens from baseline to 4 months, while there was no significant change in the Fe group over time [35] (Fig. 20.4). In contrast to the trial using a 12.5 mg iron dose daily [34], the 5 mg iron dose used in this study did not significantly increase fecal calprotectin [35].

A small study in 6-month-old infants living in rural western Kenya reported similar findings [36]. Infants received either an MNP without iron (-FeMNP group, n = 13), an MNP containing 12.5 mg iron as ferrous fumarate (+FeMNP group, n = 13), or a placebo (control group, n = 7) daily for 3 months [36]. While the relative abundance of *Escherichia/Shigella* decreased from baseline to 3 months in the -FeMNP and the control groups, it did not decrease in the +FeMNP group. Moreover, *Bifidobacterium* abundance decreased in the +FeMNP and the control group but not in the –FeMNP group. In contrast to the results of the trial using the same iron dose of

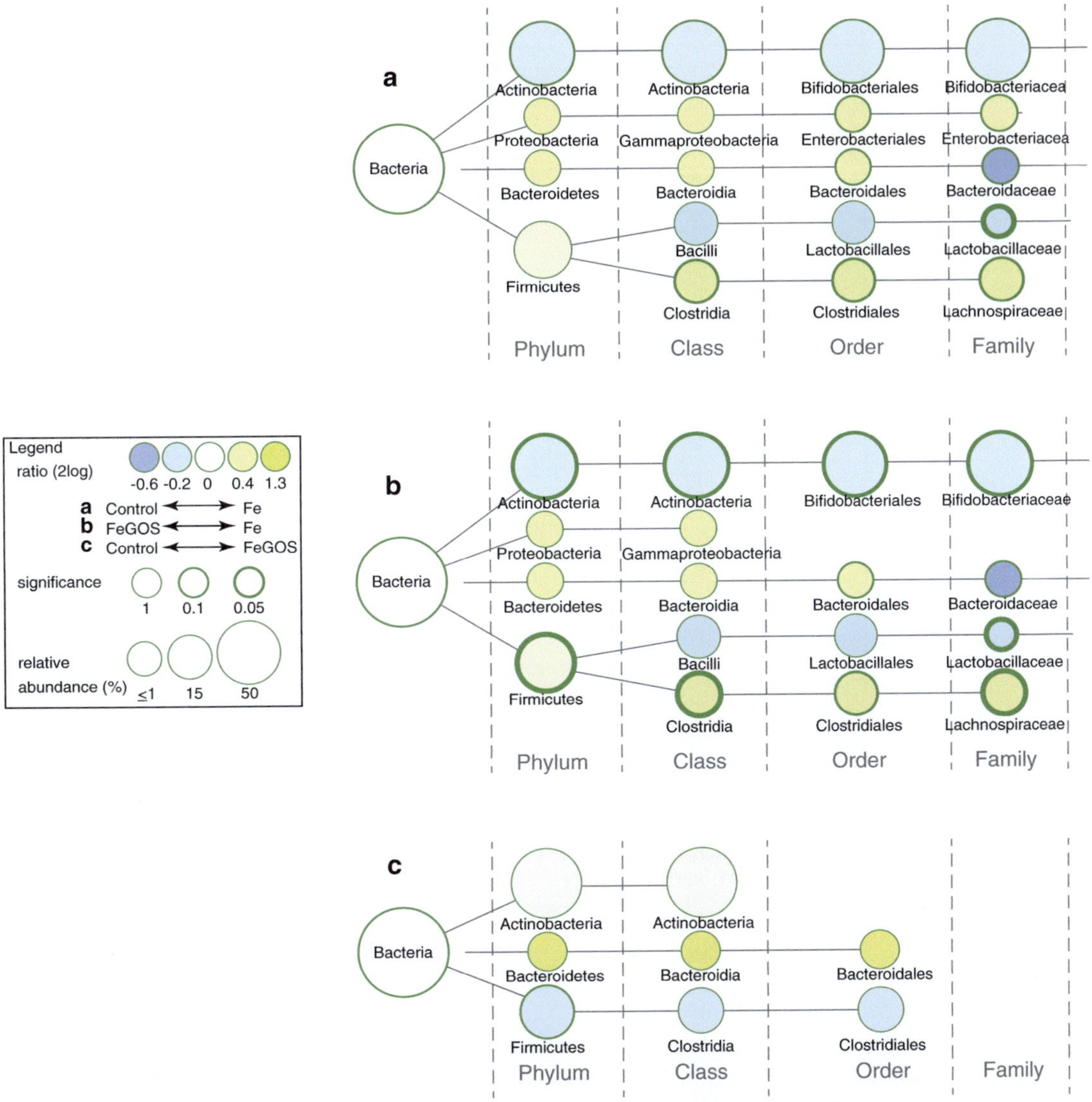

Fig. 20.3 Differences in the gut microbiota composition among Kenyan infants ($n = 155$) after receiving daily for 4 months a micronutrient powder without iron (Control group), with 5 mg of iron (Fe group), or with 5 mg iron and 7.5 g galacto-oligosaccharides (FeGOS group). Circles represent different taxa; the circle-sizes correspond to the relative taxa abundance (%), the green circle-borders represent the level of statistical significance. The fold difference is calculated as the 2log of the ratio of the relative abundance between groups (represented with the different circle-filling; yellow filling meaning more abundant in the group standing on the right side of the arrow in the legend, blue filling meaning more abundant in the group standing on the left side of the arrow in the legend). Mann-Whitney U test was used for statistical comparisons. (**a**) Control versus Fe group; (**b**) FeGOS versus Fe group; (**c**) Control versus FeGOS group. Adapted from [35]

12.5 mg [34], in this study, there was no between group difference or change over time in fecal calprotectin [36].

Besides diet, antibiotics are another factor that can have major impact on the infant gut microbiota. Antibiotics are prescribed to infants early and often; in low-resource settings, children <2 years of age receive an average of 4.9 antibiotic courses per child year [37]. Peak antibiotic use is between 6 and 12 months of age [37]; the age when many infants also receive iron fortificants to treat or prevent iron deficiency anemia

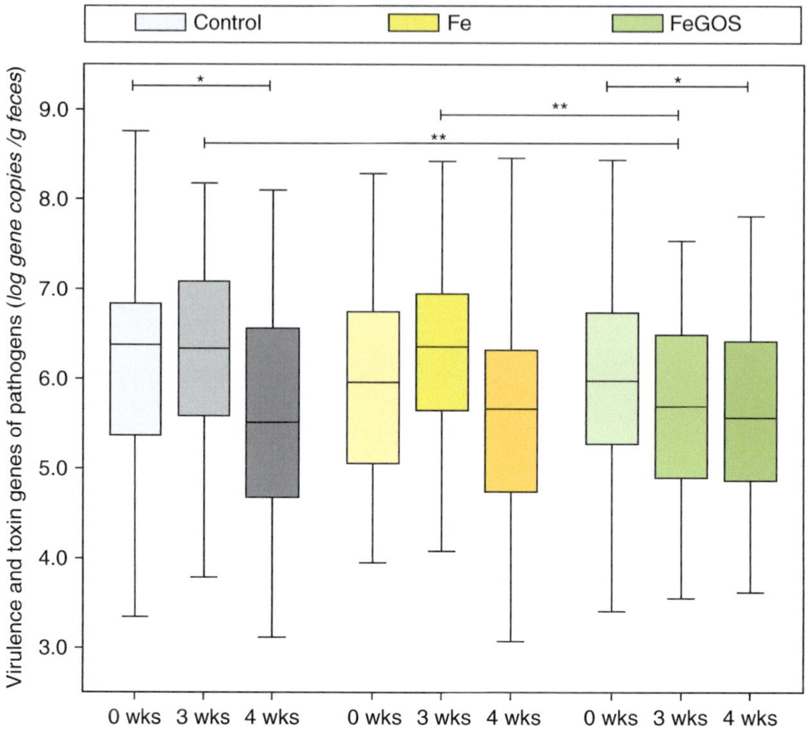

Fig. 20.4 Abundances of the sum of virulence and toxin genes of 10 pathogens at baseline (0 wks), 3 weeks (3 wks), and 4 months (4 mo), by group in Kenyan infants (n = 155) consuming daily a micronutrient powder containing either no iron (control); 5 mg of iron (Fe); or 5 mg of iron and 7.5 g of galacto-oligosaccharides (FeGOS). Significance is expressed as the p value of a Wilcoxon rank-sum test, $*p < 0.05$, $**p < 0.01$. Boxes show the median and 25th and 75th percentiles; whiskers show the range. Adapted from [35]

[38]. Therefore, the potential interaction between iron and antibiotics on the gut microbiota is important in these settings. A controlled intervention trial conducted in rural Kenya (n = 29) investigated the effects of this interaction in infants consuming MNPs with (+FeMNP) or without iron (–FeMNP) [39]. The trial showed that in infants receiving antibiotics and the –FeMNP, there was a significant decrease in abundance of pathogenic *E. coli* after antibiotic treatment, suggesting efficacy of antibiotics against potential enteropathogens. In contrast, in infants receiving antibiotics and the +FeMNP, there was no significant decrease in pathogenic *E. coli* after antibiotic treatment, suggesting iron fortification blunted the efficacy of the antibiotic to reduce potential enteropathogens [39], possibly because the increase in colonic iron supported continued growth of enteropathogens. Moreover, in infants receiving antibiotics and the +FeMNP, there was a significant decrease in abundance of *Bifidobacterium*, while infants receiving antibiotics and the -FeMNP maintained greater abundance of *Bifidobacterium* [39]. This study was limited by a low sample size and needs confirmation by larger trials.

Contrasting data came from a study in 6-month-old Malawian infants (n = 213) who were randomly assigned to receive (a) no intervention, (b) micronutrient-fortified corn-soya blend (providing 5.5 mg iron/day), (c) micronutrient-fortified lipid-based nutrient supplements with milk protein base (providing 6.0 mg iron/day), or (d) micronutrient-fortified lipid-based nutrient supplements with soya protein base (providing 6.0 mg iron/day) [40]. This trial showed no significant differences between the four intervention groups in the gut microbiota composition after 12 months of intervention. Recently another trial from rural Malawi showed only moderate effects of iron on the gut microbiota [41]. In this trial, pregnant women ($n = 869$) were randomized to receive daily either: (a) a multiple micronutrient supplement (MMN group); (b) an iron and folic acid supplement (IFA group); or (c) a lipid-based nutrient supplement (LNS group) daily during pregnancy and 6 months postpartum [41]. Infants from mothers in the LNS group received daily LNS (6 mg iron/day) from 6–18 months of age; infants from the other two groups did not receive supplements. There were no differences in the infant microbiota alpha-diversity (alpha diversity quantifies richness, evenness, and diversity within a sample) or microbiota maturation (defined as microbiota-for-age z scores (MAZ)) between the IFA and MMN groups. However, infant microbiota alpha-diversity was significantly higher in the LNS group at 18 months compared to the IFA and MMN groups together [41]. These studies in rural Malawi did not investigate specific VTGs of enteropathogens nor fecal calprotectin. Therefore, it is uncertain whether baseline colonization of the infant gut microbiota and gut inflammation were as high as in the infant studies conducted in Kenya [34, 35]. In addition, age-related differences in the gut microbiota composition, differences in complementary feeding patterns, iron dose and iron compound given, intervention duration as well as methodological differences in characterization of the gut microbiota may have contributed to the different findings from the studies.

Two studies looking at the effect of iron fortification or supplementation on the gut microbiota have been done in high-income countries. One study investigated the effect of iron fortification or supplementation on the gut microbiota in healthy, iron-sufficient Swedish infants [42]. Six-month-old infants were randomized to receive daily for 45 days either low-iron-fortified formula (1.2 mg iron/day; $n = 24$), high-iron-fortified formula (6.6 mg iron/day, $n = 24$), or no-added-iron formula with liquid ferrous sulfate ($FeSO_4$) supplementation (iron drops, 6.6 mg iron/day; $n = 24$). In agreement with the Kenyan infant studies, consumption of high-iron formula for 45 days was associated with decreased relative abundance of *Bifidobacterium* ($p < 0.001$). Moreover, in the iron drops group after the intervention, there were lower abundance of *Lactobacillus* (8% vs. 42%, $p < 0.007$) but higher abundance of *Clostridium* (25% vs. 9%, $p < 0.05$) and of *Bacteroides* (1.2% vs. 0.9%, $p < 0.02$) compared to the high-iron formula group. However, there was no effect on abundance of pathogenic bacteria or on fecal calprotectin [42]. Of note, all formulas in this study contained 3.3 g/L of GOS, which may have partially mitigated the adverse effects of iron on the gut microbiota (discussed below) and may have protected from an increase in pathogenic bacteria and fecal calprotectin.

The second study was a small trial in US infants and toddlers aged 9–24 months [43]. Participants were randomized to receive $FeSO_4$ syrup alone (6 mg iron/kg/day) ($n = 22$) or with vitamin E (18 mg/d) ($n = 14$) for 2 months [43]. There were no significant changes over time or between groups in gut inflammation as assessed by fecal calprotectin. In both intervention groups, there was a decrease in the abundances of *Escherichia* spp. over time with no group differences and there was no decrease in beneficial commensals, such as *Lactobacillus* spp. [43]. However, both intervention groups received iron, making it difficult to draw conclusions on the effects of iron on the gut microbiota.

In contrast to the findings from Kenya, these studies in Swedish and US infants found no effect of additional dietary/supplemental iron on enteropathogens or on fecal calprotectin. Thus, it appears the adverse effects of iron may be particularly pronounced in settings with poor hygiene and a high burden of infection and inflammation, such as in rural Africa. Notably, baseline mean calprotectin concentrations were ca. 50 μg/g in the study in US infants [43], while in the Kenyan infants, the mean baseline calprotectin concentration was much higher, at 200–300 μg/g [34, 35].

Controlled Studies of Iron Fortification and Supplementation in Children

Two trials conducted in African school children investigated the effect of iron fortification and supplementation on the gut microbiota. The first was a randomized, double-blind, controlled trial in 6–14-year-old children ($n = 139$) in Côte d'Ivoire [44]. Children consumed either iron-fortified biscuits containing 20 mg iron as electrolytic iron/day (iron group) or nonfortified biscuits (control group) 4 times/week for 6 months. After 6 months of intervention, there was a significant increase in the number of enterobacteria ($p < 0.005$) and a decrease in the number of *Lactobacilli* ($p < 0.0001$) in the iron group, compared to the control group [44]. Moreover, in the iron group, compared to the control group, there was a significant increase in fecal calprotectin ($p < 0.01$) [19] (Fig. 20.5), which also correlated with the increase in the abundance of enterobacteria ($p < 0.05$) [44]. The study was conducted in a setting with poor hygiene conditions, which likely explained the unfavorable ratio of enterobacteria to bifidobacteria and lactobacilli at baseline that was aggravated by iron fortification [44].

The second study was a randomized, placebo-controlled intervention trial examining the effects of higher dose iron supplementation on the gut microbiota and gut inflammation in 6–11-year-old children living in South Africa. In this study, the children were randomized to receive either oral tablets containing 50 mg iron as $FeSO_4$ ($n = 22$) or placebo ($n = 27$) for 38 weeks [45]. At the end of the intervention, there were no significant group differences in the gut microbiota composition and inflammation (as measured by fecal calprotectin) [45]. Compared to the setting in the Côte d'Ivoire study [44], this study was conducted in an area with improved water supply, better hygiene, and a lower risk of contaminated foods.

The contrasting findings of these two studies [44, 45] suggest that the adverse effects of iron on the gut microbiota of children may be context-specific and more pronounced in settings with poor hygiene conditions where the gut microbiota is colonized by opportunistic enteropathogens. The two studies did not analyze the gut microbiota for specific VTGs of enteropathogens, which would have provided insight into their findings. To our knowledge, there are no studies published looking at the effects of iron on the gut microbiota of school aged children living in high-income countries with high hygienic standards.

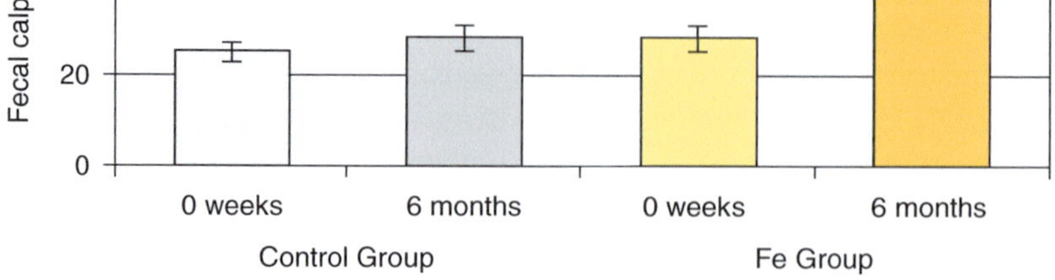

Fig. 20.5 Fecal calprotectin at baseline and 6 months, by group in Ivorian children ($n = 139$) consuming either iron-fortified biscuits containing 20 mg iron as electrolytic iron/day (Fe group) or nonfortified biscuits (Control group) 4 times/week for 6 months. Values without a common letter are significantly different ($p < 0.01$); 2-factor ANOVA with post hoc t tests was used to compare groups. Adapted from [44]

Controlled Studies of Iron Fortification and Supplementation in Adults

Women of reproductive age (nonpregnant and pregnant) are at risk of developing iron deficiency anemia. Although the WHO recommends daily oral iron supplementation for nonpregnant women of reproductive age in settings with a prevalence of anemia ≥40% and for pregnant women [46], little is known on its effects on the gut microbiota. A recent study in pregnant women examined the effect of iron supplements comparing a low-iron group with intakes of 0–10 mg iron per day ($n = 94$) versus a high-iron group with intakes ≥60 mg iron per day ($n = 65$) [47]. There were no between-group differences in microbiota alpha-diversity or in gut microbiota taxa [47]. However, the gut microbiota of the women consuming the low-iron supplements had higher abundances of bacteria producing short-chain fatty acids (SCFAs); the authors suggested this may be beneficial to maintain gut barrier integrity [47]. A recent study reported the gut microbiota of lactating women living in rural Kenya, an area with poor hygiene conditions, was highly colonized by enteropathogens [48]. This unfavorable gut microbiota composition might be particularly vulnerable to adverse effects of iron supplements. Studies in women of reproductive age and particularly in pregnant women living in low-resource settings would therefore be valuable.

Iron deficiency anemia is common in patients with inflammatory bowel disease (IBD) and often requires oral or intravenous iron therapy [49]. A recent open-labeled trial in adults with and without IBD assessed the impact on the gut of 300 mg $FeSO_4$ tablets given twice a day for 3 months compared to intravenous iron therapy [50]. Iron did not have a major effect on the gut microbiota composition in patients with IBD and did not overrule sample clustering based on IBD, characterized by a significant drop in taxa richness, versus healthy patients [50]. However, results suggested the gut microbiota of IBD patients was more sensitive to iron: phylogenetic distances (distances between within-subject samples before and after therapy) were greater in patients with IBD than in healthy controls [50]. Comparing oral and intravenous iron therapy, after oral iron treatment, there were lower abundances of *Colinsella aerofacies*, *Faecalibacterium prausnitzii*, *Ruminococcus bromii,* and *Dorea* spp., but higher abundances of *Bifidobacterium*. The authors concluded that intravenous iron therapy may be preferable for patients with IBD with an unstable gut microbiota [50].

Increasing Iron Intakes and Risk of Diarrhea

Provision of iron supplements and iron-containing MNPs to infants and children in low-resource settings may increase risk of diarrhea. A recent systematic review reported a 15% increased risk of diarrhea (RR 1.15; 95% CI: 1.06–1.26) with iron supplementation or MNP fortification when providing at least 80% of the WHO recommended dietary allowance (daily iron dose for 6–24-month-old infants: 12.5 mg; and for 2–5-year-old children: 20 mg) [51]. This is concerning, considering diarrheal disease is among the two leading causes of mortality among children under 5 years of age, accounting for 17% of the 10.4 million deaths among children under 5 years of age [52]. A recent review summarized the evidence linking oral iron to diarrhea [53]. The adverse effects of iron on the infant gut microbiota described above, and particularly the increase in *Escherichia/Shigella* spp. and pathogenic *E. coli* with iron fortification, provide a plausible mechanism that may explain the increase in diarrhea. The Global Enteric Multicentre Study investigating the etiology of diarrhea in infants in developing countries reported ETEC and *Shigella* to be two of the four pathogens that were significantly associated with diarrhea [54].

Strategies to Balance the Need for Iron and the Risk of Adverse Effects

One approach to mitigate the adverse effects of iron on the gut microbiota could be to reduce the amount of unabsorbed iron entering the colon by decreasing the iron dose given and increasing its bioavailability to maintain efficacy. This effect is evident in recent studies in Kenyan infants comparing the effects of MNPs containing 5 mg iron and 12.5 mg of iron. The 5 mg iron dose was clearly efficacious in reducing iron deficiency anemia, and the improvement of hemoglobin levels and decrease of anemia prevalence [35] compared favorably to results from a 12.5 mg iron dose [38]. Although the 5 mg iron dose negatively affected the infant gut microbiota [35], the adverse effects were less pronounced compared to a dose of 12.5 mg [34]. In contrast to the 12.5 mg iron dose, the 5 mg iron dose did not increase the abundance of the sum of all enteropathogens and pathogenic *E. coli* and did not increase fecal calprotectin levels, suggesting a lower iron dose might not trigger gut inflammation [34, 35].

Another promising strategy to reduce the adverse effects of iron on the gut microbiota is the coprovision of prebiotic GOS. As nondigestible carbohydrates, prebiotics enter the colon intact, where they can selectively enhance the growth of beneficial commensal bifidobacteria and lactobacilli [55]. Prebiotics may protect from colonization and overgrowth of potential enteric pathogens by increasing colonization resistance, increasing production of SCFAs, and decreasing intestinal luminal pH [56, 57]. A 4-month trial in Kenyan infants (study design is described earlier in this chapter) showed that the addition of GOS to a low-dose iron MNP (5 mg iron) mitigated most of the adverse effects of iron on the infant gut microbiota [35]. After 4 months of intervention, compared to the Fe group, in the FeGOS group, there was higher abundance of *Bifidobacterium* and *Lactobacillus* and lower abundance of *Clostridiales* (Fig. 20.3b). Remarkably, there were no significant differences in the abundances of *Bifidobacterium*, *Lactobacillus*, *Enterobacteriaceae*, *Clostridiales*, and *Bacteroidetes* between the control and FeGOS groups (Fig. 20.3c). After 3 weeks of intervention, there were lower abundances of the sum of VTGs of all pathogens in the FeGOS group compared with both the control and Fe group (Fig. 20.4). Also there were significantly lower abundances of the sum of VTGs of pathogenic *E. coli* in the FeGOS group compared to the control group. While there was a significant decrease in the abundances of pathogens from baseline to 4 months in the FeGOS group, there was no significant change in the Fe group (Fig. 20.4). At 4 months, plasma intestinal fatty acid-binding protein (I-FABP, a biomarker of enterocyte damage) was significantly higher in the Fe group compared to the control group but was not higher in the FeGOS group when compared to the control group [35]. Another study that suggests prebiotic GOS may be protective against the adverse effects of iron was conducted in Swedish infants described above [42]. While the authors reported effects of iron fortification and supplementation on abundances of *Bifidobacterium*, *Lactobacillus*, *Clostridium*, and *Bacteroides*, there were no effects on pathogenic bacteria or on fecal calprotectin [42]. All formulas contained 3.3 g/L of GOS and the authors suggested that the coprovision of GOS might have partially mitigated the adverse effects of iron on gut pathogens and fecal calprotectin.

Conclusions and Perspectives

More research is needed to better understand the underlying mechanisms and the effects of dietary iron on the gut microbiota in infants, school-aged children, and adults from low- and high-income countries. In low-income countries, future research should define the lowest effective doses of iron and GOS (and other prebiotics) that can be added to MNPs to offset the adverse effects of iron. The use of lactoferrin in iron-fortified infant formula is associated with a reduced incidence and duration of diarrhea [58]. The benefits of adding this iron-binding protein to iron-containing MNPs to mitigate the adverse effects of iron on the infant gut warrant investigation. In industrialized countries, the effect of high- versus low-iron formulas on the infant gut microbiota should be studied, while defining more clearly the potential benefits of addition of GOS in these settings.

References

1. Sangkhae V, Nemeth E. Regulation of the iron homeostatic hormone hepcidin. Advances in nutrition (Bethesda, Md). 2017;8(1):126–36. https://doi.org/10.3945/an.116.013961.
2. Prentice AM, Mendoza YA, Pereira D, Cerami C, Wegmuller R, Constable A, et al. Dietary strategies for improving iron status: balancing safety and efficacy. Nutr Rev. 2017;75(1):49–60. https://doi.org/10.1093/nutrit/nuw055.
3. Puntarulo S. Iron, oxidative stress and human health. Mol Asp Med. 2005;26(4–5):299–312. https://doi.org/10.1016/j.mam.2005.07.001.
4. Brittenham GM, Andersson M, Egli I, Foman JT, Zeder C, Westerman ME, et al. Circulating non-transferrin-bound iron after oral administration of supplemental and fortification doses of iron to healthy women: a randomized study. Am J Clin Nutr. 2014;100(3):813–20. https://doi.org/10.3945/ajcn.113.081505.
5. Tondeur MC, Schauer CS, Christofides AL, Asante KP, Newton S, Serfass RE, et al. Determination of iron absorption from intrinsically labeled microencapsulated ferrous fumarate (sprinkles) in infants with different iron and hematologic status by using a dual-stable-isotope method. Am J Clin Nutr. 2004;80(5):1436–44. https://doi.org/10.1093/ajcn/80.5.1436.
6. Cook JD, Reddy MB. Efficacy of weekly compared with daily iron supplementation. Am J Clin Nutr. 1995;62(1):117–20. https://doi.org/10.1093/ajcn/62.1.117.
7. Nemeth E, Tuttle MS, Powelson J, Vaughn MB, Donovan A, Ward DM, et al. Hepcidin regulates cellular iron efflux by binding to ferroportin and inducing its internalization. Science (New York, NY). 2004;306(5704):2090–3. https://doi.org/10.1126/science.1104742.
8. Kortman GA, Raffatellu M, Swinkels DW, Tjalsma H. Nutritional iron turned inside out: intestinal stress from a gut microbial perspective. FEMS Microbiol Rev. 2014;38(6):1202–34. https://doi.org/10.1111/1574-6976.12086.
9. Andrews SC, Robinson AK, Rodríguez-Quiñones F. Bacterial iron homeostasis. FEMS Microbiol Rev. 2003;27(2–3):215–37. https://doi.org/10.1016/s0168-6445(03)00055-x.
10. Kramer J, Ozkaya O. Bacterial siderophores in community and host interactions. 2020;18(3):152–63. https://doi.org/10.1038/s41579-019-0284-4.
11. Aisen P, Listowsky I. Iron transport and storage proteins. Annu Rev Biochem. 1980;49:357–93. https://doi.org/10.1146/annurev.bi.49.070180.002041.
12. Carrano CJ, Raymond KN. Ferric ion sequestering agents. 2. Kinetics and mechanism of iron removal from transferrin by enterobactin and synthetic tricatechols. J Am Chem Soc. 1979;101(18):5401–4.
13. Bjarnason J, Southward CM, Surette MG. Genomic profiling of iron-responsive genes in salmonella enterica serovar typhimurium by high-throughput screening of a random promoter library. J Bacteriol. 2003;185(16):4973–82. https://doi.org/10.1128/jb.185.16.4973-4982.2003.
14. Troxell B, Hassan HM. Transcriptional regulation by ferric uptake regulator (Fur) in pathogenic bacteria. Front Cell Infect Microbiol. 2013;3:59. https://doi.org/10.3389/fcimb.2013.00059.
15. Kortman GA, Boleij A, Swinkels DW, Tjalsma H. Iron availability increases the pathogenic potential of salmonella typhimurium and other enteric pathogens at the intestinal epithelial interface. PLoS One. 2012;7(1):e29968. https://doi.org/10.1371/journal.pone.0029968.
16. Rivera-Chavez F, Mekalanos JJ. Cholera toxin promotes pathogen acquisition of host-derived nutrients. Nature. 2019;572(7768):244–8. https://doi.org/10.1038/s41586-019-1453-3.
17. Ho TD, Ellermeier CD. Ferric uptake regulator fur control of putative iron acquisition systems in Clostridium difficile. J Bacteriol. 2015;197(18):2930–40. https://doi.org/10.1128/jb.00098-15.
18. Berges M, Michel AM, Lassek C, Nuss AM, Beckstette M, Dersch P, et al. Iron regulation in Clostridioides difficile. Front Microbiol. 2018;9:3183. https://doi.org/10.3389/fmicb.2018.03183.
19. Konikoff MR, Denson LA. Role of fecal calprotectin as a biomarker of intestinal inflammation in inflammatory bowel disease. Inflamm Bowel Dis. 2006;12(6):524–34.
20. Nakashige TG, Zhang B, Krebs C, Nolan EM. Human calprotectin is an iron-sequestering host-defense protein. Nat Chem Biol. 2015;11(10):765–71. https://doi.org/10.1038/nchembio.1891.
21. Flo TH, Smith KD, Sato S, Rodriguez DJ, Holmes MA, Strong RK, et al. Lipocalin 2 mediates an innate immune response to bacterial infection by sequestrating iron. Nature. 2004;432(7019):917–21. https://doi.org/10.1038/nature03104.
22. Weinberg ED. The lactobacillus anomaly: total iron abstinence. Perspect Biol Med. 1997;40(4):578–83.
23. Vazquez-Gutierrez P, Lacroix C, Jaeggi T, Zeder C, Zimmerman MB, Chassard C. Bifidobacteria strains isolated from stools of iron deficient infants can efficiently sequester iron. BMC Microbiol. 2015;15:3. https://doi.org/10.1186/s12866-014-0334-z.
24. Vazquez-Gutierrez P, de Wouters T, Werder J, Chassard C, Lacroix C. High iron-sequestrating

bifidobacteria inhibit enteropathogen growth and adhesion to intestinal epithelial cells in vitro. Front Microbiol. 2016;7:1480. https://doi.org/10.3389/fmicb.2016.01480.

25. Pandey A, Bringel F, Meyer J. Iron requirement and search for siderophores in lactic acid bacteria. Appl Microbiol Biotechnol. 1994;40:735–9.
26. Valdebenito M, Crumbliss AL, Winkelmann G, Hantke K. Environmental factors influence the production of enterobactin, salmochelin, aerobactin, and yersiniabactin in Escherichia coli strain Nissle 1917. Int J Med Microbiol. 2006;296(8):513–20. https://doi.org/10.1016/j.ijmm.2006.06.003.
27. Deriu E, Liu JZ, Pezeshki M, Edwards RA, Ochoa RJ, Contreras H, et al. Probiotic bacteria reduce salmonella typhimurium intestinal colonization by competing for iron. Cell Host Microbe. 2013;14(1):26–37. https://doi.org/10.1016/j.chom.2013.06.007.
28. Sassone-Corsi M, Nuccio SP, Liu H, Hernandez D, Vu CT, Takahashi AA, et al. Microcins mediate competition among Enterobacteriaceae in the inflamed gut. Nature. 2016;540(7632):280–3. https://doi.org/10.1038/nature20557.
29. Bessman NJ, Mathieu JRR, Renassia C, Zhou L, Fung TC. Dendritic cell-derived hepcidin sequesters iron from the microbiota to promote mucosal healing. Science. 2020;368(6487):186–9. https://doi.org/10.1126/science.aau6481.
30. Ganz T, Nemeth E. Iron homeostasis in host defence and inflammation. Nat Rev Immunol. 2015;15(8):500–10. https://doi.org/10.1038/nri3863.
31. Das NK, Schwartz AJ, Barthel G, Inohara N, Liu Q, Sankar A, et al. Microbial metabolite signaling is required for systemic iron homeostasis. Cell Metab. 2020;31(1):115–30.e6. https://doi.org/10.1016/j.cmet.2019.10.005.
32. Shanmugam NK, Trebicka E, Fu LL, Shi HN, Cherayil BJ. Intestinal inflammation modulates expression of the iron-regulating hormone hepcidin depending on erythropoietic activity and the commensal microbiota. J Immunol (Baltimore, Md : 1950). 2014;193(3):1398–407. https://doi.org/10.4049/jimmunol.1400278.
33. WHO. Guideline: use of multiple micronutrient powders for home fortification of foods consumed by infants and children 6–23 months of age. Geneva: World Health Organization; 2011.
34. Jaeggi T, Kortman GA, Moretti D, Chassard C, Holding P, Dostal A, et al. Iron fortification adversely affects the gut microbiome, increases pathogen abundance and induces intestinal inflammation in Kenyan infants. Gut. 2015;64(5):731–42. https://doi.org/10.1136/gutjnl-2014-307720.
35. Paganini D, Uyoga MA, Kortman GAM, Cercamondi CI, Moretti D, Barth-Jaeggi T, et al. Prebiotic galacto-oligosaccharides mitigate the adverse effects of iron fortification on the gut microbiome: a randomised controlled study in Kenyan infants. Gut. 2017;66(11):1956–67. https://doi.org/10.1136/gutjnl-2017-314418.
36. Tang M, Frank DN, Hendricks AE, Ir D, Esamai F, Liechty E, et al. Iron in micronutrient powder promotes an unfavorable gut microbiota in Kenyan infants. Nutrients. 2017;9(7). https://doi.org/10.3390/nu9070776.
37. Rogawski ET, Platts-Mills JA, Seidman JC, John S, Mahfuz M, Ulak M, et al. Use of antibiotics in children younger than two years in eight countries: a prospective cohort study. Bull World Health Organ. 2017;95(1):49–61. https://doi.org/10.2471/blt.16.176123.
38. De-Regil LM, Suchdev PS, Vist GE, Walleser S, Pena-Rosas JP. Home fortification of foods with multiple micronutrient powders for health and nutrition in children under two years of age (review). Evid Based Child Health. 2013;8(1):112–201. https://doi.org/10.1002/ebch.1895.
39. Paganini D, Uyoga MA, Kortman GAM, Cercamondi CI, Winkler HC, Boekhorst J, et al. Iron-containing micronutrient powders modify the effect of oral antibiotics on the infant gut microbiome and increase post-antibiotic diarrhoea risk: a controlled study in Kenya. Gut. 2019;68(4):645–53. https://doi.org/10.1136/gutjnl-2018-317399.
40. Cheung YB, Xu Y, Mangani C, Fan YM, Dewey KG, Salminen SJ, et al. Gut microbiota in Malawian infants in a nutritional supplementation trial. Trop Med Int Health. 2016;21(2):283–90. https://doi.org/10.1111/tmi.12650.
41. Kamng'ona AW, Young R, Arnold CD, Patson N, Jorgensen JM, Kortekangas E, et al. Provision of lipid-based nutrient supplements to mothers during pregnancy and 6 months postpartum and to their infants from 6 to 18 months promotes infant gut microbiota diversity at 18 months of age but not microbiota maturation in a rural Malawian setting: secondary outcomes of a randomized trial. J Nutr. 2020;150(4):918–28. https://doi.org/10.1093/jn/nxz298.
42. Simonyte Sjodin K, Domellof M, Lagerqvist C, Hernell O, Lonnerdal B, Szymlek-Gay EA, et al. Administration of ferrous sulfate drops has significant effects on the gut microbiota of iron-sufficient infants: a randomised controlled study. Gut. 2019;68(11):2095–7. https://doi.org/10.1136/gutjnl-2018-316988.
43. Tang M, Frank DN, Sherlock L, Ir D, Robertson CE, Krebs NF. Effect of vitamin E with therapeutic iron supplementation on iron repletion and gut microbiome in US iron deficient infants and toddlers. J Pediatr Gastroenterol Nutr. 2016;63(3):379–85. https://doi.org/10.1097/mpg.0000000000001154.
44. Zimmermann MB, Chassard C, Rohner F, N'Goran EK, Nindjin C, Dostal A, et al. The effects of iron fortification on the gut microbiota in African children: a randomized controlled trial in cote d'Ivoire. Am J Clin Nutr. 2010;92(6):1406–15. https://doi.org/10.3945/ajcn.110.004564.
45. Dostal A, Baumgartner J, Riesen N, Chassard C, Smuts CM, Zimmermann MB, et al. Effects of iron

supplementation on dominant bacterial groups in the gut, faecal SCFA and gut inflammation: a randomised, placebo-controlled intervention trial in south African children. Br J Nutr. 2014;112(4):547–56. https://doi.org/10.1017/s0007114514001160.

46. WHO. Nutritional anaemias: tools for effective prevention and control. Geneva: World Health Organization; 2017.
47. Dekker Nitert M, Gomez-Arango LF, Barrett HL, McIntyre HD, Anderson GJ, Frazer DM, et al. Iron supplementation has minor effects on gut microbiota composition in overweight and obese women in early pregnancy. Br J Nutr. 2018;120(3):283–9. https://doi.org/10.1017/s0007114518001149.
48. Paganini D, Uyoga MA, Kortman GAM, Boekhorst J, Schneeberger S, Karanja S, et al. Maternal human milk oligosaccharide profile modulates the impact of an intervention with iron and galacto-oligosaccharides in kenyan infants. Nutrients. 2019;11:11. https://doi.org/10.3390/nu11112596.
49. Goldberg ND. Iron deficiency anemia in patients with inflammatory bowel disease. Clin Exp Gastroenterol. 2013;6:61–70. https://doi.org/10.2147/ceg.s43493.
50. Lee T, Clavel T, Smirnov K, Schmidt A, Lagkouvardos I, Walker A, et al. Oral versus intravenous iron replacement therapy distinctly alters the gut microbiota and metabolome in patients with IBD. Gut. 2017;66(5):863–71. https://doi.org/10.1136/gutjnl-2015-309940.
51. Neuberger A, Okebe J, Yahav D, Paul M. Oral iron supplements for children in malaria-endemic areas. Cochrane Database Syst Rev. 2016;2:CD006589. https://doi.org/10.1002/14651858.CD006589.pub4.
52. WHO. The global burden of disease: 2004 update. Geneva: World Health Organization. p. 2008.
53. Paganini D, Uyoga MA, Zimmermann MB. Iron fortification of foods for infants and children in low-income countries: effects on the gut microbiome, gut inflammation, and diarrhea. Nutrients. 2016;8(8) https://doi.org/10.3390/nu8080494.
54. Kotloff KL, Nataro JP, Blackwelder WC, Nasrin D, Farag TH, Panchalingam S, et al. Burden and aetiology of diarrhoeal disease in infants and young children in developing countries (the global enteric multicenter study, GEMS): a prospective, case-control study. Lancet (London, England). 2013;382(9888):209–22. https://doi.org/10.1016/s0140-6736(13)60844-2.
55. Gibson GR, Roberfroid MB. Dietary modulation of the human colonic microbiota: introducing the concept of prebiotics. J Nutr. 1995;125(6):1401–12. https://doi.org/10.1093/jn/125.6.1401.
56. Hopkins MJ, Macfarlane GT. Nondigestible oligosaccharides enhance bacterial colonization resistance against Clostridium difficile in vitro. Appl Environ Microbiol. 2003;69(4):1920–7. https://doi.org/10.1128/aem.69.4.1920-1927.2003.
57. Roberfroid M, Gibson GR, Hoyles L, McCartney AL, Rastall R, Rowland I, et al. Prebiotic effects: metabolic and health benefits. Br J Nutr. 2010;104(Suppl 2):S1–63.
58. Chen K, Chai L, Li H, Zhang Y, Xie HM, Shang J, et al. Effect of bovine lactoferrin from iron-fortified formulas on diarrhea and respiratory tract infections of weaned infants in a randomized controlled trial. Nutrition (Burbank, Los Angeles County, Calif). 2016;32(2):222–7. https://doi.org/10.1016/j.nut.2015.08.010.

Safety of Interventions to Reduce Nutritional Anemia

21

Andrew M. Prentice, Carla Cerami,
Martin N. Mwangi, and Hans Verhoef

Keywords

Iron · Anemia prevention · Safety · Malaria
Bacteria · Viruses

Introduction

As a general class, iron compounds are probably the most widely distributed pharmacological intervention worldwide, with the need for therapy most commonly indicated by anemia. For individual patients, the physician should investigate and treat the underlying cause of iron deficiency (ID) and iron deficiency anemia (IDA), administer supplemental iron together with dietary advice, and monitor the response to treatment. At the community level, a similar pathway would be desirable but is often not feasible, thus requiring more general approaches to each of the steps including population assessment of prevalence, general assumptions about likely etiological factors, community-wide treatment of underlying causes in vulnerable subgroups (e.g., mass deworming of children), community-wide efforts to improve dietary iron supply and uptake, and group-wide administration of iron (e.g., to pregnant women, children, and adolescent girls).

Among the range of possible interventions against iron deficiency, there tends to be a reciprocity between efficacy and safety. One the one hand, promotion of dietary diversity is safe but constrained by the cost and availability of iron-rich foods and by cultural norms. Biofortification to create iron-rich staples is a highly promising innovation but will never be a complete solution by itself. Nationally mandated iron fortification of staple foods is constrained by the high cost of the best absorbed forms of iron, poor absorption of cheaper versions, and by the pro-oxidant effects of iron on food. Delayed cord-clamping is efficacious and safe but requires further advocacy to encourage its use in clinical practice in most settings. Water, sanitation, and hygiene interventions (WASH) are safe but hard to implement and of modest efficacy against ID and anemia. On the

A. M. Prentice (✉) · C. Cerami
MRC Unit The Gambia at London School of Hygiene and Tropical Medicine, Banjul, The Gambia
e-mail: andrew.prentice@lshtm.ac.uk; ccerami@mrc.gm

M. N. Mwangi
Training and Research Unit of Excellence (TRUE), Blantyre, Malawi

School of Public Health and Family Medicine, College of Medicine, Kamuzu University of Health Sciences (KUHES), Blantyre, Malawi
e-mail: mmwangi@true.mw

H. Verhoef
Division of Human Nutrition and Health, Wageningen University, Wageningen, The Netherlands
e-mail: hans.verhoef@wur.nl

C. D. Karakochuk et al. (eds.), *Nutritional Anemia*, Nutrition and Health,
https://doi.org/10.1007/978-3-031-14521-6_21

other hand, direct administration of supplemental iron is affordable and implementable, and is generally more efficacious. However, supplementation has been associated with worrying evidence of adverse outcomes in several randomized trials leading to more generalized safety concerns, a conundrum for international policy makers, and a challenge for national health departments. These concerns are most prominent in low-income countries where the burden of iron deficiency (ID), and its consequent anemia (IDA), is highest. Extensive reviews of safety issues pertaining to iron administration in pregnancy [1] and childhood [2] are published elsewhere.

In this chapter, we briefly review the biochemical pathways contributing to the host-pathogen battle for iron, and summarize the published evidence for adverse outcomes in humans together with the implications for the design of interventions that could circumvent the safety risks. We restrict our review to exclude studies of parenteral administration of iron. We conclude that concerns about the safety of iron supplementation are real, but can be ameliorated, and that the benefits of combatting ID and IDA generally outweigh the concerns in many settings. The risk-benefit balance could be made even more favorable by the design of future iron supplements and supplementation regimens with fewer side effects and greater efficacy while remaining affordable for low-income countries. These aims constitute a persisting challenge for the field.

Mechanisms by Which Iron May Promote Infections

Iron requirements by microorganisms and viruses: Like humans, virtually all bacteria, fungi, protozoa, and helminths need iron for basic biochemical processes [3]. For example, iron is an indispensable cofactor for enzymes that are critical in nucleic acid synthesis and oxidative phosphorylation, the metabolic pathway used by almost all aerobic organisms to produce adenosine triphosphate (ATP) as the primary intracellular source of energy. In contrast, viruses do not inherently have their own metabolism. They replicate only inside living cells of their host organism, and require these cells to be iron-replete to allow copying of the viral genome and synthesis of viral proteins. Some viruses use transferrin receptors expressed on the outer surface of cell membranes as a portal to recognize and enter host cells [4].

Sources of iron for microorganisms: In the natural environment, microorganisms must access iron that is ubiquitous but occurs mostly precipitated as insoluble ferric oxides or ferric complexes. Invading microbes also need access to iron bound to tissue- or site-specific host proteins, that is, hemoglobin (blood); myoglobin (skeletal muscle); transferrin, haptoglobin, hemopexin (plasma); ferritin and hemosiderin (intracellularly, particularly in hepatocytes and macrophages); and lactoferrin (secretory fluids such as milk, saliva, tears, nasal and vaginal secretions, and extracellular fluids where lactoferrin is deposited by neutrophils as part of the innate immune response).

In the human gut, microorganisms compete for dietary iron that occurs as heme (virtually all animal-derived) or in nonheme forms (mostly bound to phytates from plant seeds, and to a lesser extent incorporated in ferritin from liver and other animal sources). In contrast, iron from oral supplements or food fortificants is in forms that do not occur naturally (or at least in these amounts) with a normal diet: ferrous salts (e.g., ferrous sulfate, ferrous fumarate, ferrous gluconate), ferric salts (e.g., ferric citrate, ferric sodium ethylenediaminetetraacetate [NaFeEDTA]), or the elemental metal (e.g., electrolytic iron, hydrogen-reduced iron). Much supplemental iron or fortificant iron (typically >80%) is unabsorbed in the duodenum and passes into the large intestine. Industrial iron fortification is probably safer than iron supplementation, because the lower amount of iron added to industrially fortified foods is closer to the physiological situation [5].

Point-of care fortificants recommended by the World Health Organization contain iron in amounts similar to the daily dose of iron recommended for oral supplementation in children aged 4–23 months (10–12.5 mg).

Iron acquisition mechanisms in microorganisms: Fig. 21.1 summarizes some of the complex mechanisms by which microorganisms acquire iron. Microorganisms have evolved several mechanisms to scavenge host iron [13]. More than 90% of the iron in mammals occurs intracellularly and is not accessible for extracellular pathogens unless it can be liberated from host cells. Bacterial toxins cause cell lysis or damage, leading to the release of hemoglobin or ferritin from host cells. Most bacteria and fungi secrete and resorb small proteins (siderophores) that bind extracellular iron in the environment or competitively "steal" iron from host proteins. The soluble siderophore–Fe^{3+} complexes thus formed are recognized by receptors at the bacterial surface and taken up by active transport mechanisms. Some bacteria are able to utilize siderophores that are produced by other bacterial species (xenosiderophores). Other bacterial pathogens and some parasites (e.g., *Trypanosoma brucei*, *Trichomonas vaginalis*, *Schistosoma mansoni*) acquire iron through receptor-mediated uptake of transferrin, lactoferrin, hemopexin, hemoglobin, or hemoglobin-haptoglobin complexes.

Many pathogenic species have evolved multiple iron acquisition systems that allow them to occupy a variety of niches within the host, with diverse amounts and forms of available iron. For example, *Staphylococcus aureus* is a commensal Gram-positive bacterium that is found in normal skin flora, in the nostrils, and in the lower reproductive tract of women. Upon breaching the epithelium, it can also become an opportunistic extracellular pathogen colonizing nearly every organ, being a common cause of skin infections and abscesses but also causing bacteremia, pneumonia, osteomyelitis, endocarditis, and septic shock. To survive in these varied host environments, *S. aureus* can obtain iron from circulating or transudated transferrin or lactoferrin using siderophores (staphyloferrin A and B) or it can obtain hemoglobin iron in blood or abscesses by lysing erythrocytes through the secretion of hemolysins. To prevent oxidative damage and to limit iron availability to pathogens, the host counters by binding free hemoglobin to haptoglobin in plasma. *S. aureus* is nonetheless able to access this iron by stripping heme from the haptoglobin-hemoglobin complex by hemoprotein receptors on the surface of the cell wall, followed by receptor-mediated transport across the cell wall, protein-mediated transport across the cell membrane, and intracellular release of iron by heme-degrading enzymes [14]. The extraordinary molecular tools that are available to bacteria and their hosts in this example illustrate and result from their ongoing evolutionary battle for iron.

Host's iron-withholding response to infections: Following infection, plasma iron concentrations rapidly decrease, a mechanism that probably developed evolutionarily to deny host iron to invading extracellular pathogens. As part of the host response, which is mediated by hepcidin under influence of proinflammatory cytokines ([15] and Chap. 2), both iron recycling by macrophages from phagocytosed senescent erythrocytes and intestinal absorption of iron are impaired. This leads in turn to a reduced supply of iron to bone marrow erythroid precursors and reduced erythropoiesis. The resulting anemia of inflammation is a "price" paid by the host for the protection offered by the iron-withholding response. By diverting iron from serum toward macrophages, however, the host provides an iron-rich intracellular environment that possibly favors the proliferation of pathogens for which replication in macrophages is a predominant or critical component of the species' pathogenic lifestyle [16]. Bacteria in this group encompass diverse species of great public health importance such as *Mycobacterium tuberculosis* (causing tuberculosis), *Salmonella* species (typhoid fever, gastroenteritis), *Brucella melitensis* (brucellosis), *Coxiella*

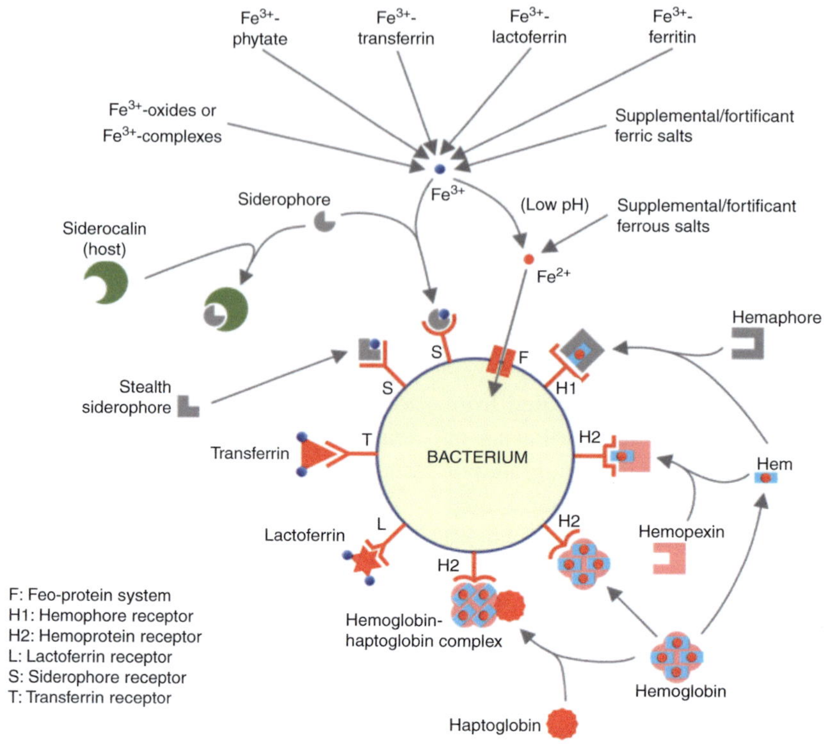

Fig. 21.1 Iron availability and acquisition by microorganisms in natural and various host environments. Under aerobic conditions as prevailing in the natural environment, iron occurs mostly precipitated as insoluble ferric oxides or ferric complexes. Microorganisms can access this iron by secreting small iron-chelating compounds ("siderophores") into the environment. The Fe^{3+}-siderophore complex is then actively re-internalized by transport across the cell membrane through specific receptors and transporters and released as a nutrient for the microorganism. In food, iron mostly occurs as ferric iron bound to phytate (in plant foods) or contained in ferritin (mostly animal foods), or ferrous iron bound to hems in hemoglobin or myoglobin (animal foods). In the stomach, gastric acid and ascorbic acid promote release and solubilization of ferric iron from dietary plant sources, or of ferrous iron from poorly soluble supplemental ferrous salts (e.g., ferrous fumarate; [6]). In the duodenum, the prevailing pH favors the reduction of ferric iron to the ferrous form, and the reformation of Fe^{2+}- or Fe^{3+}-ligand complexes. The entry of elemental iron and Fe^{3+}-salts from iron supplements and fortificants into the common nonheme iron pool is limited by their solubility. Supplemental ferrous salts given in doses to prevent or treat iron deficiency anemia produce a bolus of soluble ferrous iron that does not normally occur with food sources. Ferrous iron can be acquired by bacteria through several mechanisms, including uptake by Feo proteins [7]. In the colon, the Fe^{3+}-phytate and Fe^{3+}-ferritin complexes can be made accessible by enzymatic degradation or removal of iron by siderophores [8]. As part of the immune response to infection, the host can produce proteins ("siderocalins") that specifically bind to a particular siderophore, thus preventing its use for bacterial iron acquisition. Several bacteria species outmaneuver this host immune response by producing structural variant siderophores ("stealth siderophores") that are not recognized and thus preclude binding by siderocalin (e.g., [9–11]). Invading microbes need access to iron bound to tissue- or site-specific host proteins: hemoglobin (blood); myoglobin (skeletal muscle); transferrin, haptoglobin, hemopexin (plasma); ferritin and hemosiderin (intracellularly, particularly in hepatocytes and macrophages); and lactoferrin (secretory fluids and extracellular fluids where lactoferrin is deposited by neutrophils). Most iron occurs intracellularly and is not accessible for extracellular pathogens unless it can be liberated from host cells. Bacterial toxins cause cell lysis or damage, leading to the release of hemoglobin or ferritin from host cells. In blood plasma, hemoglobin that is released as a result of natural lysis or bacterial toxin-induced lysis of erythrocytes is oxidized into met-hemoglobin, which then further disassociates into free heme along with the globin chains. Free hemoglobin or heme are toxic and are rapidly sequestered to the host proteins haptoglobin and hemopexin, respectively. Bacterial pathogens and some parasites acquire iron through receptor-mediated uptake of transferrin, lactoferrin, hemopexin, hemoglobin, or hemoglobin-haptoglobin complexes. In addition, microbes use siderophores to "steal" iron from host proteins. Some bacteria are able to utilize siderophores that are produced by other bacterial species ("xenosiderophores"). Secreted hemophores, which show functional analogy with siderophores, can remove heme from heme-binding proteins (hemoglobin, hemopexin, or hemoglobin-haptoglobin) and deliver it to bacterial cells through binding with hemophore receptors [12]

burnetii (Q fever), *Burkholderia pseudomallei* (melioidosis), *Listeria monocytogenes* (gastroenteritis, bacteraemia), and *Chlamydia trachomatis* (trachoma, pelvic inflammatory disease).

In mucosal tissues, iron is bound to lactoferrin and, to a lesser degree, by transudated transferrin and ferritin. Lactoferrin has unusually strong affinity for iron. In breast milk, where it constitutes 15–20% of protein, lactoferrin is largely unsaturated with iron [17]. Human milk has a powerful bacteriostatic effect on *Escherichia coli*, which is abolished if the iron-binding proteins are saturated with iron [18]. The iron-binding capacity of lactoferrin is enhanced in weakly acidic environments. This property facilitates the transfer of iron from transferrin to lactoferrin during inflammation, when the pH in tissues decreases due to accumulation of lactic acid and other acids [19]. Lactoferrin works in tandem with *Lactobacilli* to protect the female genital tract from pathogenic infections [20].

Iron and Risk of Malaria Infection

We start with malaria, since this is the infection that has driven policy uncertainty in the past 15 years, following the premature termination of a large trial on Pemba Island, Tanzania, due to an excess of serious adverse events (SAEs) in the two trial arms that were receiving iron [21]. A very similar concurrent trial in a nonmalarious region of Nepal found no such association; so, despite there being uncertainty about the precise causes of the SAEs in Pemba, it was assumed that malaria (*Plasmodium falciparum*) was key. Much has been written about this trial and the policy aftermath [22]. What follows is a brief update on subsequent research and the best evidence on which current policy can be based.

There is now good epidemiological and experimental evidence that anemia protects against *P falciparum* malaria in both children (e.g., [23]) and pregnant women (e.g., [24]). In addition to the Pemba Trial, there is evidence from other trials indicating that administration of iron can increase the risk of malaria (e.g., [25]) though these associations are by no means universal [22].

The Pemba results stimulated numerous studies searching for the specific mechanism by which iron stimulated malaria infections. Candidate mechanisms included increased iron supply to hepatocytes and/or red blood cells (RBCs) [22], and increased levels of unbound plasma iron [26], but strong experimental evidence proved elusive.

Our group developed novel bar-coded FACS methods to study the *in vitro* invasion, growth, and sporozyte formation of *P. falciparum* in fresh RBCs drawn from Gambian mothers and children with different grades of anemia, and their response to iron supplementation [27, 28]. Figure 21.2 summarizes some of these results. The upper left panel shows that in RBCs from children, parasite growth was strongly inhibited by anemia when compared to the growth in RBCs from nonanemic controls. The panel below shows that parasite growth was greatly increased after 49 days of oral iron supplementation. The right-hand panels replicate these data in pregnant women and show that growth was stimulated after only 14 days of iron therapy (note that the children were not sampled at 14 days). Our prior work had shown that, as was already known for *P. vivax*, *P. falciparum* preferentially invades young, large erythrocytes, especially reticulocytes [27]. We believe that this is the primary mechanism by which iron supplementation promotes the risk of malaria.

These results have clear policy implications. Given that correction of anemia will always require an increase in reticulocyte production, any effective hematological response to iron will inevitably create a period of vulnerability to malaria. Fortunately, the reticulocytosis is transient and hence that elevated malaria risk is also transient (see Fig. 21.3). These findings align with the WHO advice that, in malarious areas, iron supplements should be accompanied by effective measures to prevent, detect, and treat malaria [30].

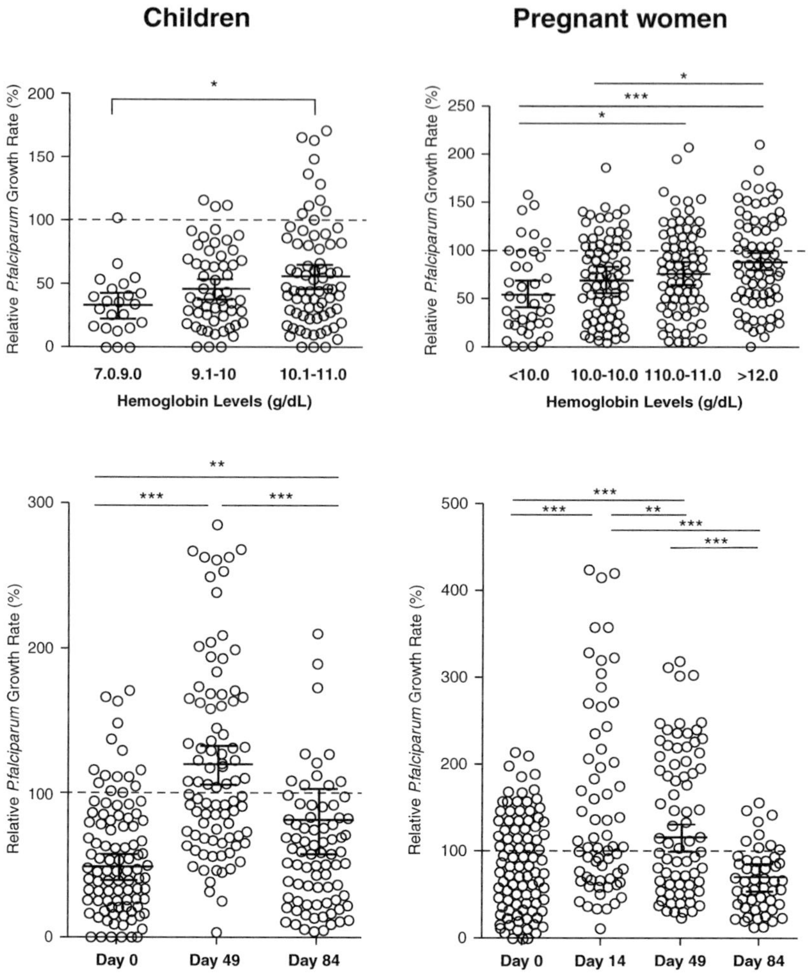

Fig. 21.2 *In vitro* growth of *P. falciparum* in fresh RBCs drawn from Gambian mothers and children with different grades of anemia and their response to iron supplementation. Upper panels show relative parasite growth rates according to levels of anemia. Lower panels show response to iron supplementation. Data redrawn from Bah et al. [29] and Goheen et al. [28]

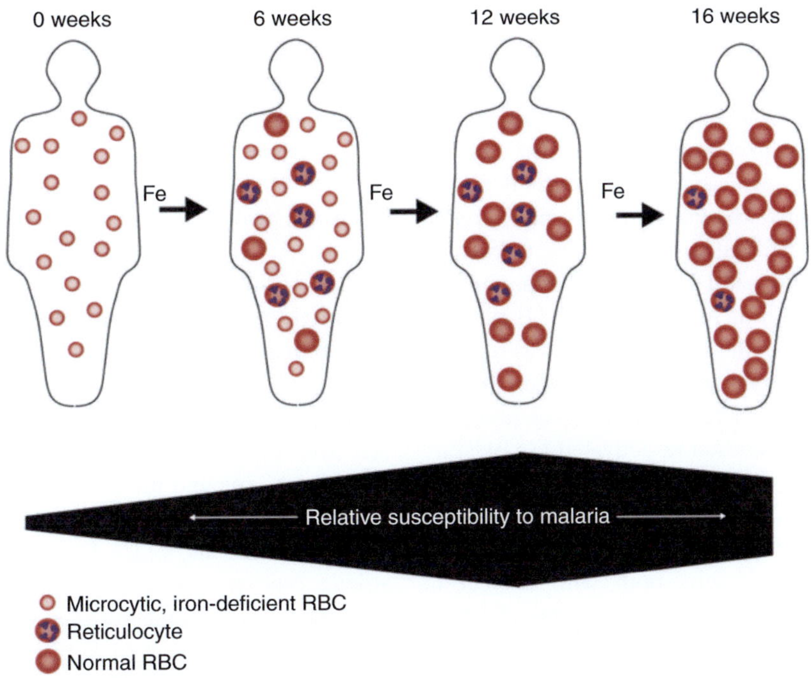

Fig. 21.3 Schematic representation of increased susceptibility to *P. falciparum* malaria caused by the transient reticulocytosis caused by iron supplementation in individuals with iron deficiency anemia (after [28])

Iron and Other Infections

There is widespread evidence that "iron-loaded" individuals (e.g., as a consequence of hemochromatosis) are more susceptible to infections, especially bacterial infections [16]. Patients with disturbed iron redistribution as a consequence of infections and inflammation also appear to have poor outcomes. For instance, high iron status at the time of entry into a longitudinal cohort of Gambian HIV patients independently predicted a greater likelihood of incident TB and of accelerated mortality [31, 32]. These and other studies confirm that excess body iron can drive infections, but do not directly address the issue of iron supplementation.

Animal studies conducted over many decades show that sublethal inoculation with numerous pathogenic bacteria become rapidly lethal if coadministered with iron (from various sources) [33, 34]. More recent studies have revealed an important role for hepcidin in protecting against bacterial infections; hepcidin-deficient mice are highly susceptible to a range of organisms that are well tolerated by wild-type mice (see Chap. 2 and associated citations).

In humans, *ex vivo* studies using "sentinel" bacteria representative of different modes of iron acquisition clearly demonstrate that iron-loaded serum in the hours following oral iron supplementation supports a much faster rate of bacterial growth. Experiments in adult men showed that oral iron did not affect the growth in postdose plasma of *Staphylococcus aureus*, a species that preferentially scavenges heme iron, but led to markedly elevated growth of *Escherichia coli*, *Yersinia enterocolitica*, *Salmonella enterica* serovar Typhimurium, and *Staphylococcus epidermidis* [35]. However, in pregnant women, the growth of *S. aureus* was augmented as well as the growth of *E. coli* and *S. enterica* [29]. Similar experiments in young Gambian children showed no increase in the growth of *S. aureus, E. coli,* or *S. enterica* after 49 of iron supplementation, but the plasma was drawn 24 h after the last iron dose. On Day 84 of supplementation, when plasma was drawn 4 h after the last iron dose, the growth of *E. coli* and *S. enterica* was significantly faster [36].

In vivo observations in humans support the contention that iron administration can enhance the growth of a wide range of potentially pathogenic organisms. The Parisian physician Armand Trousseau is credited with publishing the first of these observations in 1872, when he reported that supplementing iron in the diets of TB patients hastened their death [37]. This topic was reawakened a century later by another quasi-interventional study in Somali nomads reporting that iron administration re-activated pre-existing malaria, brucellosis, and tuberculosis [38].

Formal RCTs in which iron is administered (with or without additional micronutrients) have yielded variable results both with respect to malaria (see above) and other infections. Perhaps the most concerning results emerged from a large cluster-randomized trial in Pakistan which reported that episodes of chest indrawing (indicative of pneumonia) in children aged 6–18 m was higher in the two intervention groups receiving food fortified with iron-containing micronutrient powders than in the nonsupplemented control group [39]. In children aged 18–24 months, there were too few episodes to establish whether this pattern was maintained. This trial also reported an increase in the number of episodes of bloody diarrhea (see below for discussion).

While many iron-supplementing RCTs reveal no evidence of safety concerns, there are sufficient instances of trials that do flag safety signals to warrant attention and caution. For example, in a cluster-randomized trial among Ghanaian children aged 6–35 months, point-of-care fortification of foods with iron-containing micronutrient powers resulted in a 23% increase in the number of hospital admissions during the 5 months of active intervention [40]; this may have been attributable to diarrhea. A post-hoc analysis of a physician-prescribed RCT of an iron-containing multiple micronutrient supplement in 1100 Gambian children revealed an excess of return clinic visits in the first few weeks after the supplements were issued compared to the placebo group [41]. In these and other instances (see above for malaria), it is noteworthy that the adverse outcomes seem to appear in the first few weeks of iron administration, although the reverse was true in the Pemba trial [21].

Additional instances of adverse safety signals arising from the gut and vaginal microbiome are discussed below.

Iron Interventions and the Gut Microbiome

Several studies suggest that iron supplementation and iron fortification can lead to changes in the gut microbiome and increase the abundance and virulence of enteric pathogens (see also Chap. 18 in this volume, and [42]). In a randomized trial among Ivorian children aged 6–14 years [43], consumption of biscuits fortified with poorly soluble electrolytic iron (4 times per week for 6 months) resulted in an increase in the number of enterobacteria and a decrease in the *Lactobacilli* population. The *Enterobacteriaceae* include, along with many commensal and non-pathogenic symbionts (e.g., non-pathogenic *E. coli*), many pathogens such as *Salmonella*, pathogenic *E. coli*, *Shigella,* and *Klebsiella*. After 6 months, the prevalence of *Salmonella* colonization in the iron group was higher than in the control group (23.3% vs. 16.6%), but the statistical evidence was weak ($p > 0.05$). Iron fortification also led to marked increases in fecal calprotectin concentrations, which were also associated with changes in the number of enterobacteria, suggesting that the iron-associated increases in enterobacteria may have contributed to an increase in gut inflammation.

In two randomized placebo-controlled trials among 6-month-old Kenyan infants consuming maize porridge daily for 4 months, point-of-care fortification with iron (2.5 mg as NaFeEDTA or 12.5 mg iron as ferrous fumarate) increased enterobacteria as assessed by pyrosequencing, particularly *Escherichia*/*Shigella*, the enterobacteria/bifidobacteria ratio, and *Clostridium* spp. [44]. Using qPCR, iron fortification led to increased pathogenic *E. coli* strains. Iron fortification almost doubled fecal calprotectin concentrations [44]. There was no compelling evidence that iron fortification increased the frequency of diarrhea.

In contrast, a randomized trial in iron-deficient South African children aged 6–11 years administered oral supplements for 4 days per week for 38 weeks containing either 50 mg iron as ferrous sulfate or placebo (see Chap. 18). Iron supplementation improved iron status in iron-deficient children, but there was no evidence that it increased fecal calprotectin concentration, or that it affected the change in fecal bacterial load over time, or fecal concentrations of short-chain fatty acids.

Nonanemic or mildly anemic, predominantly breastfed, Kenyan infants aged 6 months were randomized to consume foods that were fortified with micronutrient powders containing 12.5 mg iron, micronutrient powders without iron, or no micronutrient powders (daily, for 3 months) (see Chap. 18). There were some indications that iron may have adversely affected the colonization of beneficial microbes and attenuated the decrease of potential pathogens, but the study was small, and comparisons were done within groups over time instead of between-intervention groups.

In healthy, nonanemic Swedish infants, consumption of high-iron formula was associated with reduced abundance of bifidobacteria compared with low-iron formula, and administration of liquid ferrous sulfate as drops, even in an iron dose comparable with the daily iron requirement and for a short time, led to decreased relative abundance of *Lactobacilli* [45]. There was some but conflicting evidence that it resulted in increased susceptibility to bacterial infection, and no statistical support for increased fecal calprotectin concentration.

A small trial in Kenyan infants ($n = 28$) indicated that iron fortification can reduce the efficacy of concurrently administered broad-spectrum antibiotics against potential enteropathogens, particularly pathogenic *E. coli*, and may increase risk for diarrhea (see Chap. 18).

In an open-label randomized trial among anemic Nigerian toddlers, there was no evidence that consumption of 200–600 mL multinutrient-fortified dairy-based drink supplying 2.2 mg, 4.5 mg, and 6.7 mg of iron as ferrous sulfate per day caused an increase in the pathogenic gut bacteria [46]. Likewise, in a trial among Bangladeshi children, there was no evident difference in gut microbiota profile/composition between children who received daily micronutrient powder supplementation with low-iron (2.5 mg) versus standard-dose iron (12.5 mg) [47].

An analysis of stool samples collected at 12 and 24 m from a small subset of children in the aforementioned cluster-randomized trial by Soofi et al. [39] in Pakistan provides preliminary evidence that iron and/or vitamin may promote disruptive protozoal and fungal communities in the gut, an effect ameliorated by zinc [48].

A normal gut microbiome composition is highly effective in resisting colonization by potentially pathogenic invaders. Loss of the normal microbiota or a shift in the balance of these microorganisms can lead to their replacement by Gram-negative aerobic bacteria or other pathogenic organisms. From this perspective, it is of concern that several studies suggest that supplementation or fortification with iron can lead to such disturbances, or to growth of pathogenic taxa in vulnerable populations. These results should nonetheless be interpreted with caution, for several reasons.

First, contrary to high-income countries, asymptomatic gut infections by pathogenic microorganisms are extremely common in many low-income countries, from a young age onward. For example, in GEMS, a large study in seven sites in Africa and Asia, the prevalence of *Shigella*, *Cryptosporidium*, and heat-labile enterotoxigenic *E. coli* by qPCR was 27%, 21%, and 29% in controls without diarrhea in the second year of life [49]. A large birth cohort study at eight sites in Africa, Asia, and South America (MAL-ED) showed similar results [50]. Thus, the question arises to what extent a mild or moderate increase in enteropathogen carriage, as suggested by some studies that evaluated the effect of iron, will lead to increased morbidity and mortality associated with diarrhea. For many of these enteropathogen infections, current knowledge about their epidemiology in various settings and subpopulations in low-income country is inadequate to answer that question. Intensive community surveillance for diarrhea in the MAL-ED study showed no evidence that three frequently detected pathogens (entero-aggregative *E. coli*, *Giardia* species, and atypical enteropathogenic *E. coli*) were associated with diarrhea for any age group, site, or diarrheal syndrome. Evidence from epidemiological studies indicates that coinfections involving *G. duodenalis* may even be associated with a protective effect against enteropathogen-driven diarrhea in low-income countries, as indicated by several reports that children infected with *Giardia* present with reduced frequency of diarrheal illness and reduced serum inflammatory scores [51].

A second reason for caution is that any effect of iron, if extant, may be trivial in comparison to disturbances in gut microbiota composition and effects on enteropathogens caused by the frequent use of antibiotics. Nationally representative facility-based and household-based surveys in eight low-income countries showed that children received on average 24.5 antibiotic prescriptions for respiratory tract infection or fever during their first 5 years of life (range: 7·1 in Senegal to 59·1 in Uganda), and most of these prescriptions were deemed inappropriate [52]. The actual number of antibiotic treatments is likely to be even higher, because a substantial proportion of antibiotic treatments are purchased from private providers, without prescription (e.g., [53]).

Iron Interventions and Diarrhea

Increased iron intakes can theoretically increase the risk of diarrhea by causing a dysbiosis of the gut microbiome (including enteropathogen colonization and invasion) or through other mechanisms such as increased permeability of the small intestine, formation of free radicals and increased oxidative stress in the intestinal lumen, or by impairing the immune response to pathogens [42]. In a systematic review of 19 randomized controlled trials of oral iron supplementation or iron fortification that reported diarrheal outcomes in children aged 4–59 months, most studies (12 of 19) failed to show an effect of iron on diarrheal incidence or found such an effect only within a specific subgroup of the population (3 studies), while only 4 studies showed an increase in overall diarrhea incidence [54]. Absent or variable case definitions for diarrhea made meta-analysis impossible. Two studies [39, 55] suggest that iron can lead to an increased incidence of acute bloody diarrhea (dysentery). Although alarming, it cannot be excluded that these effects were due to prescription of cefdinir, an antibiotic that produces a red color when coadministered with iron [54]. The reasons for which different meta-analyses draw different conclusions as to whether iron supplements increase the incidence of diarrhea have been the topic of recent debate (e.g., [56]).

Iron Interventions and the Vaginal Microbiome

Increased iron availability can theoretically disturb the delicate equilibrium within the vaginal microbiome, and lead to a microbiota composition that is associated with premature birth, pelvic inflammatory disease, and acquisition of sexually transmitted infections such as HIV [57, 58]. To our knowledge, however, compelling *in vivo* evidence for these effects is yet to be provided. In a randomized controlled trial among healthy nulliparous, nonpregnant women aged 15–24 years in Burkina Faso, iron-deficient women were more likely to have normal vaginal flora at baseline than their iron-replete peers [59]. There was no evidence that weekly iron influenced the prevalence of bacterial vaginosis and *T. vaginalis* and microbiota profiles at trial endpoints (first scheduled antenatal visit for women who become pregnant, and at 18 months for women remaining nonpregnant). On the other hand, iron-supplemented nonpregnant women received more antibiotic treatments for nongenital infections (mainly gastrointestinal infections), antifungal treatments for genital infections and analgesics, even though there was no evidence that iron supplementation affected the prevalence of iron deficiency [59].

Administration of Iron with Prebiotics and Probiotics

There is some evidence, mostly from animal studies, that gut microbiota modulation through intake of prebiotics (food compounds that induce the growth or activity of beneficial microorganisms) and probiotics (live microorganisms that provide health benefits when ingested, generally by improving or restoring gut microbiota composition) can increase iron absorption. Thus, when administered in conjunction with iron, prebiotics and probiotics can theoretically improve iron status while mitigating potential adverse effects of oral iron on pathogenic infections and gut inflammation (see Chap. 18 in this volume which includes human studies).

Conclusions

While by no means universal, there is widespread evidence ranging from cellular mechanistic research, through animal studies, and to large-scale real-life human intervention studies that the administration of iron can cause a range of adverse outcomes ranging from the inconvenient (gastric pain) to death. National and regional decision-making must try to assess the net benefit or harm that will accrue in any given setting. Pasricha et al. [60] attempted to model the cost-benefit balance in 78 countries using microsimulation. They concluded that there could be net benefit in 54 countries, but net harm in 24 (22 of which were in Africa). Though limited by the available data for conducting such simulations (e.g., there was an absence of data on potential benefits on cognitive function), this analysis emphasizes that context is critical in assessing the optimal route to ameliorating iron deficiency. It is not possible to provide a universal prescription except to recommend that iron administration is an important intervention and can be given safely if other relevant precautions are taken. This remains the current approach recommended by WHO [30].

References

1. Mwangi MN, Prentice AM, Verhoef H. Safety and benefits of antenatal oral iron supplementation in low-income countries: a review. Br J Haematol. 2017;177:884–95.
2. Mwangi MN, Mzembe G, Moya E, Verhoef H. Iron deficiency anaemia in sub-Saharan Africa: a review of current evidence and primary care recommendations for high-risk groups. Lancet Haematol. 2021;8:e732–43.
3. Andrews SC, Robinson AK, Rodríguez-Quiñones F. Bacterial iron homeostasis. FEMS Microbiol Rev. 2003;27:215–37.
4. Wessling-Resnick M. Crossing the iron gate: why and how transferrin receptors mediate viral entry. Annu Rev Nutr. 2018;38:431–58.
5. Hurrell RF. Iron Fortification Practices and Implications for Iron Addition to Salt. J Nutr. 2021;151(Suppl 1):3S–14S.
6. García-Casal MN, Layrisse M. The effect of change in pH on the solubility of iron bis-glycinate chelate and other iron compounds. Arch Latinoam Nutr. 2001;51(1 Suppl 1):35–6.
7. Lau CKY, Krewulak KD, Vogel HJ. Bacterial ferrous iron transport: the Feo system. FEMS Microbiol Rev. 2016;40:273–98.
8. Kortman GAM, Raffatellu M, Swinkels DW, Tjalsma H. Nutritional iron turned inside out: intestinal stress from a gut microbial perspective. FEMS Microbiol Rev. 2014;38:1202–34.
9. Abergel RJ, Wilson MK, Arceneaux JEL, et al. Anthrax pathogen evades the mammalian immune system through stealth siderophore production. Proc Natl Acad Sci U S A. 2006;103:18499–503.
10. Golonka R, San Yeoh B, Vijay-Kumara M. The iron tug-of-war between bacterial siderophores and innate immunity. J Innate Immun. 2019;11:249–62.
11. Raffatellu M, Bäumler AJ. Salmonella's iron armor for battling the host and its microbiota. Gut Microbes. 2010;1:70–2.
12. Wandersman C, Delepaire P. Haemophore functions revisited. Mol Microbiol. 2012;85:618–31.
13. Skaar EP. The battle for iron between bacterial pathogens and their vertebrate hosts. PLoS Pathog. 2010;6:e1000949.
14. Hammer ND, Skaar EP. Molecular mechanisms of Staphylococcus aureus iron acquisition. Annu Rev Microbiol. 2011;65:129–47.
15. Ganz T. Iron and infection. Int J Hematol. 2018;107:7–15.
16. Drakesmith H, Prentice AM. Hepcidin and the iron-infection axis. Science. 2012;338:768–72.
17. Lönnerdal B. Excess iron intake as a factor in growth, infections, and development of infants and young children. Am J Clin Nutr. 2017;106(Suppl 6):1681S–7S.

18. Bullen JJ, Rogers HJ, Leigh L. Iron-binding proteins in milk and resistance to Escherichia coli infection in infants. Br Med J. 1972;1:69–75.
19. De Sousa M, Brock JH, editors. Iron in immunity, cancer, and inflammation. New York: John Wiley & Sons; 1989.
20. Valenti P, Rosa L, Capobianco D, Stefania Lepanto M, Schiavi E, Cutone A, Paesano R, Mastromarino P. Role of lactobacilli and lactoferrin in the mucosal cervicovaginal defense. Front Immunol. 2018;9:376.
21. Sazawal S, Black RE, Ramsan M, Chwaya HM, Stoltzfus RJ, Dutta A, Dhingra U, Kabole I, Deb S, Othman MK, Kabole FM. Effects of routine prophylactic supplementation with iron and folic acid on admission to hospital and mortality in preschool children in a high malaria transmission setting: community-based, randomised, placebo-controlled trial. Lancet. 2006;367:133–43.
22. Spottiswoode N, Fried M, Drakesmith H, Duffy PE. Implications of malaria on iron deficiency control strategies. Adv Nutr. 2012;3:570–8.
23. Gwamaka M, Kurtis JD, Sorensen BE, et al. Iron deficiency protects against severe *Plasmodium falciparum* malaria and death in young children. Clin Infect Dis. 2012;54:1137–44.
24. Kabyemela ER, Fried M, Kurtis JD, Mutabingwa TK, Duffy PE. Decreased susceptibility to *Plasmodium falciparum* infection in pregnant women with iron deficiency. J Infect Dis. 2008;198:163–6.
25. Veenemans J, Milligan P, Prentice AM, Schouten LRA, Inja N, van der Heijden AC, de Boer LCC, Jansen EJS, Koopmans AE, Enthoven WTM, et al. Effect of supplementation with zinc and other micronutrients on malaria in Tanzanian children: a randomised trial. PLoS Med. 2011;8:e1001125.
26. Clark M, Fisher NC, Kasthuri R, Cerami Hand C. Parasite maturation and host serum iron influence the labile iron pool of erythrocyte stage Plasmodium falciparum. Br J Haematol. 2013;161:262–9.
27. Goheen MM, Wegmüller R, Bah A, Darboe B, Danso E, Affara M, Gardner D, Patel JC, Prentice AM, Cerami C. Anemia offers stronger protection than sickle cell trait against the erythrocytic stage of falciparum malaria and this protection is reversed by iron supplementation. EBioMedicine. 2016;14:123–30.
28. Goheen MM, Bah A, Wegmüller R, Verhoef H, Darboe B, Danso E, Prentice AM, Cerami C. Host iron status and erythropoietic response to iron supplementation determines susceptibility to the RBC stage of falciparum malaria during pregnancy. Sci Rep. 2017;7:17674.
29. Bah A, Muhammad AK, Wegmuller R, Verhoef H, Goheen MM, Sanyang S, Danso E, Sise EA, Pasricha SR, Armitage AE, Drakesmith H, Cross JH, Moore SE, Cerami C, Prentice AM. Hepcidin-guided screen-and-treat interventions against iron-deficiency anaemia in pregnancy: a randomised controlled trial in The Gambia. Lancet Glob Health. 2019;7:e1564–74.
30. World Health Organization. WHO guideline: use of multiple micronutrient powders for point-of-use fortification of foods consumed by infants and young children aged 6–23 months and children aged 2–12 years. Geneva: World Health Organization; 2016.
31. McDermid JM, van der Loeff MF, Jaye A, Hennig BJ, Bates C, Todd J, Sirugo G, Hill AV, Whittle HC, Prentice AM. Mortality in HIV infection is independently predicted by host iron status and SLC11A1 and HP genotypes, with new evidence of a gene-nutrient interaction. Am J Clin Nutr. 2009;90:225–33.
32. McDermid JM, Hennig BJ, van der Sande M, Hill AV, Whittle HC, Jaye A, Prentice AM. Host iron redistribution as a risk factor for incident tuberculosis in HIV infection: an 11-year retrospective cohort study. BMC Infect Dis. 2013;13:48.
33. Schaible UE, Kaufmann SH. Iron and microbial infection. Nat Rev Microbiol. 2004;2:946–53.
34. Weinberg ED. Iron and susceptibility to infectious disease. Science. 1974;184:952–6.
35. Cross JH, Bradbury RS, Fulford AJ, Jallow AT, Wegmüller R, Prentice AM, Cerami C. Oral iron acutely elevates bacterial growth in human serum. Sci Rep. 2015;5:16670.
36. Wegmüller R, Bah A, Kendall L, Goheen MM, Sanyang S, Danso E, Sise EA, Jallow A, Verhoef H, Jallow MW, Wathuo M, Armitage AE, Drakesmith H, Pasricha SR, Cross JH, Cerami C, Prentice, AM. Hepcidin-guided screen-and-treat interventions for iron-deficiency anaemia in young children: a proof-of-concept, randomised controlled trial in The Gambia. Lancet Global Health, 2022, in press.
37. Trousseau A. True, false chlorosis. Lectures on clinical medicine. Philadelphia, PA: Lindsay and Blakiston; 1872.
38. Murray MJ, Murray AB, Murray MB, Murray CJ. The adverse effect of iron repletion on the course of certain infections. BMJ. 1978;2:1113–5.
39. Soofi S, Cousens S, Iqbal SP, Akhund T, Khan J, Ahmed I, Zaidi AKM, Bhutta ZA. Effect of provision of daily zinc and iron with several micronutrients on growth and morbidity among young children in Pakistan: a cluster-randomised trial. Lancet. 2013;382:29–40.
40. Zlotkin S, Newton S, Aimone AM, Azindow I, Amenga-Etego S, Tchum K, Mahama E, Thorpe KE, Owusu-Agyei S. Effect of iron fortification on malaria incidence in infants and young children in Ghana: a randomized trial. JAMA. 2013;310:938–47.
41. Unger SA, Drammeh S, Hasan J, Ceesay K, Sinjanka E, Beyai S, Sonko B, Dondeh BL, Fulford AJ, Moore SE, Prentice AM. Impact of fortified versus unfortified lipid-based supplements on morbidity and nutritional status: A randomised double-blind placebo-controlled trial in ill Gambian children. PLoS Med. 2017;14:e1002377.
42. Paganini D, Uyoga MA, Zimmermann MB. Iron fortification of foods for infants and children in low-income countries: effects on the gut microbiome, gut inflammation, and diarrhea. Nutrients. 2016;8:494.
43. Zimmermann MB, Chassard C, Rohner F, N'goran EK, Nindjin C, Dostal A, Utzinger J, Ghattas H,

Lacroix C, Hurrell RF. The effects of iron fortification on the gut microbiota in African children: a randomized controlled trial in Cote d'Ivoire. Am J Clin Nutr. 2010;92:1406–15.

44. Jaeggi T, Kortman GAM, Moretti D, Chassard C, Holding P, Dostal A, Boekhorst J, Timmerman HM, Swinkels DW, Tjalsma H, Njenga J, Mwangi A, Kvalsvig J, Lacroix C, Zimmermann MB. Iron fortification adversely affects the gut microbiome, increases pathogen abundance and induces intestinal inflammation in Kenyan infants. Gut. 2015;64:731–42.
45. Sjödin KS, Domellöf M, Lagerqvist C, Hernell O, Lönnerdal B, Szymlek-Gay EA, Sjödin A, West CE, Lind T. Administration of ferrous sulfate drops has significant effects on the gut microbiota of iron-sufficient infants: a randomised controlled study. Gut. 2019;68:2095–7.
46. Owolabi AJ, Senbanjo IO, Oshikoya KA, Boekhorst J, Eijlander RT, Kortman GAM, Hageman JHJ, Samuel F, Melse-Boonstra A, Schaafsma A. Multi-nutrient fortified dairy-based drink reduces anaemia without observed adverse effects on gut microbiota in anaemic malnourished Nigerian toddlers: a randomised dose–response study. Nutrients. 2021;13:1566.
47. Rahman S, Kortman GAM, Boekhorst J, Lee P, Khan MR, Ahmed F. Effect of low-iron micronutrient powder (MNP) on the composition of gut microbiota of Bangladeshi children in a high-iron groundwater setting: a randomized controlled trial. Eur J Nutr. 2021;60:3423–36.
48. Popovic A, Bourdon C, Wang PW, Guttman DS, Soofi S, Bhutta ZA, Bandsma RHJ, Parkinson J, Pell LG. Micronutrient supplements can promote disruptive protozoan and fungal communities in the developing infant gut. Nat Commun. 2021;12:6729.
49. Liu J, Platts-Mills JA, Juma J, Kabir F, Nkeze J, Okoi C, Operario DJ, Uddin J, Ahmed S, Alonso PL, Antonio M, Becker SM, Blackwelder WC, Breiman RF, Faruque ASG, Fields B, Gratz J, Haque R, Hossain A, Hossain MJ, Jarju S, Qamar F, Talat Iqbal N, Kwambana B, Mandomando I, McMurry TL, Ochieng C, Ochieng JB, Ochieng M, Onyango C, Panchalingam S, Kalam A, Aziz F, Qureshi S, Ramamurthy T, Roberts JH, Saha D, Sow SO, Stroup SE, Sur D, Tamboura B, Taniuchi M, Tennant SM, Toema D, Wu Y, Zaidi A, Nataro JP, Kotloff KL, Levine MM, Houpt ER. Use of quantitative molecular diagnostic methods to identify causes of diarrhoea in children: a reanalysis of the GEMS case-control study. Lancet. 2016;388:1291–301.
50. Amour C, Gratz J, Mduma E, Svensen E, Rogawski ET, McGrath M, Seidman JC, McCormick BJJ, Shrestha S, Samie A, Mahfuz M, Qureshi S, Hotwani A, Babji S, Rengifo Trigoso D, Lima AAM, Bodhidatta L, Bessong P, Ahmed T, Shakoor S, Kang G, Kosek M, Guerrant RL, Lang D, Gottlieb M, Houpt ER, Platts-Mills JA, Etiology, Risk Factors, and Interactions of Enteric Infections and Malnutrition and the Consequences for Child Health and Development Project (MAL-ED). Network Investigators. Epidemiology and impact of *Campylobacter* infection in children in 8 low-resource settings: results from the MAL-ED study. Clin Infect Dis. 2016;63:1171–9.
51. Fekete E, Allain T, Siddiq A, Sosnowski O, Buret AG. Giardia spp. and the gut microbiota: dangerous liaisons. Front Microbiol. 2021;11:618106.
52. Fink G, D'Acremont V, Leslie HH, Cohen J. Antibiotic exposure among children younger than 5 years in low-income and middle-income countries: a cross-sectional study of nationally representative facility-based and household-based surveys. Lancet Infect Dis. 2020;20:179–87.
53. Do NTT, Vu HTL, Nguyen CTK, Punpuing S, Khan WA, Gyapong M, Poku Asante K, Munguambe K, Gómez-Olivé FX, John-Langba J, Tran TK, Sunpuwan M, Sevene E, Nguyen HH, Ho PD, Abdul Matin M, Ahmed S, Mahbubul Karim M, Cambaco O, Afari-Asiedu S, Boamah-Kaali E, Ali Abdulai M, Williams J, Asiamah S, Amankwah G, Pomaa Agyekum M, Wagner F, Ariana P, Sigauque B, Tollman S, Rogier van Doorn H, Sankoh O, Kinsman J, Wertheim HFL. Community-based antibiotic access and use in six low-income and middle-income countries: a mixed-method approach. Lancet Glob. Health. 2021;9:e610–9.
54. Ghanchi A, James PT, Cerami C. Guts, germs, and iron: a systematic review on iron supplementation, iron fortification, and diarrhea in children aged 4–59 months. Curr Dev Nutr. 2019;3:nzz005.
55. Mitra AK, Akramuzzaman SM, Fuchs GJ, Rahman MM, Mahalanabis D. Long-term oral supplementation with iron is not harmful for young children in a poor community of Bangladesh. J Nutr. 1997;127:1451–5.
56. Suchdev PS, Jefferds ME, Dewey KG, Zlotkin S, Aguayo VM, de Pee S, Kraemer K, Greig A, Arabi M, De-Regil LM, Home Fortification Technical Advisory Group. Micronutrient powders and diarrhoea risk in infants and young children. Lancet Child Adolesc Health. 2021;5:e28–9.
57. Srinivasan S, Fredricks DN. The human vaginal bacterial biota and bacterial vaginosis. Interdiscip Perspect Infect Dis. 2008;750479
58. Superti F, De Seta F. Warding off recurrent yeast and bacterial vaginal infections: lactoferrin and *Lactobacilli*. Microorganisms. 2020;8:130.
59. Brabin L, Roberts SA, Gies S, Nelson A, Diallo S, Stewart CJ, et al. Effects of long-term weekly iron and folic acid supplementation on lower genital tract infection - a double blind, randomised controlled trial in Burkina Faso. BMC Med. 2017;15:1–13.
60. Pasricha SR, Gheorghe A, Sakr-Ashour F, Arcot A, Neufeld L, Murray-Kolb LE, Suchdev PS, Bode M. Net benefit and cost-effectiveness of universal iron-containing multiple micronutrient powders for young children in 78 countries: a microsimulation study. Lancet Glob Health. 2020;8:e1071–80.

Novel Approaches to Oral Iron Supplementation

22

Diego Moretti and Nicole U. Stoffel

Iron Deficiency

Anemia affects more than one billion people globally, a substantial part of which is caused by iron deficiency [1]. Iron deficiency anemia develops when requirements for growth and basal metabolism cannot be met by the amount of iron absorbed from the diet [2]. Iron deficiency without anemia is even more common [3]. The concepts of functional and absolute iron deficiency [4] allow the differentiation between individuals with low total body iron (absolute iron deficiency) and individuals with adequate total body iron, but impaired metabolic iron mobilization, such as during infection and inflammation (functional iron deficiency). In low and middle-income countries, absolute iron deficiency is common, caused by insufficient iron in the diet, and the inability to cover the requirements due to basal metabolism, growth as well as potential losses. In this case, the first-line treatment is oral iron, while preventive approaches include optimizing dietary iron intake and bioavailability and treating/minimizing losses (e.g., intestinal parasites) or malabsorption [4]. Absolute iron deficiency often coexists with functional iron deficiency both in high-income and low-income countries: in these more complex situations, treatment of the underlying disease should be prioritized and iron should be provided when indicated [4].

Although iron deficiency anemia is a leading cause of morbidity worldwide, the first cause for disability in women [3], and one the most frequent conditions found in hospitalized populations [5], there is a lack of agreement on the optimal treatment schedules for oral iron supplementation. In this chapter, we will focus on settings where oral iron administration is clearly indicated, analyze factors that may affect iron bioavailability and side effects, and discuss recent studies and guidelines.

Balancing Iron Absorption and Tolerability

When iron deficiency is diagnosed [6], the first-line treatment usually is oral iron supplementation [7]. Recommended oral iron supplementation regimens for the treatment of iron deficiency range from 100 to 200 mg of elemental iron per day either as single dose or

D. Moretti (✉)
Department of Health, Nutrition Group, Swiss Distance University of Applied Sciences (FFHS), Zürich, Switzerland

Department of Health, Nutrition Group, University of Applied Sciences and Arts of Southern Switzerland (SUPSI), Zürich, Switzerland
e-mail: diego.moretti@ffhs.ch

N. U. Stoffel
Laboratory of Human Nutrition, Department for Health Sciences and Technology (D-HEST), Institute of Food, Nutrition and Health (IFNH), ETH Zürich, Zürich, Switzerland

C. D. Karakochuk et al. (eds.), *Nutritional Anemia*, Nutrition and Health,
https://doi.org/10.1007/978-3-031-14521-6_22

Table 22.1 Examples of iron supplements available in the United Kingdom in 2021 (adapted from [8])[a]

Iron compound	Dose (mg)	Elemental iron (mg)	Relative cost per 28 days[b]	Relative bioavailability[c]
Ferrous sulfate tablets	200	65	1 (reference)	100 (reference)
Ferrous sulfate drops	125 mg/125 mL	25 mg/mL	60	100
Modified release tablet ferrous sulfate	325	105	2.6	Variable
Modified release capsule ferrous sulfate	150	48	3.9	Variable
Ferrous gluconate	300	37	2.2	89
Ferrous fumarate	210	69	1.3	100
Ferric maltol	30	30	47	Variable
Multivitamins with iron	Variable	Variable	Up to 14	100

[a] Further compounds described in the literature include carbonyl iron, which has a relative bioavailability of 5–20 compared to ferrous sulfate. Ferrous glycine chelates have been reported to elicit less side effects than ferrous sulfate
[b] Once daily dosing 50–100 mg iron daily
[c] Adapted from Stoffel et al. [17]. Relative bioavailability measured in foods may not be directly equivalent to the relative bioavailability from supplements

split into multiple doses spread over the day for 3–6 months [7]. This corresponds to 1–4 mg elemental iron/day per kg body weight in adults [7]. Oral iron supplements differ in their chemical composition, iron concentration, and release mechanism (Table 22.1) which can affect bioavailability and the gastrointestinal (GI) side effect profile [8].

Bioavailability from Oral Iron Supplements

A common definition of nutrient bioavailability is the relative amount of ingested nutrient which is subsequently used for normal physiological function [9]. Iron bioavailability is defined as the amount of iron reaching red blood cells, the tissue which contains the highest amount of iron in the body [3]. In an early iron bioavailability study in young women, fractional iron absorption from a 50 mg dose of ferrous sulfate was 0.5–13% when given with a meal consisting of rice and beans, but was 1.2–28% when given without food, depending on the subject's iron status [10]. Iron bioavailability from oral iron supplements is low, even in fasted iron-depleted subjects using iron sulfate ($FeSO_4$). Iron is predominately absorbed in the duodenum [2] and there is limited evidence for iron absorption in the distal ileum or the colon. It is likely that the decreasing iron solubility with increasing pH in the duodenal environment, as well as the fact that iron must be in its reduced Fe(II) form to be absorbed through the gut mucosa, are rate limiting steps for iron bioavailability in general and from iron supplements in particular.

Side Effects from Oral Iron

A recent meta-analysis of randomized controlled trials identified a significant association between iron given as ferrous sulfate and GI side effects when compared to placebo (OR: 2.32, 95% CI: 1.74–3.08, $p < 0.0001$) or to intravenous iron formulations (OR: 3.05, 95% CI: 2.07–4.48, $p < 0.0001$) [11]. These GI side effects can result non-adherence in 30–70% of patients [11]. GI side effects are likely caused by gastric and duodenal mucosa irritation caused by soluble iron Fe(II) and the generation of reactive oxygen species (ROS) mediated toxicity [3]. More recently, another physiological mechanism potentially contributing to GI side effects and a reason of concern in infants and young children living in areas with poor hygiene and sanitation has been reported. Unabsorbed colonic iron from iron supplements and micronutrient powders (MNPs) causes detrimental changes in the gut microbiota by promoting opportunistic pathogens at the detriment of commensal species [12].

The most frequently reported side effects of oral iron supplements are nausea, black stools, epigastric pain, constipation, heartburn, and diarrhea. A study comparing side effects using ferrous sulfate, −gluconate or -fumarate, or placebo suggests that side effects are not significantly influenced by the iron compound [13]. In the study, 22–31% of the subjects reported side effects [13]. A further systematic review and meta-analysis suggests that "slow release" formulations may cause less side effects than conventional formulations [14], even if substantial heterogeneity between the trials was identified [14]. This observation was not confirmed by the meta-analysis including only randomized, double-blind studies [11]. Furthermore, slow release formulations may have the disadvantage of lower bioavailability [14].

Intermittent Iron Supplementation

A recent meta-analysis assessed the efficacy and tolerability of intermittent iron supplementation, defined as the intake of iron on non-consecutive days once, twice, or three times a week. Intermittent iron supplementation was reported to cause less side effects than daily iron supplementation (RR 0.41, 95% CI 0.21–0.82) [15], with a similar response in hemoglobin, but a lower response in ferritin [15].

Weekly iron supplementation was originally thought to improve iron absorption based on the concept that an earlier supplement dose would block absorption from a following dose. This concept had its origins in early experiments in animals and suggested that the gut mucosa's absorptive capacity would be blocked after an initial iron dose, giving raise to the "mucosal block." Thus, iron from following doses could only be absorbed after 5–7 days, the time required for the gut mucosal lining to renew. The "mucosal block" was identified in animals and subsequently studied in humans, albeit with contradicting results [16, 17]. Cook and Reddy (1995) found iron absorption from a single dose to be 9.8% (50 mg Fe as $FeSO_4$), while when supplements were given for six consecutive days the average absorption was 8.5% [10]. Similar results were reported by Olivares et al. suggesting no difference in fractional absorption between weekly and daily iron administration [18].

Advances in Understanding of Iron Biology and Iron Supplementation

Early studies in the 1960s [19, 20] suggested that iron absorption may be regulated by a humoral factor. However, there was no clear evidence until 2001, when three different research groups reported the discovery of a small peptide, synthesized in the liver (hepcidin), which later became clearly defined as the central regulatory hormone for iron metabolism [21–24]. Hepcidin inhibits iron entry into plasma either through internalization and degradation of ferroportin [25], the only known cellular iron exporter, or through occlusion of the iron export site [26]. Consequently, hepcidin is a predictor of iron absorption [27]. Hepcidin is synthesized in response to iron status but also in response to systemic iron availability, following an inverse correlation with transferrin saturation [28]. In addition, hepcidin is increased in response to an oral iron challenge [28]. In four fasting subjects with serum ferritin between 120 and 168 µg/L who received 60 mg iron as ferrous sulfate, hepcidin continuously increased in the following 4 h in three out of four subjects, while a dose of 3.5 mg Fe did not cause a significant increase in hepcidin [27]. In another early small study assessing urinary hepcidin, the peak urinary hepcidin concentration was reached at 12 h after oral iron administration, while the hepcidin increase was detectable for up to 40 h in three out of six subjects [28]. These results are not inconsistent with the previous study, as urinary hepcidin is expected to peak later than serum hepcidin, reflecting kidney excretion. Furthermore, individual subject factors such as iron status may affect hepcidin response to an iron challenge [28].

Studies in Young Women with and without Anemia

To investigate whether the duration and magnitude of the iron-induced hepcidin rise would be relevant in the context of iron supplementation, we investigated these questions systematically in generally healthy, iron-depleted young women (serum ferritin <20 μg/L). Concomitantly with hepcidin measurements, we assessed iron absorption from supplemental oral iron (as $FeSO_4$) doses using stable iron isotopes. Serum hepcidin was significantly increased at 24 h after the intake of ≥60 mg oral iron, but not at 48 h. [29]. The hepcidin increase at 24 h was associated with a significant decrease in fractional iron absorption by 30–45%. Our studies further showed that fractional iron absorption decreased with increasing iron dose, whereas absolute absorption increased: a sixfold increase in iron dose resulted only in a threefold increase in iron absorption ([29], Fig. 22.1). These studies focused on single and consecutive day doses and while the hepcidin profiles were consistent with a benefit in alternate day dosing over daily dosing (fractional absorption), longer term studies with multiple administrations were needed to confirm these findings [29].

Dividing high oral iron doses into multiple doses spread over the day is common in daily practice [7]. We found that administering 60 mg Fe in the morning, in the afternoon and on the following day did not benefit the total amount of iron absorbed [29], suggesting iron administration in the afternoon following a morning dose, at the time when serum hepcidin is highest [29], to be of limited benefit. In a follow-up study, iron bioavailability was similar from a single dose of 120 mg and a twice daily dose of 60 mg iron as $FeSO_4$ [30].

To investigate long-term benefit of alternate day administrations, iron-depleted young women were randomized to receive iron supplements (60 mg Fe as $FeSO_4$) either daily for 14 days or

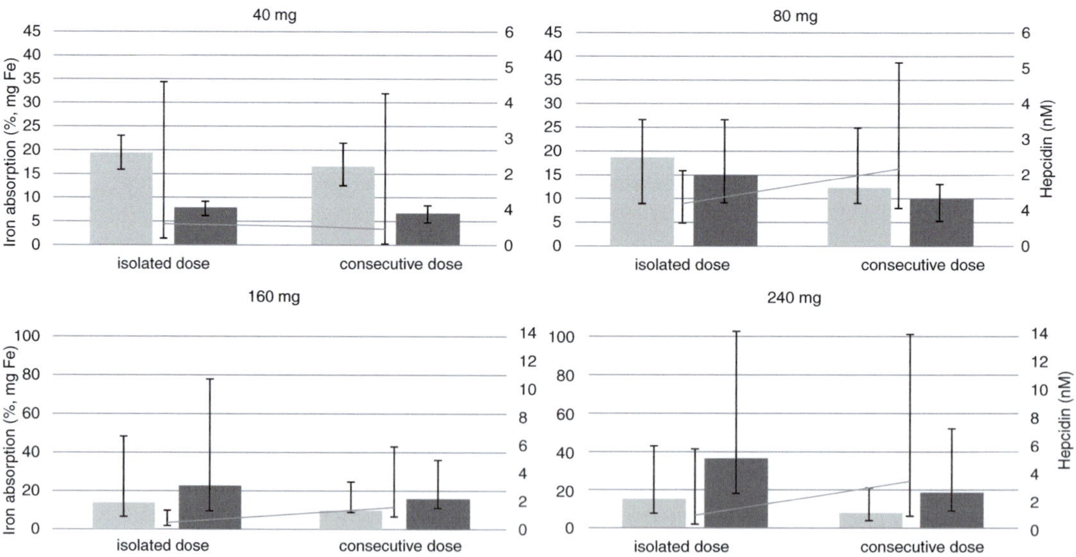

Fig. 22.1 Fractional (%) and total iron absorption (mg Fe) using single vs. consecutive day dosing in iron depleted fasted women (morning). Supplements were given either on 2 following days (consecutive dose) or as a single dose. Fractional iron absorption shown in the light bars, total iron absorption shown in the dark bars. The increase in hepcidin (nM) after consecutive day dosing is shown by the line. Fractional and total absorption differed between single and consecutive day doses in all administered doses ($P < 0.05$): Hepcidin concentrations differed at 80, 160, and 240 mg ($P < 0.05$) but not at 40 mg Fe doses. Please note the different scale between panels for 40 and 80 mg Fe and 160 and 240 mg. Adapted from [29]

every other day for 28 days. All doses were labelled with stable iron isotopes. The average fractional iron absorptions (+SD, -SD) were 16·3% (9.3, 28.8) using consecutive-day dosing and 21.8% (13.7, 34.6) using alternate-day dosing (p = 0.0013). The cumulative total iron absorption was 131.0 mg (71.4, 240.5) versus 175.3 mg (110.3, 278.5; $P < 0.01$) after 14 days (consecutive day dosing) and 28 days (alternate day dosing), respectively. During the first 14 days, serum hepcidin was increased in the group receiving iron supplements on consecutive days compared to the alternate day supplementation group ($P < 0.01$) [30].

A limitation of this study was that only a small number of the iron-deficient subjects were anemic. As it is well known that hepatic hepcidin expression is suppressed by hypoxia and during increased erythropoietin stimulation (such as during anemia), the study was repeated in recent blood donors with mild iron deficiency anemia. Serum hepcidin was lower and there was a less pronounced iron-induced increase in hepcidin in subjects with anemia compared to non-anemic subjects [31]. However, even in mild anemia, alternate day dosing with 100 or 200 mg resulted a significant increase in fractional iron absorption by 40–50% compared to daily dosing [31]. A further interesting finding from these studies was that there was no residual absorption inhibition at 48 h post-administration, suggesting there is no "mucosal block" lasting up to 5 or 6 days [31].

Alternate day dosing results in a 30–50% increase in fractional absorption compared to consecutive day dosing. However, the 50% increase in fractional iron absorption does not fully offset the halving of the iron dose. To compensate for the lower total iron dose per unit time, a potential option would be to provide twice the daily iron dose on alternate days [32]. In a secondary analysis of published studies, Stoffel et al. report that alternate day dosing of twice the daily dose resulted in higher total iron absorption compared to consecutive day dosing for total doses of 80, 120, 160, 200, and 240 mg (Table 22.2, [17]). Thus, this practice appears to compensate for the lower overall dosage of alternate day administration on the total amount of iron absorbed. While in this analysis we did not detect a difference in absorption between 200 and 2 × 100 mg Fe [17], a study in athletes undergoing altitude training found a single nightly 200 mg Fe dose to be superior to a split dose (2 × 100 mg) in increasing hemoglobin mass [33].

Table 22.2 Comparison of alternated day and consecutive day iron absorption modified from Stoffel et al. [17]

	Total iron absorption (mg)[a]		
Dose	Alternate day	Consecutive day	P-value[b]
2 × 40	15.4 (10.3, 22.8)		0.214
1 × 80		12.1 (9.4, 15.6)	
2 × 60	16.6 (12.3, 22.3)		0.018
1 × 120		22.7 (15.5 27.9)	
2 × 80	20.4 (15.0. 27.9)		0.058
1 × 160		34.6 (20.1, 59.5)	
2 × 100	21.8 (12.0, 39.4)		0.496
1 × 200		20.9 (12.6, 34.9)	
2 × 120	28.1 (19.7, 39.9)		0.571
1 × 240		31.7 (16.7, 60.1)	

[a] Measured by erythrocyte incorporation of stable isotopic labelled $FeSO_4$- supplements administered in the morning in fasting state. Data adjusted for a serum ferritin of 15 μg/L [43]

[b] Probability for a difference in total iron absorbed comparing alternate and consecutive dosing. Tested with independent sample t-test, except 200 mg comparison (dependent sample t-test)

Studies in Infants and Young Children

Would the iron-induced hepcidin rise be of relevance also in infants and young children, and would it be advisable to recommend alternate day micronutrient powder (MNP) administration? To answer this question, Uyoga et al. [34] performed a stable iron isotope study administering maize porridge and MNPs containing 12 mg Fe as $FeSO_4$ to 6–12-month-old Kenyan infants, which were predominantly iron-deficient anemic (65%). Hepcidin was increased beyond 24 h after a first oral iron dose, and iron absorption was decreased by 10–15%, compared to alternate day or every third day iron administration [34]. Overall, the authors concluded that in contrast to studies in adults, MNP consumed with food, even at a comparable supplemental iron dose of 1–1.5 mg/kg bodyweight, appear to elicit a less pronounced response in hepcidin and a less dramatic decrease in iron absorption. This could have several reasons: (1) a higher baseline hepcidin due to a higher prevalence of mild infections among Kenyan infants, which may have superseded the iron-induced hepcidin increase; (2) the slightly more pronounced anemia in the infant population relative to other comparable studies in adults conducted to date on this subject; and (3) the fact that MNPs are consumed with foods, blunting the acute increase in transferrin saturation, which is likely instrumental for the iron-induced hepcidin rise. Overall, this study suggest that in infant populations living in areas with a high prevalence of infection and inflammation, it would not appear to be advantageous to space dosages of MNPs on alternate days [34].

Studies Investigating Side Effects from Intermittent and Daily Iron Supplementation

Whether side effects are dose dependent is uncertain [11], but they may be less common at doses ≤45 mg/day in adults [35], which is also the upper limit for iron intake as defined by the Institute of Medicine based on side effects from iron supplements.

It has been suggested that changing the administration schedule to alternate day supplementation bears the potential to improve the tolerability of iron supplements [3], and support for this hypothesis is provided by a recent meta-analysis comparing intermittent and daily iron supplementation [15]. In contrast, a meta-analysis which included iron supplementation studies with a dose range of 20–222 mg of ferrous sulfate (median 120 mg, average 121 mg) and did only include randomized controlled studies, did not identify an effect of dose on the prevalence of side effects from iron supplementation [11]. In a study in elderly patients, Rimon et al. reported different numbers of side effects between 15 mg/day and 50 mg/day for abdominal discomfort, diarrhea, constipation, and darkened stools. When comparing iron doses of 15 and 150 mg/day, the number of reports for abdominal discomfort, nausea/vomiting, diarrhea, constipation, darkened stools, and drop-outs were lower in the group receiving 15 mg/day. When comparing groups receiving doses of 50 mg and 150 mg iron per day, less cases of darkened stools and nausea/vomiting were reported in the group receiving 50 mg iron per day [36].

The efficacy in improving iron status and the side effect profile of varying iron supplementation schedules has been studied recently and is summarized in Table 22.3. Three studies in iron-deficient anemic subjects identified less side effects of alternate day schedules compared to daily schedules, and all three studies provided half of the iron dose during the alternate day supplementation schedule. Efficacy in improving iron status was reported for both schedules, in particular regarding hemoglobin increase, while one study reported a higher increase in serum ferritin with 2 × 80 mg Fe given daily [37] compared to alternate day schedules. One study reported similar efficacy in improving iron status when comparing similar total dose (but different durations of the supplementation schedule) [38]. Kaundal et al. [38] concluded that the choice of the ideal schedule should be patient specific and should depend on the severity of the anemia and the rapidity of the desired hematological response. A limitation of studies shown in Table 22.3 is that they were generally small and tested a variety of different iron compounds as supplements, without a double-blind design.

Table 22.3 Recent studies assessing side effects of alternated day supplementation vs. consecutive day supplementation and of single vs. split dosages in prospective studies

Author	Population	Compound/dose	Design	Results: iron status	Results: side effects
Karakoc et al. [44]	Iron-deficient anemic pregnant women ($n = 264$)	100 mg Fe/day as ferrous fumarate	Open label, two parallel groups: Daily ($n = 124$) vs. alternate day treatment ($n = 140$)	Higher increase in Hb in alternate day group, comparable increase in SF.	Gastrointestinal side effects in 47 of 264 women. Lower number alternate day supplementation (41.4% vs. 15.1%, $P = 0.0057$)
Kaundal et al. [38]	Iron-deficient anemic patients ($n = 31$ per arm)	120 mg Fe on alternate days or 60 mg Fe twice a day	Randomized trial comparing twice daily iron (2 × 60 mg) for 3 weeks vs. alternate day iron (120 mg) over 6 weeks	Similar Hb between the groups at 6 weeks, but higher Hb in the twice daily arm at 3 weeks	Increase in reports for nausea in the twice daily arm ($P = 0.03$)
McCormick et al. [45]	Athletes with suboptimal iron status defined as serum ferritin <50 μg/L ($n = 31$)	105 mg Fe as ferrous sulfate with 500 mg of ascorbic acid	8-week intervention either on alternate day or daily supplementation	Similar increase in serum ferritin in both groups	Seven complaints of side effects in the daily group, 1 complaint in the alternate day group
Hall et al. [33]	Elite runners ($n = 24$), male ($n = 8$) and female ($n = 14$); all iron sufficient (serum ferritin >30 μg/L)	1 × 200 mg (9–10 PM) vs. 2 × 100 mg (7–8 am and 9–10 pm) Fe as ferrous fumarate	Randomized, stratified by iron status, investigating effect on Hb mass and GI side effects over 3 weeks	Higher increase in Hb mass in the single dose arm ($P = 0.048$)	Overall, GI tolerability similar over 3 weeks. But higher scores for GI distress in weeks 1 and 2 combined in the single dose treatment arm
Metha et al. [46]	Iron-deficient anemic patients ($n = 50$, divided in two groups, each group with 20 subjects with IDA)	Oral iron supplements were given on alternate days and daily (60 mg as ferrous sulphate)	Assessment of hepcidin, reticulocyte Hb content, and Hb increase	Increase in Hb in the alternate day group, but not in the daily group after 21 days	No statistically significant differences
Oflas et al. [37]	150 women with IDA, aged between 18 and 50 years of age	Group1: 2 × 80 mg vs. group 2: 80 mg / day vs. group 3: 80 mg every other day. Fe as ferrous sulfate: Supplements contained mucoproteose and ascorbic acid	Open label, randomized 1-month study. Total iron dose: Group 1: 4800 mg; group 2: 2400 mg; group 3: 1200 mg	Similar increase in Hb but higher serum ferritin increases in the 2 × 80 mg group	Nausea and stomachache most frequent side effect. Frequency after 1 month: Group 1: 34/50; group 2: 12/50; group 3: 5/50. Significant difference between groups ($P = 0.001$)

Recommendations for Iron Supplementation

As a preventive strategy, in areas where the prevalence of anemia in women of reproductive age is >20% the WHO recommends supplementation of 60 mg of Fe once per week, followed by 3 months without supplementation. In areas where anemia in menstruating women and adolescents is >40%, the WHO recommends supplementation of daily 30–60 mg Fe to be given during three consecutive months in the course of a year [39, 40].

More recent guidelines suggest that excessive iron supplementation doses may be counterproductive by decreasing fractional iron absorption and increasing side effects [41]. It should be recommended to take iron on alternate days, and to avoid more than one iron dose per day [41]. In contrast, some patients may choose daily regiments for ease of use or tolerability [41]. Recent UK guidelines for the management of iron deficiency in pregnancy recommend the use 40–80 mg Fe as ferrous salt, employing daily or alternate day schedules and avoiding twice-daily dosing [42]. The British Society of Gastroenterology recommends once daily dosing of 50–100 mg of elemental iron in case of confirmed iron deficiency anemia. If this dose is tolerated, treatment should be continued for 3–4 months provided an adequate hematological response is detectable after 2–4 weeks. If not tolerated, alternate day supplementation should be recommended [8].

Doses of ≥60 mg Fe in iron depleted, non-anemic women and of 100 mg Fe in anemic women trigger a hepcidin increase that persists for 24 h, subsiding by 48 h. This suggests that optimal dosages to maximize absorption are ≤40 mg iron as ferrous salts daily or ≥ 60 mg iron as ferrous salts every other day [17].

Despite the fact that smaller studies suggest a benefit of alternate day supplementation, and the concept that dose reduction and spacing may result in less side effects [41], data from large prospective, randomized double-blind studies assessing the efficacy and side effects of alternate day and consecutive day schedules are needed. In general, patient preference and previous history of iron tolerability should be considered when defining a personalized supplementation schedule, which should also consider the magnitude of the iron deficit and the rapidity of the response desired. A long-term research agenda to further optimize oral iron supplementation regimens could include [17]:

1. Large prospective studies investigating efficacy and side effects profile of alternate vs. consecutive day supplementation regimens, in different population groups, including more severely anemic populations and pregnant women.
2. Comparing intravenous iron formulations to oral iron in high and lower resource settings, including outcomes on efficacy and cost-effectiveness.
3. Even with alternate day supplementation, side effects to iron therapies may remain a limiting factor, thus the development of low-cost iron formulations with optimal fractional absorption but improved safety profile compared to ferrous sulfate appears warranted.
4. Iron absorption is not fully explained by hepcidin and iron status. The interplay between systemic and enterocyte regulation affecting iron absorption during iron deficiency deserves further study.
5. In Africa and other areas were malaria and genetic hemoglobinopathies (e.g., sickle cell disease or hemoglobin E variants) have been historically endemic, these factors may affect

Conclusion and Future Directions

Increased fractional absorption of lower iron dose and alternate day dosing is likely to improve the efficacy and the side effect profile of iron supplementation schedules [41]. While the WHO has recommended intermittent iron supplementation [39], recent data suggests that 48 h in between doses are sufficient in both women and children for absorption and hepcidin to normalize [31]. The practice of spacing iron doses for more than 48 h appears unnecessary from the point of view of iron bioavailability.

iron status and biomarkers in ways that may cloud common diagnostic paradigms.

6. The decision of giving iron is dictated by the diagnostic portfolio available and improving field-friendly diagnostic tools to identify individuals who would benefit the most from iron supplementation appears a key further priority.

References

1. Petry N, Olofin I, Hurrell RF, Boy E, Wirth JP, Moursi M, et al. The proportion of anemia associated with iron deficiency in low, medium, and high human development index countries: a systematic analysis of national surveys. Nutrients. 2016;8(11):693.
2. Zimmermann MB, Hurrell RF. Nutritional iron deficiency. Lancet. 2007;370(9586):511–20.
3. Camaschella C. Iron deficiency. Blood. 2019;133(1):30–9.
4. Pasricha S-R, Tye-Din J, Muckenthaler MU, Swinkels DW. Iron deficiency. Lancet. 2021;397(10270):233–48.
5. Theurl I, Aigner E, Theurl M, Nairz M, Seifert M, Schroll A, et al. Regulation of iron homeostasis in anemia of chronic disease and iron deficiency anemia: diagnostic and therapeutic implications. Blood. 2009;113(21):5277–86.
6. Lynch S, Pfeiffer CM, Georgieff MK, Brittenham G, Fairweather-Tait S, Hurrell RF, et al. Biomarkers of nutrition for development (BOND)—iron review. J Nutr. 2018;148(suppl_1):1001S–67S.
7. Brittenham G. Iron deficiency and overload. In: Hematology: basic principles and practice. 7th ed. Philadelphia, PA: Elsevier; 2018. p. 478–90.
8. Snook J, Bhala N, Beales ILP, Cannings D, Kightley C, Logan RP, et al. British Society of Gastroenterology guidelines for the management of iron deficiency anaemia in adults. Gut. 2021;70(11):2030.
9. Fairweather-Tait S, Hurrell RF. Bioavailability of minerals and trace elements: members of EC flair concerted action no. 10: measurements of micronutrient absorption and status. Nutr Res Rev. 1996;9(1):295–324.
10. Cook JD, Reddy MB. Efficacy of weekly compared with daily iron supplementation. Am J Clin Nutr. 1995;62(1):117–20.
11. Tolkien Z, Stecher L, Mander AP, Pereira DIA, Powell JJ. Ferrous sulfate supplementation causes significant gastrointestinal side-effects in adults: a systematic review and meta-analysis. PLoS One. 2015;10(2):e0117383.
12. Paganini D, Zimmermann MB. The effects of iron fortification and supplementation on the gut microbiome and diarrhea in infants and children: a review. Am J Clin Nutr. 2017;106(suppl_6):1688S–93S.
13. Hallberg L, Ryttinger L, Sövell L. Side-effects of oral iron therapy: a double-blind study of different iron compounds in tablet form. Acta Med Scand. 1966;180(S459):3–10.
14. Cancelo-Hidalgo MJ, Castelo-Branco C, Palacios S, Haya-Palazuelos J, Ciria-Recasens M, Manasanch J, et al. Tolerability of different oral iron supplements: a systematic review. Curr Med Res Opin. 2013;29(4):291–303.
15. Fernández-Gaxiola A, De-Regil L. Intermittent iron supplementation for reducing anaemia and its associated impairments in adolescent and adult menstruating women. Cochrane Database Syst Rev [Internet]. 2019;(1) https://doi.org/10.1002/14651858.CD009218.pub3.
16. Hallberg L. Combating iron deficiency: daily administration of iron is far superior to weekly administration. Am J Clin Nutr. 1998;68(2):213–7.
17. Stoffel NU, von Siebenthal HK, Moretti D, Zimmermann MB. Oral iron supplementation in iron-deficient women: how much and how often? Iron Health Dis. 2020;75:100865.
18. Olivares M, Pizarro F, Walter T, Arredondo M, Hertrampf E. Bioavailability of iron supplements consumed daily is not different from that of iron supplements consumed weekly. Nutr Res. 1999;19(2):179–90.
19. Fischer DS, Price DC. A possible humoral regulator of iron absorption. Proc Soc Exp Biol Med. 1963;112(1):228–9.
20. MacDermott RP, Greenberger NJ. Evidence for a humoral factor influencing iron absorption. Gastroenterology. 1969;57(2):117–25.
21. Park CH, Valore EV, Waring AJ, Ganz T. Hepcidin, a urinary antimicrobial peptide synthesized in the liver. J Biol Chem. 2001;276(11):7806–10.
22. Nemeth E, Valore EV, Territo M, Schiller G, Lichtenstein A, Ganz T. Hepcidin, a putative mediator of anemia of inflammation, is a type II acute-phase protein. Blood. 2003;101(7):2461–3.
23. Nicolas G, Chauvet C, Viatte L, Danan JL, Bigard X, Devaux I, et al. The gene encoding the iron regulatory peptide hepcidin is regulated by anemia, hypoxia, and inflammation. J Clin Invest. 2002;110(7):1037–44.
24. Pigeon C, Ilyin G, Courselaud B, Leroyer P, Turlin B, Brissot P, et al. A new mouse liver-specific gene, encoding a protein homologous to human antimicrobial peptide hepcidin, is overexpressed during iron overload*. J Biol Chem. 2001;276(11):7811–9.
25. Elizabeta N, Tuttle MS, Julie P, Vaughn MB, Adriana D, McVey WD, et al. Hepcidin regulates cellular iron efflux by binding to Ferroportin and inducing its internalization. Science. 2004;306(5704):2090–3.
26. Aschemeyer S, Qiao B, Stefanova D, Valore EV, Sek AC, Ruwe TA, et al. Structure-function analysis of ferroportin defines the binding site and an alternative mechanism of action of hepcidin. Blood. 2018;131(8):899–910.
27. Zimmermann MB, Troesch B, Biebinger R, Egli I, Zeder C, Hurrell RF. Plasma hepcidin is a modest

predictor of dietary iron bioavailability in humans, whereas oral iron loading, measured by stable-isotope appearance curves, increases plasma hepcidin. Am J Clin Nutr. 2009;90(5):1280–7.

28. Lin L, Valore EV, Nemeth E, Goodnough JB, Gabayan V, Ganz T. Iron transferrin regulates hepcidin synthesis in primary hepatocyte culture through hemojuvelin and BMP2/4. Blood. 2007;110(6):2182–9.
29. Moretti D, Goede JS, Zeder C, Jiskra M, Chatzinakou V, Tjalsma H, et al. Oral iron supplements increase hepcidin and decrease iron absorption from daily or twice-daily doses in iron-depleted young women. Blood. 2015;126(17):1981–9.
30. Stoffel NU, Cercamondi CI, Brittenham G, Zeder C, Geurts-Moespot AJ, Swinkels DW, et al. Iron absorption from oral iron supplements given on consecutive versus alternate days and as single morning doses versus twice-daily split dosing in iron-depleted women: two open-label, randomised controlled trials. Lancet Haematol. 2017;4(11):e524–33.
31. Stoffel NU, Zeder C, Brittenham GM, Moretti D, Zimmermann MB. Iron absorption from supplements is greater with alternate day than with consecutive day dosing in iron-deficient anemic women. Haematologica. 2020;105(5):1232–9.
32. Schrier SL. So you know how to treat iron deficiency anemia. Blood. 2015;126(17):1971.
33. Hall R, Peeling P, Nemeth E, Bergland D, McCluskey WTP, Stellingwerff T. Single versus Split dose of iron optimizes hemoglobin mass gains at 2106 m altitude. Med Sci Sports Exerc. 2019;51(4). https://journals.lww.com/acsm-msse/Fulltext/2019/04000/Single_versus_Split_Dose_of_Iron_Optimizes.18.aspx
34. Uyoga MA, Mikulic N, Paganini D, Mwasi E, Stoffel NU, Zeder C, et al. The effect of iron dosing schedules on plasma hepcidin and iron absorption in Kenyan infants. Am J Clin Nutr. 2020;112(4):1132–41.
35. Institute of Medicine (US) Panel on Micronutrients. Iron. In: Dietary reference intakes for vitamin a, vitamin k, arsenic, boron, chromium, copper, iodine, iron, manganese, molybdenum, nickel, silicon, vanadium, and zinc [Internet]. Washington, DC: National Academies Press (US); https://www.ncbi.nlm.nih.gov/books/NBK222309/
36. Rimon E, Kagansky N, Kagansky M, Mechnick L, Mashiah T, Namir M, et al. Are we giving too much iron? Low-dose iron therapy is effective in octogenarians. Am J Med. 2005;118(10):1142–7.
37. Düzen Oflas N, Demircioğlu S, Yıldırım Doğan N, Eker E, Kutlucan A, Doğan A, et al. Comparison of the effects of oral iron treatment every day and every other day in female patients with iron deficiency anaemia. Intern Med J. 2020;50(7):854–8.
38. Kaundal R, Bhatia P, Jain A, Jain A, Nampoothiri RV, Mishra K, et al. Randomized controlled trial of twice-daily versus alternate-day oral iron therapy in the treatment of iron-deficiency anemia. Ann Hematol. 2020;99(1):57–63.
39. World Health Organization. Intermittent iron and folic acid supplementation in menstruating women [internet]. Geneva; 2011. https://www.ncbi.nlm.nih.gov/books/NBK179900/
40. World Health Organization. Guideline: daily iron supplementation in adult women and adolescent girls [internet]. Geneva: World Health Organization; 2016. https://apps.who.int/iris/handle/10665/204761
41. Auerbach M. Treatment of iron deficiency anemia in adults [internet]. UpToDate; 2021. https://www.uptodate.com/contents/treatment-of-iron-deficiency-anemia-in-adults
42. Pavord S, Daru J, Prasannan N, Robinson S, Stanworth S, Girling J, et al. UK guidelines on the management of iron deficiency in pregnancy. Br J Haematol. 2020;188(6):819–30.
43. Cook JD, Dassenko SA, Lynch SR. Assessment of the role of nonheme-iron availability in iron balance. Am J Clin Nutr. 1991;54(4):717–22.
44. Karakoc G, Orgul G, Sahin D, Yucel A. Is every other day iron supplementation effective for the treatment of the iron deficiency anemia in pregnancy? J Matern Fetal Neonatal Med. 2021;1–5
45. McCormick R, Dreyer A, Dawson B, Sim M, Lester L, Goodman C, et al. The effectiveness of daily and alternate day Oral iron supplementation in athletes with suboptimal iron status (part 2). Int J Sport Nutr Exerc Metab. 2020;30(3):191–6.
46. Metha S, Bhavani S, Gulati S, Sharma N, Goyal L, Metha S. A prospective, randomized, interventional study of Oral iron supplementation comparing daily dose with alternate day regimen using hepcidin as a biomarker in iron deficiency anemia. J Assoc Physicians India. 2020;68:39–41.

Cognitive and Behavioral Consequences of Iron Deficiency

23

Laura E. Murray-Kolb and Amrita Arcot

Keywords

Iron deficiency · Cognition · Behavior · Affect Neurophysiology · Women · Children Neurobiology

Introduction

Iron deficiency is the most prevalent single nutrient deficiency worldwide primarily affecting infants, children, and women of reproductive age [1]. Although individuals of all ages and classes are susceptible to iron deficiency, those who are poor and less educated are most vulnerable. Iron deficiency has been identified as a biological risk factor for the failure of >250 million children in reaching their full developmental potential, resulting in reductions in economic productivity [2]. The association between iron status and brain functioning has been examined through investigations of central nervous system biochemical changes using animal studies and through the assessment of cognitive functioning and behavior in humans. There is clear evidence from animal studies that iron is critical for myelination, neuronal morphology, neuronal metabolic activity, and the synthesis of monoamines [3]. In humans, the evidence points to cognitive, motor, behavioral, and affective alterations in iron-deficient individuals [4]. In most age groups, iron repletion appears to ameliorate these alterations. The exception is infancy where the negative consequences of iron deficiency seem to persist despite iron repletion, perhaps indicating critical periods of development during which a deficiency in iron leads to irreversible effects.

A heterogeneous distribution of iron exists in the human brain with differential patterns in children versus adults [5]. The accumulation of iron in different brain regions is a function of the stage of brain development [6]. The highest concentrations of brain iron are found in the substantia nigra, deep cerebellar nuclei, the red nucleus, the nucleus accumbens, and portions of the hippocampus [7, 8]. Dopaminergic, serotonergic, and noradrenergic systems have been identified as sensitive to brain iron status [9].

This chapter summarizes cognitive and behavioral alterations resulting from iron deficiency and iron deficiency anemia in children and women of reproductive age. Multiple reviews have been published on these topics [10, 11], so here we focus on reviewing randomized controlled studies published in the past decade,

The original version of this book was revised. An erratum to this book can be found at https://doi.org/10.1007/978-3-031-14521-6_28

L. E. Murray-Kolb (✉)
Department of Nutrition Science, Purdue University, West Lafayette, IN, USA
e-mail: lmurrayk@purdue.edu

A. Arcot
Department of Nutritional Sciences, The Pennsylvania State University, University Park, PA, USA
e-mail: avr5374@psu.edu

C. D. Karakochuk et al. (eds.), *Nutritional Anemia*, Nutrition and Health,
https://doi.org/10.1007/978-3-031-14521-6_23

examining both the short- and long-term cognitive and behavioral consequences of iron deficiency. Studies where the control group contained approximately the same levels of iron as the treatment group (for instance, control group given a multiple micronutrient (MMN) treatment or comparing oral iron to intravenous iron) were excluded from evaluation.

Effects of Iron Deficiency on Cognition and Behavior in Children

Most studies examining the association between iron status and cognitive/behavioral outcomes have been conducted in infants and young children. Over 40 years of accumulated evidence from infant studies reveals that iron deficiency anemia is associated with impaired performance on developmental tests as well as behavioral differences such that iron-deficient anemic infants are more wary, hesitant, and clingy when compared to their iron-sufficient counterparts [12]. During the preschool years, iron deficiency anemia has been associated with impairments in learning and language acquisition; motor development; and in school-aged children, iron deficiency anemia has been shown to be related to impaired academic performance (especially on verbal and math tests) and memory [13]. Many of the recent studies on the association between iron status and cognition/behavior have focused on the long-term consequences of early-life iron treatment. The studies that we include here were conducted in apparently healthy children; we have divided the studies by primary outcome of interest (cognitive or behavioral outcomes).

Effects of Iron Treatment on Child Cognitive Outcomes

Ten recent publications were identified in which children or adolescents received iron treatment or a true control to assess cognitive outcomes [14–23]. Sample sizes across all ten studies ranged from 140 to 1933 with supplementation periods ranging from 4.5 to 8.5 months. As far as vehicle of supplementation, four provided iron supplements (drops or tablets) [14, 16, 19, 21], three provided iron via infant formula [15, 22, 23], and three provided iron through either fortification [17, 18] or biofortification [20] of food. Five of the studies assessed outcomes immediately following the end of the treatment period [14, 17, 18, 20, 21] and the other five assessed outcomes several years later [15, 16, 19, 22, 23]. As far as data analysis, eight used the original randomized groups [14–20, 23] while two ran the analyses with children stratified by iron status in infancy [22] or by iron status in the fetal-neonatal and infancy periods [21]. All studies used multiple biomarkers specific to iron to determine iron status although the 3.5-year follow-up study conducted in Sweden [16] did not measure iron status. Since iron status at follow-up may have affected the interpretation of the findings, contextualization of those results are more difficult. Of note, the study in China included measures of serum ferritin concentrations but did not collect a measure of inflammation and, therefore, ferritin levels were not adjusted [21].

Table 23.1 summarizes the main outcome variables and findings from these studies. Full scale intelligence quotient (IQ), memory, and motor function were the main outcome domains assessed using both manual and computerized tasks. Of the eight studies which used the original randomized groups, three reported no significant differences between the intervention and the control group at endline or follow-up [16, 17, 19]. Two of these studies provided supplementation (iron drops) to infants in Sweden [16, 19] while the other used fortified biscuits, provided to Moroccan school-aged children [17]. All three of these studies used measures of cognition that require highly trained administrators and that are subjective in nature. In addition, these measures were developed and standardized in a Western context. As such, using Western-based standardized scores may not have been appropriate for the study conducted in Morocco. Three other studies which ran analyses using the original randomization groups reported improvements in cognition favorable to the iron treatment group, and there was indication that those with a lower iron status

Table 23.1 Studies examining the effects of iron treatment on cognitive domains in children and adolescents (2010–2020)

Location	*n*	Age at enrollment into original study	Intervention duration (months)	Age at follow-up (years)	Control group	Intervention group(s)	Outcome domain	Analyses groups	Main findings
South Africa (2012) [14]	321[a]	6–11 years	8.5	Same range as enrollment (immediately after 8.5-month intervention)	Placebo	Iron (50 mg iron sulfate) plus DHA/EPA (420/80 mg) or Iron (50 mg iron sulfate) plus placebo or Placebo plus a mixture of DHA/EPA (420/80 mg)	Memory Visuospatial cognition	As per original randomization	• Iron supplemented groups had higher memory scores compared to placebo group; subanalyses reveal this is likely driven by the children who were anemic at baseline • DHA/EPA supplemented group had lower memory scores compared to placebo group • A significant difference in baseline scores were seen between children who were iron-deficient and iron-deficient anemic with the anemic children having lower scores
Chile (2012) [15]	573	6 months	6	10	Formula with 2.3 mg/L iron	Formula with 12.7 mg/L iron	Intelligence quotient (IQ) Spatial memory Achievement (math) Visual perception and motor coordination	As per original randomization	• Spatial memory and visual motor integration were significantly higher in the low-iron formula group than the high-iron formula group • When accounting for hemoglobin level at enrollment, higher scores were seen with high-iron formula consumption in children with the lowest hemoglobin levels but lower scores for children with the highest hemoglobin levels

(continued)

Table 23.1 (continued)

Location	*n*	Age at enrollment into original study	Intervention duration (months)	Age at follow-up (years)	Control group	Intervention group(s)	Outcome domain	Analyses groups	Main findings
Sweden (2013) [16]	285[a] (birth weight between 2000 and 2500 g)	1.5 months	4.5 (until child was 6 months of age)	3.5	0 mg/kg/d iron drops	1 mg/kg/d iron drops or 2 mg/kg/d iron drops	Intelligence quotient (IQ)	As per original randomization	• No significant differences in IQ between control and intervention groups nor between the two intervention groups
Morocco (2016) [17]	457[a]	Third-sixth graders (~7 years on average)	7 (2 or 3 biscuits per day for 6 days/week)	Same range as enrollment (immediately after 7-month intervention)	Placebo biscuits	Biscuits containing the following: ~8 mg Fe as ferrous sulfate or ~8 mg Fe as sodium iron EDTA that contained ~41 mg EDTA or ~41 mg sodium EDTA	Memory Manual activity Visuospatial cognition	As per original randomization	• No significant improvement was found on cognitive outcomes, with iron or EDTA
Cambodia (2018) [18]	1933	6–16 years	6 (during school days, 6 days/week excluding national holiday)	Same range as enrollment (immediately after 6-month intervention)	Local conventional rice	UltraRice original (10.7 mg Fe/100 g) or UltraRice new (7.6 mg Fe/100 g) or NutriRice (7.5 mg Fe/100 g)	Fluid and crystalized intelligence	As per original randomization	• The UltraRice original group improved in fluid intelligence to a greater degree than the placebo group • No differences found between the UltraRice new and placebo groups nor between the NutriRice and placebo groups

Sweden (2018) [19]	285[a] (birth weight between 2000 and 2500 g)	1.5 months	4.5 (until child was 6 months of age)	7	0 mg/kg/d iron drops	1 mg/kg/d iron drops or 2 mg/kg/d iron drops	Intelligence quotient (IQ)	As per original randomization	• No significant differences in IQ between control and intervention groups nor between the two intervention groups
India (2018) [20]	140[a]	12–16 years	6	Same range as enrollment (immediately after 6-month intervention)	Conventional pearl millet (21 ppm Fe from baseline-4 mo: 52 ppm Fe from 4–6 mo)	Iron biofortified pearl millet (86 ppm Fe)	Attention Memory	As per original randomization	• Biofortified group improved in attention and memory to a greater degree than the control group
China (2018) [21]	1482	1.5 months	7.5	9 months	Placebo (in utero, mom received 0.40 mg folate/d or 300 mg Fe and 0.40 mg folate/d)	Iron (~1 mg/kg of elemental iron/d) (in utero, mom received 0.40 mg folate/d or 300 mg Fe and 0.40 mg folate/d)	Motor	• Iron-deficient in both fetal-neonatal and infancy periods • Fetal-neonatal iron deficiency only • Infancy iron deficiency only • No iron deficiency	• Fetal-neonatal and/or infancy iron deficiency groups had lower motor scores than children without iron deficiency
Chile (2019) [22]	875[b]	6 months	6 (until child was 12 months of age)	5.5 and 10	Formula with no added iron	Formula with 2.3 mg/L iron or Formula with 12.7 mg/L iron	Language	• Iron sufficient in infancy • Iron deficient in infancy • Iron deficient anemic in infancy[b]	• More severe iron deficiency in infancy related to lower language abilities at 5 and 10 years of age (resulting from higher child dull affect/social reticence and parental unresponsiveness at 5 years)

(continued)

Table 23.1 (continued)

Location	*n*	Age at enrollment into original study	Intervention duration (months)	Age at follow-up (years)	Control group	Intervention group(s)	Outcome domain	Analyses groups	Main findings
Chile (2019) [23]	405[b]	6 months	6 (until child was 12 months of age)	16	Formula with 2.3 mg/L iron	Formula with 12.7 mg/L iron	Cognitive ability Visual-motor Memory Achievement (math, vocabulary, and comprehension)	As per original randomization	• Lower memory and achievement (math and comprehension) scores for those randomized to the higher iron formula vs. the lower iron formula • For visual-motor outcome, group who consumed higher iron formula had better scores if hemoglobin was low at 6 months and lower scores if hemoglobin was high at 6 months, compared to group who consumed lower iron formula

[a]Children who were severely anemic at enrollment were excluded from the study
[b]Children identified as anemic during infancy were treated with iron

at baseline experienced the greatest gains in terms of cognitive scores [14, 18, 20]. It may be noteworthy that supplementation occurred during the school years in these studies and not during the infancy period, when supplementation was not related to improvements in cognition [16, 19]. The study conducted in India [20] used computerized tests which are less subjective and allow for a finer assessment of cognition (for instance, measuring time in milliseconds). Nevertheless, two studies [14, 18] used more subjective measures, similar to those used in the Sweden and Morocco studies described above and yet, reported significant differences after supplementation. Again, timing of supplementation may be at play, but it may also be important to consider the way in which the cognitive test scores were calculated. The study in Cambodia used raw scores for the three administered tests (Raven's Colored Progressive Matrices and the Block Design and Picture Completion subtests from the Wechsler Intelligence Scale for Children III), citing that no standardized scores appropriate to that setting were available [18]. The study in South Africa used Western standardized scores for some of the outcomes (subscales of the Kaufman Assessment Battery for Children) and raw scores for others (where no standardized scores exist; Hopkins Verbal Learning Test) [14]. Interestingly, the differences between groups were only seen for tests where the authors used raw scores. Whether or not a lack of association when using Western-based standardized scores is an indication that applying these scores in these contexts is inappropriate is a question that remains to be answered. One final possibility should be mentioned here. The iron treatments used in the studies conducted in Cambodia [18] and India [20] provided higher levels of other micronutrients (such as vitamin B12 or zinc) compared to the placebo groups. The possibility that these nutrients positively influenced cognition cannot be ruled out. Of the remaining studies that conducted analyses using the original randomization groups, both reported worse cognitive outcomes for children who had been treated with higher iron formula vs. those treated with a low iron formula during infancy [15, 23]. These follow-up studies assessed children at 10 and 16 years of age and used cognitive assessments that require a highly trained administrator. Interestingly, when accounting for hemoglobin levels at enrollment, both studies reported higher scores (for spatial memory assessed with the Kaufman Assessment Battery for Children at 10 years of age and for visual motor integration assessed with the Beery-Buktenica Developmental Test of Visual-Motor Integration at both 10 and 16 years of age) after iron treatment for those children whose hemoglobin was low at baseline (6 months of age) but lower scores after iron treatment for those children whose hemoglobin was high at baseline.

The two studies that ran analyses based on iron status in infancy both reported lower scores (motor or language) in children who were iron deficient during the fetal/neonatal and/or infancy periods [21, 22]. One of these studies assessed outcomes immediately at the end of the treatment (9 months of age) [21] while the other assessed outcomes several years after the treatment ended (at 5.5 and 10 years of age) [22].

Overall, results from recent studies, which assessed the association between iron and cognition in children and adolescents, are mixed. In general, the studies point to an association between poor iron status and lower cognitive scores. However, the benefits of treating with iron on cognitive outcomes are not clearly established. Studies that provided iron treatment during infancy seem to indicate no benefit or even worse outcomes with higher doses of iron. Alternatively, studies that provided the iron treatment during the school-age years appear to show a benefit of the supplementation. Given the findings that early life iron deficiency may have irreversible effects, it appears that preventing iron deficiency in infancy should be a top priority. While a limited number of observational studies that assess the association between iron status in children and adolescents and neurophysiology exist, no such randomized controlled trials were found in our assessment of articles published in the past decade. Additional studies are needed to better understand the role of timing, duration, and severity of iron deficiency on cognitive outcomes and neurophysiology as well as the effect of timing, duration, dose, and vehicle of supplementation on these outcomes in children. Type of testing conducted and manner in which the tests are scored may also affect the findings.

Long-Term Effects of Iron Treatment in Early Life on Child Behavioral and Affective Outcomes

Over the past decade, seven publications were identified in which children had received iron treatment or a control during infancy and were then followed up at later ages during childhood to assess behavioral and affective (outward expression of an individual's internal emotions) outcomes [16, 19, 24–28]. The seven included studies represent follow-up from three original studies [29–31] with follow-up sample sizes ranging from 161 to 1116 and supplementation periods of approximately 6 months for six of the studies [16, 18, 25–28] and 12–20 months for one [24]. As far as the vehicle for supplementation, Chun-Ming et al. provided a sachet of multiple micronutrients to be added to complementary foods (comparison group received a sachet of rice flour and vegetable oil), Berglund et al. provided iron drops (1 or 2 mg/kg body weight/day with comparison group receiving 0 mg/kg body weight/day), and Lozoff et al. provided a high or low-iron formula (12.7 mg/L and 2.3 mg/L, respectively; comparison group received a formula with no added iron). Chun-Ming and colleagues only measured hemoglobin and, as such, there is no indication of whether or not the anemia measured in their study was due to iron deficiency. At baseline [29], no child was excluded due to their hemoglobin concentration while at follow-up [24], the authors excluded individuals who were anemic. The studies conducted by Berglund et al. and Lozoff et al. used multiple biomarkers which are specific for iron status and, as such, were able to classify the children as iron-sufficient, iron-deficient, and iron-deficient anemic. Of importance, the 3.5-year follow-up [16] conducted by Berglund et al. did not assess iron status at follow-up; as such, the interpretation of the findings is less clear. The study conducted by Berglund et al. excluded anemic children at baseline [30] and the study conducted by Lozoff et al. [31] was a prevention trial, randomizing children who were iron sufficient or iron deficient but not anemic but supplementing all children who were anemic at baseline. Age of children at follow up ranged from 3.5 to 17 years. Of the seven follow-up studies assessing behavior, four analyzed the data by using the original randomized groups [16, 19, 25, 27]. The others ran the analyses with the children stratified by iron status in infancy (iron-sufficient, iron-deficient, or iron-deficient anemic [26, 28] or by whether or not the deficiency was corrected by the original treatment [24]) to assess the impact of early-life iron status on later behavioral outcomes.

Table 23.2 summarizes the main outcome variables and findings from these follow-up studies. Affect, behavior, and social difficulties were the three main outcome domains assessed through researcher observation, parental report, and/or child self-report, depending on the study. The studies that utilized the original randomization groups in their analyses reported a higher prevalence of behavioral problems (overall behavior as assessed with the Child Behavior Checklist (CBCL), externalizing problems (CBCL), and conduct disorder (CBCL)) in the control group (no additional iron provided), vs. the groups who received iron when behavior was assessed through parental report [16, 19, 27], and more positive affect in children who received iron vs. those who did not when assessed via observer rating [25]. These studies assessed the children years after the original supplementation (at 3.5, 7, 10, and 14 years of age). However, when behavior was assessed through child self-report (at ~14 years of age), higher scores on the ADHD symptoms subscale were found in the groups who received iron vs. the group who did not [27]. As only one study used child self-report to assess behavior, this finding will need to be replicated in future studies before it can be properly interpreted. All of the remaining analyses assessed the association of early-life iron status to later behavioral/affective outcomes (regardless of randomization group although they controlled for group) and reported that iron deficiency ane-

Table 23.2 Long-term follow-up of studies examining the effect of iron treatment in infancy on child and adolescent behavior and affect (2010–2020)

Location	*n*	Age at enrollment into original study (months)	Intervention duration (months)	Age at follow-up (years)	Control group	Intervention group(s)	Outcome domain	Analyses groups	Main findings
China (2011) [24]	161	4–12	12–20 months (until child was 24 months of age)	4	Sachet of rice flour + vegetable oil (matched total energy of treatment sachet)	Sachet of 6 mg iron, 4.1 mg zinc, 385 mg calcium, 0.2 mg vit B_2, 7 ug vit D, 3.8 g protein)	Affect and behavior	• Chronic IDA[a] (anemic in infancy and not corrected with treatment) • Corrected IDA[a] (anemia in infancy that was corrected by 24 months) • Non-IDA in infancy and at 24 months[a]	• Chronic IDA children showed less positive affect, less frustration tolerance, more passive behavior and more physical self-soothing compared to non-IDA in infancy children • The behavior and affect of children in the corrected IDA group did not differ from those in the non-IDA in infancy group
Sweden (2013) [16]	285[b] (birth weight between 2000 and 2500 g)	1.5	4.5 (until child was 6 months of age)	3.5	0 mg/kg/d iron drops	1 mg/kg/d iron drops or 2 mg/kg/d iron drops	Behavior	As per original randomization	• Higher behavioral problem scores in control group vs. all other groups
Chile (2014) [25]	1032	6	6 (until child was 12 months of age	10	Formula with no added iron	Formula with 2.3 mg/L iron or Formula with 12.7 mg/L iron	Affect and behavior	As per original randomization comparing any (high + low iron formula) vs. no iron formula	• Iron supplemented children were more cooperative, confident, persistent, coordinated, direct, and worked harder after praise compared to non-supplemented children • In a positive affect task, iron supplemented children spent more time laughing/smiling with their mothers compared to non-supplemented children • In a social stress task, the iron supplemented children smile/laughed more and required less prompting compared to non-supplemented children

(continued)

Table 23.2 (continued)

Location	n	Age at enrollment into original study (months)	Intervention duration (months)	Age at follow-up (years)	Control group	Intervention group(s)	Outcome domain	Analyses groups	Main findings
Chile (2017) [26]	873	6	6 (until child was 12 months of age)	5.5, 10, ~14	Formula with no added iron	Formula with 2.3 mg/L iron or Formula with 12.7 mg/L iron	Social difficulties and behavior	• Iron sufficient in infancy • Iron deficient in infancy • Iron deficient anemic in infancy[c]	• Iron-deficient anemic in infancy related to child dull affect and maternal unresponsiveness at 5.5 years which, in turn, related to higher child peer rejection at 10 years and subsequent problem behaviors and deviant friends in adolescence (~14 years)
Sweden (2018) [19]	285[b] (birth weight between 2000 and 2500 g)	1.5	4.5 (until child was 6 months of age)	7	0 mg/kg/d iron drops	1 mg/kg/d iron drops or 2 mg/kg/d iron drops	Behavior	As per original randomization but combining the two iron supplemented groups	• Lower externalizing problems in iron supplemented groups vs. control group
Chile (2018) [27]	1116	6	6 (until child was 12 months of age)	11–17 (mean: ~ 14 years)	Formula with no added iron	Formula with 2.3 mg/L iron or Formula with 12.7 mg/L iron	Social difficulties and behavior	As per original randomization comparing any (high + low iron formula) vs. no iron formula and comparing high vs. low iron formula groups AND by iron status in infancy: • Iron sufficient in infancy • Iron deficient in infancy • Iron deficient anemic in infancy[c]	• Lower conduct problems in iron formula vs. no iron formula groups • Higher ADHD symptoms in iron formula vs. no iron formula groups • No differences when comparing high vs. low iron formula groups • Both iron-deficient and iron-deficient anemic infants in infancy had higher adolescent behavior problems compared to iron sufficient in infancy

Chile (2018) [28]	1116	6	6 (until child was 12 months of age)	11–17 (mean: ~14 years)	Formula with no added iron	Formula with 2.3 mg/L iron or Formula with 12.7 mg/L iron	Behavior	• Iron sufficient in infancy • Iron deficient in infancy • Iron-deficient anemic in infancy[c]	• Iron-deficient anemic in infancy related to excessive alcohol use and risky sexual behavior in adolescence (resulting from poor emotional regulation at 10 years) • Iron-deficient anemic in infancy related to higher risk taking in adolescence (resulting from attention control deficits at 10 years)

[a]Although the authors classify the children as chronic IDA (iron-deficient anemic), corrected IDA, or non-IDA, hemoglobin was the only biomarker assessed. Anemic children at follow-up (4 years of age) were excluded

[b]Children who were anemic at enrollment were excluded from the study

[c]Children identified as anemic during infancy were treated with iron

mia in infancy was related to worse affect (less positive affect, more dull affect) and worse behavior (higher externalizing problems, excessive alcohol use, risky sexual behavior) even after controlling for possible confounders (such as SES, maternal education, maternal depressive symptoms, child sex, family stressors, the home environment) when compared to children who were iron sufficient in infancy [24, 26, 28]. One study compared children whose anemia was corrected in infancy to those who were never anemic in infancy and found no differences in behavior or affect at the 4-year follow-up [24]. Another study found that children who were iron deficient (but not anemic) in infancy had higher adolescent behavior problems compared to children who were iron sufficient in infancy [28].

Together, these studies indicate negative consequences of iron deficiency and iron deficiency anemia in infancy on behavior and affect, years later. The differences reported among adolescents who were formerly iron deficient are especially troubling, given the serious potential consequences of the behaviors (excessive alcohol consumption and risky sexual behaviors). The finding that behavioral differences might persist in children who were iron deficient, but not anemic, in infancy is cause for concern as the prevalence of iron deficiency without anemia is high and iron deficiency, in the absence of anemia, typically goes undetected. Whether or not iron supplementation in early life can reverse these negative consequences is still in question since few randomized controlled trials exist and most of the long-term studies have assessed the outcomes based on early-life status as opposed to randomization group.

Effects of Iron Deficiency on Cognition and Behavior in Women of Reproductive Age

While decades of research indicate an association between iron status and cognitive/behavioral outcomes in infants and young children, few studies have been conducted in adults. This was due to the belief that the brain was resistant to changes in iron once the blood–brain barrier reached maturity [32]. However, animal studies revealed that the uptake of iron into the brain is dependent on iron status, as there is an increased rate with low iron status and a decreased rate with high iron status [33]. Furthermore, the uptake process is not reflective of overall blood–brain barrier permeability [34, 35]. Since this knowledge emerged, there has been an increased interest in understanding the association between iron status and cognition/behavior in adults, particularly in women of reproductive age, given their susceptibility to iron deficiency. Studies conducted prior to the past 10 years included both observational and intervention designs and most were conducted in developed countries. The observational studies suggested a relation between iron status and cognition such that higher iron levels are associated with better cognitive functioning, specifically, spatial ability, attention, memory, and executive functioning. These studies also report a relation between iron status and affect such that higher iron levels are associated with fewer depressive symptoms and a higher quality of life [4]. All of the intervention studies assessing cognition as the outcome, reported an improvement in cognitive functioning with iron supplementation. Likewise, in intervention studies assessing affect as the outcome, improvements were reported following iron supplementation with the greatest improvements found among women who had poor baseline iron status. However, few studies were randomized controlled trials and few studies specifically examined the effect of iron deficiency, in the absence of anemia, on cognition, behavior, or affect. Here, we focus on recent randomized controlled studies that examined the association between iron supplementation and cognition/behavior in women of reproductive age.

Effects of Iron Treatment on Cognitive and Neurophysiological Outcomes in Women of Reproductive Age

Four manuscripts, representing three randomized controlled trials, of the effects of iron treatment on cognition in adult women of reproductive age have been published over the past decade [36–39]. Three recruited university-attending women as the participants [36, 38, 39] and one recruited women who worked on a tea plantation [37]. The vehicle for supplementation was beef in one study (comparison group received non-beef foods), provided for 16 weeks [36], double-fortified salt (comparison group received single-fortified salt), provided for 10 months [37], and biofortified beans (comparison group received conventional beans), provided for 18 weeks [38, 39]. All studies included multiple iron status biomarkers which were assessed at baseline and endline and the study in Rwanda was restricted to women with a ferritin ≤20 ng/mL at baseline. The studies analyzed the data using an intent to treat approach and also included secondary data analysis approaches.

Table 23.3 summarizes the main outcome variables and findings from these randomized controlled trials. The main outcome domains were memory and attention and one study also used electroencephalogram (EEG) measurements to assess electrophysiology [39]. The study conducted in the United States did not find any difference in cognitive outcomes between the groups at endline [36]. Both groups improved their iron status over time but changes in cognitive outcomes did not differ by group. On the other hand, when classifying the women as those who had a positive change in ferritin vs. those who did not, the authors report greater improvements in all three cognitive domains tested (memory, attention, spatial planning) in the "ferritin responders" vs. the "ferritin non-responders." In contrast, the studies conducted in India and Rwanda found significant differences between groups at endline on the cognitive domains tested (memory, attention, perception) with women in the treatment arms having greater improvements [37, 38]. Although the exact tests given differed in these studies, all studies utilized computerized cognitive tests. The study in Rwanda was limited to women who were iron deficient at baseline, the study in India included only the subgroup of women who had the lowest ferritin values from the larger parent trial, and the study conducted in the United States did not limit enrollment based on ferritin concentrations. Indeed, at baseline, the mean ferritin concentrations of those in the US study were nearly four times higher than the mean ferritin concentrations of those in the Rwanda study and almost 40% higher than those in the India study. It is possible that women with a lower iron status at baseline experience a greater benefit of increased iron status. The Rwanda study also included measures of electrophysiology and found greater improvements in EEG amplitude and spectral power in the group who consumed the biofortified beans vs. those who consumed the conventional beans [39]. An important contribution of this study is the finding that changes in brain activity (EEG) mediate the relation between changes in iron biomarkers and changes in cognition (memory and attention). Studies which use electrophysiological measurements and relate the findings to changes in cognition are especially helpful in terms of providing a link between the mechanistic studies conducted with animal models and the behavioral and affective outcomes that are typically measured in human studies.

Recent observational studies (not reviewed in-depth here) are supportive of an association between iron status and cognitive functioning in women of reproductive age, indicating that better executive functioning and attention scores are found in women who are iron sufficient vs. those who are deficient [40–42]. Two recent observational studies have also examined the association between iron status and neurobiology. One revealed differences in left EEG alpha activity in prefrontal regions between iron-deficient (non-anemic) and iron-sufficient women of reproductive age [43]. The other study found differences in brain connectivity (using functional magnetic resonance imaging) between women who had been iron-deficient anemic in infancy vs. controls (iron sufficient or mild iron deficiency in infancy) [44]. Specifically, formerly iron deficient anemic subjects had decreased connectivity from the posterior Default Mode Network (DMN) to the left posterior cingulate cortex (PCC) and increased connectivity from the anterior DMN to the right PCC. They also exhibited differences in the left medial frontal gyrus.

Table 23.3 Randomized controlled trials assessing the effect of iron treatment on cognition and neurophysiology in women of reproductive age (2010–2020)

Location	*n*	Participant age (years)	Intervention duration	Control group	Intervention group(s)	Outcome domain	Analyses groups	Main findings
USA (2014) [36]	43	18–30	16 weeks	Non-beef foods containing levels of calories and protein similar to the beef lunches	Beef lunches (3 oz., 3 times per week; approximately 2.4 mg iron/3 oz. of beef)	Memory, attention, and spatial planning	As per original randomization and comparing ferritin responders vs. non-responders	• No differences on any cognitive outcomes between original randomization groups • Ferritin responders had greater improvements in working memory, attention, and spatial planning compared to ferritin non-responders
India (2017) [37]	126	18–55	10 months	Iodized salt (47 mg potassium iodate/kg)	Double fortified salt (47 mg potassium iodate/kg and 3.3 mg microencapsulated ferrous fumarate/g)	Memory, attention, and perception	As per original randomization and assessing association between change in iron biomarker and change in cognitive performance	• Greater improvements on memory, attention, and perception tasks for the double fortified salt vs. the iodized only salt group • Increases in ferritin were significantly related to better performance on all three domains tested
Rwanda (2017) [38]	150[a]	18–27	18 weeks	Conventional beans (50.1 ppm iron)	Biofortified beans (86.1 ppm iron)	Memory and attention	As per original randomization and assessing association between change in iron biomarker and change in cognitive performance	• Greater improvements on attention and memory tasks for the biofortified group vs. the conventional group • Increases in ferritin were significantly related to better performance on the attention and memory tasks
Rwanda (2019) [39]	55[a]	18–27	18 weeks	Conventional beans (50.1 ppm iron)	Biofortified beans (86.1 ppm iron)	EEG	As per original randomization	• Greater improvements in measures of EEG amplitude and spectral power for the biofortified group vs. the conventional group

[a]Only included women with a ferritin ≤20 ng/mL. The larger, parent trial included 195 women

Although these observational studies are supportive of a relation between iron and cognition in women of reproductive age, the number of recent randomized controlled trials assessing the effects of iron treatment on cognition in this population is extremely limited. While the studies provide evidence that iron deficiency is related to cognitive alterations and changes in electrophysiology, more work is needed to fully understand these associations in this age group. Optimal cognitive functioning is necessary for performing day-to-day duties. Alterations in maternal cognitive functioning may have significant implications for maternal–child interactions with subsequent negative effects on child development, as women are often the primary caregiver for children. It is therefore crucial that these types of studies continue to be conducted in women of reproductive age.

Effects of Iron Treatment on Behavioral and Affective Outcomes in Women of Reproductive Age

Three recent randomized controlled trials were identified in which women of reproductive age received iron treatment or a control and behavioral/affective variables were assessed as the outcomes of interest [45–47]. Two of the studies were conducted in developed countries [45, 46] and the other was conducted in Iran [47], a semi-developed country. Sample sizes ranged from 70–198 with intervention periods ranging from 2 weeks (intravenous iron) to 12 weeks. As for the vehicle for supplementation, the study conducted in Switzerland utilized intravenous iron (comparison group received intravenous placebo) while the other two provided oral iron supplements as tablets (with comparison groups receiving oral placebo tablets). As far as iron status assessment and inclusion criteria, all of the studies included multiple iron status biomarkers which were assessed both at baseline and endline and all of the studies excluded women who were anemic at baseline. Additionally, the studies conducted in Switzerland and France included only women whose baseline ferritin levels were ≤ 50 ng/mL and the study conducted in Iran included only women with postpartum depression. All of the studies analyzed the data using an intent to treat approach and it is important to note that the study conducted in France was observer blinded while the other studies were double blinded.

Table 23.4 summarizes the main outcome variables and findings from the randomized controlled trials conducted over the past decade. The main outcome domains were affect (specifically, anxiety, depression, and quality of life) and fatigue. In both studies where fatigue was assessed, the authors found significantly larger decreases in fatigue in the women who received iron vs. those who received a placebo [45, 46]. For one of these studies, this association was only true for women whose ferritin concentrations were ≤ 15 ng/mL at baseline [45]. For the studies that assessed affect, one reported no significant differences between groups on measures of anxiety, depression, or quality of life [46]. The other study reported significant improvements in depression scores in women who were treated with iron compared to those treated with placebo (improvement rate of 42.8% vs. 20.0% for iron vs. placebo treated, respectively; $p = 0.03$) [47]. Several differences exist between these studies which may contribute to the discrepant finding: (1) different instruments were used to assessed depression, (2) participants in the Iran study were all 1-week postpartum while the participants in France were not in the postpartum period, and (3) the study conducted in Iran only enrolled women who had been diagnosed with postpartum depression.

Although the number of randomized controlled trials assessing iron status and behavior in women of reproductive age is limited, the studies provide evidence that iron status is related to behavior and that iron repletion may ameliorate the negative findings. Of importance, all of these studies excluded anemic women and, therefore, the findings indicate alterations in behavior in those who are iron deficient but not anemic. In other words, mild iron deficiency has behavioral and affective consequences in women of repro-

Table 23.4 Randomized controlled trials assessing the effect of iron treatment on behavior and affect in women of reproductive age (2010–2020)

Location	*n*	Participant age (years)	Intervention duration	Control group	Intervention group(s)	Outcome domain	Analyses groups	Main findings
Switzerland (2011) [45]	90[a]	≥18	2 weeks (outcomes assessed at 6 weeks)	Intravenous placebo for 2 weeks (4 infusions with 200 mL of 0.9% saline, period of 10 min each)	800 mg of iron (cumulative dose) as iron (III)-hydroxide sucrose for 2 weeks (4 infusions containing 200 mg of solution) in 200 mL of 0.9% saline, period of 10 min each)	Fatigue	As per original randomization	• Fatigue decreased significantly more in IV iron vs. placebo group; this was true only for those whose baseline ferritin levels were ≤ 15 ng/mL
France (2012) [46]	198[a]	18–53	12 weeks	Placebo	80 mg iron/d (prolonged release ferrous sulfate)	Affect and fatigue	As per original randomization	• Fatigue decreased significantly more in iron vs. placebo group • No significant difference between groups on anxiety, depression, or quality of life scores
Iran (2017) [47]	70[b]	20–40	6 weeks	Placebo	50 mg elemental iron/d (ferrous sulfate)	Affect	As per original randomization	• Significant improvement in depression scores in iron treated vs. placebo group

[a]Only included women with a ferritin ≤50 ng/mL and hemoglobin ≥120 g/L
[b]Only included mothers with postpartum depression and who were not anemic

ductive age. As mentioned above in our review of the findings in children, this is especially concerning, given the lack of identification of iron deficiency in the absence of anemia, in most settings.

Conclusion

The brief review provided in this chapter reveals an association between iron deficiency (with and without anemia) and alterations in cognition and behavior for both children and women of reproductive age. Findings of this association in the absence of anemia are particularly troubling, given the magnitude of iron deficiency without anemia and the fact that it goes largely undetected. The findings of long-term cognitive and behavioral consequences of iron deficiency in infancy despite iron repletion are also of particular concern. Finally, the fact that higher iron doses used for repletion may be related to worse outcomes when supplementation occurs in infancy needs to be further investigated. These findings indicate that preventing iron deficiency in infancy should be a top priority. The magnitude of cognitive and affective changes reported with iron deficiency vary by study but, in general, indicate levels that are likely to impact daily activities. Although studies of the functional consequences of iron deficiency continue, there is a clear need for well-designed randomized controlled studies in order to better understand the effects of timing, duration, and severity of the deficiency as well as the optimal treatment timing, duration, and dose. Studies that link changes in neurophysiology to changes in these cognitive and behavioral outcomes are especially needed.

References

1. Kassebaum NJ, Jasrasaria R, Naghavi M, Wulf SK, Johns N, Lozano R, Regan M, Weatherall D, Chou DP, Eisele TP, Flaxman SR, Pullan RL, Brooker SJ, Murray CJL. A systematic analysis of global anemia burden from 1990 to 2010. Blood. 2014;123:615–24.
2. Lu C, Black MM, Richter LM. Risk of poor development in young children in low-income and middle-income countries: an estimation and analysis at the global, regional, and country level. Lancet Glob Health. 2016;4:e916–22.
3. Murray-Kolb LE. Iron and brain functions. Curr Opin Clin Nutr Metab Care. 2013;16:703–7.
4. McClung JP, Murray-Kolb LE. Iron nutrition and premenopausal women: effects of poor iron status on neuropsychological and physical performance. Annu Rev Nutr. 2013;33:271–88.
5. Beard JL, Connor JR, Jones BC. Iron in the brain. Nutr Rev. 1993;51:157.
6. Pinero DJ, Li NQ, Connor JR, Beard JL. Alterations in brain iron metabolism in response to dietary iron changes. J Nutr. 2000;130:254–63.
7. Aoki S, Okada Y, Nishimura K, Barkovich AJ, Kjos BO, et al. Normal deposition of brain iron in childhood and adolescence: MR imaging at 1.5 T. Radiology. 1989;172:381–5.
8. Hill JM. The distribution of iron in the brain. In: Youdim MBH, editor. Brain iron: neurochemistry and behavioural aspects. London: Taylor & Francis; 1988. p. 1–24.
9. Beard JL, Connor JR. Iron status and neural functioning. Annu Rev Nutr. 2003;23:41–58.
10. Pivina L, Semenova Y, Doşa MD, Dauletyarova M, Bjørklund G. Iron deficiency, cognitive functions, and neurobehavioral disorders in children. J Mol Neurosci. 2019;68:1–10.
11. Ferreira A, Neves P, Gozzelino R. Multilevel impacts of iron in the brain: the cross talk between neurophysiological mechanisms, cognition, and social behavior. Pharmaceuticals (Basel). 2019;12:126.
12. Lozoff B, Klein NK, Nelson EC, McClish DK, Manuel M, Chacon ME. Behavior of infants with iron-deficiency anemia. Child Dev. 1998;69:24–36.
13. Grantham-McGregor S, Ani C. A review of studies on the effect of iron deficiency on cognitive development in children. J Nutr. 2001;131(2S-2):649S–66S; discussion 666S–668S
14. Baumgartner J, Smuts CM, Malan L, Kvalsvig J, van Stuijvenberg ME, Hurrell RF, Zimmermann MB. Effects of iron and n-3 fatty acid supplementation, alone and in combination, on cognition in school children: a randomized, double-blind, placebo-controlled intervention in South Africa. Am J Clin Nutr. 2012;96:1327–38.
15. Lozoff B, Castillo M, Clark MK, Smith BJ. Iron-fortified vs low-iron infant formula: developmental outcome at 10 years. Arch Pediatr Adolesc Med. 2012;166:208.
16. Berglund SK, Westrup B, Hägglöf B, Hernell O, Domellöf M. Effects of iron supplementation of LBW infants on cognition and behavior at 3 years. Pediatrics. 2013;131:47–55.
17. Bouhouch RR, El-Fadeli S, Andersson M, Aboussad A, Chabaa L, Zeder C, Kippler M, Baumgartner J, Sedki A, Zimmermann MB. Effects of wheat-flour biscuits fortified with iron and EDTA, alone and in combination, on blood lead concentration, iron status,

and cognition in children: a double-blind randomized controlled trial. Am J Clin Nutr. 2016;104:1318–26.
18. Fiorentino M, Perignon M, Kuong K, de Groot R, Parker M, Burja K, Dijkhuizen MA, Sokjom S, Chamnan C, Berger J, Wieringa FT. Effect of multi-micronutrient-fortified rice on cognitive performance depends on premix composition and cognitive function tested: results of an effectiveness study in Cambodian schoolchildren. Public Health Nutr. 2018;21:816–27.
19. Berglund SK, Chmielewska A, Starnberg J, Westrup B, Hägglöf B, Norman M, Domellöf M. Effects of iron supplementation of low-birth-weight infants on cognition and behavior at 7 years: a randomized controlled trial. Pediatr Res. 2018;83:111–8.
20. Scott SP, Murray-Kolb LE, Wenger MJ, Udipi SA, Ghugre PS, Boy E, Haas JD. Cognitive performance in Indian school-going adolescents is positively affected by consumption of iron-biofortified pearl millet: a 6-month randomized controlled efficacy trial. J Nutr. 2018;148:1462–71.
21. Santos DCC, Angulo-Barroso RM, Li M, Bian Y, Sturza J, Richards B, Lozoff B. Timing, duration, and severity of iron deficiency in early development and motor outcomes at 9 months. Eur J Clin Nutr. 2018;72:332–41.
22. East P, Delker E, Blanco E, Encina P, Lozoff B, Gahagan S. Effect of infant iron deficiency on children's verbal abilities: the roles of child affect and parent unresponsiveness. Matern Child Health J. 2019;23:1240–50.
23. Gahagan S, Delker E, Blanco E, Burrows R, Lozoff B. Randomized controlled trial of iron-fortified versus low-iron infant formula: developmental outcomes at 16 years. J Pediatr. 2019;212:124–130.e1.
24. Chang S, Wang L, Wang Y, Brouwer ID, Kok FJ, Lozoff B, Chen C. Iron-deficiency anemia in infancy and social emotional development in preschool-aged Chinese children. Pediatrics. 2011;127:e927–33.
25. Lozoff B, Castillo M, Clark KM, Smith JB, Sturza J. Iron supplementation in infancy contributes to more adaptive behavior at 10 years of age. J Nutr. 2014;144:838–45.
26. East P, Lozoff B, Blanco E, Delker E, Delva J, Encina P, Gahagan S. Infant iron deficiency, child affect, and maternal unresponsiveness: testing the long-term effects of functional isolation. Dev Psychol. 2017;53:2233–44.
27. Doom JR, Richards B, Caballero G, Delva J, Gahagan S, Lozoff B. Infant iron deficiency and iron supplementation predict adolescent internalizing, externalizing, and social problems. J Pediatr. 2018;195:199–205.
28. East P, Delker E, Lozoff B, Delva J, Castillo M, Gahagan S. Association among infant iron deficiency, childhood emotion and attention regulation, and adolescent problem behaviors. Child Dev. 2018;89:593–608.
29. Chun-Ming C, Wang Y, Chang S. Effect of in-home fortification of complementary feeding on intellectual development of Chinese children. Biomed Environ Sci. 2010;23:83–91.
30. Berglund S, Westrup B, Domellöf M. Iron supplements reduce the risk of iron deficiency anemia in marginally low birth weight infants. Pediatrics. 2010;126:e874–83.
31. Lozoff B, DeAndraca I, Castillo M, Smith JB, Walter T, Pino P. Behavioral and development effects of preventing iron-deficiency anemia in health full-term infants. Pediatrics. 2003;112:846–54.
32. Murray-Kolb LE. Iron status and neuropsychological consequences in women of reproductive age: what do we know and where are we headed? J Nutr. 2011;141:747S–55S.
33. Taylor EM, Crowe A, Morgan EH. Transferrin and iron uptake by the brain: effects of altered iron status. J Neurochem. 1991;57:1584–92.
34. Malecki EA, Cook B, Devenyl AG, Beard JL, Connor JR. Transferrin is required for normal distributions of ^{59}Fe and ^{54}Mn in mouse brains. J Neurol Sci. 2000;170:112–8.
35. Pinero DJ, Jones B, Beard JL. Alterations in brain iron metabolism in response to dietary iron changes. J Nutr. 2000;130:254–63.
36. Blanton C. Improvements in iron status and cognitive function in young women consuming beef or non-beef lunches. Nutrients. 2014;9:90–110.
37. Wenger MJ, Murray-Kolb LE, Nevins JEH, Venkatramanan S, Reinhart GA, Wesley A, Haas JD. Consumption of a double-fortified salt affects perceptual, attentional, and mnemonic functioning in women in a randomized controlled trial in India. J Nutr. 2017;147:2297–308.
38. Murray-Kolb LE, Wenger MJ, Scott SP, Rhoten SE, Lung'aho MG, Haas JD. Consumption of iron-biofortified beans positively affects cognitive performance in 18 to 27-year-old Rwandan female college students in an 18-week randomized controlled efficacy trial. J Nutr. 2017;147:109–17.
39. Wenger MJ, Rhoten SE, Murray-Kolb LE, Scott SP, Boy E, Gahutu JB, Haas JD. Changes in iron status are related to changes in brain activity and behavior in Rwandan female university students: results from a randomized controlled efficacy trial involving iron-biofortified beans. J Nutr. 2019;149:687–97.
40. Blanton CA, Green MW, Kretsch MJ. Body iron is associated with cognitive executive planning function in college women. Br J Nutr. 2013;109:906–13.
41. Scott SP, Murray-Kolb LE. Iron status is associated with performance on executive functioning tasks in nonanemic young women. J Nutr. 2016;146:30–7.
42. Cook RL, O'Dwyer NJ, Parker HM, Donges CE, Cheng HL, Steinbeck KS, Cox EP, Franklin JL, Garg ML, Rooney KB, O'Connor HT. Iron deficiency anemia, not iron deficiency, is associated with reduced attention in healthy young women. Nutrients. 2017;9:1216.
43. Dziembowska I, Kwapisz J, IZdebski P, Zekanowska E. Mild iron deficiency may affect female endurance and behavior. Physiol Behav. 2019;205:44–50.

44. Algarin C, Karunakaran KD, Reyes S, Morales C, Lozoff B, Peirano P, Biswal B. Differences on brain connectivity in adulthood are present in subjects with iron deficiency anemia in infancy. Front Aging Neurosci. 2017;9:54.
45. Krayenbuehl PA, Battegay E, Breymann C, Furrer J, Schulthess G. Intravenous iron for the treatment of fatigue in non-anemic, premenopausal women with low serum ferritin concentrations. Blood. 2011;118:3222–7.
46. Vaucher P, Druais PL, Waldvogel S, Favrat B. Effect of iron supplementation on fatigue in nonanemic menstruating women with low ferritin: a randomized controlled trial. CMAJ. 2012;184:1247–54.
47. Sheikh M, Hantoushzadeh S, Shariat M, Farahani Z, Ebrahiminasab O. The efficacy of early iron supplementation on postpartum depression, a randomized double-blind placebo-controlled trial. Eur J Nutr. 2017;56:901–8.

Part VI

Program and Policy

24 Strengthening Fortification Markets to Reduce Iron Deficiency Anemia

Dipika Matthias and Penjani Mkambula

Keywords

Fortification markets · Fortification incentives Fortification quality · Fortification compliance · Industrial fortification · Fortification systems · Fortification programs Fortification partnerships · Fortification monitoring · Fortification innovations

Introduction

Food fortification holds strong potential for making a major contribution to the prevention of iron deficiency anemia. As a broad, population-based intervention requiring no change in consumption and adding little cost to staple foods that consumers are already purchasing, it is no surprise that over 90 countries globally have included iron in their wheat, rice, maize, and/or salt fortification standards [1].

Building on this legislative base, governments, donors, and NGOs focus their resources on the development and refinement of programs, including assessments of consumption patterns to ensure standards are adjusted appropriately over time [2], impact studies on effectiveness of fortified foods [3], regulatory and industry capacity-building, and program evaluations [4]. Yet, despite the progress since the 1990s when salt iodization was first expanded into low- and middle-income countries (LMICs), fortification has not reached its potential, particularly for cereal staples.

This is due, in part, to the fact that food fortification is one of the few public health interventions that is largely delivered by private sector actors, from micronutrient manufacturers to premix suppliers, millers, wholesalers, and retailers. Accordingly, a market lens is needed for improving its effectiveness.

Why Have Fortification Markets Largely Failed Us?

In general, markets tend to work best when strong demand meets a robust capacity to supply with appropriate government oversight. For fortified foods, these fundamental pillars often break down. Demand for added micronutrients tends to be missing, as consumers make their purchasing decisions largely based on taste, brand (as a proxy for quality), and/or cost. Therefore, supply chains lack a business incentive to comply with government mandates. Additionally, as low-margin commodities, there is little incentive to

D. Matthias (✉)
Formerly with the Bill and Melinda Gates Foundation, Washington, USA

P. Mkambula
Global Alliance for Improved Nutrition, Geneva, Switzerland

C. D. Karakochuk et al. (eds.), *Nutritional Anemia*, Nutrition and Health,
https://doi.org/10.1007/978-3-031-14521-6_24

develop value-added products. Further, while all food processors are concerned about food safety because it creates an immediate liability, the same cannot be said for sub-standard fortification quality. Finally, in many countries, government leadership does not send a strong enough signal on the importance of fortification for the private sector to invest in the necessary equipment and raw materials. An aggregation of coverage data from 16 fortification assessment coverage toolkit (FACT) surveys revealed that while 41% of households had access to fortifiable wheat flour, only 15% consumed fortified wheat flour, highlighting non-adherence to legislation [5].

Beyond weak incentives, fortification programs tend to over-rely on constrained governments systems for enforcement. A review by Osendarp et al. (2018) [6] found that often government regulatory oversight was inadequate. Combined with the lack of transparency around fortification quality, particularly of their competitors, there is a perception held by industry that the playing field is not level and their actions to be good stewards of the government's fortification programs could result in a loss of market share or simply added costs without consequent improvement in market positioning. In a semi-quantitative survey with industry representatives from 13 countries on key barriers for fortification compliance, 75% cited premix prices and 60% competition with non-fortifying producers as two top barriers [7]. We posit that concerns over premix prices may recede if the latter issue—the lack of a level playing field—were effectively addressed. Studies demonstrate a price premium that varies between 0.5% and 4% above the cost of the non-fortified commodity [8–10] and is generally passed on to the consumer. Some studies have found that even higher premiums are tolerated [11].

How Do we Make Fortification Markets more Functional?

Ensuring better functioning markets for fortified foods requires an understanding of the industry structures and dynamics. For iron, those tend to be the cereal staples, mainly rice, wheat, and maize due to their daily consumption, nominal sensory impact from low inclusion of iron relative to quantities consumed, and minimal incremental costs. However, these industries in some cases are dominated by small- and medium-sized enterprises (SMEs) without the capacity for fortification. Other iron-carrying vehicles are also emerging, such as double fortified salt (DFS), multiple fortified salt (MFS), bouillon cube, seasoning powders, and fish and soy sauces. Although these markets are not as fragmented, several technical and programmatic bottlenecks need addressing, including micronutrients interactions and sensory changes from the enhanced concentrations needed for the smaller quantities consumed, as well as higher incremental costs for inclusion of iron relative to cereals [12, 13]. In addition, these vehicles often face political obstacles, as governments are simultaneously implementing sugar and salt reduction strategies to reduce the risk of diseases such as diabetes and hypertension.

Public–private partnerships (PPP) with a few dominant players has come to serve as the primary means by which to addresses dysfunctional global health markets. However, in staple cereal markets, these traditional structures tend to be used less regularly, as there is often an absence of dominant players to engage, and many nutritionally vulnerable consumers tend to purchase from lower cost regional brands and local mills. Furthermore, partnerships with leading players may not create a demonstration effect for the SMEs. This is because SME investments in fortification may not be rewarded through an improvement in market position, as consumers tend to lack understanding and interest in fortification, even when promoted through social marketing campaigns [14, 15]. Additionally, SMEs face different barriers from the larger players, such as access to premix and dosifers. Thus, mandatory legislation rather than PPPs tends to be a key mechanism for influencing the full range of players in commodity industries, particularly in LMICs where there are few examples of successful fortification programs without mandated standards.

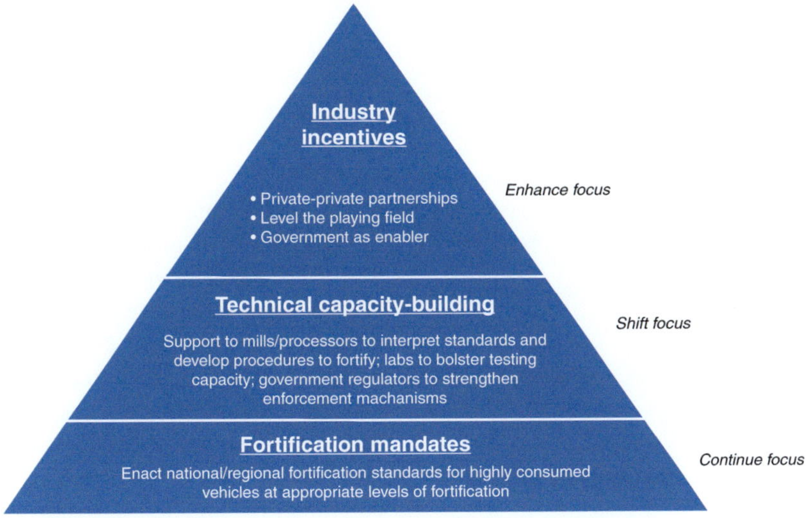

Fig. 24.1 Layered system capabilities for the development of fortified food markets

However, the use of mandatory legislation is insufficient for achieving fortification goals of coverage and quality. It follows that governments and development partners tend to focus on technical approaches to achieving compliance with mandates, but underneath these capacity-building efforts is a fundamentally failed incentive structure that undermines the goals. There are weak incentives on both the supply and demand sides of the market for fortified foods, requiring a fundamental rethinking about how development partners might support the cultivation of industry incentives to both augment and shift the current approach.

As depicted in Fig. 24.1, all three elements, fortification mandates, technical capacity-building, and industry incentives have the potential to result in more functional markets. Mandates will continue as the bedrock of fortification programs, as they create a market pull that is difficult to replicate through alternative means in commodity markets. Technical capacity building is also still needed but could be provided more effectively by fortification input suppliers than governments and development partners. Finally, industry incentives could be directly cultivated through several emerging approaches: (1) broadening fortification to additional private sector players along the value chain and encouraging more partnerships between them (private–private partnerships); (2) leveling the playing field through automated collection of quality data, transparency that engenders industry self-regulation, and new business innovations to remove barriers to fortification; and (3) repositioning government as an enabler, beyond their regulatory function.

Strengthening Market Forces for Industry Engagement in Fortification

Private–Private Partnerships to Broaden Business Opportunities

There is a growing interest in *private–private* partnerships as a mechanism for driving sustainable development goals, particularly when other constructs, such as traditional public–private partnerships, are not as well suited for the particular development challenge [16]. This concept applies well to fragmented commodity markets and may be one key to leveraging competitive dynamics along the value chain to enhance the coverage of fortified foods.

Table 24.1 below depicts various business incentives that could be exploited through pri-

Table 24.1 Exploiting industry incentives to fortify through private–private partnerships

Current technical approach	Expanded industry-oriented approach	Incentive exploited
Focus on industrial mills, where fortification takes place	Broadening fortification opportunities to others in the value chain: Premix suppliers, wholesale buyers, and retailers	Other value chain players can claim higher quality products and/or fortification-related services as an integral part of their business propositions
Capacity-building of millers is largely supported by NGOs and their donors	Creative partnership structures to enable premix or other input suppliers to offer capacity-building services to millers	New service offering can enhance the input suppliers' value proposition to millers to help expand business
Access to fortified foods is limited to the production and distribution footprint of millers who fortify	Intentional expansion of fortified products into rural markets through retail partnerships	Urban retailers expand revenue opportunities to additional markets. Rural retailers increase foot traffic through enhanced quality of offerings to consumers

vate–private constructs. The key principle is to broaden active participation to other players, including upstream micronutrient and premix suppliers and downstream wholesalers and retailers. Partnerships anchored in concrete business opportunities which can pull fortification along as an added benefit have a strong opportunity for success. For instance, to enhance their competitive positioning, premix suppliers could offer capacity-building services to millers. In this emerging model, premix suppliers sign long-term contracts with their miller clients, which enables them to secure lower prices from their global micronutrient suppliers. They then leverage these savings to provide value-added services at no additional charge to millers. Beyond generating business value, these private–private partnerships may help transform the role of donors and development partners from capacity-builders of industry to catalyzers of within-industry partnerships, thereby increasing the chances of sustainability once development partners exit.

As another opportunity, private–private partnerships between urban and rural retailers with non-overlapping markets, hold strong potential, as they exploit the incentive of both partners to cultivate new markets. For example, in India, many of the cereal staple commodities that are fortified in industrialized facilities are sold in urban markets, and therefore do not reach rural populations. This is because most wheat and rice commodities sold through fair price shops in rural areas under the country's Public Distribution System tend to be those supplied by the peri-urban and rural millers, where it is more difficult to fortify. In 2015, the Government of Rajasthan introduced *Anapurna Bhandar* [17], an innovative program that brokered partnerships between urban and rural retailers to support the pull of branded and healthy products, including fortified foods, into rural markets [18]. In the state of Rajasthan, there are over 26,000 fair price shops, from where approximately 85% of the population obtain their basic staples. In the pilot phase, they turned 5000 of these otherwise dilapidated shops into modern retail stores. The scheme involved shipping goods from urban retailers to rural fair price shops, where products were sold on consignment, with rebates associated with each sale. This enabled urban retailers to add branded, vitamin A-fortified edible oil in their basket of goods at the same cost as unfortified oil. As a result, unfortified oil was eventually phased out, placing additional pressure on non-conforming producers to fortify [19–21]. This model worked because it was anchored in business fundamentals: urban retailers expanded into rural markets, rural retailers generated additional income from increased foot traffic, and rural consumers were provided a more aspirational shopping experience without the added cost or travel time to urban centers.

Leveling the Playing Field through Process Data, Transparency, and New Business Innovations

Industry's overriding concern is that weak government enforcement of mandatory standards may enable competitors to get away with low-quality or no fortification at all, since fortification is designed to confer no change in sensory attributes to the underlying staple food and is therefore difficult to detect without specialized tests. This places those who comply at a perceived disadvantage in highly competitive markets. Therefore, the importance of a level playing field, where all entities are held to the same quality standards (i.e., rules) and have access to the same fortification inputs (i.e., opportunities) cannot be overemphasized.

Table 24.2 depicts three broad approaches towards a level playing field. The first is a change in emphasis from *where* and by *whom* the quality data is captured. At present, government regulators are responsible for quality monitoring and focus primarily on *end-product* testing at production sites and/or through products sampled in markets. Both are costly and time consuming and therefore not frequently assessed. A paradigm-shift towards *process* data that can be captured through automated, digital systems within *industry settings* and transmitted directly to government may not only simplify government oversight and reduce budget pressures, but also ensure more immediate feedback to millers to control their internal quality.

Secondly, if fortification quality data were also made transparent to downstream buyers, millers may be further incentivized to fortify. Wholesale buyers, re-packagers, and retailers may select for products of higher fortification quality, creating a market pull for fortification and ultimately a self-regulating supply chain. Transparency would also support private–private partnerships around a quality advantage, as described in earlier. Finally, a level playing field requires that all players have equitable access to needed fortification inputs. Developing new business innovations can serve this need, particularly for SMEs, who are at a significant disadvantage compared to the larger players due to their lack of access to capital.

Table 24.2 Exploiting industry incentives to fortify by leveling the playing field

Current technical approach	Expanded industry-oriented approach	Incentive exploited
Focuses on end-product data (in production sites and markets)	Generate automated quality data within milling environments and transmit directly to government to enable effective oversight over all industry players	Real-time feedback and course corrections reduce the miller's cost of re-fortifying commodities to meet standards
Fortification quality data is known only to the industry partner and government regulator	Stronger self-regulation made possible by sharing quality data with downstream buyers	Millers incentivized to fortify to enhance their competitive positioning with downstream buyers
Inequitable access to fortification inputs across industry not explicitly addressed	New business innovations that enable local access to high-quality, affordable premix and dosifiers	Enables SMEs to more effectively compete with larger players. Unleashes the competitive dynamics for quality products in regional markets that did not have prior access to fortification inputs

The following sections describes each of these three levers in more detail and provides case studies of progress along these lines.

Leveling the Playing Field through Process Data Captured within Industry Settings

Evolution from manual records to "smart dosifiers or microfeeders": Fortified foods processors use "micro-feeders" or "dosifiers" for dosing the premix into their products such as flour. To date, most equipment does not automatically collect or store fortification data on premix volume used during food processing. Food producers rely on a "systems-based approach" [22] to compliance, which in part involves premix reconciliation calculations that are undertaken to provide an indication on whether the fortification *process* is adequately dosing the targeted levels of micronutrients to the volume of fortified food produced, in line with the country's fortification standards. Errors cannot be discounted as the system depends on production personnel manually recording information correctly. Smart dosifiers, which automatically collect and transmit this data to the internet, are not in widespread use in fortification programs, but have been effectively leveraged by some development partners in limited settings. For example, in Tanzania, Sanku have deployed smart dosifiers in 300 small-scale mills and are able to monitor their usage remotely through a *cellular link. Based on the information transmitted,* they can arrange visits to mills if the premix to food commodity ratio is off, dosifiers are not in use/require repairs, or premix supply needs re-stocking. A similar concept can be extended to larger, industrialized mills in urban areas, enabling data to be written to a centralized database, accessible to both the individual company and government regulator that could lead to timely corrective action. Given regulatory resource constraints in LMICs and the criticality of credible oversight to a level playing field, such an approach could be one of the linchpins to more effective fortification programs. The cost of upgrading dosifiers in larger mills with smart functions may vary by capacity, brand and type of milling equipment, and other factors. At present, a Sanku dosifier is approximately US$2500 [23].

Future opportunities also exist for real time, in-line monitoring through Process Analytical Technologies (PAT). For instance, various spectroscopic and computer image analysis technologies can now measure various parameters in foods, such as total ash, moisture, protein, starch, fiber, and particle size in flour. Based on real-time data, production operators can take corrective action to achieve the targeted quality, reducing production variation, and overall costs of production [24]. Building on current parameters analyzed, future R&D could advance solutions for in-process micronutrient analysis.

Leveling the Playing Field Through Transparency and Self-Policing

The concept of self-policing has been used effectively, albeit in limited settings, to drive an incentive to fortify. For example, to address low compliance with mandatory salt iodization legislation in Kyrgyzstan in 2002, the Swiss Agency for Development and Cooperation (SDC) supported a program to empower retailers with rapid test kits (RTKs) to test for iodine in the salt they purchased from wholesale markets. After 18 months, non-iodized salt was largely driven out and continued demand for iodized salt incentivized retailers to sustain the program [11]. As an added benefit, the increased demand for potassium iodate by salt producers catalyzed its local availability through a national premix model (see Decentralized Premix Facilities section below), further enabling access to iodized salt and creating a virtuous flywheel effect of self-perpetuation [25].

Food manufacturers could also create market pull by checking the fortification quality of their incoming raw material ingredients, such as salt, wheat, maize, and oil. Some nudging by third parties may be required to make such practices the norm. One such organization, Changing Markets Foundation (CMF) started their food fortification advocacy work in Mexico, which mandated wheat and maize fortification with iron, zinc, folic acid, and other B vitamins in 1999. CMF independently purchased 61 different wheat and maize flour brands from the market and tested them through accredited labs. Results showed only 7% of the wheat flour while none of the maize samples were adequately fortified. Another key finding was that food processors were using not using recommended iron compounds [26]. The work catalyzed government regulatory action. Such findings have the potential to also be shared with food manufacturers and food service businesses to encourage demand for fortified ingredients from their suppliers. In turn, this has the potential to shift focus away from the miller's compliance with fortification standards towards their incentive to comply with customer requirements.

Leveling the Playing Field Through New Business Innovations

A level playing field requires that all entities that are mandated to comply with fortification standards have access to the necessary fortification inputs. New business innovations can help address these critical gaps, particularly for the less industrialized, smaller millers, which respectively represent 70% of maize, 20% of wheat, and 46% of rice processors globally [27]. In line with WHO/FAO guidance, small mills are classified as those producing less than 20MT per day [28]. Often, these entities do not have access to the foreign exchange required to purchase premix and dosifiers from global suppliers, the working capital to cover import lead times (e.g., can be up to 6 weeks or more), nor the leverage to obtain volume pricing discounts on premix. Business incentives to fortify are also weak because none of the local competitors have access to fortification inputs. Developing new business-focused models can remove these barriers while also creating an incentive for SME engagement. The medium and larger mills (>20 MTs/day) also benefit from new business innovations by reducing the cost and complexity of fortification, supporting broader industry participation. Several new innovations are emerging to fill this niche, as described below.

Cost of goods economics: As also referenced in the section above, Sanku is a social enterprise serving the technology and business model needs of SME cereal producers, starting with maize millers in the Morogoro region of Tanzania. Maize consumed in the country is predominantly produced in small-scale mills, making it difficult to fortify [29]. Sanku examined the problem from a business lens. Specifically, they determined that maize flour bags were the most expensive input for the smaller millers, so they aggregated demand and negotiated a lower price point with the bag supplier. Millers are now able to purchase premix plus the bags for the same price they were previously paying for the bags alone. Sanku has also leveraged the bags for strong branding in bright pink lettering, signaling quality, catalyzing consumer demand, and incentivizing additional millers to engage in the program [30–32]. Since expansion drives economies in their model, this is yet another example of a flywheel effect that can further drive the market [25].

Decentralized premix facilities: Production of premixes is concentrated in a few countries in Asia (mainly India and China), EU, and North America. In Africa, the premix industry is still in infancy, so most countries import premix. For fortified food producers, premix is a recurring and significant cost driver for fortification. Various barriers exist with premix supply chains including quality premix, accessing suppliers and price volatility [33]. Other barriers include, currency volatility, foreign exchange shortages, long lead times, minimum order quantities (MOQs), and access to finance for upfront payments by SMEs [34].

Given these challenges, national availability of premix is critical for sustainable food fortification programs. Various models are in operation or have shown promise in increasing local availability and access to premix. These include: local revolving funds, consignment models, informal pooled mechanisms, commercial/sales agents, government exclusive supplies, and time-limited subsidized supply models.

As an example, in Kyrgyzstan, where salt iodization has been mandatory since 2001, a consignment model for centralized Potassium Iodate (KIO_3) procurement was established by the Kyrgyz Association of Salt Producers (KASP) in 2010. A key barrier to salt producers was consistent availability of KIO_3 but also appropriate packaging configurations for SMEs (i.e., 1 kg, 5 kg). As shown in Fig. 24.2, in partnership with the GAIN Premix facility, KASP aggregates demand and imports KIO_3 for distribution to its members.

Key benefits realized by KASP members include bulk volume discounts, just-in-time local supplies, price stability, access to credit, and procurement in local currency.

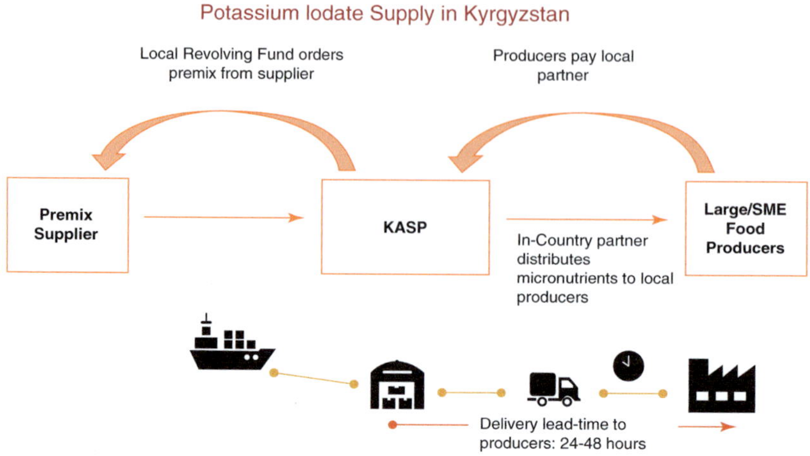

Fig. 24.2 Local premix model in Kyrgyzstan

Government as an Enabler of Fortification Programs

Trust between the regulator and private sector is essential for program scale up and compliance. Regulatory authorities are empowered to apply penalties as outlined in law, and where necessary, they should be leveraged to improve industry compliance. However, leadership at the political, policy and program levels must recognize both the power of a stick and carrot. Beyond the regulatory measures, government has a crucial role as an *enabler* of fortification as a private sector-driven public health intervention.

Table 24.3 describes three broad mechanisms through which the government's design of fortification programs and the nature of their involvement can play a strong role in industry's incentive to engage. Most compliance programs rely on scarce human resources and small budgets. In a future scenario, if industry process data could be collected through smart dosifiers, handheld devices, or other IoT [35] mechanisms, they would be in better control of their quality data. Government could then shift their role to more of an evaluator rather than collector of data. With less government need for periodic market checks of fortification quality, industry then reduces their risk of a potential discrepancy and improves

Table 24.3 Exploiting industry incentives to fortify by transforming government into an enabler

Current technical Approach	Expanded industry-oriented approach	Incentive exploited
Reliance on scarce human resource capacity and small government budgets to enforce compliance	Millers are in control of their quality data; government positioned as more of an evaluator than a collector of data	Reduces industry's risk of a discrepancy with independent assessments of fortification quality by government or third parties
Fortification advanced as a stand-alone program	Fortification embedded into food quality and safety agenda to strengthen program	Millers incentivized to invest in equipment, raw materials, and processes if fortification is more strongly tied to industry priorities
Compliance with mandatory legislation as the primary means for government to engage industry	Shifting government focus to supporting communications campaigns and engaging more proactively with industry	Value-added services from government can lower investment risk for millers and increase potential for compliance with standards, even if only voluntary

their defense if there is one. Additionally, recognizing that producers and consumers alike value quality over fortification per se, government could better integrate fortification into the food quality and safety agenda, so that quality is defined by both safety and nutrition. In turn, this could incentivize manufacturers to invest in inputs (e.g., premix, dosing, and analysis equipment). Finally, at present, compliance tends to be the center of government and industry interaction. Shifting the focus to supportive government policies, such as communications campaigns (which may elicit a stronger response from industry players along the value chain than consumers per se), and proactive technical assistance, can position government as a value-added supporter of industry. This may further lower their investment risk and increase compliance.

The Food Safety and Standards Office of India (FSSAI), the government's nodal agency for food fortification, is a good example of government that has embraced the enabler role. The FSSAI established the Food Fortification Resource Centre (FFRC) [36] as a multisector platform for scaling-up food fortification. Positioning themselves as a value-added service to industry, FFRC publishes a reference list of premix suppliers and provides a variety of technical resources, such as training modules, analytical methods, and capacity-building services to industry. They also launched the Eat Right India movement, which reinforces the importance of fortification within the context of a healthy diet. In short, FSSAI plays a dual role; as an enabler and regulator for fortification.

Conclusion

Iron deficiency is one of the most pervasive nutritional challenges in the developing world. To date, despite the proven evidence [37], food fortification programs have not made a significant contribution to ameliorating the condition globally, particularly for rural populations whose access to iron-rich foods is most limited. The traditional components of fortification programs, including legislative mandates, technical capacity-building of industry, and periodic regulatory oversight, are unlikely to yield better results without due attention to industry's incentive to engage. By cultivating the right incentives and structures, we have the potential to leverage the competitive dynamics of the industry to propel us towards better functioning programs.

This approach would leverage more players along the value chain for fortified foods, as well as an expanded set of millers/processors that serve more regional markets. Private–private partnerships and new business innovations may help industry to leverage fortification as an added dimension of quality. In doing so, it could encourage competitors to engage and ultimately broaden responsibility for fortification to an expanded set of parties.

Fundamental shifts are also required for the monitoring of fortification programs. Placing the onus on industry for automatic collection of quality data through internet-connected devices will strengthen the credibility of regulatory monitoring, give industry an opportunity to leverage the data for comparative advantage and may ultimately lead to self-policing along the value chain if the data were made transparent by industry themselves or through third parties. Finally, a stronger government commitment to fortification would reduce investment risk for industry and increase their engagement. In combination with a movement towards the automatic collection of quality data through industry, government could more easily focus on their enabler role.

Fortification programs have been conceived as a seemingly simple intervention—adding inexpensive micronutrients to foods that the population is already regularly consuming to improve micronutrient status and reduce the downstream sequela associated with these deficiencies. However, their implementation is anything but simple, and the proposed constructs are no exception. But they do lay forth a vision to better leverage industry incentives to drive coverage and compliance, and in doing so, create a virtuous cycle that will ultimately better serve the most vulnerable populations whom fortification programs were designed to most benefit. The development community can play a strong role in catalyzing this vision.

References

1. Global Fortification Data Exchange. Number of food vehicles with standards. https://fortificationdata.org/map-number-of-food-vehicles. Accessed 21 May 2020.
2. Wirth JP, Laillou A, Rohner F, Northrop-Clewes CA, Macdonald B, Moench-Pfanner R. Lessons learned from national food fortification projects: experiences from Morocco, Uzbekistan, and Vietnam. Food Nutr Bull. 2012;33(4:3):S281–92. https://doi.org/10.1177/15648265120334S304.
3. Gera T, Sachdev HS, Boy E. Effect of iron-fortified foods on hematologic and biological outcomes: systematic review of randomized controlled trials. Am J Clin Nutrit. 2012;96(2):309–24. https://doi.org/10.3945/ajcn.111.031500.
4. Neufeld LM, Baker B, Garrett GS, Haddad L. Coverage and utilization in food fortification programs: critical and neglected areas of evaluation. J Nutr. 2017;147(5):1015S–9S. https://doi.org/10.3945/jn.116.246157.
5. Mkambula P, Mbuya MNN, Rowe LA, Sablah M, Friesen VM, Chadha M, et al. The unfinished agenda for food fortification in low- and middle-income countries: quantifying progress, gaps and potential opportunities. Nutrients. 2020;12(2):354. https://doi.org/10.3390/nu12020354.
6. Osendarp SJM, Martinez H, Garrett GS, Neufeld LM, De-Regil LM, Vossenaar M, Darnton-Hill I. Large-scale food fortification and biofortification in low- and middle-income countries: a review of programs, trends, challenges, and evidence gaps. Food Nutr Bull. 2018;39(2):315–31. https://doi.org/10.1177/0379572118774229.
7. Luthringer CL, Rowe LA, Vossenaar M, Garrett GS. Regulatory monitoring of fortified foods: identifying barriers and good practices. Global Health Sci Pract. 2015;3:446–61.
8. Global Alliance for Improved Nutrition. Study on the cost of the fortification cost of wheat flour (Atta) and edible oil in Pakistan, USAID/GAIN Pakistan Regional Food Fortification Project. 2017. https://www.gainhealth.org/sites/default/files/publications/documents/gain-usaid-study-on-the-fortification-costing-of-wheat-flour-and-edible-oil-pakistan-2017.pdf
9. Muthayya S, Hall J, Bagriansky J, Sugimoto J, Gundry D, Mattias D, et al. Rice fortification: an emerging opportunity to contribute to the elimination of vitamin and mineral deficiency worldwide. Food Nutr Bull. 2012;33(4):296–307.
10. Laviolette L. Financing and sustainability of food fortification programs. In: Mannar MGV, Hurrell R, editors. Food Fortification in a globalized world. San Diego, CA: Academic Press; 2018. p. p93–5. https://doi.org/10.1016/B978-0-12-802861-2.00009-2.
11. Schüth T, Jamangulova T, Janikeeva S, Tologonov T. Power from below: enabling communities to ensure the provision of iodated salt in Kyrgyzstan. Food Nutr Bull. 2005;26(4):366–75. https://doi.org/10.1177/156482650502600406.
12. Mannar MGV. Salt. In: MGV M, Hurrell R, editors. Food fortification in a globalized world. San Diego, CA: Academic Press; 2018. p. 143–51.
13. Chavasit V, Photi J. Sauces and condiments. In: Mannar MGV, Hurrell R, editors. Food fortification in a globalized world. San Diego, CA: Academic Press; 2018. p. 153–7.
14. Goh CC. Combating iodine deficiency: lessons from China, Indonesia, and Madagascar. Food Nutr Bull. 2002;23:280–91.
15. Milani P, Spohrer R, Garrett G, Kreis K. Piloting a commercial model for fortified rice in Brazil. Food Nutr Bull. 2016;37(3):290–302.
16. Moser H, Lowes S. Catalyzing private-private partnerships for social impact. Centre for Strategic and International Studies. 2017. https://csis-website-prod.s3.amazonaws.com/s3fs-public/publication/170501_Moser_CatalyzingPrivatePrivatePartnerships_Web.pdf
17. Anapurna "Giver of food and nourishment in Sanskrit". https://en.wikipedia.org/wiki/Annapurna_(goddess). Accessed 1 June 2021.
18. Raje Launces Anapurna Bhandar Yojna. Times of India. 2015 Nov 01. https://timesofindia.indiatimes.com/city/jaipur/Raje-launches-Annapurna-Bhandar-Yojna/articleshow/49614023.cms,
19. Agarwa S. Principal secretary. Food & Civil Supplies Department, Government of Rajasthan; 2016.
20. GAIN, unpublished case study: Annapurna Bhandar Yojna: An initiative to revamp the Public Distribution System in Rajasthan, June 2019.
21. GAIN. Unpublished case study: Annapurna Bhandar Yojna: an initiative to modernize the public distribution system in Rajasthan; 2019.
22. Global Alliance for Improved Nutrition (GAIN) & Project Healthy Children (PHC). Regulatory monitoring of national food fortification programs: a policy guidance document. Global Fortification Technical Advisory Group (GF-TAG). 2018. https://www.gainhealth.org/sites/default/files/publications/documents/regulatory-monitoring-policy-guidance-doc-2018.pdf
23. Personnel communications with Felix brooks-church. CEO Sanku; 2019.
24. Hitzman B, Hauselmann R, Niemoeller A, Sangi D, Traenkle J, Glassey J. Process analytical technologies in food industry – challenges and benefits: a status report and recommendations. Biotechnol J. 2015;10:1095–100.

25. Collins J. How does your flywheel turn? A Good to Great Strategic Tool; 2017. https://www.jimcollins.com/article_topics/articles/the-flywheel-effect.html
26. Changing Markets Foundation. The grain of truth: industry compliance on flour fortification in Mexico. 2019. https://changingmarkets.org/wp-content/uploads/2019/02/The-Grain-of-Truth-English-web-double-page.pdf
27. Food Fortification Initiative. Annual report. 2019. https://static1.squarespace.com/static/5e1df234eef02705f5446453/t/5f32fd64070da6660ca46563/1597177212373/FFI_2019AnnualReport_Spreads_2s_FINAL.pdf
28. WHO, FAO. Guidelines on food fortification with micronutrients. World Health Organization; 2006.
29. FAO. The Maize Value Chain in Tanzania; 2015.
30. https://www.thelifeyoucansave.org/best-charities/project-healthy-children/
31. https://www.givewell.org/charities/project-healthy-children
32. Personal communication with Felix Brooks-church. CEO Sanku; 2019.
33. Guinot P, Jallier V, Blasi A, Guyondet C, Van Ameringen M. GAIN premix facility: an innovative approach for improving access to quality vitamin and mineral premix in fortification initiatives. Food Nutr Bull. 2012;33(4):s381–9. https://journals.sagepub.com/doi/pdf/10.1177/15648265120334S314
34. Garrett GS, Luthringer CL, Mkambula P. Improving nutritious food systems by establishing national micronutrient premix supply systems. Sight Life. 2016;30(1):62–8. https://sightandlife.org/wp-content/uploads/2016/02/SAL_Mag-Food-Systems_2016_Improving-Nutritious-Food-Systems-by-Establishing-National-Micronutrient-Premix-Supply-Systems.pdf
35. Internet of Things. https://en.wikipedia.org/wiki/Internet_of_things. Accessed 1 June 2021.
36. Food Safety and Standards Authority of India. https://ffrc.fssai.gov.in/. Accessed 1 June 2021.
37. Keats EC, Neufield LM, Garrett GS, Mbuya MNN, Bhutta ZA. Improved micronutrient status and health outcomes in low- and middle-income countries following large-scale fortification: evidence from a systematic review and meta-analysis. Am J Clin Nutr. 2019;109(6):1696–708. https://doi.org/10.1093/ajcn/nqz023.

25 Food-Based Approaches for Combating Iron Deficiency

Kristina D. Michaux, Jennifer K. Foley, and Erick Boy

Keywords

Iron deficiency · Anemia · Nutrition-specific Fortification · Home fortification Micronutrient powders · Small-quantity lipid-based nutrient supplements · Nutrition-sensitive agriculture · Biofortification Homestead food production

Introduction

Iron deficiency (ID) is the most widespread nutrient deficiency and the main cause of anemia globally [1]. It affects population groups across low- and high-income countries and is linked to the growing problem of income inequity and the transition to monotonous diets, dominated by highly processed micronutrient-poor foods. Infants, young children, adolescent girls, and pregnant women are the predominant high-risk population groups because of their high dietary iron needs required for rapid growth and development, and losses during menstruation [2].

There are a myriad of nutrition interventions that are designed to prevent and treat ID and ID anemia (IDA). Nutrition-specific interventions target the immediate causes of ID, such as poor diet, while nutrition-sensitive programs target the underlying causes, such as poverty, infection, and disease. Nutrition-specific intervention programs include supplementation, industrial fortification, and home fortification [3]. Nutrition-sensitive strategies address multi-faceted issues to support nutritional health, including infectious disease control, livelihoods and social safety net programs, early childhood development and education programs, and agricultural interventions, such as biofortification and Hellen Keller's enhanced Homestead Food Production (HFP) program [4].

This chapter will discuss the efficacy—the impact under ideal and controlled conditions—of the most widely implemented food-based strategies that improve the availability, access to, and consumption of vitamin- and mineral-rich foods, including iron, as a means to combat ID in vulnerable population groups. Observational studies are also reviewed when no controlled studies are available and effectiveness studies—the impact under "real world" settings—are referenced in the instances they have been completed. Specific indicators of iron status are described in studies where they have been measured, otherwise, anemia status or hemoglobin

K. D. Michaux
HarvestPlus, International Food Policy Research Institute (IFPRI), Washington, DC, USA

Faculty of Pharmaceutical Sciences, University of British Columbia, Vancouver, BC, Canada
e-mail: kristina.michaux@ubc.ca

J. K. Foley · E. Boy (✉)
HarvestPlus, International Food Policy Research Institute (IFPRI), Washington, DC, USA
e-mail: J.Foley@cgiar.org; e.boy@cgiar.org

C. D. Karakochuk et al. (eds.), *Nutritional Anemia*, Nutrition and Health,
https://doi.org/10.1007/978-3-031-14521-6_25

(Hb) concentration are reported, though the fundamental limitations of using them as a proxy for ID are acknowledged.

Review of Evidence

Food Fortification

Introduction

Food fortification is a nutrition-specific strategy designed to prevent micronutrient deficiencies by increasing the micronutrient content of staple foods and/or condiments during processing. Food fortification with one or more micronutrients has been successfully implemented globally and is recognized as having wider reach and greater return on investment than some other nutrition interventions, such as supplementation [5].

According to its intended reach, food fortification is classified as "mass" (or "universal") for the general population, "targeted" for specific at-risk groups, and "market-driven" for specific consumer groups [6]. This chapter addresses mass fortification of staple foods and condiments with iron, alone or in combination with other micronutrients.

A minimum daily dose of elemental iron needs to be delivered by a fortified food to achieve population level nutritional impact. It was supposed that an additional intake of at least 60% of the estimated average requirement (EAR) of iron from a fortified food was needed to improve iron stores, and at least 90% EAR to decrease nutritional anemia [7]. Data from multiple efficacy studies encompassing a variety of fortificants was consequently used to establish the minimal incremental iron dose from fortified wheat flour required to improve women's iron status: 7.1 mg iron as ferrous sulfate or fumarate, 4.6 mg as NaFeEDTA, or 10.0 mg as electrolytic iron [8]. At the highest indiscernible fortification levels, intakes below 75 g of flour a day were deemed unlikely to demonstrate impact [9].

A lack of data on the prevalence and principal cause(s) of ID, non-normal distribution of population iron requirements, unacceptable organoleptic changes to foods, and inherently poor iron bioavailability of some fortificants [10] make fortification with iron more challenging than with other nutrients (e.g., salt with iodine or wheat flour with folic acid) [11].

Efficacy of Mass Iron Fortification

A systematic review of 60 randomized controlled trials (RCTs) with fortified staples and condiments in predominantly low- and middle-income countries (LMIC) demonstrated unambiguously that iron-fortification reduced the risk of ID by 52% and increased mean serum ferritin (SF) concentration by an average of 1.36 μg/L [12].

Yet, later systematic reviews of fortified cereal flour efficacy trials, with different fortificants and extraction grades, concluded that there is no certainty that maize flour (fortified with iron in combination with other micronutrients) or wheat flour (fortified with iron-alone or in combination with other micronutrients) can reduce ID in the general population over 2 years of age [13, 14]. For wheat flour, the latest meta-analysis found fortification with iron, either alone or with other micronutrients, had little or no effect on average risk of ID relative to the flour without iron (iron-alone: RR 0.43, 95% CI 0.17–1.07; and iron + micronutrients vs. micronutrients without iron: RR 0.42, 95% CI 0.18–0.97).

Condiments are appealing vehicles for dietary iron: consumed extensively and regularly in various target populations, they can be added to multiple foods or combined with fortified staple foods. Iron-fortified dry and wet seasonings (e.g., table salt [15–17], sugar [18], curry powder [19], and soy sauce [20]) have been shown to signifcanlty improve SF and reduce ID, particularly in populations with marginally deficient baseline iron status [21]. Nonetheless, favorable consumption characteristics mean condiments are prone to overconsumption and therefore carry the risk of excessively increasing iron intake—a concern not thoroughly assessed [11].

Effectiveness of Mass Iron Fortification Programs

Low levels of ID in industrialized nations have been attributed to fortified foods and improved overall life conditions; however, program effectiveness data are scarce, especially for children of relevant ages.

A systematic review of 13 national cereal flour fortification programs (all designed and evaluated prior to the 2006 World Health Organization (WHO) fortification guidelines) assessed iron status and/or anemia indicators among women of reproductive age (WRA) and children 2–15 years old [22]. Impact on children's iron status was limited, and only occurred in children above 5 years of age. In women, all relevant studies showed significant improvement in SF and/or ID prevalence.

Although the data suggest that more consistent, positive benefits of fortified cereals are realized mainly in women, a national anemia control program in Costa Rica demonstrated significant improvements in children's iron status is achievable when multiple program elements are considered, including a plausible impact pathway, political will, rigorous monitoring and evaluation, and multiple appropriate fortification vehicles. By 2008–9, the prevalence of IDA in Costa Rican children 1–7 years old was undetectable, down from 6.5% in 1996 [23]; ID was also reduced from 26.9% to 6.8% in this period. These improvements were attributed to fortified wheat flour and milk, which contributed equally to the delivery of 3.3 mg (median) elemental iron daily.

An effectiveness study of soy sauce fortified with iron (in the form of NaFeEDTA) in nine Chinese villages (n = 14,000 aged 3 years and older) showed that after 12 months, participants who consumed foods with iron-rich soy sauce experienced significantly higher and sustained SF concentration relative to baseline levels; however, only children aged 7–18 years and adult males aged 19–54 years had significantly higher SF concentration compared to controls (mean difference among male groups: +1.87–6.79 μg/L; mean difference among female groups: +0.39 μg/L) [20]. However, caution should be applied when generalizing these findings as it is challenging to estimate coverage of this type of predominantly market-driven condiment; there are no published estimates of their total global reach, with the notable exception of iodine-fortified salt, which is mandatory in most LMIC [24].

Summary

Mass fortification with iron can maintain adequate iron status and prevent or decrease ID in children 5 years of age or older and non-pregnant, non-lactating WRA. When ID is the major cause of anemia, iron-fortified foods can also prevent IDA or decrease anemia prevalence. For consistent and sustained impact, iron fortification interventions and programs should be designed, implemented, monitored, and evaluated according to international guidelines [10] and combined with nutrition-sensitive agricultural interventions and sanitation and hygiene measures.

Home Fortification

Introduction

Home fortification is a direct food-based strategy primarily used to improve child nutrition. Otherwise called "at-home fortification" or "point-of-use-fortification," it describes two main products that increase the nutrient density of foods and aim to prevent and treat nutritional anemia: micronutrient powders (MNP) and small quantity lipid-based nutrient supplements (SQ-LNS) [25, 26].

Micronutrient Powders

MNP are single-serving packages containing a powdered blend of micronutrients in a dose specific to the needs of the target population.

Conceived in 1996 as an alternative to traditional iron supplementation for infants and young children (6–23 months old) in LMIC [27], MNP are sprinkled on and stirred into semi-solid foods immediately before consumption at home, or in an institutional setting (e.g., school).

In 2018, 54 countries were reportedly implementing MNP interventions, reaching an estimated 11 million children under 5 years of age; more than half of these programs were national or subnational [28].

Efficacy of MNP in Infants and Young Children

MNP have been extensively tested across population groups, settings, and contexts [29–32]. Initial studies used MNP formulations with 1–5 micronutrients (with at least iron) because of the known impact on nutritional anemia [33]. Subsequent formulations were expanded to address coexisting micronutrient deficiencies and dietary intake gaps. Most programs now use a mix of 15 micronutrients, including 2.5–30 mg of elemental iron [34].

Consistent with findings from a prior systematic review and meta-analysis [25], a systematic review of the efficacy of MNP in children 6–23 months old found that MNP reduced the risk of ID by 53% and anemia by 18% compared with placebo or no intervention [31]. MNP were also shown to significantly increase mean SF concentration by an average of 12.93 μg/L and mean Hb concentration by an average of 2.74 g/L [31]. When compared to iron supplementation interventions, there were no significant differences in the risk of anemia or mean Hb concentration between the MNP and iron supplementation groups; however, these results are based on only two RCTs and thus should be interpreted with caution.

Efficacy of MNP in Preschool and School-Aged Children

A 2017 systematic review of the effect of MNP on the nutritional status and health of preschool and school-aged children (2–12 years old) was conducted; however, the randomized controlled studies included varied greatly in the age of participants, study duration, and MNP formulation used (i.e., number of micronutrients included, and amount and type of iron provided). Nevertheless, the review found that MNP were associated with a lower risk of ID (65%) and anemia (34%), and higher average mean Hb concentration (3.37 g/L) compared to no intervention or placebo [32]. No significant effect was observed for mean SF concentration.

Efficacy of MNP in Pregnant and Lactating Women

The success of MNP interventions with infants and young children encouraged their use in broader populations, including pregnant women who have increased needs for iron for fetal growth and development. A systematic review compared the effects of MNP to the current antenatal standard of care (i.e., daily or intermittent supplementation with iron and folic acid (IFA) tablets containing 30-60 mg of elemental iron and 0.4 mg of folic acid) and to multiple micronutrient supplementation (MMS) [30]. When compared to IFA supplementation, MNP were associated with a higher rate of moderate anemia (Hb concentration 70–99 g/L) and lower Hb concentration at 32 weeks' gestation; no significant differences were observed for mild anemia (Hb concentration 100–109 g/L) or anemia of any severity. When compared to MMS with the same composition, no difference in the prevalence of anemia was observed between the MNP and MMS groups at 34 weeks' gestation. Neither study reported on specific measures of iron status.

A subsequent cluster RCT that evaluated whether MNP or MMS could be used instead of fortified foods (*Nutrivida* for women and *Nutrisano* for children) to prevent anemia in Mexican pregnant and lactating women and young children found all three interventions reduced baseline anemia prevalence and increased Hb concentration; no significant group differences were observed for women at 37 weeks' gestation, 1- or 3-months post-partum, or for children after 10 months of supplementation [35]. While MNP and MMS were preferred over fortified food by women, MNP were not as well liked as MMS due to difficulty with their preparation and unfavorable taste changes to some of the food in which they were mixed [36].

Small-Quantity Lipid-Based Nutrient Supplements

Lipid-based nutrient supplements (LNS) are pastes that provide energy (mainly as fat), protein, and essential micronutrients. LNS can either be added to food before consumption, or consumed directly by target population groups (e.g., infants, young children, and pregnant and lactating women) [26]. LNS, otherwise called ready-to-use supplementary foods, were initially used to treat severe acute malnutrition and were designed to provide ~200 kcal/kg/day of energy. In 2001, SQ-LNS were developed as a home fortification strategy [37] and thus are reviewed here. SQ-LNS are small, single serving sachets (< 20 g) that provide 110–120 kcal/day together with essential micronutrients [26].

There are two main SQ-LNS formulations: one for pregnant and lactating women that provides close to the United Nations International Multiple Micronutrient Antenatal Preparation (UNIMMAP) formulation, including 20 mg of iron/day [38]; and one for infants and young children (aged 6–23 months) that provides at least 15 essential micronutrients, including 5.8 mg of iron [39]. The formulations used for each group, however, can vary.

Efficacy of SQ-LNS

A systematic review of the effect of LNS with complementary foods on the nutritional status and health of children less than 2 years of age found a 21% lower risk of anemia and a 5.78 g/L average improvement in mean Hb concentration compared to no intervention or placebo [40]. Two subsequent studies examined the impact of SQ-LNS and nutrition education on ID and anemia in infants and young children. In the Democratic Republic of Congo, SQ-LNS and a maternal nutrition education program were associated with a 11% lower adjusted anemia and a smaller decline in mean Hb concentration (2.6 g/L) in 6- to 12-month-old infants compared to the standard of care with no SQ-LNS [41]. In Madagascar, SQ-LNS given to infants (aged 6–18 months) were associated with a 40% lower risk of anemia and 25% lower risk of IDA compared to children who received no SQ-LNS [42].

A recent systematic review examined the effect of SQ-LNS during pregnancy on maternal nutritional status and found SQ-LNS were associated with an increase in anemia prevalence at or near term compared to IFA supplementation or MMS (SQ-LNS vs. IFA: RR 2.35; 95% CI 1.67–3.30; SQ-LNS vs. MMS: RR 1.40; 95% CI 1.07–1.82) [43].

Summary

The evidence suggests that home fortification with MNP is an efficacious strategy to control ID and IDA in infants and young children. MNP are recommended by the WHO for children 6 months to 12 years of age where anemia prevalence is greater than 20% [44, 45]. To promote and sustain impact, implementers must remain mindful of the cultural, practical, and logistical challenges of MNP programs, including maternal and child acceptability and compliance, possible color and smell changes in food, supply and quality management, and training of already overburdened healthcare workers. While there are less available data on the efficacy of SQ-LNS for preventing IDA in infants and young children, findings are promising. For pregnant women, however, current evidence does not support the use of either MNP or SQ-LNS to control or prevent ID or anemia and should not be recommended as an alternative to more effective IFA and MMS programs.

Nutrition-Sensitive Agricultural Interventions

Introduction

Improving micronutrient status by increasing the production, consumption, and diversity of nutrient-rich foods is a long-term strategy to combat micronutrient deficiencies. It is thought to be more sustainable, accessible, and culturally appropriate than more direct strategies, such as supplementation or home fortification. Numerous studies and reviews have examined the nutritional and health impacts of plant- and animal-based agricultural interventions, with generally inconsistent results. Data on the impact on iron status are limited, except in the instance of biofortification, where the evidence base for impact on ID is building [46–49]. The most common agricultural-nutrition strategies to combat ID and IDA are reviewed here.

Biofortification

Biofortification uses conventional and transgenic breeding methods, as well as agronomic approaches to increase the density of micronutrients, including iron, in staple food crops. These methods have been shown to be an effective way to use plant-based foods to deliver more iron to malnourished populations [50].

To date, progress on iron biofortification has been achieved largely through conventional breeding of high-iron pearl millet and beans [51–53], but iron biofortification is also applicable to other cereals including rice [54] and wheat, and pulses like peas and lentils [55].

The breeding targets for iron in biofortified crops are intentionally modest. They are not designed to deliver doses at the levels provided by supplementation or fortification. Instead biofortified crops aim to provide an additional 30% of the EAR for iron for non-pregnant, non-lactating WRA and young children (1–6 years)[1] when consumed as a main part of the diet [56]. One of the advantages of biofortification is its cost-effectiveness: after an initial investment in plant breeding and the mainstreaming of the micronutrient trait(s) into national and international agricultural programs, recurrent investment is minimal [56, 57].

Efficacy of Biofortification in Children, Adolescents, and Women

Four randomized controlled studies have demonstrated the efficacy of three iron-biofortified crops on improving iron status and associated functional outcomes: iron beans in Mexico; iron pearl millet in India; iron beans in Rwanda; and iron rice in the Philippines.

In Mexico, school-aged children (5–12 years old, of whom, 18% were anemic [Hb < 115 g/L for <12 years old and Hb < 120 g/L for ≥12 years old] and 16% were iron deficient [SF <15.0 μg/L, adjusted for inflammation]) were fed iron-biofortified or control beans (95 mg Fe/kg vs. 55 mg Fe/kg control) for 6 months. The iron beans did not significantly improve iron status compared to control beans; all children experienced improvements in Hb, SF, sTfR, and total body iron (TBI) at endline [52]. However, because of unanticipated reductions in feeding days (i.e., the medium number of days children were fed was 68 of the planned 120) the *a priori* assumptions for adequate power to test significant intervention effects were not met. Nonetheless, improvements by both groups indicate the potential for benefits of a food-based intervention in this population.

In India, adolescent children (12–16 years old, of whom, 41% were iron deficient [SF <15.0 μg/L], 28% were anemic [Hb < 120 g/L], and 21% had negative TBI at baseline) experienced a significant improvement in SF and TBI after consuming flat bread made with iron-pearl millet (86.3 mg Fe/kg vs. 21.8–52.1 mg Fe/kg control) daily for 4 months. By 6 months, children who were ID at baseline and who ate biofortified foods were 64% more likely to have their ID resolved compared to the control group [51],

[1]Assuming 7% bioavailability and after accounting for processing losses and other inhibitory effects

and they experienced cognitive improvements in memory and attention [58].

In Rwanda, women (aged 18–27 years) who were iron depleted (SF <20.0 μg/L at baseline) experienced a significant increase in Hb, SF, and TBI after consuming iron-biofortified beans (86.1 mg Fe/kg vs. 50 mg Fe/kg control) daily for 4.5 months (here, most anemia within the subjects was due to ID) [53]. In addition, women experienced improvements to their brain activity [59], memory and attention [60], and physical work efficiency [61].

In the Philippines, non-anemic religious sisters (aged 18–45 years) experienced a modest increase in SF and TBI after consuming iron-biofortified rice (3.21 mg Fe/kg vs. 0.57 mg Fe/kg control) daily for 9 months [54]. While the intervention resulted in a small increase in dietary iron, there was a significant positive dose response and women with the lowest baseline iron status benefitted the most from the intervention.

Three of the iron biofortification efficacy studies were analyzed in two meta-analyses (excluding Mexico, which was not published before the review) [47, 62]. Both meta-analyses concluded that daily consumption of iron-biofortified crops significantly improved SF and TBI as continuous outcome variables, with a greater effect size observed in participants with poor baseline iron status. The more recent meta-analysis, based on the same pooled data, showed the SF and TBI improvements did not generate significant changes in iron status when the outcome was defined as a categorical variable, prevalence of ID or anemia. This finding was attributed to an effect size too small to shift the population distribution sufficiently, which could be addressed by a larger sample size and/or longer duration feeding trial.

Other Agricultural Interventions to Combat Iron Deficiency

The impact of 36 household agricultural programs, including small animal husbandry, dairy production, and promotion of home gardens, in LMIC on the nutritional status of women and children was systematically reviewed in 2012 [46]. Only three studies reported on anemia, all of which were impact evaluations of Helen Keller's HFP program. This program combines technical assistance and inputs for year-round home gardening together with small animal husbandry and/or fish farming, nutrition education, and women's empowerment training [63]. Two studies observed a significant reduction in anemia prevalence among women and children. The quality of evidence on anemia reduction, however, was poor: the studies had dissimilar interventions and comparison groups at baseline, the rates of decline in anemia prevalence between treatment groups was not reported, and there was no control for confounding in the analyses.

A subsequent review examined 16 impact evaluations of nutrition-sensitive agricultural interventions on women's and children's health [48]. Of these studies, two HFP programs (one in Burkina Faso and the other in Nepal), and a dairy value chain program that was used to distribute fortified yoghurt to pastoralists in Senegal, generated a significant and positive impact on infant and child (aged 6–59 months) anemia status and Hb concentration; the HFP programs in Nepal also showed a significant reduction on maternal anemia. Despite implementation in different settings and with different project components, the plausibility of the studies' findings are supported by significant improvements in outcomes along the impact pathway from agriculture to improved nutrition. These include increased access to and production of nutrient-rich foods, improvements in some infant and young child feeding practices, and improved dietary diversity.

A systematic review of the relationship between animal agricultural and anemia among women and children in LMIC examined the benefits, in terms of increased consumption of micronutrient-rich animal source foods, and potential harm of animal agriculture by increased exposure to pathogens [49]. Of 23 included studies, nine were intervention evaluations, of which three examined the impact of small-scale fish farming and six evaluated HFP in different settings; the impact on anemia in both women and children was either small or not significant. In the 14 observational studies (which examined the relationship between animal agriculture and anemia or infection), the authors found no consistent relationship between participation in animal agriculture and anemia or iron status, nor increased risk of infection.

Summary

Whether agricultural interventions that increase production and consumption of animal- and plant-based foods can combat ID remains an open discussion, biofortification aside. Biofortification studies to date demonstrate that eating iron-biofortified foods—without changing other aspects of the diet—can combat ID. The impact of biofortification will rely on multiple factors, including adoption by farmers and consumer acceptance. Thus far, the data on prolonged adoption [64], alongside high consumer favorability across continents, superior yield, and no visible trait differences from conventional varieties, suggest that iron biofortified crops are sustainably and successfully being scaled-up for long-term impact [65, 66].

As for the impact of other agricultural interventions on ID, it is challenging to differentiate between the effects of the agricultural components and other project components (such as behavior change communication). It is not known if an increase in production and consumption of micronutrient-rich foods from these interventions leads to increased micronutrient intake and a change in biochemical status. For example, an HFP evaluation in Cambodia observed higher iron intakes, lower prevalence of iron inadequacy [67], and a significant reduction in anemia prevalence among women in intervention groups compared to control [68]. However, because IDA in this population is low (1.5–14%) [69, 70], it is unclear if increased iron intake drove the reduction in anemia or if it was due to other factors.

Ultimately, there is a need for more well-designed controlled trials of integrated agricultural programs that include specific outcome indicators of iron status, rather than only Hb, and that objectively measure which project components (or combination of components) lead to improvements in these indicators.

Program Considerations for Controlling ID

The evidence on food-based approaches to reduce ID leads to a lingering question: why do efficacy trial results not translate consistently into programmatic effectiveness?

A pervasive weakness in published research is the incorrect assumption that anemia is synonymous with ID; using Hb and anemia prevalence as the basis for iron interventions is not good science. Iron deficiency, even in the absence of anemia, is known to impair brain development and learning capacity, and inhibit physical performance, among other negative functional effects [60, 62]. The fraction of anemia attributable to ID varies by geography, ethnicity, culture, life stage, and socioeconomic status, among other determinants of insufficient intake of bioavailable dietary iron. Iron deficiency is the cause of <50% of anemia cases in countries where anemia prevalence is >40% [1], and the contribution of sickle cell disease [71] and other chronic diseases [72]—of which many do not respond to iron interventions—in the etiology of anemia is higher than previously thought [73]. It is therefore necessary when planning, designing, and monitoring ID control programs to ascertain the baseline prevalence of ID and monitor the impact of interventions in a timely manner. Measuring iron-specific biomarkers and acute phase proteins has become much more affordable and should complement the use of Hb for program planning and evaluation.

Despite their efficacy, the technologies used to decrease ID still have issues related to cultural and financial sustainability, which determine compliance and coverage [74]. The solutions to these constraints require continuous improvements based on program process and impact indicators.

Adding iron to staples and condiments for mass consumption, and blanket home fortification programs, can raise due concern about safety because of adverse health events among iron replete infants and children living in malaria-endemic regions who consumed iron supplements and hereditary disorders that cause progressive iron overload; these concerns have been addressed in depth in Chap. 21. Even though the risk of adverse effects is much lower when iron is delivered in food throughout the day [75], screening for these conditions in specific populations should be the norm.

Suggestions to Improve Food-Based ID Control Program Effectiveness

1. Single or multiple micronutrient fortification with iron should only be relied upon in "real world" conditions to meet the iron requirements of populations affected by ID and not by anemia from other causes.
2. The fortificant and food vehicle combinations must simultaneously optimize acceptability, coverage, compliance, and an effective dose of bioavailable iron.
3. Foods that have been fortified with iron (either through industrial or home fortification) should be combined with safe water, adequate sanitation, hygiene education, and infection prevention through immunization and treatment (as well as obesity reduction) to free the hepcidin-induced downregulation of iron absorption associated with inflammation and infection.
4. Maintenance of adequate iron reserves prior to rapid growth phases (i.e., 6–23 months of age, adolescence, and pregnancy) should be accompanied by public health measures including delayed umbilical cord clamping, exclusive breastfeeding, family planning, and oral contraceptives (to increase interpregnancy intervals and decrease menstrual blood loss).
5. Fortification and anemia prevention programs should be designed, implemented, monitored, and evaluated in accordance with the international evidence-based guidelines and best practices addressed comprehensively by WHO [2, 10].

In summary, effective programs address several important determinants of ID concurrently, as demonstrated by multiple industrialized and LMIC, like Costa Rica [23]. A thorough situation analysis should be used within each context to dictate the essential elements of an integrated solution for entire population groups, as well as specific population segments that require a more nuanced mix of interventions.

Conclusions

ID is a complex health issue: reducing its global burden requires complementary strategies that simultaneously consider efficacy, acceptability, sustainability, and safety. The most successful approach to increasing consumption of micronutrient-rich foods is likely a combined strategy that addresses both increased production and consumption of diversified foods, yet efforts to improve and maintain dietary quality take a long time and specific groups require particular attention [10, 46]. Together, fortification, biofortification, and other food-based interventions that enhance or improve dietary diversification play a critical role in alleviating ID. Advantages of food-based strategies include improved intakes of specific nutrients, as well as overall improved diets, health status, productivity, cognitive function, and livelihoods [76].

Acknowledgement We sincerely thank Dr. Jere D. Haas for his contribution as an editorial reviewer.

References

1. Petry N, Olofin I, Hurrell RF, Boy E, Wirth JP, Moursi M, et al. The proportion of anemia associated with iron deficiency in low, medium, and high human development index countries: a systematic analysis of national surveys. Nutrients. 2016;8:1–17.
2. WHO. Nutritional anaemias: tools for effective prevention. Geneva: World Health Organization; 2017.

3. da Silva LK, Takemoto Y, Garcia-Casal MN, Ota E. Nutrition-specific interventions for preventing and controlling anaemia throughout the life cycle: an overview of systematic reviews. Cochrane Database Syst Rev. 2018;8
4. Ruel MT, Alderman H. Nutrition-sensitive interventions and programmes: how can they help to accelerate progress in improving maternal and child nutrition? Lancet. 2013;382:536–51.
5. Horton S, Mannar V, Wesley A. Best practice paper: food fortification with iron and iodine. Copenhagen Consensus Centre Working Paper Copenhagen; 2008.
6. Blanco-Rojo R, Vaquero MP. Iron bioavailability from food fortification to precision nutrition. A review. Innov Food Sci Emerg Technol. 2019;51:126–38.
7. Dary O. The importance and limitations of food fortification for the management of nutritional anemias. In: Kraemer K, Zimmermann MB, editors. Nutritional anemia. Basel: Sight Life Press; 2007. p. 315–36.
8. Hurrel RF, Egli IM. Fortification of food: principles and practice. In: Means RTJ, editor. Nutritional anemia: scientific principles, clinical practice, and public health. Cambridge: Cambridge University Press; 2019. p. 16–30.
9. Hurrell R, Ranum P, De Pee S, Biebinger R, Hulthen L, Johnson Q, et al. Revised recommendations for iron fortification of wheat flour and an evaluation of the expected impact of current national wheat flour fortification programs. Food Nutr Bull. 2010;31
10. Allen L, de Benoist B, Dary O, Hurrell RF. Guidelines on food fortification with micronutrients. World Health Organization and Food and Agriculture Organization of the United Nations. 2006.
11. García-Casal MN. Planning and implementing food fortification programs to combat micronutrient malnutrition: iron. Food Nutr Sci. 2014;05:880–8.
12. Gera T, Singh Sachdev H, Boy E. Effect of iron-fortified foods on hematologic and biological outcomes: systematic review of randomized controlled trials. Am J Clin Nutr. 2012;96:309–24.
13. Garcia-Casal MN, Peña-Rosas JP, De-Regil LM, Gwirtz JA, Pasricha SR. Fortification of maize flour with iron for controlling anaemia and iron deficiency in populations. Cochrane Database Syst Rev. 2018;12(12):CD010187.
14. Field MS, Mithra P, Estevez D, Peña-Rosas JP. Wheat flour fortification with iron for reducing anaemia and improving iron status in populations. Cochrane Database Syst Rev. 2020;7:CD011302.
15. Haas JD, Rahn M, Venkatramanan S, Marquis GS, Wenger MJ, Murray-Kolb LE, et al. Double-fortified salt is efficacious in improving indicators of iron deficiency in female Indian tea pickers. J Nutr. 2014;144:957–64.
16. Andersson M, Thankachan P, Muthayya S, Goud RB, Kurpad AV, Hurrell RF, et al. Dual fortification of salt with iodine and iron: a randomized, double-blind, controlled trial of micronized ferric pyrophosphate and encapsulated ferrous fumarate in southern India. Am J Clin Nutr. 2008;88:1378–87.
17. Wegmüller R, Camara F, Zimmermann MB, Adou P, Hurrell RF. Salt dual-fortified with iodine and micronized ground ferric pyrophosphate affects iron status but not hemoglobin in children in Côte d'Ivoire. J Nutr. 2006;136:1814–20.
18. Viteri FE, Alvarez E, Batres R, Torún B, Pineda O, Mejía LA, et al. Fortification of sugar with iron sodium ethylenediaminotetraacetate (FeNaEDTA) improves iron status in semi rural Guatemalan populations. Am J Clin Nutr. 1995;61:1153–63.
19. Ballot DE, MacPhail AP, Bothwell TH, Gillooly M, Mayet FG. Fortification of curry powder with NaFe(111)EDTA in an iron-deficient population: report of a controlled iron-fortification trial. Am J Clin Nutr. 1989;49:162–9.
20. Chen J, Zhao X, Zhang X, Yin S, Piao J, Huo J, et al. Studies on the effectiveness of NaFeEDTA-fortified soy sauce in controlling iron deficiency: a population-based intervention trial. Food Nutr Bull. 2005;26:177–86.
21. Waller AW, Andrade JE, Mejia LA. Performance factors influencing efficacy and effectiveness of iron fortification programs of condiments for improving anemia prevalence and iron status in populations: a systematic review. Nutrients. 2020;12
22. Pachón H, Spohrer R, Mei Z, Serdula MK. Evidence of the effectiveness of flour fortification programs on iron status and anemia: a systematic review. Nutr Rev. 2015;73:780–95.
23. Martorell R, Ascencio M, Tacsan L, Alfaro T, Young MF, Addo OY, et al. Effectiveness evaluation of the food fortification program of Costa Rica: impact on anemia prevalence and hemoglobin concentrations in women and children. Am J Clin Nutr. 2015;101:210–7.
24. Hoogendoorn A, Luthringer C, Parvanta I, Garrett GS. Food fortification global mapping study 2016: technical assistance for strengthening capacities in food fortification; 2016.
25. Tam E, Keats E, Rind F, Das J, Bhutta A. Micronutrient supplementation and fortification among children under-five in low- and middle-income countries: a systematic review and meta-analysis. Nutrients. 2020;12
26. Arimond M, Zeilani M, Jungjohann S, Brown KH, Ashorn P, Allen LH, et al. Considerations in developing lipid-based nutrient supplements for prevention of undernutrition: experience from the international lipid-based nutrient supplements (iLiNS) project. Matern Child Nutr. 2015;11:31–61.
27. Zlotkin S, Arthur P, Antwi KY, Yeung G. Treatment of anemia with microencapsulated ferrous fumarate plus ascorbic acid supplied as sprinkles to complementary (weaning) foods. Am J Clin Nutr. 2001;74:791–5.
28. UNICEF. NutriDash 2.0. 2018 [cited 2020 Sep 1]. https://www.unicefnutridash.org/surveyreports
29. Nyhus Dhillon C, Sarkar D, Klemm RDW, Neufeld LM, Rawat R, Tumilowicz A, et al. Executive summary for the micronutrient powders consultation: les-

sons learned for operational guidance. Matern Child Nutr. 2017;13:1–9.
30. Suchdev PS, Peña-Rosas JP, De-Regil LM. Multiple micronutrient powders for home (point-of-use) fortification of foods in pregnant women. Cochrane Database Syst Rev. 2015;6
31. Suchdev PS, Jefferds MED, Ota E, da Silva LK, De-Regil LM. Home fortification of foods with multiple micronutrient powders for health and nutrition in children under two years of age. Cochrane Database Syst Rev. 2020;2
32. De-Regil LM, Jefferds MED, Peña-Rosas JP. Point-of-use fortification of foods with micronutrient powders containing iron in children of preschool and school-age. Cochrane Database Syst Rev. 2017;11
33. Zlotkin SH, Schauer C, Christofides A, Sharieff W, Tondeur MC, Ziauddin Hyder SM. Micronutrient sprinkles to control childhood anaemia: a simple powdered sachet may be the key to addressing a global problem. PLoS Med. 2005;2:0024–8.
34. Home Fortification Technical Advisory Group. Programmatic guidance brief on use of micronutrient powders. 2011.
35. Neufeld LM, García-Guerra A, Quezada AD, Théodore F, Bonvecchio Arenas A, Islas CD, et al. A fortified food can be replaced by micronutrient supplements for distribution in a Mexican social protection program based on results of a cluster-randomized trial and costing analysis. J Nutr. 2019;20:2302S–9S.
36. Young SL, Blanco I, Hernandez-Cordero S, Pelto GH, Neufeld LM. Organoleptic properties, ease of use, and perceived health effects are determinants of acceptability of micronutrient supplements among poor Mexican women. J Nutr. 2010;140:605–11.
37. Briend A. Highly nutrient-dense spreads: a new approach to delivering multiple micronutrients to high-risk groups. Br J Nutr. 2001;85:S175.
38. UNICEF, WHO, University UN. Composition of a multi-micronutrient supplement to be used in pilot programmes among pregnant women in developing countries. New York, NY; 1999.
39. Smuts CM, Matsungo TM, Malan L, Kruger HS, Rothman M, Kvalsvig JD, et al. Effect of small-quantity lipid-based nutrient supplements on growth, psychomotor development, iron status, and morbidity among 6-to 12-mo-old infants in South Africa: a randomized controlled trial. Am J Clin Nutr. 2019;109:55–68.
40. Das JK, Salam RA, Hadi YB, Sheikh SS, Bhutta AZ, Prinzo ZW, et al. Preventive lipid-based nutrient supplements given with complementary foods to infants and young children 6 to 23 months of age for health, nutrition, and developmental outcomes. Cochrane Database Syst Rev. 2019;5
41. Addo OY, Locks LM, Jefferds ME, Nanama S, Albert B, Sandalinas F, et al. Combined infant and young child feeding with small-quantity lipid-based nutrient supplementation is associated with a reduction in anemia but no changes in anthropometric status of young children from Katanga Province of the Democratic Republic of Congo. Am J Clin Nutr. 2020;1–12
42. Stewart CP, Fernald LCH, Weber AM, Arnold C, Galasso E. Lipid-based nutrient supplementation reduces child anemia and increases micronutrient status in Madagascar: a multiarm cluster-randomized controlled trial. J Nutr. 2020;150:958–66.
43. Das JK, Hoodbhoy Z, Salam RA, Bhutta AZ, Valenzuela-Rubio NG, Weise Prinzo Z, et al. Lipid-based nutrient supplements for maternal, birth, and infant developmental outcomes. Cochrane Database Syst Rev. 2018;2018
44. WHO. Guideline: use of multiple micronutrient powders for home fortification of foods consumed by infants and children 6–23 months of age. Geneva: World Health Organization; 2011.
45. WHO. WHO guideline: use of multiple micronutrient powders for point-of-use fortification of foods consumed by infants and young children aged 6–23 months and children aged 2–12 years. Geneva: World Health Organization; 2016.
46. Girard AW, Self JL, McAuliffe C, Olude O. The effects of household food production strategies on the health and nutrition outcomes of women and young children: a systematic review. Paediatr Perinat Epidemiol. 2012;26(Suppl 1):205–22.
47. Finkelstein JL, Haas JD, Mehta S. Iron-biofortified staple food crops for improving iron status: a review of the current evidence. Curr Opin Biotechnol. 2017;44:138–45.
48. Ruel MT, Quisumbing AR, Balagamwala M. Nutrition-sensitive agriculture: what have we learned so far? Glob Food Sec. 2018;17:128–53.
49. Lambrecht NJ, Wilson ML, Jones AD. Assessing the impact of animal husbandry and capture on anemia among women and children in low- and middle-income countries: a systematic review. Adv Nutr. 2019;10:331–44.
50. Vasconcelos MW, Gruissem W, Bhullar NK. Iron biofortification in the 21st century: setting realistic targets, overcoming obstacles, and new strategies for healthy nutrition. Curr Opin Biotechnol. 2017;44:8–15.
51. Finkelstein JL, Mehta S, Udipi SA, Ghugre PS, Luna SV, Wenger MJ, et al. A randomized trial of iron-biofortified pearl millet in school children in India. J Nutr. 2015;145:1576–81.
52. Finkelstein JL, Mehta S, Villalpando S, Mundo-Rosas V, Luna SV, Rahn M, et al. A randomized feeding trial of iron-biofortified beans in school children in Mexico. Nutrients. 2019;11:381.
53. Haas JD, Luna SV, Lung'aho MG, Wenger MJ, Murray-Kolb LE, Beebe S, et al. Consuming iron biofortified beans increases iron status in Rwandan women after 128 days in a randomized controlled feeding trial. J Nutr. 2016;146:1586–92.
54. Haas JD, Beard JL, Murray-Kolb LE, del Mundo AM, Felix A, Gregorio GB. Iron-biofortified rice improves

the iron stores of nonanemic Filipino women. J Nutr. 2005;135:2823–30.
55. Kumar S, Pandey G. Biofortification of pulses and legumes to enhance nutrition. Heliyon. 2020;6:4–9.
56. Bouis HE, Saltzman A. Improving nutrition through biofortification: a review of evidence from HarvestPlus, 2003 through 2016. Glob Food Sec. 2017;12:49–58.
57. Meenakshi JV, Johnson NL, Manyong VM, De Groote H, Javelosa J, Yanggen DR, et al. How cost-effective is biofortification in combating micronutrient malnutrition? An ex ante assessment. World Dev. 2010;38:64–75.
58. Scott SP, Murray-Kolb LE, Wenger MJ, Udipi SA, Ghugre PS, Boy E, et al. Cognitive performance in Indian school-going adolescents is positively affected by consumption of iron-biofortified pearl millet: a 6-month randomized controlled efficacy trial. J Nutr. 2018;148:1462–71.
59. Wenger MJ, Rhoten SE, Murray-Kolb LE, Scott SP, Boy E, Gahutu J-B, et al. Changes in iron status are related to changes in brain activity and behavior in Rwandan female university students: results from a randomized controlled efficacy trial involving iron-biofortified beans. J Nutr. 2019;149:687–97.
60. Murray-Kolb LE, Wenger MJ, Scott SP, Rhoten SE, Lung'aho MG, Haas JD. Consumption of iron-biofortified beans positively affects cognitive performance in 18- to 27-year-old Rwandan female college students in an 18-week randomized controlled efficacy trial. J Nutr. 2017;147:2109–17.
61. Luna SV, Pompano LM, Lung'aho M, Gahutu JB, Haas JD. Increased iron status during a feeding trial of iron-biofortified beans increases physical work efficiency in Rwandan women. J Nutr. 2020:1093–9.
62. Finkelstein JL, Fothergill A, Hackl LS, Haas JD, Mehta S. Iron biofortification interventions to improve iron status and functional outcomes. Proc Nutr Soc. 2019;78:197–207.
63. Iannotti L, Cunningham K, Ruel M. Improving diet quality and micronutrient nutrition: homestead food production in Bangladesh. Washington, DC: International Food Policy Research Institute; 2009.
64. Asare-Marfo D, Herrington C, Alwang J, Birachi E, Birol E, Tedla Diressie M, et al. Assessing the adoption of high iron bean varieties and their impact on iron intakes and other livelihood outcomes in Rwanda: listing exercise report. Washington, DC: HarvestPlus; 2016.
65. Birol E, Meenakshi JV, Oparinde A, Perez S, Tomlins K. Developing country consumers' acceptance of biofortified foods: a synthesis. Food Secur. 2015;7:555–68.
66. Saltzman A, Birol E, Oparinde A, Andersson MS, Asare-Marfo D, Diressie MT, et al. Availability, production, and consumption of crops biofortified by plant breeding: current evidence and future potential. Ann N Y Acad Sci. 2017;1390:104–14.
67. Verbowski V, Talukder Z, Hou K, Sok Hoing L, Michaux K, Anderson V, et al. Effect of enhanced homestead food production and aquaculture on dietary intakes of women and children in rural Cambodia: a cluster randomized controlled trial. Matern Child Nutr. 2018;14:1–9.
68. Michaux KD, Hou K, Karakochuk CD, Whitfield KC, Ly S, Verbowski V, et al. Effect of enhanced homestead food production on anaemia among Cambodian women and children: a cluster randomized controlled trial. Matern Child Nutr. 2019;15 Suppl 3(Suppl 3):e12757.
69. Karakochuk CD, Whitfield KC, Barr SI, Lamers Y, Devlin AM, Vercauteren SM, et al. Genetic hemoglobin disorders rather than iron deficiency are a major predictor of hemoglobin concentration in women of reproductive age in rural Prey Veng, Cambodia. J Nutr. 2015;145:134–42.
70. Wieringa FT, Sophonneary P, Whitney S, Mao B, Berger J, Conkle J, et al. Low prevalence of iron and vitamin a deficiency among Cambodian women of reproductive age. Nutrients. 2016;8:2–9.
71. Wastnedge E, Waters D, Patel S, Morrison K, Goh MY, Adeloye D, et al. The global burden of sickle cell disease in children under five years of age: a systematic review and meta-analysis. J Glob Health. 2018;8:1–9.
72. Weiss G, Ganz T, Goodnough LT. Anemia of inflammation. Blood. 2019;133:40–50.
73. Kassebaum NJ, Jasrasaria R, Naghavi M, Wulf SK, Johns N, Lozano R, et al. A systematic analysis of global anemia burden from 1990 to 2010. Blood. 2015;123:615–25.
74. Pelletier D, DePee S. Micronutrient powder programs: new findings and future directions for implementation science. Matern Child Nutr. 2019;15:1–10.
75. Prentice AM, Mendoza YA, Pereira D, Cerami C, Wegmuller R, Constable A, et al. Dietary strategies for improving iron status: balancing safety and efficacy. Nutr Rev. 2017;75:49–60.
76. Thompson B, Amoroso L. Improving diets and nutrition: food-based approaches. Food and Agriculture Organization of the United Nations and CABI; 2015.

Food Fortification with Iron: Policy Considerations

26

Greg S. Garrett

Keywords

Nutrition · Iron · Anemia · Deficiency Malnutrition · Fortification · Micronutrients Public health · Policy · Food quality Standards · Staple foods

Overview of Food Fortification with Iron

Food systems too often fail to deliver foods sufficiently rich in iron and other micronutrients. Where this gap exists for large parts of the population, food fortification—the practice of adding one or more essential nutrients to food—can enhance the nutritional quality of the food supply and help address micronutrient deficiencies [1].

Food fortification can take various forms. These include targeted fortification as well as large-scale mandatory or voluntary fortification. Targeted fortification aims to increase the nutrient intake of specific target population groups, for example, through complementary foods for infants, rather than for all population groups. Mandatory large-scale food fortification (LSFF) sets legislation which requires all large-scale food industry to fortify by adding one or more micronutrients to foods commonly consumed by large parts of the population as part of efforts to address deficiencies. Voluntary fortification, legislation permitting but not requiring fortification, is also practiced but its impact has been less studied. This chapter primarily reviews and discusses the policy considerations which are related to mandatory LSFF with iron. Mandatory LSFF with iron aims to increase regular intake of iron that is otherwise not sufficiently obtained in the diets of populations. It is therefore not a stand-alone solution for addressing iron deficiency. Rather, effective and relevant policy ensures that food fortification with iron can provide a cost-effective, public health approach that complements other long-term nutrition-specific and nutrition-sensitive strategies to address iron deficiency.

History and Status of Food Fortification with Iron

Food fortification with iron has a significant history of public health sucess. In the 1940s, programs for wheat flour fortification with iron were introduced nationally in the United Kingdom and the United States in order to target widespread anemia. Following these mandates, LSFF with iron was rapidly adopted in these countries, and aided by targeted advocacy from the nutritionist community as well as a wartime climate which tapped a patriotic incentive to improve the health and well-being of the population [2].

G. S. Garrett (✉)
ThinkWell, Geneva, Switzerland
e-mail: greg.garrett@accesstonutrition.org

C. D. Karakochuk et al. (eds.), *Nutritional Anemia*, Nutrition and Health,
https://doi.org/10.1007/978-3-031-14521-6_26

Dozens of countries throughout Latin America, Africa, and Asia started to mandate iron fortification of cereal grains in the 1990s and early 2000s. Wheat flour, maize flour, and rice are the most common food vehicles selected for mandatory LSFF with iron (Table 26.1).

Table 26.1 The most common food vehicles used for large-scale iron fortification programs

Food vehicle	Number of countries with mandate
Wheat flour	84
Maize flour	16
Rice	7

Today, iron fortification of wheat flour is mandatory in 84 countries (Fig. 26.1), iron fortification of maize flour is mandated in 16 countries (Fig. 26.2) and of iron fortificaiton of rice is manadated in seven countries (Fig. 26.3) (GFDx, 2020; [3]).

To ensure optimal impact of iron fortification programs, it is critical that there is an appropriate selection of food vehciles coupled with effective compliance mechanisms [4]. Most policy evidence which has been generated to date on iron fortification is based on programs fortifying wheat flour, maize flour, and rice. Iron fortifica-

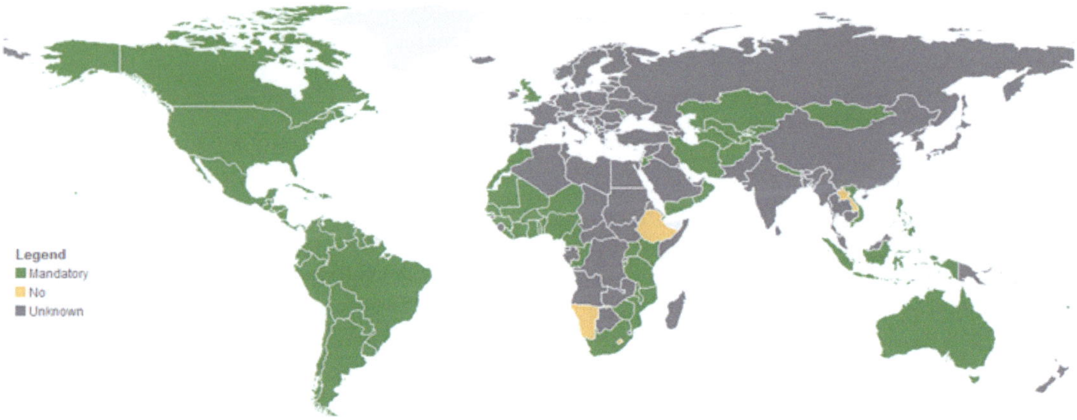

Fig. 26.1 Legislation for the fortification of wheat flour with iron (GFDx, 2020 [3]; permission for reproduction not required). ('Mandatory' signifies that the country has mandated all registered mills to fortify. 'No' signifies that the country has fortification standards but does not require fortification. 'Unknown' signifies that the GFDx has yet to verify the existence of any standards or legislation)

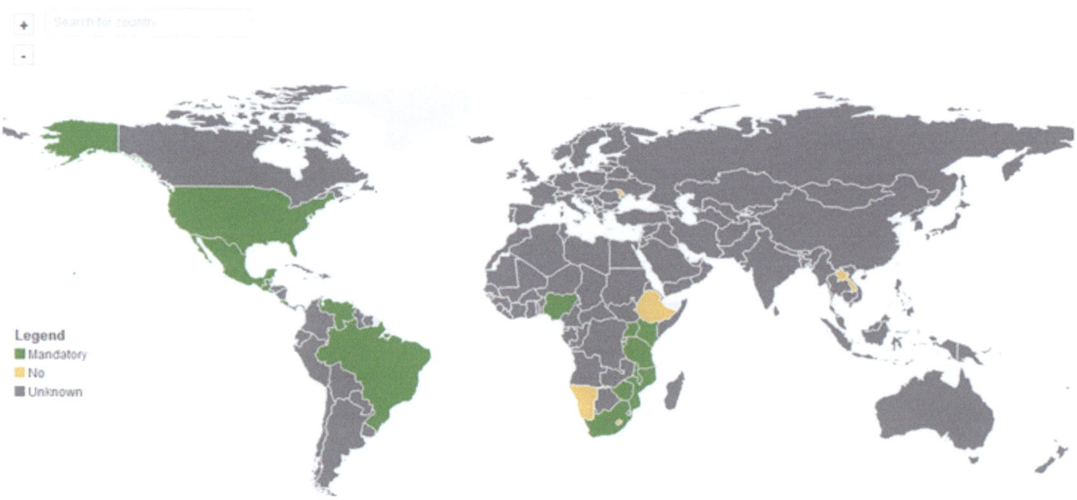

Fig. 26.2 Legislation for the fortification of maize flour with iron. (GFDx, 2020 [3]; permission for reproduction not required)

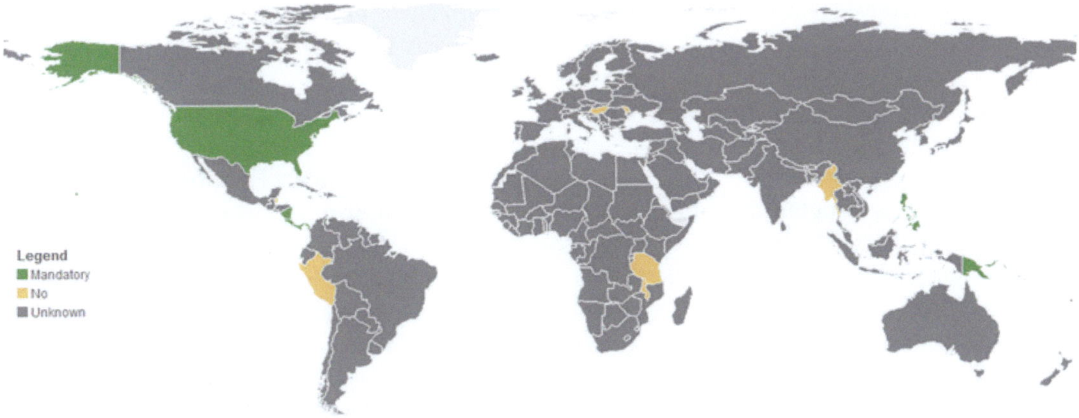

Fig. 26.3 Legislation for the fortification of rice with iron (GFDx, 2020 [3]; permission for reproduction not required)

tion using wheat flour is the most advanced practice, relative to the other food vehicles, and has the highest potential for impact in the short- to medium-term in countries where wheat flour is consumed as a staple [5].

Other than wheat flour, maize flour and rice, there are a handful of other widely consumed food vehicles under consideration for iron fortification. The most notable include bouillon cubes and salt (the latter through double fortified salt with iodine and iron). Although bouillon cubes are widely consumed in many regions, especially West Africa—and despite the fact that some large industries are already manufacturing or selling fortified bouillon cubes on a voluntary basis—little policy related to safety standards, technical guidance, and mandates for fortifying bouillon cubes has been developed.

Similarly, double fortified salt with iodine and iron has been an attractive proposition under consideration for several decades due to the success of salt iodization and the near universal consumption of salt. However, while India has been successful in incorporating double fortified salt into much of its safety net system, there remain several technical and financial issues that require resolution before this intervention can go to scale. The technical issues needing to be resolved include the adverse interaction of micronutrients, nutrient homogeneity, quality production parameters, and organoleptic changes. In terms of cost, the extra margin created by adding iron to salt remains a barrier in many low-income contexts unless it can be subsidized by governments. These issues are being systematically reviewed by the nutrition community through recent consultations [6].

Lastly, unlike most other micronutrients, iron can cause unacceptable sensory changes to foods. This has meant that the development of efficacious iron fortified foods has been more challenging than developing efficacious foods fortified with other micronutrients [5]. When added to many foods the more bioavailable, soluble iron compounds often cause unacceptable organoleptic changes, whereas the less soluble iron compounds, which are much less well absorbed, are more acceptable organoleptically. Many of these issues have been largely overcome by developing acceptable iron forms or fortification technologies (e.g., extrusion technology for rice) [7].

Impact to Date Through Food Fortification with Iron

When designed, delivered, and monitored well, LSFF with iron can be expected to improve or sustain adequate iron status. A 2019 systematic review and meta-analysis of 50 studies on the impact of large-scale fortification programs in low- and middle-income countries (LMIC) found that there was a 34% reduction in anemia from improved iron stores due to iron fortification [8]. The study also revealed that while all age groups benefited from iron fortification, those most at risk of deficiency benefited the most, such as women of reproductive age (WRA) and pregnant women (ibid).

Lastly, LSFF is a highly cost-effective intervention for all essential vitamins and minerals, and this is the case for iron as well. Following a review of 40-plus interventions, the Copenhagen Consensus ranked micronutrient interventions as one of the top development priorities ranking higher than water and sanitation and immunization coverage. More specifically, in ten LMIC with high anemia prevalence, a review found that the cost of iron fortification against future benefits related to cognitive improvements amounted to a benefit-cost ratio of 8.7:1 [9].

Effective Policy for Food Fortification with Iron

When policy is well designed and implemented, LSFF with iron can lead to sustained, positive impacts in iron intakes at the population level. There are therefore specific policy considerations which need to be addressed by policymakers to (1) design, (2) implement and improve; and (3) monitor iron fortification programming. Here we summarize these considerations to help countries to effectively deliver their iron food fortification programs leading towards sustained impact.

Policy Considerations to Design National Iron Fortification Programs

There are several guidelines available to support effective design and implementation of LSFF programs. These include the 2006 WHO/FAO Guidelines on food fortification with micronutrients [10], which covers all aspects of programming, and the 2018 policy guidance document, "Regulatory Monitoring of National Food Fortification Programs" [11]. The latter document specifically provides guidance on quality assurance and control. These manuals, alongside the principles of the Codex Alimentarius, form a solid basis for designing national iron fortification programs.

Setting Mandatory Fortification Legislation and Standards

During design, policymakers need to look at the advantages of mandatory fortification over voluntary fortification. Voluntary fortification is less likely than mandatory fortification to deliver a widespread, favorable public health outcome of increased intakes of iron across entire populations [10]. Voluntary fortification is typically aimed for populations who are not at-risk. Because fortified, as well as unfortified products, will be available in markets, voluntary fortification requires brand differentiation and consumer choice to purchase the fortified product, which is often more costly than the unfortified version.

Therefore, mandatory fortification is more relevant therefore in contexts where there is significant public health need or risk [10]. Mandatory fortification should create increased parity among the relevant industry players. It helps guarantee that all packaged varieties of a fortifiable food vehicle are fortified, thus facilitating greater access to fortified foods without necessitating significant changes in consumption habits. Importantly, fortification mandates provide the legal basis for enforcement [12].

To ensure that mandatory iron fortification policy will be effective it should cover four key principles on adding essential nutrients to foods found in the Codex Alimentarius, a set of globally recognized food standards developed by the Codex Alimentarius Commission.[1] The four principles are: (1) addressing documented nutritional needs; (2) selecting food(s) which are regularly consumed in sufficient amounts by the target population; (3) setting the levels of added fortification so that they provide a biologically effective contribution of the nutrient without this

[1] In 1963 by the Food and Agriculture Organization and World Health Organization established the Codex Alimentarius Commission.

resulting in excess intakes; and (4) using fortificants which are stable and bioavailable [13].

Thus, during design of an iron fortification program, the critical first step is to identify if there is a gap in dietary iron adequacy. This should be established using the most up-to-date data and information available on current iron status and population-level dietary intake of iron. If data are not available, new dietary intake studies among the population may be required [14].

Second, if a gap has been identified, the food to be fortified needs to be identified. The food vehicle should be selected based on regular consumption patterns (based on per capita consumption), industry consolidation, the feasibility of fortification at the processing stage, and the economics or cost-effectiveness of fortifying that food. As noted, wheat flour, maize flour, and rice to date have been the most frequently selected vehicles for iron fortification based on consumption, industry layout, and feasibility. Bouillon cubes and salt have also been under consideration as prospective vehicles in several contexts, especially West Africa and India, respectively.

Third, the standards for iron fortification need to be developed and set by government. Standards should be based on WHO's guidance on Tolerable Upper Intake Level (UL) [10]. UL is the highest average intake which is used as a reference value for determining whether the micronutrient intakes of subgroups in the population are safe and do not create a risk of excessive intake that would lead to adverse health effects. In other words, standards should set the minimum and maximum levels for the addition of iron to the food vehicle to achieve their intended purpose [13]. In practice, the amount of iron that can be added to the selected food is dictated by safety concerns for those at the top end of consumption of the chosen food vehicle. Therefore, based on consumption levels of the selected food vehicle, and considering the presence of other iron interventions that are addressing iron deficiency, the UL should help set recommended iron levels that provide, for example, 20–50% of the Estimated Average Requirement, EAR [10]. Periodic assessment of coverage and utilization is critical to reassess risk of excessive intake—taking into consideration iron from all dietary sources [11].

Lastly, standards need to specify which iron fortificants should be used based on bioavailability, lack of adverse interaction with other food constituents and nutrients, organoleptic acceptability, and availability of the compound at an acceptable cost [7]. There are many compounds which have been considered for iron fortification. The WHO/FAO fortification guidelines [10] lists 19 iron compounds together with their relative absorption in humans. Currently, there are about seven acceptable and relevant iron compounds regularly deployed in food fortification programs. These are ferrous fumarate, ferrous sulfate, ferrous gluconate, ferric pyrophosphate (FPP), sodium iron ethylenediaminetetraacetic acid (NaFeEDTA), ferrous bisglycinate (FBG), and elemental iron powders.

Policy Considerations to Implement and Improve Iron Fortification Programs

Policies to Aid in Coordinating National Efforts

Fortification programs are successful when driven by a final public health objective and when trust is built between the public and private sector actors [15]. To build this trust, not unlike other multi-sectoral programs, iron fortification programs require clear lines of responsibility from design through to monitoring. It is important that governments help establish mechanisms to coordinate all stakeholders, and hold each accountable, so as to deliver an impactful fortification program.

One such mechanism that has been successful to improve national efforts for fortification programs in at least two dozen countries is national food fortification alliances (NFFAs) [15]. NFFAs are useful mechanisms to establish clear roles, foster collective decision-making and to help establish trust between governments, industry, and civil society.

A 2016 review of nine NFFAs identified several policies and clear government roles that lead to better coordination within fortification programs [16]. These government roles include: overall leadership provided by the Ministry of Health or Ministry of Industry (NB: these ministries often host a dedicated fortification project management); clear mandates for the federal and/or subnational food control authorities to monitor the quality of domestically produced fortified foods; robust monitoring of imported foods by custom officials; and lastly, nutrition surveillance units that routinely monitor the public health impact of the fortification program.

Lastly, the private sector takes on the lion's share of the fortification processes. It also works to ensure markets expand and to enhance their respective brand value through improving quality. NFFAs can help to foster the ongoing motivation of all parties to complete their responsibilities and to work together for the success of national fortification efforts [16].

Policies Related to Regulatory Monitoring

According to the WHO/FAO, regulatory monitoring of fortified foods is defined as the process of "continuous collection, review, and use of information on program implementation activities, for the purpose of identifying problems, such as non-compliance, and informing corrective actions so as to fulfil stated objectives." [10].

Regulatory monitoring and enforcement of iron fortification thus requires supportive policies and appropriate budgetary allocations for government institutions charged with these tasks. There are several policies which need to be put in place to implement strong quality control and enforcement of iron fortification programs. In the case of mandatory fortification, all production facilities under legislation must conform to the relevant iron fortification standards and any other food requirements. Specifically, these policies should set forth the rules related to labelling and nutrition claims, as well as setting applicable penalties [17]. For the former, national iron fortification standards should stipulate the information to be included on iron-fortified food packaging and labels, such as how much iron the product contains, the lot or batch number (or other traceability data) and dates of manufacture.

For the latter on penalties, it is critical for policymakers to ensure standards which stipulate clear actionable limits that express the iron specification as a target value within an acceptable range of lower and upper parameters for test results. If a sample collected from the fortified food production sites falls outside of this range it would be considered noncompliant [11]. This range can be determined based on mean value from standardized sampling procedures [11].

To enhance effectiveness, regulatory monitoring of fortification should be part of the national or subnational food safety system. Food safety systems are important because they play a role in maintaining consumer safety and overall satisfaction. They are usually improved over time and incorporate standard management systems focused on food quality and safety. To ensure compliance of iron fortified foods along the entire supply chain, food safety systems need to routinely conduct external monitoring activities at food production facilities and border control sites. Periodic monitoring within the marketplace complements the data collected at other points in the supply chain. The inspection guidelines should emphasize the need for audits of food production facilities coupled with less frequent, yet critical, quantitative testing at certified laboratories. This places attention on the fortification process and leverages the internal monitoring activities being conducted by food manufacturers [11].

Lastly, because the cost of the fortificant (iron included) is the most substantial recurring input cost for fortification programs, it is often a barrier to industry fortifying appropriately [18]. To enhance the cost-effectiveness of premix procurement and distribution, governments should remove fortificant-related customs taxes and value-added taxes, and support the selection of verified supply agents who can deliver quality-assured fortificants in line with national standards [19].

Policy Considerations to Support Monitoring of Iron Fortification Programming

Monitoring iron fortification programs and then assessing their potential for impact within a population requires regular consumption information to determine the extent to which iron fortified foods are being consumed by the population and among subgroups. Consumption monitoring can be defined as the periodic assessment of household coverage and consumption of fortified foods and the additional micronutrient content provided to a population via the fortified food [20]. Related, because iron fortification programs often exist for dozens of years, it is important to assess whether other nutrition or food programs are providing iron through other sources and to recalibrate the program as needed.

Monitoring information can help policymakers to decide whether an iron fortification program should be enhanced, course corrected or even terminated, identify if there is a different strategy to improve iron status which could have greater impact, or if dietary gaps no longer exist among the population.

Lastly, thorough impact evaluations should be undertaken which look at the impact of iron fortification programs on biological (i.e., iron status) and functional (e.g., anemia, child development) outcomes. However, because these assessments are expensive, they should be done only when there is adequate reason to believe that there has been impact.

Conclusion

Mandatory, large-scale food fortification of staple foods and condiments with iron is an evidence-based, cost-effective intervention that can help address iron deficiency in a sustainable way. Its benefits can extend over the entire life cycle of humans. However, achieving impact often takes many years for countries to achieve [4]. It is therefore important that countries use evidence-based policy as summarized here which helps design, implement, improve, and monitor iron fortification programs. This will help ensure that the program is integrated within the context of a country's overall micronutrient strategy and delivered effectively via the food system. Moving forward, countries should garner the necessary resources and political commitment required to put in place the policies outlined here and to optimize their iron fortification programs for sustained health impact.

References

1. Bhutta ZA, Das JK, Rizvi A, Gaffey MF, Walker N, Horton S, Webb P, Lartey A, Black RE. Evidence-based interventions for improvement of maternal and child nutrition: what can be done and at what cost? Lancet. 2013;382:452–77.
2. Bishai D, Nalubola R. The history of food fortification in the United States: its relevance for current fortification efforts in developing countries. Econ Dev Cult Change. 2002;51:37–53. https://jhu.pure.elsevier.com/en/publications/the-history-of-food-fortification-in-the-united-states-its-releva-3
3. Global Fortification Data Exchange. Global Fortification Data Exchange | GFDx – Providing actionable food fortification data all in one place. 2018 [cited 2021 Jun 1]. https://fortificationdata.org/
4. Neufeld LM, Baker S, Garrett GS, Haddad L. Coverage and utilization in food fortification programs: critical and neglected areas of evaluation. J Nutr. 2017;147:1015S–9S. https://creativecommons.org/
5. Hurrell RF. The potential of iodine and iron double-fortified salt compared with iron-fortified staple foods to increase population iron status. J Nutr. 2021;151:47S–63S. https://doi.org/10.1093/jn/nxaa204.
6. Drewnowski A, Garrett GS, Kansagra R, Khan N, Kupka R, Kurpad AV, Mannar V, Martorell R, Zimmermann MB, Houston R. Key considerations for policymakers - iodized salt as a vehicle for iron fortification: current evidence, challenges, and knowledge gaps. J Nutr. 2021;151:64S–73S.
7. Hurrell R. Efficacy and Safety of Iron Fortification. Food Fortification in a Globalized World - 1st Edition [Internet]. London: Academic Press; 2018. [cited 2021 Jun 1]. 196–212 p. https://www.elsevier.com/books/food-fortification-in-a-globalized-world/mannar/978-0-12-802861-2
8. Keats EC, Neufeld LM, Garrett GS, Mbuya MNN, Bhutta ZA. Improved micronutrient status and health outcomes in low-and middle-income countries following large-scale fortification: evidence from a systematic review and meta-analysis. Am J Clin Nutr. 2019;109:1696–708.

9. Wessells KR, Brown KH. Estimating the global prevalence of zinc deficiency: results based on zinc availability in national food supplies and the prevalence of stunting. PLoS One. 2012;7(11):e50568.
10. Lindsay A, Bruno de B, Omar D, Richard H. Guidelines on food fortification with micronutrients [internet]. Who, Fao Un. 2006. https://www.who.int/publications/i/item/9241594012.
11. GAIN, PHC. Regulatory monitoring of national food fortification programs: A policy guidance document. 2018 [cited 2021 Jun 1]; https://s3-us-west-2.amazonaws.com/gfdx-published-files/Regulatory+Monitoring+Policy+Guidance+April+2018.pdf
12. Greiner T. Fortification of processed cereals should be mandatory [internet]. Lancet. 2007;369(9575):1766–8.
13. FAO. General principles for the addition of essential nutrition to foods. 2015.
14. Harvey PWJ, Dary O. Governments and academic institutions play vital roles in food fortification: Iron as an example. Public Health Nutr. 2012;15(10):1791–5.
15. Garrett GS. National mandated food fortification programs. In: Mannar MG, Hurrell R, editors. Food Fortification in a Globalized World - 1st Edition [Internet]. London: Academic Press; 2018. [cited 2021 Jun 1]. https://www.elsevier.com/books/food-fortification-in-a-globalized-world/mannar/978-0-12-802861-2.
16. Hafeez-ur-Rehman H, Luthringer C, Spohrer R, Timmer A, Rees A, Garrett G. National Fortification Alliances (NFAs): program guidance based on lessons learned from nine countries. Micronutrient Forum; 2016 [cited 2021 Jun 1]. https://micronutrientforum.org/abstracts/national-fortification-alliances-nfas-program-guidance-based-on-lessons-learned-from-nine-countries/
17. Marks KJ, Luthringer CL, Ruth LJ, Rowe LA, Khan NA, De-Regil LM, López X, Pachóna H. Review of grain fortification legislation, standards, and monitoring documents. Glob Heal Sci Pract. 2018;6:354–69.
18. Luthringer CL, Rowe LA, Vossenaar M, Garrett GS. Regulatory monitoring of fortified foods: identifying barriers and good practices. Glob Heal Sci Pract. 2015;3:446–61.
19. Garrett GS, Luthringer CL, Mkambula P. Improving nutritious food systems by establishing National Micronutrient Premix Supply Systems. 2016.
20. ECSA. Assessment of consumption monitoring systems fortified and nutritious foods in the east, central and southern Africa (ECSA) Region [Internet] 2017. [cited 2021 Jun 1]. https://www.gainhealth.org/resources/reports-and-publications/assessment-consumption-monitoring-systems-fortified-and

27 Designing Effective Programs for Anemia Reduction

Monica T. Kothari and Kaitlyn L. I. Samson

Keywords

Iron deficiency · Anemia · Program design Policy · Anemia prevention · Anemia reduction · Programming

Background

Progress in anemia reduction has been slow; rather, anemia prevalence has risen slightly among women of reproductive age (WRA; women aged 15–49 years) from 31.6% in 2000 to 32.8% in 2016. The World Health Assembly (WHA) has called for a 50% reduction in anemia prevalence among WRA by 2025 and, globally, no countries are currently on track to achieve this target [1, 2]. WHA targets were then also included in the 2030 development agenda and are referred to in target 2.2 of the Sustainable Development Goals. This target is based on an estimated baseline anemia prevalence of 30.3% in 2012 and an endline prevalence of 15.2% in 2030, requiring an average annual reduction rate of 3.8% [3]. It is commonly thought that iron deficiency is the most common cause of anemia in low- and middle-income countries. In 2015, the World Health Organization (WHO) estimated that iron deficiency anemia (IDA) accounted for ~50% of cases in women and ~42% of cases in children [4]. Hence, iron-focused interventions have resolved roughly half of anemia cases [5–7]. However, as the causes of anemia are multifactorial and include aspects beyond nutrition, such as infections and genetic hemoglobin disorders, programs must not *solely* focus on iron-related interventions [5, 8]. The prevalence and etiology of anemia vary widely by geography, thus programs to prevent and treat anemia must be designed accordingly.

Historical Perspective

The use of supplemental iron for the treatment of anemia has existed since the early 1900s. The ground-breaking work of Helen Mackay post-World War I led to the establishment of normal hemoglobin values for young children. Her work concluded that anemia in late infancy resulted from insufficient iron [9, 10]. Upon treating infants with iron, she noted that those who received supplements looked "healthier [and had fewer] episodes of respiratory tract infections, diarrhea and fever compared to un-supplemented infants"—thus helping to establish a clear link

M. T. Kothari (✉)
Surveys for Monitoring in Resilience and Food Security (SMRFS), International Health Division, ICF, Rockville, MD, USA
e-mail: Monica.Kothari@icf.com

K. L. I. Samson
Food, Nutrition, and Health, Faculty of Land and Food Systems, The University of British Columbia, Vancouver, BC, Canada

C. D. Karakochuk et al. (eds.), *Nutritional Anemia*, Nutrition and Health,
https://doi.org/10.1007/978-3-031-14521-6_27

between IDA and iron [9, 10]. Around the same time, the role of iron in hypochromic anemia in adults was also established—it was found that iron therapy led to positive changes in epithelial and subcutaneous structures and alleviated pallor [11]. Despite advances in defining the role of iron in the treatment and prevention of anemia in the last century, practice and policy remain a challenge. This chapter discusses program strategies and interventions for the reduction of anemia.

Consequences of Anemia and Target Populations

The devastating consequences of anemia highlight the need for effective reduction strategies. The morbidity, mortality, and economic ramifications associated with anemia are numerous, in some cases irreversible, and can have a lifelong impact [12]. During pregnancy, anemia is associated with poor maternal and birth outcomes, such as low birth weight, small for gestational age, premature birth, and maternal, perinatal, and neonatal mortality [13]. In children, iron deficiency and IDA have been linked to poor cognitive and motor development outcomes [14]. The persistence of anemia into adolescence and adulthood can negatively impact one's physical capacity, concentration, and work productivity [15]. Implementing strategies to successfully control anemia can improve children's school performance, women's work capacity, and pregnancy outcomes for mothers and infants [1]. These improvements can result in intergenerational benefits that not only improve individual health and well-being but also enhance economic potential and community development [1].

Anemia prevention and reduction programs are typically targeted towards infants and children under 2 years of age, children under 2 years of age, adolescents, and WRA (pregnant and non-pregnant). When possible, efforts should be made to consider socio-economic data for these target populations. Detailed descriptions of the increased needs of infants and young children and pregnant women can be found in Chaps. 6 and 7, respectively.

Interventions to Reduce Nutritional Anemia

Numerous interventions exist that are intended to prevent and correct nutritional anemias. These include behavior change dietary interventions, fortification of foods with micronutrients, micronutrient supplementation, and other public health measures, such as helminth control through deworming programs. The objectives of these approaches are to improve nutritional status, thus, reduce nutritional anemia. Tables 27.1 and 27.2 present some interventions that have been implemented to reduce, treat, or prevent anemia in recent years.

Nutrition-Specific Strategies to Reduce Anemia

Nutrition-specific interventions, defined in Chap. 27, act directly on the immediate nutritional causes of anemia, such as poor intake of hematopoietic nutrients (e.g., iron, folate, vitamins B12 A), infant feeding practices, and access to iron-fortified foods [2, 14]. In instances where behavior-change communication directly influences nutrition-related behaviors, it is also classified as a nutrition-specific intervention.

Micronutrient Supplementation

Intermittent iron supplementation is recommended in populations where the prevalence of anemia among non-pregnant WRA, preschool (24–59 months; 25 mg elemental iron in liquid form) or school-age (5–12 years; 45 mg elemental iron in tablet/capsule form) children is greater than 20% [16, 17]. For non-pregnant menstruating women and adolescent girls, intermittent iron supplements are recommended to also include folic acid in order to improve blood folate status and reduce the risk of neural tube defects should an unplanned pregnancy occur (60 mg elemental iron and 2.8 mg folic acid in tablet/capsule form) [17]. Intermittent supplements should be given once weekly for three consecutive months followed by 3 months of no supplementation, after which the provision of supplements can restart;

Table 27.1 Nutrition-specific interventions and strategies for anemia reduction

Program/recommendation/practice[a]	Geography/setting	Policy/ guideline available[b]	Target population(s)	Prevention (P)/ treatment (T)/ control (C)
Supplementation				
Intermittent (weekly) iron supplementation with doses varying by target population	Anemia prevalence among target population is ≥20%	Yes	All menstruating adolescent girls and women Preschool-age children (24–59 months) School-age children (5–12 years)	PTC
Intermittent iron and folic acid supplementation with 60 mg elemental iron and 2.8 mg folic acid	Anemia prevalence among target population is 20–39%	Yes	All menstruating women and adolescent girls	PTC
Daily iron supplementation with doses varying by target population	Anemia prevalence among target population is ≥40% and the diet does not provide foods fortified with iron	Yes	All low-birth-weight infants Children: 6–23 months, preschool-age (24–59 months), school-aged (5–12 years) Non-pregnant menstruating women and adolescent girls (12–49 years)	PTC
Iron and folic acid supplementation with 30–60 mg elemental iron and 0.4 mg folic acid	Recommended within the context of routine antenatal care	Yes	Pregnant women and adolescent girls	PTC
Daily oral iron and folic acid supplementation with 60 mg elemental iron and 0.4 mg folic acid	Anemia prevalence among target population is ≥40% (i.e., blood hemoglobin concentration <110 g/L)	Yes	Pregnant women and adolescent girls	PTC
Intermittent oral iron and folic acid supplementation with 120 mg elemental iron and 2.8 mg folic acid	If daily iron is not acceptable due to side effects and anemia prevalence among target population is <20%	Yes	Pregnant women	PTC
United Nations International Multiple Micronutrient Antenatal Preparation (UNIMMAP) (15 micronutrients; including 30 mg elemental iron and 0.4 mg folic acid)	Antenatal multiple micronutrient supplements that include iron and folic acid in the context of rigorous research, including implementation research	Yes	Pregnant women	PTC
Multiple micronutrient supplements during (and after) pregnancy	WHO recommends antenatal supplements containing 60 mg of elemental iron in populations where anemia prevalence is ≥40%	Yes	Pregnant women Postpartum women	PTC

(continued)

Table 27.1 (continued)

Program/recommendation/practice[a]	Geography/setting	Policy/ guideline available[b]	Target population(s)	Prevention (P)/ treatment (T)/ control (C)
Oral iron supplementation, either alone or in combination with folic acid supplementation	Gestational anemia prevalence is ≥20%	Yes	Postpartum women	PTC
Mass fortification (edible products with wide consumption)				
Rice fortification	In settings where rice is a staple food	Yes	Population	PC
Wheat/noodle fortification	In settings where wheat flour is industrially produced and consumed by large population groups	Yes	Population	PC
Maize/cornmeal fortification	In settings where maize/cornmeal is a staple food	Yes	Population	PC
Targeted fortification (addition of micronutrients to food for specific populations)				
Use of multiple micronutrient powders (sprinkles or point of use fortification)	Where the prevalence of anemia in this group is 20% or higher	Yes	Children aged 6–23 months School-age children (2–12 years)	PTC
Provision of fortified complementary foods	All settings	Yes	Children aged 6–23 months	PC
Provision of supplementary foods containing macronutrients (e.g., protein) alone or in combination with micronutrients (e.g., lipid-based nutrition supplements)	In emergency settings	Yes	Pregnant women Older infants and young children.	PC
Blanket supplementary feeding programs (BSFP) and nutritional supplement Programmes (MNP and lipid-based nutrient supplements (LNS))	In emergency settings (e.g., refugee settings)	Yes	Children aged 6–59 months Pregnant and lactating women	PTC
Biofortification				
Legumes and pulses (beans, peas, and lentils) [34–37]	Populations who produce and consume staple food crops in significant quantities, and who may not have access to other nutrition interventions such as fortification	No	At-risk populations Children: 6–59 months, school-age (5–12 years) Women: Pregnant, postpartum, WRA	PC
Iron-biofortification of rice, millet, wheat, maize, sweet potato, cassava [32, 35, 38, 39]	Populations who produce and consume staple food crops in significant quantities, and who may not have access to other nutrition interventions such as fortification	No	At-risk populations Children: 6–59 months, school-age (5–12 years) Women: Pregnant, postpartum, WRA	PC

Improving dietary diversity and quality				
Increasing food variety through nutrition education and provision of nutrient-dense foods (i.e., fruits, vegetables, and iron-rich foods)	In settings where micronutrient deficiencies (e.g., iron deficiency anemia) are caused by low dietary intakes and exacerbated by inflammation and infection	Yes	Children: 6–59 months, school-age (5–12 years) Women: Pregnant, postpartum, WRA General population	PC
Nutrition education and use of iron-pot cooking and fish-shaped iron ingots	In settings where micronutrient deficiencies (iron deficiency anemia) are caused by low dietary intakes and exacerbated by inflammation and infection	Yes	Children: 6–59 months, school-age (5–12 years) Women: Pregnant, postpartum, WRA	PC
General nutrition education and counseling (e.g., increasing the intake of micronutrient absorption factors and decreasing inhibitors of micronutrient absorption)	In settings where micronutrient deficiencies (iron deficiency anemia) are caused by low dietary intakes and exacerbated by inflammation and infection	Yes	Children: 6–59 months, school-age (5–12 years) Women: Pregnant, postpartum, WRA General population	PC
Dietary modification and diversification (to enhance the bioavailability of micronutrients)				
Increase the production and consumption of iron-rich foods, primarily animal-source foods such as meat (especially red meat), poultry, and fish, but also iron-rich plant sources such as legumes	In settings where micronutrient deficiencies (iron deficiency anemia) are caused by low dietary intakes and exacerbated by inflammation and infection	Yes, part of a guideline	Children: 6–59 months, school-age (5–12 years) Women: Pregnant, postpartum, WRA General population	PC
Increase the production and consumption of foods that are rich in vitamin A/carotenoids (e.g., green leafy vegetables and orange-fleshed sweet potatoes)	In settings where micronutrient deficiencies (iron deficiency anemia) are caused by low dietary intakes and exacerbated by inflammation and infection	Yes, part of a guideline	Children: 6–59 months, school-age (5–12 years) Women: Pregnant, postpartum, WRA General population	PC
Add fruits and vegetables that are rich in citric or ascorbic acid (e.g., citrus fruits) to the diet, to increase the absorption of non-hem iron	In settings where micronutrient deficiencies (iron deficiency anemia) are caused by low dietary intakes and exacerbated by inflammation and infection	Yes, part of a guideline	Children: 6–59 months, school-age (5–12 years) Women: Pregnant, postpartum, WRA General population	PC
Identify and promote culturally appropriate and feasible methods of food processing and preparation, to improve bioavailability and absorption	In settings where micronutrient deficiencies (iron deficiency anemia) are caused by low dietary intakes and exacerbated by inflammation and infection	Yes, part of a guideline	Children: 6–59 months, school-age (5–12 years) Women: Pregnant, postpartum, WRA General population	PC

(continued)

Table 27.1 (continued)

Program/recommendation/practice[a]	Geography/setting	Policy/ guideline available[b]	Target population(s)	Prevention (P)/ treatment (T)/ control (C)
Avoid combining known inhibitors of iron absorption with meals that are high in iron content	In settings where micronutrient deficiencies (iron deficiency anemia) are caused by low dietary intakes and exacerbated by inflammation and infection	Yes, part of a guideline	Children: 6–59 months, school-age (5–12 years) Women: Pregnant, postpartum, WRA General population	PC
Social and behavior-change communication				
Social and behavior-change communication strategies should be developed for a particular context, using formative research or ethnographic work prior to implementation	All settings	Yes	Not specified but would include policymakers and implementers, community leaders	P
Multiple social and behavior-change communication approaches and channels (e.g., interpersonal communication, media, community/social mobilization)	All settings	Yes	Not specified but would include policymakers and implementers, community leaders	P
Targeting multiple contacts in addition to the target group (e.g., targeting other caregivers) has a greater effect	All settings	Yes	Not specified but would include policymakers and implementers, community leaders	P

[a] Additional information regarding nutrition-specific interventions to prevent and control anemia can be found in the World Health Organization's report *Nutritional Anaemias: Tools for Effective Prevention and Control* [14]

[b] World Health Organization guidelines are available from: https://www.who.int/publications/who-guidelines

Table 27.2 Nutrition-sensitive interventions and strategies for anemia reduction

Program/recommendation/practice[a]	Geography/setting	Policy/ guideline available[b]	Target population(s)	Prevention (P)/ treatment (T)/ control (C)
Treatment of infections (malaria, helminth infections, and other infections)				
Intermittent preventive treatment of malaria in pregnancy (IPTp) and infants (SP- IPTi)	In malaria-endemic areas (areas with moderate to high malaria transmission)	Yes	Infants Pregnant women	PC
Seasonal malaria chemoprevention	In areas with highly seasonal malaria transmission	Yes	Children <6 years	PC
Insecticide-treated nets (ITNs) and indoor residual spraying (IRS)	In malaria-endemic areas	Yes	General population	PC
Case management of malaria	In malaria-endemic areas	Yes	General population	PC
Deworming	Baseline prevalence of any soil-transmitted infection among target population is ≥20% Baseline prevalence of hookworm and/or *T. trichiura* infection is ≥20% among pregnant women and (ii) anemia prevalence is ≥40% among pregnant women	Yes	Children: 12–23 months, preschool (24–59 months), school-age (5–12 years) Non-pregnant adolescent girls (10–19 years) and WRA Pregnant women	PC
Reproductive health practices				
Delayed cord clamping	All countries, all settings	Yes	Postpartum women Newborns	PC
Early initiation and exclusive breastfeeding for infants	All countries, all settings	Yes	Children aged 0–6 months	PC
Delaying the age of first pregnancy [14]	All settings	No	WRA	PC
Screening for anemia	All settings	Yes	Pregnant women	PC
Prevention of postpartum hemorrhage	All settings	Yes	Postpartum women	PTC
Birth spacing [8, 14, 48]	All settings	No	WRA	—
Blood transfusion [49]	Active bleeding and postpartum hemorrhage	No	Not specified	T
Water, sanitation, and hygiene (WASH)				
Promote optimal hand washing	Populations that face structural and environmental barriers to access safe WASH services	Yes	Communities and vulnerable populations	P
Promote treatment of water and safe storage of drinking water in the household	Populations that face structural and environmental barriers to access safe WASH services	Yes	Communities and vulnerable populations	—

(continued)

Table 27.2 (continued)

Program/recommendation/practice[a]	Geography/setting	Policy/ guideline available[b]	Target population(s)	Prevention (P)/ treatment (T)/ control (C)
Promote safe, hygienic methods of sanitation/feces management	Populations that face structural and environmental barriers to access safe WASH services	Yes	Communities and vulnerable populations	P
Promote wearing of shoes (for control of soil-transmitted helminths)	Populations that face structural and environmental barriers to access safe WASH services	Yes	Communities and vulnerable populations	—
Discourage standing in rivers/lakes to play or wash clothes (for schistosomiasis control)	Populations that face structural and environmental barriers to access safe WASH services	Yes	Communities and vulnerable populations	P
Intersectoral actions				
Improving gender equality and women's empowerment [14, 50, 51]	Emphasized for developing/low-income settings or countries	No	WRA	P
Supporting educational opportunities for girls and women [8, 14, 52]	Emphasized for developing/low-income settings or countries	No	Adolescent girls (10–19 years) WRA	P
Supporting income-generating activities for women [8, 14]	Emphasized for developing/low-income settings or countries	No	WRA	P
Raising awareness among policymakers and communities [1, 8, 14, 51]	Emphasized for developing/low- and middle-income settings or countries	No	Policymakers and implementers community leaders	—

[a] Additional information regarding nutrition-sensitive interventions to prevent and control anemia can be found in the World Health Organization's report *Nutritional Anaemias: Tools for Effective Prevention and Control* [14]

[b] World Health Organization guidelines are available from: https://www.who.int/publications/who-guidelines

alternatively, in a school setting, supplementation can follow the school or calendar year. Intermittent iron and folic acid supplements are also recommended for non-anemic pregnant women (120 mg elemental iron and 2.8 mg folic acid in tablet/capsule form) in settings where the prevalence of anemia among pregnant women is less than 20%. This strategy is recommended when daily iron supplementation is poorly tolerated and should commence as early in pregnancy as possible [18].

Alternatively, daily iron supplementation is recommended for three consecutive months per year in settings where the prevalence of anemia among infants and young children (6–23 months; 10–12.5 mg elemental iron in liquid form), preschool-age children (30 mg elemental iron in liquid or tablet form), school-aged children (30–60 mg elemental iron), or non-pregnant WRA is greater than 40% (30–60 mg elemental iron) [19, 20].

Daily iron (30–60 mg elemental iron) and folic acid supplementation is also recommended throughout pregnancy for women and adolescent girls as part of routine antenatal care [18]. In the context of rigorous research, including implementation research that uses high-quality methods appropriate to the specific research questions, antenatal multiple micronutrient supplements containing iron and folic acid are an alternative option [23]. One such example is the United Nations International Multiple Micronutrient Antenatal Preparation (UNIMMAP) which contains 30 mg of elemental iron and 14 other micronutrients [23]. However, the WHO recommends a higher dose of iron (e.g., 60 mg) in populations where the prevalence of anemia is greater than 40% among pregnant women [18, 23]. Following pregnancy, in settings where gestational anemia is a public health concern (>20%), daily supplementation with iron (with or without folic acid) can be provided to postpartum women for 6–12 weeks following delivery to reduce their risk of anemia [24]. In malaria-endemic regions, iron supplementation, regardless of regimen or folic acid content, should be delivered in tandem with adequate measures to prevent, diagnose, and treat malaria [14].

Low-birth-weight infants (birth weight between 1.5 and 2.5 kg) and very-low-birth-weight infants who are fed human milk (birth weight between 1.0 and 1.5 kg) should receive daily iron supplementation from 2 to 23 months of age (2 mg/kg body weight per day) and from 2 weeks to 6 months of age (2–4 mg/kg body weight per day), respectively [21, 22].

Fortification

Universal fortification, or mass fortification, is appropriate when a large proportion of a population is at risk of specific micronutrient deficiencies [25], such as those that are implicated in the etiology of anemia (e.g., B12, folate, iron, vitamin A, and zinc). For universal fortification to be successful, the target population must consume large quantities of industrially processed foods (e.g., cereals) [26]. Alternatively, targeted fortification can be used to increase the nutrient intake of specific subsets of the population without increasing the intake of the general population [21]. This intervention is often used when the nutrient needs of a population subset are high and unlikely to be met through universal fortification [14]. For instance, complementary foods fortified with iron are recommended for children aged 6–23 months in all settings [27]. In populations where the prevalence of anemia is greater than 20% among children young children, targeted (home or point-of-use) fortification with micronutrient powders is recommended for children aged 6–23 months and 2–12 years [28, 29]. In emergency settings, iron and other micronutrient-fortified blended foods (e.g., the World Food Programme's S"per Cereal and Super Cereal Plus) can be provided to pregnant women, older infants, and young children [30, 31].

Populations who produce and consume staple food crops in significant quantities, and who may not have access to other nutrition interventions like fortification, may benefit from biofortification interventions. Crops that have been successfully biofortified with micronutrients include pulses, legumes, rice, millet, wheat, maize, sweet potato, and cassava [14, 32]. A detailed description of food-based strategies for combatting iron deficiency and anemia can be found in Chap. 26.

Improving Dietary Diversity and Quality

Nutrition education can also be used to promote the consumption of the key nutrients required for red blood cell synthesis and, ultimately, anemia prevention and control. Ensuring the appropriate intake of iron, folate, vitamin B_{12}, vitamin A, and other hematopoietic nutrients is paramount for the prevention of nutritional anemia. General nutrition education and counseling should promote the consumption of a variety of nutrient-dense foods and highlight techniques that promote the absorption of micronutrients and limit known absorption inhibitors (e.g., consuming vitamin C to enhance iron absorption) [14]. A detailed discussion about the dietary sources of iron and its bioavailability can be found in Chapts. 10 and 11, respectively.

Social and Behavior-Change Communication

Social and behavior-change communication should accompany nutrition-specific interventions that aim to prevent and treat anemia [14]. Social and behavior-change strategies need to be developed for a specific context using formative research or ethnographic work; utilize multiple communication channels and approaches instead of a singular approach; and should also aim to reach groups that are peripheral to the intended target group [33].

Nutrition-Sensitive Strategies to Reduce Anemia

Nutrition-sensitive interventions, defined in Chap. 27, indirectly address nutrition by targeting the underlying and basic causes of anemia that can occur at the household and societal levels [2]. These interventions span numerous sectors but common strategies focus on infection control; water, sanitation and hygiene (WASH) practices; and poverty reduction and eliminating gender norms [14].

Treatment and Control of Infections (Malaria, Helminth Infections, and Other Infections).

Globally, malaria is one of the primary causes of anemia [40, 41], thus it is important to also implement interventions for its control and treatment. In malaria-endemic regions, long-lasting insecticidal nets or indoor residual spraying should be delivered at high coverage as a means of vector control [42]. Areas with high rates of transmission are recommended to use chemoprevention strategies for pregnant women and infants while seasonal malarial chemoprevention is recommended for children aged 3–59 months who live in areas with high seasonal malaria transmission within the Sahel subregion [41, 43, 44]. Soil-transmitted helminth (hookworm) infections and schistosomiasis are other parasitic infections that contribute to the global burden of anemia. Periodic deworming is recommended among at-risk populations for the control of both soil-transmitted helminth infections and schistosomiasis [45]. However, long-term solutions to soil-transmitted helminth infections and schistosomiasis require improved WASH access and practices to break the cycle of infection and re-infection [14].

Water, Sanitation, and Hygiene (WASH)

Adequate WASH access and practices help to lower the odds of schistosomiasis and soil-transmitted helminth infection, primarily through access to safe water [46]. Further, poor WASH access and practice may lead to increased gut permeability and reduced absorptive and barrier capacity in the small intestine as a result of environmental enteric dysfunction (EED) [47]. WASH strategies should aim to promote proper handwashing and food hygiene practices, treatment of water and the safe storage of drinking water; safe, hygienic methods of sanitation/feces management, and the wearing of shoes to control soil-transmitted helminth infection [14]. Moreover, standing in rivers/lakes to play or wash clothes should be discouraged as a means for schistosomiasis control [46].

Reproductive Health Practices

Intervention strategies related to reproductive health and pregnancy may also lower the risk of anemia among adolescent girls and WRA. Some strategies include delaying the age of first pregnancy, ensuring access to quality prenatal and postnatal care, and increasing the interval of time between births. These strategies reduce the risk of anemia for not only the mother but also her child [14].

Intersectoral Actions

Limited access to healthcare, nutrition, education, and household income among women is associated with poor nutritional status and an increased risk of anemia [14]. Thus, multiple sectors, in addition to the health sector, require engagement to improve gender equality and women's empowerment; support educational opportunities for girls and women; support income-generating activities for women; and raise awareness about the consequences of anemia among policymakers and communities [14].

Strategies for the Treatment of Iron Deficiency Anemia

Specific nutrient deficiencies should be confirmed before oral supplementation is initiated. For uncomplicated IDA, oral iron supplements are recommended daily for 3 months accompanied by the monitoring of red cell indices [15]. In situations where oral iron supplementation is unsuccessful or poorly tolerated, or in instances of iron malabsorption, parenteral/intravenous iron therapy may be indicated [15]. Red blood cell transfusions may be required in cases of severe IDA or scenarios with serious complications, such as during postpartum hemorrhage [49].

Development of Programs for Anemia Reduction

The development of programs for effective anemia reduction requires a comprehensive understanding of the determinants of anemia within a region or population. Understanding the primary causes and distribution of anemia among affected populations will allow for the selection of appropriate intervention strategies. Moreover, a comprehensive understanding allows engagement and coordination among relevant partners and stakeholders. Following implementation, programs should be monitored and evaluated to ensure program adjustment, maintenance, expansion, or termination as needed [14]. Important elements for developing anemia reduction programs are outlined in Fig. 27.1. Select examples of current and past National Anemia Action Programs can be found in Table 27.3.

Role of Policy in Anemia Reduction

Policy has an important role to play in the successful implementation of anemia interventions.

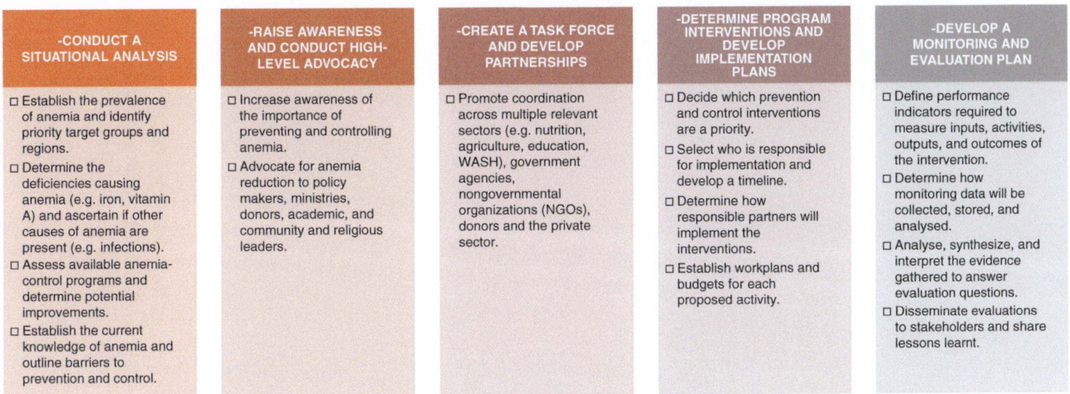

Fig. 27.1 Key elements for developing anemia reduction programs (adapted from *Nutritional Anaemias: Tools for Effective Prevention and Control*) [14]

Table 27.3 Examples of current and past national anemia action plans

Country	WHO estimated anemia prevalence among vulnerable groups (2016)[a]	National anemia action plans	Interventions	Target populations	Delivery platforms
India	Children <5 years: 57.3% Non-pregnant women: 51.5% Pregnant women: 50.1% WRA: 51.4%	Anemia Mukt Bharat (Anemia Free India) 2018–2022 [53]	1. Iron–folic acid supplementation 2. Deworming 3. Year-round behavior change communication 4. Therapeutic management of anemia 5. Mandatory provision of iron and folic acid fortified foods in government-funded health programs 6. Screening and treatment for following non-nutritional causes of anemia with special focus on malaria, hemoglobinopathies, and fluorosis	Young children (6–59 months) School-age children (5–9 years) Adolescent boys and girls (10–19 years) WRA (20–24 years) Pregnant and lactating women	Village health and nutrition day Anganwadi centers Schools Antenatal contact points
Peru	Children <5 years: 31.9% Non-pregnant women: 18.1% Pregnant women: 25.8% WRA: 18.5%	National Plan for the Reduction of Chronic Malnutrition in Children and the Prevention of Anemia in the Country 2014–2016 [54]	1. Promote scientifically proven interventions: (a) Iron and folic acid supplementation for pregnant women (b) Delayed cutting of the umbilical cord (c) Exclusive breastfeeding (d) Supplementary feeding (e) Multimicronutrient (MMN) supplementation for girls and boys from 6–35 months (f) Handwashing with soap and water 2. Intensify interventions in districts with a high prevalence of anemia and a high number of children <3 years 3. Universalize supplementation with MMN in children 6–35 months 4. Monitor children <3 years from online newborn identification 5. Transversal approach to interculturality and gender 6. Management agreements with regional governments	Pregnant mothers Children <5 years with emphasis on children <3 years	Health services: Prenatal controls, institutional delivery, and growth and development control Home counseling Demonstration sessions

[a] Estmates obtained from the World Health Organization's Global Health Observatory. Global Health Observatory estimates for WRA and children <5 years were obtained from population-representative data sources. Data collected from 1990 to 2016 were used and a Bayesian hierarchical mixture model was used to estimate hemoglobin distributions and account for missing data, nonlinear time trends, and representativeness of data sources

Even though IDA is extensively researched, from the molecular to the population level, its treatment has not achieved an effective intervention coverage compared with other micronutrients, such as iodine and vitamin A. This is also partly due to the fact that not all anemia is due to iron, and it is important to find causes of anemia before drafting blanket policies for iron or multiple micronutrient supplementation.

We have adequate information on what needs to be done, but there is a lack of political commitment to improve mechanisms at the country level for effective program implementation. For instance, from a review of 167 countries, the World Health Organization found that only 57% of national policies included goals, targets, or indicators related to anemia [55]. Box and Fig. 27.1 provide information about the minimum requirements and key elements that can inform the design of a program to prevent, control, and treat anemia. In the last decade, countries have started developing stand-alone anemia reduction strategies (Table 27.3) or include anemia reduction as one of the strategic objectives in their broader multisectoral national nutrition policies and/or health plans (Table 27.4).

Table 27.4 Examples of current and past multisectoral national nutrition plans that include anemia-related objectives and strategies

Country	Multisectoral national nutrition plans	Strategic objectives	Select anemia-related strategies
Oman	National Nutrition Strategy—Strategic Study 2014—2050 [57]	1. Reduce the prevalence of overweight and obesity through exercise and a balanced diet of fresh vegetables and fruits 2. Reduce levels of stunting and low birth weight through improvement of all women's health and nutrition before, during, and after pregnancy 3. Raise exclusive breastfeeding rates at 6 months to improve nutritional and cognitive potential of children 4. Reduce anemia and all micronutrient deficiencies through consumption of appropriate micronutrient-rich foods 5. Increase diet of non-obesogenic fresh fruits and vegetables by reducing importation of cardiotoxic processed through cooperative agreements with regional suppliers and increase regulation and import tariffs on unhealthy foods 6. Increase local food self-sufficiency and dietary diversity through organically grown vegetables and fruits by introducing high-tech rural and urban gardens in 80% of all households 7. Improve physical fitness of the population at all ages through promotion of aerobic heart-friendly exercise 8. Create urban green spaces and pedestrian transport routes in all cities	**Strategic objective two**[a] (a) Focus health and nutrition programs primarily on pre-pregnant, prenatal, and lactating women to improve potential for normal height and cognitive development (b) Collaborate with other ministries who reach adolescent girls and women in the community (e.g., education, agriculture) (c) Reduce unmet need for contraception and increase birth spacing; continue progress on reduction of TFR to reach replacement rates **Strategic objective three** (a) Strengthen education and assessment of all hospitals and clinics so that 100% are baby friendly (b) Ensure adequate space for continued breastfeeding in all workplaces **Strategic objective four**[a] (a) Develop and promote biofortified foods (including increasing bioavailability of iron) to provide adequate micronutrients **Strategic objective six** (a) Scale-up rural and urban agriculture using water and nutrient efficient technologies (e.g., hydroponics, aquaponics) to facilitate local production of vegetable and, fruits (and fish) (b) Develop vertical farms in all new urban structures

(continued)

Table 27.4 (continued)

Country	Multisectoral national nutrition plans	Strategic objectives	Select anemia-related strategies
United Republic of Tanzania	National Multi-sectoral Nutrition Action Plan (2016–2021) [58]	1. Scaling up maternal, infant, young child, and adolescent nutrition (MIYCAN) 2. Scaling up prevention and management of micronutrient deficiencies 3. Scaling up integrated management of acute malnutrition (IMAM) 4. Scaling up prevention and management of diet-related non-communicable diseases 5. Scaling up multisectoral nutrition-sensitive interventions (agriculture and food security; health and HIV; WASH; education; social protection; and environment and climate change) 6. Strengthening multisectoral nutrition governance 7. Establishing a multisectoral nutrition information system	**Strategic objective one** (a) Increased coverage and quality of MIYCAN services at the community level (b) Improved quality of MIYCAN services at the health facilities level (c) MIYCAN is promoted at all levels through mass media and the use of new technologies (d) Improved MIYCAN law enforcement through advocacy and capacity building of key institutions **Strategic objective two**[a] (a) Increased access to food fortification (home and mass) for children aged 6–23 months, pregnant women, and WRA (b) Children receive regular supplementation of vitamin A and deworming (c) Children and women utilize improved services for anemia reduction, reflected by an increased proportion of WRA who took IFA supplementation during pregnancy **Strategic objective five** (a) Communities have access to a diverse range of nutritious foods throughout the year (b) Communities regularly use quality maternal health, family planning prevention services, and treatment of HIV and malaria (c) Communities and schools access adequate WASH services (d) Girls complete primary and secondary education (e) Poorest households benefit from conditional cash transfers, cash for work, and nutrition education during the community sessions

[a] Strategic objective directly relates to anemia

Box 27.1: Following Are the Minimum Requirements for Effective Prevention and Control of Iron Deficiency Anemia[a]

Essential elements of a policy:

- Define a **goal** to reduce iron deficiency in children and women by X percentage as per WHA targets.
- Define **strategy** with a commitment to the goal and resources to support a program to achieve the goal.
- A well-defined and effective strategy and capacity for sustained **operationalization** of the policy.

Major policy and program components:

- Communications: policy support and advocacy.
- Research & Development: Define the strategy; Define the service delivery content; Define the delivery mechanism (feasibility).
- Program operations: Funding; Promotion (social marketing); Defined service or product provider.

Types of evidence needed to inform the essential elements of policy: Evidence of disease burden; consequences of disease; health impact; human resource development; economic assessment; evidence of feasibility for intervention; technical feasibility; operational feasibility.

[a]Adapted from *Prevention and control of iron deficiency: policy and strategy issues* [56]

Conclusion

The reduction of anemia requires the implementation of context-specific, evidence-informed interventions [14]. It is imperative to identify, measure, and understand the burden and etiology of anemia in a given context in order to select appropriate nutrition-specific and nutrition-sensitive interventions for the intended target groups. Leveraging existing platforms and coordinating partners and stakeholders helps to ensure success—however, comprehensive policies and plans need to be developed to facilitate an enabling environment. The policies have to be appropriately funded, ideally through domestic funds, to support these programs. Finally, monitoring and evaluation plans must be in place for accountability. Program outputs and impacts have to be actively monitored, allowing implementers to learn from past experiences and ensure that future programs are evidence-based and effective [14].

References

1. World Health Organization. Global nutrition targets 2025: anaemia policy brief (WHO/NMH/NHD/14.4). Geneva: World Health Organization; 2014.
2. Development Initiatives. 2018 global nutrition report: shining a light to spur action on nutrition. Bristol: Development Initiatives; 2018.
3. World Health Organization, UNICEF. The extension of the 2025 Maternal, Infant and Young Child nutrition targets to 2030 [Internet]. 2019. https://www.who.int/nutrition/global-target-2025/discussion-paper-extension-targets-2030.pdf
4. World Health Organization, United Nations Children's fund, United States Agency for International Development. Improving nutrition outcomes with better water, sanitation and hygiene: practical solutions for policy and programmes. Geneva: World Health Organization; 2015.
5. Wirth JP, Woodruff BA, Engle-Stone R, Namaste SM, Temple VJ, Petry N, et al. Predictors of anemia in women of reproductive age: biomarkers reflecting inflammation and nutritional determinants of anemia (BRINDA) project. Am J Clin Nutr. 2017;106(Suppl 1):416S–27S.
6. Ngure FM, Reid BM, Humphrey JH, Mbuya MN, Pelto G, Stoltzfus RJ. Water, sanitation, and hygiene (WASH), environmental enteropathy, nutrition, and early child development: making the links. Ann N Y Acad Sci. 2014;1308:118–28.
7. Engle-Stone R, Aaron GJ, Huang J, Wirth JP, Namaste SM, Williams AM, et al. Predictors of anemia in preschool children: biomarkers reflecting inflammation and nutritional determinants of anemia (BRINDA) project. Am J Clin Nutr. 2017;106(Suppl 1):402S–15S.

8. World Health Organization. Global anaemia reduction efforts among women of reproductive age: impact, achievement of targets and the way forward for optimizing efforts. Geneva: World Health Organization; 2020.
9. Poskitt EME. Early history of iron deficiency. Br J Haematol. 2003;122(4):554–62.
10. Mackay HM. Nutritional anaemia in infancy with specific reference to iron deficiency. MRC Special Report no. 157. HMSO, London; 1931.
11. Davies DT. Simple achlorhydric anaemia. Lancet. 1931;2:385–91.
12. Walter T. Effect of iron-deficiency anemia on cognitive skills and neuromaturation in infancy and childhood. Food Nutr Bull. 2003;24(4 Suppl):S104–10.
13. Rasmussen K. Is there a causal relationship between iron deficiency or iron-deficiency anemia and weight at birth, length of gestation and perinatal mortality? J Nutr. 2001;131:590S–603S.
14. World Health Organization. Nutritional anaemias: tools for effective prevention and control. Geneva: World Health Organization; 2017.
15. Lopez A, Cacoub P, Macdougall IC, Peyrin-Biroulet L. Iron deficiency anaemia. Lancet. 2016;387(10021):907–16.
16. World Health Organization. Guideline: intermittent iron supplementation in preschool and school-age children. Geneva; 2011.
17. World Health Organization. Guideline: intermittent iron and folic acid supplementation in menstruating women. Geneva: World Health Organization; 2011.
18. World Health Organization. WHO recommendation on antenatal care for positive pregnancy experience. WHO Recommendation on Antenatal care for positive pregnancy experience. Geneva; 2016.
19. World Health Organization. Guideline: daily iron supplementation in infants and children. Geneva; 2016.
20. World Health Organization. Guideline: daily iron supplementation in adult women and adolescent girls. Geneva: World Health Organization; 2016.
21. United Nations Children's Fund. Iron deficiency anaemia assessment, prevention, and control: a guide for programme managers. Geneva; 2001.
22. World Health Organization. Guidelines on optimal feeding of low birth-weight infants in low- and middle-income countries. Geneva: World Health Organization; 2011.
23. World Health Organization. WHO antenatal care recommendations for a positive pregnancy experience: nutritional interventions update: multiple micronutrient supplements during pregnancy. Geneva: World Health Organization; 2020.
24. World Health Organization. Guideline: iron supplementation in postpartum women. Geneva: World Health Organization; 2016.
25. Allen L, de Benoist B, Dary O, Hurrell R. Guidelines on food fortification with micronutrients. Geneva: World Health Organization, Food and Agricultural Organization of the United Nations; 2006.
26. Hurrell R, Ranum P, de Pee S, Biebinger R, Hulthen L, Johnson Q, et al. Revised recommendations for iron fortification of wheat flour and an evaluation of the expected impact of current national wheat flour fortification programs. Food Nutr Bull. 2010;31(1 Suppl):S7–21.
27. World Health Organization. Guiding principles for complementary feeding of the breastfed child. Washington, DC: Pan American Health Organization; 2003.
28. World Health Organization. Guideline: use of multiple micronutrient powders for point-of-use fortification of foods consumed by pregnant women. Geneva: World Health Organization; 2016.
29. Zlotkin SH, Schauer C, Christofides A, Sharieff W, Tondeur MC, Hyder SMZ. Micronutrient sprinkles to control childhood anaemia. PLoS Med. 2005;2(1):e1.
30. Style S, Tondeur M, Wilkinson C, Oman A, Spiegel P, Kassim IAR, et al. Operational guidance on the use of special nutritional products in refugee populations. Food Nutr Bull. 2014;34(4):420–8.
31. United Nations High Commissioner for Refugees. UNHCR Strategic Plan for Anaemia Prevention, Control and Reduction: Reducing the Global Burden of Anaemia in Refugee Populations 2008–2010. 2008.
32. World Health Organization. Biofortification of staple crops [Internet]. 2021 [cited 2021 Feb 10]. https://www.who.int/elena/titles/biofortification/en/
33. Lamstein S, Stillman T, Koniz-Booher P, Aakesson A, Collaiezzi B, Williams T, et al. Evidence of Effective Approaches to Social and Behavior Change Communication for Preventing and Reducing Stunting and Anemia: Findings from a Systematic Literature Review. Arlington, VA: USAID/Strengthening Partnerships, Results, and Innovations in Nutrition Globally (SPRING) Project; 2014.
34. Finkelstein JL, Haas JD, Mehta S. Iron-biofortified staple food crops for improving iron status: a review of the current evidence. Curr Opin Biotechnol. 2017;44:138–45.
35. Garg M, Sharma N, Sharma S, Kapoor P, Kumar A, Chunduri V, et al. Biofortified crops generated by breeding, agronomy, and transgenic approaches are improving lives of millions of people around the world. Front Nutr. 2018;5
36. Mutwiri LN, Kyallo F, Kiage B, Van der Schueren B, Matthys C. Can improved legume varieties optimize iron status in low- and middle-income countries? A systematic review. Adv Nutr. 2020;11(5):1315–24.
37. Prentice AM, Mendoza YA, Pereira D, Cerami C, Wegmuller R, Constable A, et al. Dietary strategies for improving iron status: balancing safety and efficacy. Nutr Rev. 2017;75(1):49–60.
38. Jongstra R, Mwangi MN, Burgos G, Zeder C, Low JW, Mzembe G, et al. Iron absorption from iron-biofortified Sweetpotato is higher than regular Sweetpotato in Malawian women while iron absorption from regular and iron-biofortified potatoes is high in Peruvian women. J Nutr. 2020;150(12):3094–102.

39. Kodkany BS, Bellad RM, Mahantshetti NS, Westcott JE, Krebs NF, Kemp JF, et al. Biofortification of pearl millet with iron and zinc in a randomized controlled trial increases absorption of these minerals above physiologic requirements in young children. J Nutr. 2013;143(9):1489–93.
40. Stevens G, Finucane M, De-Regil L, Paciorek C, Flaxman S, Branca F, et al. Global, regional, and national trends in haemoglobin concentration and prevalence of total and severe anaemia in children and pregnant and non-pregnant women for 1995–2011: a systematic analysis of population-representative data. Lancet Glob Heal. 2013;1:E16–25.
41. World Health Organization. World malaria report 2019. Geneva: World Health Organization; 2019.
42. World Health Organization. WHO guidance for countries on combining indoor residual spraying and long-lasting insecticidal nets. Geneva: World Health Organization; 2014.
43. World Health Organization. WHO policy brief for the implementation of intermittent preventive treatment of malaria in pregnancy using sulfadoxine-pyrimethamine (IPTp-SP). Geneva: World Health Organization; 2014.
44. World Health Organization. Seasonal malaria chemoprevention with sulfadoxine-pyrimethamine plus amodiaquine in children. A field guide. Geneva: World Health Organization; 2013.
45. World Health Organization. Guideline: preventive chemotherapy to control soil-transmitted helminth infections in at-risk population groups. Geneva: World Health Organization; 2017.
46. World Health Organization. Water sanitation and hygiene for accelerating and sustaining progress on neglected tropical diseases. A global strategy 2015–2020. Geneva: World Health Organization; 2015.
47. Humphrey JH. Child undernutrition, tropical enteropathy, toilets, and handwashing. Lancet. 2009;374(9694):1032–5.
48. Afeworki R, Smits J, Tolboom J, van der Ven A. Positive effect of large birth intervals on early childhood hemoglobin levels in Africa is limited to girls: cross-sectional DHS study. PLoS One. 2015;10(6)
49. Surbek D, Vial Y, Girard T, Breymann C, Bencaiova GA, Baud D, et al. Patient blood management (PBM) in pregnancy and childbirth: literature review and expert opinion. Arch Gynecol Obstet. 2020;301(2):627–41.
50. Gupta S, Pingali P, Pinstrup-Andersen P. Women's empowerment and nutrition status: the case of iron deficiency in India. Food Policy. 2019;88:101763.
51. Shekar M, Kakietek J, Eberwein JD, Walters D, Dayton Eberwein J, Walters D. An investment framework for nutrition: reaching the global targets for stunting, anemia, breastfeeding and wasting. Directions in development. Washington, DC: World Bank; 2016.
52. Roche ML, Bury L, Yusadiredja IN, Asri EK, Purwanti TS, Kusyuniati S, et al. Adolescent girls' nutrition and prevention of anaemia: a school based multisectoral collaboration in Indonesia. BMJ. 2018;363:k4541.
53. Ministry of Health and Family Welfare, Government of India. Intensified National Iron Plus Initiative (I-INI) - Operational Guidelines for Programme Managers; 2018.
54. World Health Organization. Policy - National Plan for the reduction of anemia and malnutrition 2014-2016 [Internet]. Global Database on the Implementation of Nutrition Action (GINA). 2014 [cited 2021 Mar 1]. https://extranet.who.int/nutrition/gina/en/node/40743
55. World Health Organization. Global nutrition policy review 2016–2017: country progress in creating enabling policy environments for promoting healthy diets and nutrition. Geneva: World Health Organization; 2018.
56. Yip R. Prevention and control of iron deficiency: policy and strategy issues. J Nutr. 2002;132(4 Suppl):802S–5S.
57. World Health Organization. Policy - National Nutrition Strategy - Strategic Study 2014–2050 [Internet]. Global Database on the Implementation of Nutrition Action (GINA). 2014 [cited 2021 Mar 1]. https://extranet.who.int/nutrition/gina/en/node/23559
58. World Health Organization. Policy - National Multisectoral Nutrition Action Plan (NMNAP) [Internet]. Global Database on the Implementation of Nutrition Action (GINA). 2016 [cited 2021 Mar 1]. https://extranet.who.int/nutrition/gina/en/node/36034

Correction to: Nutritional Anemia

Crystal D. Karakochuk, Michael B. Zimmermann,
Diego Moretti, and Klaus Kraemer

Correction to:
Chapter 6 and chapter 23 in C. Karakochuk et al. (eds.), *Nutritional Anemia*, Nutrition and Health, https://doi.org/10.1007/978-3-031-14521-6

In Chapter 6, Author name Magnus **Domelöf** has been changed to Magnus **Domellöf**. The error appears in the Table of Content, chapter opening page, and running heads throughout the chapter.

In Chapter 6, Reference 6 "Fewtrell M, Bronsky J, Campoy C, **Domellof M**, Embleton N, Fidler Mis N, et al. Complementary feeding: a position paper by the European Society for Paediatric Gastroenterology, Hepatology, and Nutrition (ESPGHAN) Committee on Nutrition. J Pediatr Gastroenterol Nutr. 2017;64(1):119–32" **has been changed to** "Fewtrell M, Bronsky J, Campoy C, **Domellöf M**, Embleton N, Fidler Mis N, et al. Complementary feeding: a position paper by the European Society for Paediatric Gastroenterology, Hepatology, and Nutrition (ESPGHAN) Committee on Nutrition. J Pediatr Gastroenterol Nutr. 2017;64(1):119–32".

In Chapter 23, Reference 30 "Berglund S, Westrup B, **Domeloff M**. Iron supplements reduce the risk of iron deficiency anemia in marginally low birth weight infants. Pediatrics. 2010;126:e874–83" **has been changed to** "Berglund S, Westrup B, **Domellöf M**. Iron supplements reduce the risk of iron deficiency anemia in marginally low birth weight infants. Pediatrics. 2010;126:e874–83".

The updated original version of these chapters can be found at
https://doi.org/10.1007/978-3-031-14521-6_6
https://doi.org/10.1007/978-3-031-14521-6_23

C. Karakochuk et al. (eds.), *Nutritional Anemia*, Nutrition and Health,
https://doi.org/10.1007/978-3-031-14521-6_28

Index

C. D. Karakochuk et al. (eds.), *Nutritional Anemia*, Nutrition and Health,
https://doi.org/10.1007/978-3-031-14521-6

MIX
Papier aus verantwortungsvollen Quellen
Paper from responsible sources
FSC® C105338

If you have any concerns about our products,
you can contact us on
ProductSafety@springernature.com

In case Publisher is established outside the EU,
the EU authorized representative is:
Springer Nature Customer Service Center GmbH
Europaplatz 3, 69115 Heidelberg, Germany

Printed by Libri Plureos GmbH
in Hamburg, Germany